Handbook of
FOOD-DRUG
INTERACTIONS

Handbook of

FOOD-DRUG
INTERACTIONS

Edited by
Beverly J. McCabe
Eric H. Frankel
Jonathan J. Wolfe

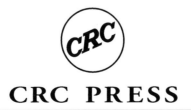

CRC PRESS

Boca Raton   London   New York   Washington, D.C.

Library of Congress Cataloging-in-Publication Data

Handbook of food-drug interactions / edited by Beverly J. McCabe, Jonathan J. Wolfe, Eric H. Frankel.
      p. cm.
    Includes bibliographical references and index.
    ISBN 0-8493-1531-X
    1. Drug-nutrient interactions—Handbooks, manuals, etc. I. McCabe, Beverly J. II. Wolfe, Jonathan James, 1944- III. Frankel, Eric H.

RM302.4.H36 2003
615′.7045—dc21   2002041312

Visit the CRC Press Web site at www.crcpress.com

Preface

As health professionals from different disciplines, we learn the basic concepts, terminology, and procedures that are central to our areas of expertise. In doing so, we become acculturated to thinking, interacting, networking, and learning with peers from the same discipline. When we begin to interact as members of healthcare teams, we bring our own jargon and mores. Often we assume that others may understand us as fully and completely as our professional peers, but we fail to grasp different meanings or focus that others may have on a given subject, case, or problem. The term multidisciplinary is used to define teams in which different disciplines are represented but tend to function in isolation of each other. Interdisciplinary means that teams combine their unique talents and knowledge to create a working unit.

This book is written by an interdisciplinary team of authors and contributors representing the fields of nutrition, pharmacy, dietetics, medicine, and technology. Each chapter and appendix was viewed from the aspect of different disciplines: "Is this something everyone knows, or is this something that one discipline is unlikely to know or is likely to view differently?" "What type of information would be helpful for all disciplines to have readily available?" The book attempts to bring the detailed and discipline-specific knowledge to other disciplines. In providing common concepts, communications among different disciplines can be improved and, in turn, improve healthcare. The authors of each chapter have worked from a perspective of generic drug names in every case. Example trade names have been provided solely for the convenience of readers. In no case do the authors or the editors intend any endorsement, or imply that the example trademark names possess any advantage over equivalent generic products.

The first six chapters introduce basic concepts from pharmacy and from nutrition for all disciplines. In jointly authored chapters involving more than one discipline, comparisons are sometimes made between the thinking and focus of one discipline with the other. For example, Chapter 6 is written by two pharmacists and a dietitian and reflects both similarities and differences in approaches.

Chapters 7 through 13 present specific detailed topics of diseases, disorders, and lifestyle choices. Chapters 14 through 17 represent guidance in planning and implementing counseling programs, meeting accreditation requirements, and application of technology. The appendices provide valuable reference materials, comprehensive summaries of drug and dietary details, and suggested tools that may aid the practitioner regardless of the discipline.

The Editors

Beverly J. McCabe, Ph.D., R.D., L.D., as a young psychiatric dietitian, began the study of food and drug interactions involving monoamine oxidase inhibitor (MAOI) drugs and pressor amines. In the following years, she found that many facilities and review articles recommend unnecessary restrictions based on ill-conceived extrapolation from one food to others. Today, with a compilation of tyremine and other pressor amine values in foods drawn from a comprehensive review of the world literature, she works closely with physicians and pharmacists to reduce the risks of adverse food and drug interactions. She has published more than 20 articles, monographs, and book chapters, and her students' abstracts now number over 50 from national and international meeting presentations in the last 18 years.

Currently, Dr. McCabe serves on the board of editors of the *Journal of the American Dietetic Association.* She has served as a reviewer for the *Journal of Clinical Psychiatry* for nutrition articles and as a national officer and on the board of directors of the American Dietetic Association. She established the list serve for the Dietetic Educators of Practitioners Dietetic Practice Group and received the first outstanding service award from this group in recognition of her contribution. More recently, she was named outstanding dietitian in Arkansas for 2002. She has also been honored by the Arkansas affiliate of the American Heart Association for state-wide workshops and presentations on nutrition in heart disease and for development of educational materials.

Dr. McCabe has been an innovator in the application of technology to the practice of nutrition counseling and dietetic education. With a federal grant, she developed an interactive compressed video program to teach healthier cooking techniques to rural food service personnel in the Arkansas delta counties. Through a grant of the Arkansas Rural Hospital Program, she also pioneered individual and group nutrition counseling of rural patients on diets for weight control, diabetes, hypertension, and other conditions using the interactive compressed video network that reaches some 50 rural hospitals and clinics. Additionally, Dr. McCabe has team counseled with pharmacy faculty using a long-distance counseling technique known as Telehealth and Telenutrition.

A dedicated educator, Dr. McCabe has made numerous presentations to lay audiences including television and radio interviews. She has been active in the National Nutrient Databank Conferences and has a strong interest in food composition and analysis. Her most recent research grant is for the study of the stability of biotin in frozen foods.

Dr. McCabe received her bachelor of science degree from the University of Arkansas at Fayetteville, her dietetic internship at the University of Kansas Medical Center, her master of science from the University of Kansas, and her Ph.D. from the University of Iowa.

Eric H. Frankel, M.S.E., Pharm.D., F.A.D.A., is the nutritional support service coordinator for Covenant Health System (formerly Methodist Hospital and St. Mary of the Plains Hospital and Rehabilitation Center) in Lubbock, Texas. He has practiced in nutritional support for 22 years. Prior to his pharmacy career, Dr. Frankel earned a bachelor of science in psychology and a master of science in education from the City College of New York, after which he taught at the secondary level for several years. Dr. Frankel received his bachelor of pharmacy degree from Arnold and Marie Schwartz College of Pharmacy in New York City and went on to earn a doctor of pharmacy degree in 1979 from Mercer University.

Still an educator, Dr. Frankel has taught in pharmacy school and served as a preceptor for doctor of pharmacy candidates and for dietetic interns. He is currently the director of a residency program for pharmacy practice specializing in nutritional support and is a clinical assistant professor for Texas Tech University Health Sciences Center School of Pharmacy, as well as an adjunct professor for the School of Human Sciences, Division of Nutrition, in Lubbock. In addition, Dr. Frankel has taught classes for physical therapists, dietitians, and respiratory therapists at Texas Tech as well as Emory University, Georgia State University, and Georgia Tech, all in Atlanta. Besides teaching, he serves as a consultant for home care patients receiving nonvolitional nutrition outside the hospital and has been appointed to represent the Texas Pharmacy Association to the U.S. Pharmacopeial Convention. He has been an author of several articles in the nutritional support and pharmacy literature, and has spoken at numerous local, state, and national meetings.

Jonathan J. Wolfe, Ph.D., R.Ph., is currently associate dean of the College of Pharmacy at the University of Arkansas for Medical Sciences in Little Rock. His teaching responsibilities within the college include professional ethics, history of pharmacy, and intravenous therapy. He also works with an interdisciplinary faculty to offer a course in death and dying. His current research interests are medication error reduction and history. He recently served as guest curator for an exhibit at the Old State House Museum in Little Rock: Medical Education at the Old State House: From Flexner to New Deal.

Dr. Wolfe was educated first as an historian, completing his doctorate at the University of Virginia in Charlottesville. After 3 years of teaching college courses, he returned to school and earned his degree in pharmacy. His practice experiences include hospital pharmacy and home infusion pharmacy. He joined the faculty at the pharmacy college full time in 1991.

His other service reflects his interest in pain treatment and end-of-life care. He was a cofounder of the Arkansas Cancer Pain Initiative and has served on the board of the American Association of State Cancer Pain Initiatives. In addition, he was appointed a delegate to the U.S. Pharmacopeia in 1995, continuing to serve in that capacity through February 2003.

Contributors

Albert Barrocas, M.D., F.A.C.S., F.A.C.N.
Pendleton Memorial Methodist
  Hospital
Tulane University
New Orleans, Louisiana

Tiffany R. Bolton, Pharm.D.
DCH Regional Medical Center
Tuscaloosa, Alabama

Nancy Carthan, Pharm.D., C.D.E.
Southeast Dallas Health Center
Dallas, Texas

Ronni Chernoff, Ph.D., R.D., F.A.D.A.
Arkansas Center on Aging
Geriatrics Research, Education and
  Clinical Center, Central Arkansas
  Veterans Healthcare System
College of Public Health
University of Arkansas for Medical
  Sciences
Little Rock, Arkansas

Howell Foster, Pharm.D.
Arkansas Poison Control Center
College of Pharmacy
University of Arkansas for Medical
  Sciences
Little Rock, Arkansas

Eric H. Frankel, M.S.E., Pharm.D., B.C.N.S.P.
Covenant Health System
Texas Tech University Health Sciences
  Center
Department of Food and Nutrition,
  College of Human Sciences
Texas Tech University
Lubbock, Texas

Paul O. Gubbins, Pharm.D.
Department of Pharmacy Practice,
  College of Pharmacy
University of Arkansas for Medical
  Sciences
Little Rock, Arkansas

Bill J. Gurley, Ph.D.
Department of Pharmaceutical
  Sciences, College of Pharmacy
University of Arkansas for Medical
  Sciences
Little Rock, Arkansas

Dorothy W. Hagan, Ph.D., R.D., L.D., F.A.D.A.
Oregon Health Sciences University
Portland, Oregon

Reza Hakkak, Ph.D.
Department of Dietetics and Nutrition,
  College of Health Related Professions
University of Arkansas for Medical
  Sciences
Little Rock, Arkansas

Jan K. Hastings, Ph.D.
Department of Pharmacy Practice,
  College of Pharmacy
University of Arkansas for Medical
  Sciences
Little Rock, Arkansas

John W. Holladay, Ph.D.
Prescription Compounding of Sumter
Sumter, South Carolina

Charles W. Jastram, Jr., Pharm.D., B.C.N.S.P.
University of Louisiana at Monroe
Medical Center of Louisiana—
  Charity Campus
New Orleans, Louisiana

Kim E. Light, Ph.D.
Department of Pharmaceutical Sciences
  and Department of Interdisciplinary
  Toxicology and Pharmacology
University of Arkansas for Medical
  Sciences
Little Rock, Arkansas

Razia Malik, Pharm.D.
Niles, Michigan

Beverly J. McCabe, Ph.D., R.D., L.D.
Department of Dietetics and Nutrition
College of Health Related Professions
  and College of Public Health
University of Arkansas for Medical
  Sciences
Little Rock, Arkansas

Beth Miller, Pharm.D.
Methodist University Pain Institute
Memphis, Tennessee

**Kathleen M. Strausburg, M.S, R.Ph.,
B.C.N.S.P.**
Lakewood, Colorado

Pete Tanguay
Rock-Pond Solutions, Inc.
Conway, Arkansas

Jonathan J. Wolfe, Ph.D., R.Ph.
Associate Dean, College of Pharmacy
University of Arkansas for Medical
  Sciences
Little Rock, Arkansas

**Fantahun Yimam, Pharm.D.,
B.C.N.S.P.**
Covenant Health System
Lubbock, Texas

Contents

CHAPTER 1

Pharmacy: Basic Concepts

Eric H. Frankel

CONTENTS

0-8493-1531-X/03/$0.00+$1.50
© 2003 by CRC Press LLC

Basic information about pharmaceutics, pharmacology, pharmacokinetics, and pharmacodynamics is discussed in this chapter. The information will allow readers to appreciate the mechanisms that can result in interactions between drugs and nutrients.

BACKGROUND VIEW OF DRUGS

Animals are dependent on food for their very existence. Man is no exception. Man, as hunter and gatherer and later as agronomist, looked to plants and animals for more than just food. Animals and plants provided tools, shelter, clothing, and transportation, as well as labor.

Early man manifested an intelligence that led him to attempt to influence the external world and to change things to his advantage. Inevitable injury and illness were treated by means influenced by logic and intelligence. The means readily available to preliterate mankind included experimentation with plant and animal materials in the immediate environment. The trial and error method, combined with oral traditions and later written record keeping, produced diverse local practices of medicinal arts.

> "The desire to take medicine is perhaps the greatest feature which distinguishes man from animals." William Osler (1849–1919), Canadian writer, lecturer, and physician.

Pharmacognosy, the study of the origin, nature, properties, and effects of natural products on living organisms, grew from such instinctive responses to disease. Pharmacology, the study of the origin, nature, properties, and effects of various substances (naturally occurring and synthetic) on living organisms, grew from roots grounded for centuries in these primitive practices. It is interesting to note that there is a recent resurgence of interest in natural products for medical use.

With this new interest in natural products, keep in mind that efficacy, purity, and active ingredient concentration of substances sold as nutritional supplements are not regulated by any arm of the U.S. federal government. Recently, the U.S. Pharmacopeial (USP) Convention began a voluntary program for the certification of purity and active ingredient concentration of nutritional supplements. The USP is a private, not-for-profit entity founded in 1820 and entirely independent from the government. Except for products certified by this process, a potential for variance still exists between manufacturers, between lots from the same manufacturer, and even within the same lot.

THE PERFECT MEDICATION

Ideally, medications should be extremely specific in their effects, have the same predictable effect for all patients, never be affected by concomitant food or other medications, exhibit linear potency, be totally nontoxic in any dosage, and require only a single dose to effect a permanent cure. Unfortunately, that "perfect" drug has yet to be discovered. The concept has fascinated pharmacists and physicians since Galen of Kos expressed it nearly 18 centuries ago.

In reality, most drugs have multiple effects on the host. Those actions may even vary among hosts, depending upon factors as diverse as genetics and local environments. A drug is usually taken for one desired pharmacological action, but this is often accompanied by other, usually undesired, reactions referred to as side effects. Even drugs genetically engineered and chemically close to an endogenous chemical may fall short of the ideal profile. Exogenous administration of a "normally occurring substance" may disturb or fail to match a particular patient's internal control mechanisms for homeostasis, the balance of physiology. Part of the interest in natural products is motivated by the wish to produce a desirable effect with fewer side effects. However, on a philosophical level, the reality of pharmacology is that all substances in high amounts, including even oxygen or water, can be toxic. From this viewpoint, drugs can be likened to poisons that may have desirable side effects. If health professionals adopt this viewpoint in using, prescribing, or recommending medications, iatrogenic drug misuse, misadventures, abuse, and nosocomial-medication-related errors could be minimized. In many cases, knowledge of both the indicated use of a product and its reported side-effect profile allow the caregiver to select among similar agents for an individual patient in order to minimize undesired side effects.

DRUG DELIVERY AND ADMINISTRATION

Prior to discussing basic pharmacology and pharmacokinetics, some exposure to pharmaceutics is helpful. This area of pharmacy knowledge focuses on dosage forms and routes of administration. Knowledge of pharmaceutics is required in order to begin to understand how drugs work.

For a medication to be effective, it first needs to reach a target location in the organism. Some type of delivery system is needed for this to occur. This requires use of a specific route of administration. Routes of administration are more numerous than people outside the medical professions would think. Thanks to technological advances, both routes for drug administration and dosage forms (a term describing the specific physical form of the drug's active and inactive ingredients) exhibit more variety today than ever before.

Three major routes are used for drug delivery: topical, enteral, and parenteral. The topical route (cutaneous) can be used to apply a drug for its local activity at the area of application. Antifungal medications, such as miconazole creams for athlete's foot, serve as examples. Drugs may also be applied topically (transcutaneous) to a site from which they can be absorbed to exert a systemic effect. Nitroglycerin ointment or patches, used to prevent angina pain, are examples of this route. Vaginal creams and suppositories are examples of topical drugs used in contact with mucous membranes rather than the epidermis. Topical drugs are also used for the eye (ophthalmic), ear (otic), and nose (intranasal). Finally, certain topical drugs can be delivered into the lung (inhalation) for both local and systemic effects.

The most common and convenient route for drug administration is via the gastrointestinal tract. The oral route (*per os,* PO) is the most common enteral route, but not the sole one. Medication may be administered sublingually (SL), using tablets formulated for SL administration. Nitroglycerin is available as a sublingual tablet. This dosage form is rapidly absorbed into the bloodstream. Medication can also be administered buccally (in contact with the oropharyngeal mucosa), as in the case of nystatin oral suspension; and rectally. When medication is given via the gastrointestinal tract, mechanisms usually involved in the absorption of nutrients are "borrowed" to transport the drug into the body. In effect, the gastrointestinal tract takes on an added function. This is possible because absorbable drugs have some chemical features in common with nutrients. This facilitates the active or passive absorption of the drug. The nasoenteric and percutaneous enteral tubes, familiar to many for delivery of nutrition, may, with appropriate precautions, also be pressed into service for enteral drug delivery.

The most invasive route for drug administration is the parenteral route. Whereas, technically, parenteral means not via the gastrointestinal tract, it is commonly used to refer to routes requiring some form of injection. Once again, a variety of routes come under this umbrella. The routes include injection into the bloodstream, most commonly intravenously (IV), or into a vein. This can be done rapidly (IV push), over a limited time (IV piggyback), or over a longer time (IV infusion). Occasionally, the blood vessel may be an artery instead of a vein. Arteries are sometimes used as the injection site for provision of intrahepatic chemotherapy. This is referred to as intraarterial injection.

Medication can be injected into the subcutaneous tissue (SQ), muscle tissue (intramuscularly, IM), or the skin (intradermal). Medication may also be injected into the spinal canal or into the dura surrounding the spinal cord. This is done mainly for pain control. The techniques here are intrathecal and subdural, respectively. Occasionally, chemotherapy for cancer or infection is given intrathecally in an attempt to decrease systemic side effects while maximizing central nervous system (CNS) effectiveness or to compensate for poor passage of many medications across the blood/brain barrier from the bloodstream into the cerebrospinal fluid. Antiinflammatory steroids, used for severe arthritis, may be injected into the space within a joint. This is called synovial injection. Occasionally medication, particularly hydration fluids, may be given by slow infusion subcutaneously rather than into a vein. This is called hypodermoclysis, and it is no longer commonly used for large volumes. Small volumes are sometimes given this way. An example of this would be insulin delivered by a pump. Medication can also be given directly into the peritoneum (intraperitoneal), directly into the wall of the heart or into one of its chambers (intracardiac), and sprayed into the trachea (intratracheal). The latter two routes may be used during cardiopulmonary resuscitation. Occasionally, drugs can be given via catheter into the ventricles of the brain. This is called intraventricular administration. During gestation, drugs may even be administered to a fetus *in utero* or into the amniotic fluid, referred to as intrauterine injection. Finally, there is a route of injection called intraosseous, where the injection is done into the bone marrow of long bones such as the tibia. This may be useful in children with poor veins and relatively soft bones.

DOSAGE FORMS

In order to take advantage of this multitude of medication administration routes, a similarly diverse number of dosage forms have been devised. Some, such as urethral bougies, are no longer in common use, while others, such as the transcutaneous patch and metered dose inhalers (MDI), are becoming increasingly popular.

Pills and Powders

When the general public thinks of an oral dosage form, the word pill is commonly used. The pill is actually an archaic dosage form. Pills consist of medication combined with inactive ingredients to form a gelatinous (doughy) mass. This mass is then divided, rolled into cylinders on a pill tile, and then cut into individual pills. The pills are then dried prior to use. Currently, few medications are truly pills. Carter's Little Liver Pills® and Lydia Pinkham's Pills® are among the last of a once popular dosage form for both manufactured and extemporaneously prepared medications. Powder papers (a small, precisely measured quantity of medication and diluent inside a folded piece of paper) were once a popular method of drug delivery. Two over-the-counter (OTC) popular medications are available in this form: BC Powders® and Goody's Powders®.

Tablets, Capsules, and High Tech

The most common dosage form is the tablet. It is prepared from a dry mixture of active and inactive ingredients (excipients). The excipients include binders, lubricants, diluents, and coloring agents. This mixture is mechanically compressed into solid tablets in various shapes. The excipients are considered inert ingredients, but can occasionally cause difficulty in individual patients. Lactose is commonly used as a diluent. The quantity is usually too small to cause adverse effects, even in a lactose intolerant individual. Tartrazine, commonly called FD&C yellow dye No. 5, is a coloring agent. Serious allergic reactions are possible to this agent and to medications colored with it. Capsules are the other most common oral dosing form. Active ingredients, diluents, and lubricants (to improve the flow of the powder through the equipment) are put into preformed, hard gelatin shells that are then mated with a second gelatin shell. Liquid medication can also be sealed into a capsular shell. Several variations on the manufacturing of tablets and capsules can result in delayed or extended medication release into the gastrointestinal tract. The absorption of the drug into the bloodstream and the pharmacological effect of the drug will be affected by this alteration in the release of the medicine. The most advanced oral dosage forms use semipermeable membranes or laser technology to produce dosage forms that release medication into the gastrointestinal tract at a controlled rate.

Some drugs may be absorbed from the capillary beds in the mouth. Nitroglycerin tablets are designed to dissolve under the tongue and will be absorbed sublingually. Recently, rapid dissolving tablets have been developed to deliver medications into the gastrointestinal tract. The medication is released in the oral cavity but is absorbed at numerous locations in the gastrointestinal tract. This results in a quicker onset of action. Rapid disintegration (RD) is frequently associated with this type of dosage form. Other medications may be designed for absorption from the inner aspect of the cheek. These are referred to as buccal dosage forms. Lozenges may be used to deliver medication into the oral cavity for both local and systemic action. Local anesthetics for treating a sore throat can be put into a lozenge. A powerful pain medication, fentanyl, is available in a lozenge on a stick form for transmucosal absorption. Cough suppressants are also available as lozenges.

Liquids

Of course, oral liquids remain a popular dosage form. This category includes solutions such as teas (infusions and decoctions), fluid extracts, syrups, drops, and tinctures, as well as emulsions and powders ready for reconstitution with water. With the popularity of "natural remedies," the use of teas and homemade preparations has increased. All oral liquids are relatively simple in comparison to oral liquid nutritional supplements. The supplements are generally oil-based solutions emulsified within water-based solutions with some of their ingredients suspended in a colloidal form.

Recently, the introduction of foods having desirable pharmacological properties has further blurred the distinction among drugs, nutritional supplements, and foods. Benecol® (contains plant stanol esters) and Take Control® (plant sterol-enriched spread) are the best examples of this, but even the marketing of oatmeal and oat bran ventures into this newly grayed area separating drugs and foods.

Rectal Dosage Forms

Other enteral dosage forms are designed for absorption in the sigmoid colon and may be solid dosage forms (suppositories), liquids (enemas), or aerosols (foams). Again, both local and systemically acting medications may be given via this route. Hemorrhoid treatments, antiemetics, laxatives, and antipyretics (medications used to treat fever) are all commonly given in these forms.

Topical Agents

Topical dosage forms are similarly diverse. Ointments (oil base) may deliver topical medications. Creams (water-soluble base), gels, and mustards (pasty substance spread on a cloth and wrapped around a body part) also do so. Shampoos, soaps, solutions, and topical patches may also deliver medication in a useful manner. Nasal, ophthalmic, and otic (for the ear) solutions and suspensions are available. Aerosols, sprays, nebulized medications, metered dose inhalers, and powders for inhalation are used to deliver medication to the respiratory tract. Intravaginal suppositories (also called vaginal tablets), creams, douches, and sponges are used to deliver medications.

Injections

Parenteral dosage forms are mainly water-based solutions, but a few novel approaches are used. These include solutions in solvents other than water, oil-in-water emulsions, and even drug-impregnated solids used as subdermal implants. Recently, drugs have even been delivered inside liposomes in a parenteral liquid.

Pharmaceutical Elegance: Coats to Disguise, Protect, and Increase Duration

Coatings have been used on tablets to hide bad tastes (e.g., E-Mycin—erythromycin). One liquid suspension (Biaxin®—clarithromycin) consists of film-coated granules. The coating again hides the taste of the medicine. Interestingly, this is a liquid medication that should not be given via a small-bore feeding tube. The granules can "logjam" at the curves in the tube and occlude it. Other coatings, referred to as enteric coatings, are used to prevent dissolution and inactivation of the drug in the stomach by gastric secretions. Extensive efforts have been made to engineer dosage forms that change the absorption of medications. The goal is usually to extend the duration of action for a drug with a relatively short half-life. Repetabs® provide an example of tablets designed to provide a quantity of quickly released medication followed by a quantity of drug released slowly over time. Capsules can contain pellets coated with varying thickness of slowly dissolving excipients to achieve a timed-release bioavailability. Since medications are sometimes crushed before administration, one needs to know why the coating was on the tablet, where the drug will enter the gastrointestinal tract, and how removing the coating will affect the bioavailability of the dosage form.

COMPOUNDING: WHAT'S OLD IS NEW AGAIN

As can be seen from the preceding information, the history of pharmacy goes back to production of medication by a pharmacist rather than a commercial manufacturer. Today, many pharmacists are entering a niche market meeting individualized needs with individualized products. Compounding of pharmaceutical products provides such an opportunity. In this area, pharmacists with knowledge of product and patient work as problem solvers to provide a solution to a medical problem not amenable to treatment with off-the-shelf approaches.

Dosage forms, which are prepared by compounding pharmacists, parallel commercial dosage forms. Capsules, topical preparations including transdermal gels with enhanced ability to penetrate the skin, ophthalmic ointments, suppositories, troches, medicinal lollipops, and oral suspensions are among the dosage forms used by compounding pharmacists. Flavoring of liquid oral preparations is another area of expertise used by these practitioners.

Dosage forms containing multiple drugs can also be prepared to increase patient compliance and alleviate problems in patients who have difficulty swallowing capsules, tablets, or liquid medications. Specially prepared lozenges that slowly dissolve and release small volumes of medications into the gastrointestinal tract are useful for this purpose. Preparations that may have a therapeutic advantage but also have limited stability, and hence require short expiration dating, are poorly suited for large-scale manufacturing operations. A compounding pharmacy may be the only source for these types of preparations.

PHARMACOKINETICS

In order to understand drug interactions and drug interactions with nutrients, one needs to have a basic knowledge of pharmacokinetics. Pharmacokinetics is a science that deals with the progressive movement and alteration of chemical substances within the body. Bioavailability is important when reviewing the effects or pharmacology of a drug. In order for a drug to have an effect, it needs to be physically present at the site where it exerts its pharmacological action. First, the drug needs to be absorbed, and then it needs to be distributed or transported to a receptor—the site of action. The drug may then exert its pharmacological effect. Subsequently, the drug may be metabolized and then excreted. The acronym ADME is used to help people remember the pharmacokinetic arenas of absorption, distribution, metabolism, and elimination.

Keep in mind that drugs are usually substances not commonly ingested. All the pharmacokinetic mechanisms for each of the four ADME processes probably did not evolve to handle drugs. Drugs can be likened to a "Trojan Horse." Most frequently, drugs enter the body via the gastrointestinal tract, a route that clearly serves the purpose of absorbing food. Drugs have to be chemically similar to food substances in order to be absorbed, but dissimilar enough to avoid digestion. For example, the reason that insulin must be injected is that it is a polypeptide. If ingested, insulin would be digested into smaller peptides and amino acids and lack the pharmacological action expected from insulin.

In order to understand drug dosing, one needs to appreciate how the amount of drug in the bloodstream changes after administration of the drug. Pharmacologists will frequently employ a graph of serum concentrations of a drug vs. time in order to describe the drug's bioavailability. The serum concentration is affected by each ADME component. The relative amount of absorbed drug compared with administered drug is referred to as the drug's bioavailability. Total bioavailability and the time course of absorption affect drug action. Even while the drug is being absorbed, the processes of distribution, metabolism, and elimination are already at work affecting serum levels. When a drug leaves the bloodstream and accumulates in another tissue, this lowers the serum level. Sometimes, this will increase the activity of the drug, particularly for drugs that exert their effects in tissues other than the bloodstream. General anesthetics and antidepressants have their effects in the CNS. Other drugs may accumulate in adipose tissue, only to be released slowly over an extended time. A graph of the serum concentration of a typically orally administered drug plotted against time is depicted in Figure 1.1.

Absorption

Many factors affect absorption. The principal factors are the route of administration, the dosage form, the chemical nature of the drug, and the local environment

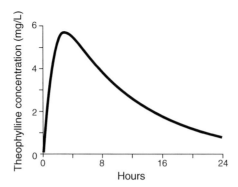

Figure 1.1   Serum concentration of a typically orally administered drug plotted against time.

at the site of absorption (i.e., pH, blood flow, physiological changes of tissue, etc.). One general principle to remember is that drugs are generally absorbed in an unionized form. Weakly acidic drugs are, therefore, generally absorbed in the stomach, while weakly basic drugs are absorbed in the small intestine. Most drugs are weakly basic. Binding to other chemicals in the gastrointestinal tract may interfere with absorption.

Distribution

Once the drug enters the body, it travels within the bloodstream. Depending on its chemical nature, the drug may preferentially concentrate in a particular tissue. Many water-soluble drugs remain in the fluid compartment. Other drugs may preferentially accumulate in adipose tissue or muscle. This affects the serum levels of the drug. Theoretically, the concentration of a drug put in a solvent should be equal to the amount of the drug divided by the volume of the solvent. If you think of the organism as the solvent for a drug, then the amount of the drug absorbed divided by the volume of the organism should equal the measured drug concentration. Since the organism is not a single solvent, this does not work. A theoretical construct called volume of distribution (Vd) is used to reconcile the measured serum level and the amount of drug absorbed. A volume of distribution of 0.6 L/kg indicates that the drug is distributed principally in the fluid compartment that accounts for about 60% of our body weight. A lower Vd would indicate that the drug is preferentially found in the bloodstream. Higher Vds indicate that the drug is sequestered in tissues other than the bloodstream (i.e., muscle, bone, CNS, etc.).

Metabolism

When a drug enters the body, it will encounter metabolic processes that may alter its chemistry. As a general rule, the metabolic processes in the body tend to decrease toxicity and enhance the elimination of foreign chemicals. These paired processes are achieved by three principal mechanisms: (1) increasing the water solubility of these chemicals, (2) decreasing the size of the foreign molecules, and

(3) binding the drugs to larger molecules (conjugation). The end products of these processes are referred to as metabolites. Metabolism can happen in the peripheral tissue of the body or in a specific organ. The liver is frequently the organ involved in this process. Many enzymes participate in drug metabolism; one group of liver enzymes responsible for much of this activity is the cytochrome P450 enzymes. Furthermore, many subgroups of enzymes exist in this class. One drug or nutrient may alter the action of these enzymes on a second drug or nutrient by binding to or having a greater affinity for the enzymes than the other substance. This may result in drug–drug or drug–nutrient interactions. Changes in liver function may also affect drug metabolism. Age alone, in the absence of liver pathology, will affect drug metabolism. This will be elaborated in later chapters of the text.

Elimination

Several organs are involved in eliminating drugs from the body. The kidneys are the most important organs in this regard. These organs of homeostasis remove drugs and drug by-products from circulation by both passive action (filtration) and by active processes involving secretion and resorption of substances from the plasma. The lungs, the liver, the skin, and various glands may also help in the elimination of chemicals from the body.

Once again, age will be a factor because renal function declines as a function of normal aging. Substances processed by the kidney may be actively or passively secreted into the urine as it traverses the nephron, which is the functional unit of the kidney. Substances can also be actively or passively reabsorbed into the bloodstream before leaving the nephron. This process can be affected by the pH of the urine and can be enhanced or inhibited by the presence of other substances in the urine or the blood. Drugs that alter urine production, such as diuretics, may also affect the urinary excretion of drug and drug metabolites, and this may result in interactions.

PHARMACODYNAMICS

The study of the actions of drugs is called pharmacodynamics. Drugs can be categorized as exerting an action in a general or a specific manner. Drugs with general, nonspecific effects may affect all body tissues and cells. Drugs with specific effects will have a target substrate that they act on, in one or more organ systems. The fewer systems affected by the drug, the more specific its action. Specifically acting drugs are generally considered better to work with from a pharmacodynamic perspective. In contrast to the serendipitous manner in which drugs were developed in the past, drug development now focuses on chemical specificity based on drug and receptor structure. Drugs or foods that interfere directly with another drug's action would cause a drug–drug or drug–nutrient interaction. Drugs with an effect similar to another drug may cause a greater than additive pharmacological effect. This type of interaction is called synergism. Drugs with opposing pharmacological effects may negate the benefits of one of the agents.

REFERENCE MATERIALS

This chapter has presented a brief overview of some ways that pharmacists tend to categorize and think about pharmacology, drugs, and drug interactions. For readers who wish to know more about these concepts, the following references provide in-depth and authoritative information.

Textbooks and References

Merck Manual, 17th edition, Beers, M.H. and Berkow, R., Eds., Merck Research Laboratories, Whitehouse Station, NJ, 1997. (A concise guide to medical science designed for the lay public, this reference generally provides quick cursory information about illness. It is a valuable tool that may rapidly provide information about unfamiliar medical conditions.)

Hansten & Horn's Drug Interactions Analysis and Management, Hansten, P.D. and Horn, J.R., Eds., Facts & Comparisons, Inc., St. Louis, MO., updated quarterly. (This text details the mechanism of various drug interactions. It is useful for someone who wants more than a superficial understanding of how drugs interact.)

Goodman and Gilman's The Pharmacological Basis of Therapeutics, 10th ed., Hardman, J.F. and Limbird, L.E., Eds., McGraw-Hill, New York, 2001. (This is the classic reference for pharmacology.)

Drugs Manuals and References

Readers who wish to know more about a particular drug or class of drugs would do well to refer to the following references.

Drug Facts and Comparisons, Facts & Comparisons, Inc., St. Louis, MO; updated monthly. (This is the drug reference most extensively used by pharmacists. It is somewhat more oriented to community practice. A loose-leaf format that is updated monthly, a hardbound format that is updated annually, and a CD-ROM are all marketed. The CD-ROM can be made accessible on a computer network. It covers over 10,000 products and includes comparison charts between similar products. Both over the counter (OTC) and prescription products are covered. It provides information about sugar-free and alcohol-free formulations. Information regarding the relative costs of drugs is included. Both FDA-approved and non–FDA-approved (off-label) uses of drugs are covered. Information is presented on a large number of, but not all, investigational agents. The monthly updates highlight product changes. Manufacturer addresses, normal lab values, and pharmaceutical abbreviations are included. It includes the information that is commonly required by practitioners about medications. Pharmacology, pharmacokinetics, adverse reactions, drug interactions, and food interactions are all covered.)

AHFS Drug Information 2003, McEvoy, G.K., Ed., American Society of Health-System Pharmacists, Bethesda, MD, 2003. (This reference provides detailed monographs on most drugs and includes both FDA-approved and non–FDA-approved (off-label) uses and information on the stability and incompatibility of drugs. Monographs cover pharmacology, pharmacokinetics, dosages, contraindications, precautions, adverse effects, and interactions. Quarterly updates are issued, but most revisions are done annually. This reference is also available in hard- and softcover editions as well as on CD-ROM and online. The soft cover edition usually gets dog-eared after a year in a busy pharmacy department. It is most commonly found in hospital pharmacy settings because the American Society of Health-System Pharmacists is the publisher. The information on each agent in this reference is more extensive than *Facts and Comparisons.* One shortcoming is that it does not include every marketed medication.)

Drug Information Handbook APhA, Lacy, C.F. et al., Eds., Lexi-Comp, Inc., Hudson, OH, 2002. (A handbook-sized but rather weighty paperback that can fit in a lab coat pocket, this reference includes concise monographs of all drugs, and it is updated annually. Comparison charts of various agents are included, and the appendix contains therapy recommendations. Useful if information is needed in a very portable form.)

Drug Interaction Facts, Tatro, D.S., Ed., Facts & Comparisons, Inc., St. Louis, MO, updated quarterly. (Providing extensive information about drug–drug and drug–food interactions, this reference examines mechanism, clinical significance, timing, and management of interactions. The information is quite clear and accessible. Case and study descriptions are provided, and the information is referenced. It is available in a hardbound format and also is computerized. Subscribers are provided with quarterly updates.)

Drug-Induced Nutrient Depletion Handbook, Pelton, R., et al., Eds., Lexi-Comp, Inc., Hudson, OH, 2001. (This unique reference is designed to assist healthcare professionals in guiding patients receiving medications on the selection of appropriate nutritional supplementation. The *Drug-Induced Nutrient Depletion Handbook* contains a complete and up-to-date listing of the drugs known to deplete the body of nutritional compounds and identifies symptoms that may result from the depletion of specific nutrients. The reference section includes summaries of selected findings organized by individual drugs.)

Drugs in Pregnancy and Lactation, Briggs, G.G., Freeman, R.K., and Yaffe, S.J., Eds., Williams & Wilkins, Baltimore, MD, 2001. (This text is a complete reference on the use of drugs in pregnancy and lactation, including classification of risk. Summaries of available studies are included, and the information is very carefully referenced.)

Evaluations of Drug Interactions, Vol. 1, II (EDI), Zucchero, F.J., et al., Eds., First DataBank, St. Louis, MO, 2002. (This book is a comprehensive reference for both prescription and OTC drug conflicts. It covers more than 34,000 drug interactions. Each interaction is outlined in a monograph format. The monographs include severity coding of the interaction, a summary of the overall effect of the interaction, and a synopsis of documented cases. Mechanisms of action and related agents that are chemically similar to the interacting drugs are discussed. Helpful recommendations, when available, of acceptable alternative therapies supported by primary literature are also included. EDI is updated six times a year.)

Geriatric Dosage Handbook, Semla, T.P., Beizer, J.L., and Higbee, M.D., Eds., Lexi-Comp, Inc., Hudson, OH, 2002. (This guide provides information on medications for the elderly. Informative monographs, compiled from current literature and clinical experiences, cover 800 commonly used drugs. The appendix includes additional clinical drug information (charts, tables, and graphs) relevant to the practice of geriatric pharmacotherapy.)

King Guide to Intravenous Admixtures, Catania, P.N., Ed., King Guide Publications, Inc., St. Louis, MO, updated quarterly. (This reference contains information on the stability and compatibility of parenteral drugs. It is in loose-leaf format and is updated quarterly. The information is presented in tabular form.)

Handbook on Injectable Drugs, 11th ed., Trissel, L.A., American Society of Health-System Pharmacists, Bethesda, MD, 2000. (*Handbook on Injectable Drugs* contains stability and compatibility information on roughly 300 drugs that are commercially available as well as investigational drugs, with references.)

Ident-A-Drug Reference, Therapeutic Research Center, Stockton, CA, 2001. (This reference, updated annually, allows you to quickly identify prescription and OTC tablets and capsules by the code number imprinted on them. The latest version has more than 25,000 drug listings. It lists the code number, physical description, dose, ingredients, National Drug Code (NDC) universal identification number, Drug Enforcement Administration (DEA) class number, and manufacturer of each drug. Brand name and generic products available in the U.S. and in Canada are covered.)

Micromedex, Greenwood Village, CO. (A multiple CD-ROM or Internet-based comprehensive drug information reference, *Micromedex* allows electronic searches of its database. Besides the information available in the printed references, it also provides citations for the primary information sources used to compile the monographs. It can be networked within an institution for availability at multiple workstations. This reference helps the user track down hard to find information without consulting the primary literature. Unapproved but literature-supported uses for medications are well documented in this reference, and the citations are included. The CD-ROM contains multiple references. A user may subscribe to all or only part of the services, as practice requirements dictate. Subscriptions are available for all the modules at additional cost. The available modules are DRUGDEX, POISINDEX, IDENTIDEX, EMERGINDEX, PDR, MARTINDALE, TOMES, and DRUG-REAX. Identidex is a feature of *Micromedex* that can help identify drugs based on the color, shape, and markings on the tablets. It is particularly helpful when trying to identify generic drugs and products of foreign origin.)

Pediatric Dosage Handbook, 8th ed., Taketomo, C.K., Hodding, J.H., and Kraus, D.M., Eds., Lexi-Comp, Hudson, OH, 2001. (This handbook is one of the best references for pediatric drug information. It includes more than 615 monographs featuring compilations of recommended pediatric doses found in the literature. Administration guidelines are provided for the proper administration of oral and parenteral medications. Directions for preparing extemporaneously compounded liquid dosage forms for oral administration are provided along with appropriate references. This may be useful for patients with feeding tubes after consulting a pharmacist about other issues. Guidelines for monitoring patients with laboratory tests and other parameters to assess the efficacy and toxicity of selected medications are provided. Food interactions, describing the interactions between the drug listed in the monograph and food or nutritional substances, are also presented. The handbook is available in soft cover and fits in a laboratory coat pocket.)

Physician's Desk Reference, Medical Economics Inc., Montvale, NJ, 2002. (Known as the PDR, this reference consists of paid advertisements placed by pharmaceutical companies. The advertisement for each drug is limited to the package labeling (package insert) approved by the Federal Food and Drug Administration (FDA). The limitations of the information exceed its benefits for health professionals. Literature-supported but unapproved uses of drugs are not covered. The information is current only as of the last time the package insert was changed (possibly when the drug was first introduced for sale in the U.S.). Drugs that are widely marketed in generic versions but no longer marketed by the originator company may not appear at all, even though they are useful and cost-effective agents (i.e., phenobarbital). One helpful feature of the PDR is the drug identification section with color pictures of dosage forms. The best thing about the PDR is that it may be readily available because it is given away to physicians and may be available on nursing units, in nursing homes, and in clinics.)

United States Pharmacopeia, Volume I, Drug Information for Health Care Professionals (USP-DI, I), U.S. Pharmacopeial Convention, Inc., Rockville, MD, 2001. (This is an excellent source of authoritative drug information. Micromedex has recently become the publisher in collaboration with the U.S. Pharmacopeial Convention. It contains monographs on most brand and generic prescription drugs including side effects, dosing, drug interactions, precautions and storage information, labeled and off-label uses, and patient counseling guidelines. Subscribers also have access to a Web site and online updates as well as online information that can be printed readily.)

United States Pharmacopeia, Volume II, Drug Information for the Patient (USP-DI, II), U.S. Pharmacopeial Convention, Inc., Rockville, MD, 1995. (This is an excellent source of simplified drug monographs, corresponding to *Drug Information for Health Care Professionals*). This reference is designed to provide direct, reassuring guidance on proper drug use for non–health professionals and may be useful to nonpharmacists as well. Information in this reference can be photocopied for patient distribution.)

Internet-Based Resources

Edmund Hayes Homepage, http://www.edhayes.com/. (Edmund Hayes, Pharm.D., R.Ph. maintains a page with multiple pharmacy, medical, and nutritional links to other Web sites. Check out the site and follow the links.)

Intelihealth for the general public, http://www.intelihealth.com/. (A Web site that provides quality medical information for the public. Includes basic drug information and also nutrition information. Patient education leaflets are included.)

CHAPTER 2

Biopharmaceutics of Orally Ingested Products

John W. Holladay

CONTENTS

The goal of this chapter is to present the fundamental concepts of biopharmaceutics and how the ingestion of food may alter the fate of orally ingested drugs. Upon entry into the stomach, food may alter the rate and/or the extent of drug absorption through a variety of direct and indirect mechanisms. A comprehensive examination of food and drug interactions should include the biopharmaceutics and pharmacokinetics viewpoints provided in this chapter. Patients should be aware that food ingestion might enhance or hinder drug action by means of changing drug absorption parameters. This discussion will begin with an overview of the pharmacokinetic parameters that are pertinent to oral drug absorption.

0-8493-1531-X/03/$0.00+$1.50

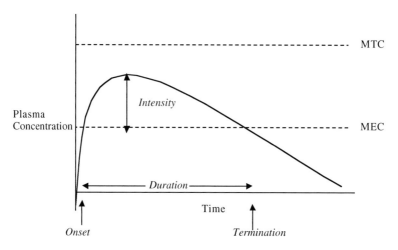

Figure 2.1   Relationship between drug plasma concentration and pharmacological/toxicological action. MTC (minimum toxic concentration), MEC (minimum effective concentration.)

PHARMACOKINETIC PARAMETERS

This discussion limits its consideration to the movement of orally ingested drugs through the gastrointestinal tract (GIT). The movement is active rather than passive. During the sequence from ingestion to elimination, a variety of active processes common to both foods and drugs play important roles. Several pharmacokinetic parameters are used to judge the clinical importance of food/drug interactions. Chapter 1 demonstrated that the appearance and disappearance of drug concentrations in whole blood or blood components (principally plasma or serum) are the primary measures of drug movement into target tissues. Pharmacologic effects occur when the drug reaches these sites in appropriate amounts. The plasma or serum drug concentration vs. time profile of a typical, immediate-release tablet is given in Figure 2.1. From this profile, several meaningful parameters can be obtained that relate the rate and extent of drug absorption from the dosage form. The rate refers to how fast the drug reaches the systemic circulation, which is generally considered to translate into the onset and intensity of the intended drug effect. The extent refers to the total exposure of the drug in the bloodstream. The extent of drug absorption is integral in determining the duration, termination, intensity, and therapeutic index of the drug.

Drugs may be absorbed by various routes and processes. For most drugs, the rate of absorption can be classified as a zero-order or first-order rate process. Although an in-depth discussion of rate orders of reactions is beyond the mission of this chapter, a general understanding of these rate orders facilitates a deeper understanding of how food may alter overall rates of drug absorption. The zero-order rate process proceeds in a constant fashion and without regard to any other factor. In terms of drug absorption, a certain amount of the drug will be absorbed in a given time period and will not change. Usually, zero-order absorption is the

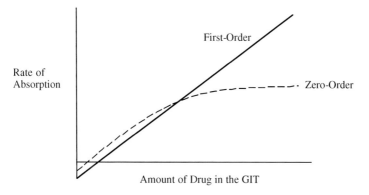

Figure 2.2   Comparative rates of drug absorption from the gastrointestinal tract (GIT).

result of specific drug carriers working at their maximal capacity. The first-order rate process differs considerably from that of a zero-order process. The first-order rate process will increase as the concentration of drug at the absorption site increases. In terms of drug absorption, the rate of drug absorption increases as the drug concentration at the absorption site increases. Figure 2.2 displays the zero- and first-order rate processes as a function of drug concentration at the absorption site.

Rate of Absorption (K_A)

The overall rate of drug absorption, K_A, represents the sum of many individual rates of processes that eventually lead to the appearance of drug in the bloodstream. These individual rates include: (1) the rate of disintegration of the dosage form, (2) the rate of dissolution (or solvation) of the drug from the disintegrated dosage form, (3) the rate of gastric emptying, (4) the rate of drug degradation in the GIT, and (5) the rate of intestinal emptying (transit). If food interferes with any of these processes, then the overall rate of absorption will be affected. Several different methods of determining the rate of absorption exist, and these methods are covered in detail in clinical pharmacokinetics textbooks. In this chapter, we will focus on the use of the K_A term, rather than its discovery from experimental data.

As explained previously, one cannot inspect a plasma-drug concentration vs. time profile and identify the component of the curve that represents K_A. K_A is determined, however, by mathematical treatment of the plasma-drug concentration vs. time data. K_A is used to calculate a tangible parameter called the time to maximal drug concentration (T_{MAX}). This parameter also corresponds to the time to peak absorption. Figure 2.3 relates T_{MAX} to other clinical pharmacokinetic parameters important in the assessment of drug absorption. When considering the implications of the magnitude of K_A, one sees that a small T_{MAX} value leads to a rapid onset of action. Thus, a rapid onset of action correlates to a small T_{MAX} value, which in turn is proportional to a rapid K_A. For certain drugs, food may enhance the rate of absorption, while the same food may substantially reduce the rate of absorption of other drugs.

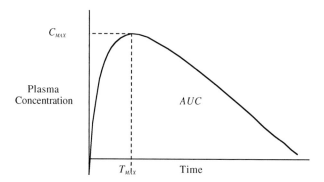

Figure 2.3   Critical pharmacokinetic parameters in the assessment of drug absorption.

Maximal Drug Concentration (C_{MAX})

The maximal concentration or peak concentration of drug in plasma after a single dose occurs at T_{MAX}. Stated differently, C_{MAX} is a function of and is inversely related to T_{MAX}. C_{MAX} directly impacts the intensity of the pharmacological and/or toxicological drug action. Therefore, circumstances that may slow the rate of absorption (and thus increase T_{MAX}) may result in a decrease in C_{MAX}. This in turn may reduce the intensity of drug action. Figure 2.3 visually demonstrates the relationship between T_{MAX} and C_{MAX}.

Area under the Plasma Concentration vs. Time Curve (AUC)

AUC is the fundamental pharmacokinetic parameter that denotes the extent of drug absorption. Many dosing regimens are based on the total systemic exposure of a drug after a given dose as measured by the plasma-drug AUC. The unusual dimension of the AUC term (mass × time/volume) is due to the formula used to derive AUC. Two (x, y) coordinates on the plasma-drug concentration vs. time curve create a trapezoid, and, as such, the area contained in that trapezoid can be calculated with elementary geometry. Thus, the "AUC" term is the sum of all the individual trapezoids formed by the drug plasma concentration vs. time data. The magnitude of the AUC value influences the intensity, duration and termination of activity (see Figure 2.1). AUC is also governed by metabolic and elimination pathways; therefore, the prediction of how food may directly alter the magnitude of AUC is confounding.

One of the main elimination routes of any drug absorbed in the GIT occurs during its first pass through the liver. As a result of this pathway that is designed to protect the body from toxins, it is quite likely that not all of the drug that is absorbed will reach the systemic circulation. The AUC value is thus used to calculate the bioavailability (F) of the drug or the percentage of the dose that reaches the systemic circulation. The following expressions describe the relationships among the parameters discussed in this section.

$$AUC \propto F$$

$$T_{MAX} \propto 1/K_A$$

$$C_{MAX} \propto K_A$$

$$C_{MAX} \propto F$$

GASTROINTESTINAL PHYSIOLOGICAL RESPONSE TO INGESTED FOOD AND LIQUIDS

The anatomy of the GIT has been well characterized by numerous texts and will not be covered in this chapter. The effects of food, however, on GIT secretions, motility, and dynamics are integral to understanding how food will affect the pharmacokinetic parameters mentioned in the previous section. The primary focus of this section will be to discuss the physiological processes mentioned in the rate of absorption section.

Gastric Emptying Rate

Arguably, the gastric (stomach) emptying rate (GER) is the most important parameter that influences the rate of drug absorption from the GIT. Since most of a drug dose is absorbed in the small intestine, the rate at which the drug is presented to the small intestine is often the rate-limiting process of drug absorption. Many factors can influence the GER, including the type and volume of meal ingested, the emotional state of the patient, the body position of the patient, and coadministered drugs.[1] Table 2.1 eloquently describes how various factors influence gastric emptying rate. The GER is slower for solids, which need more processing than do liquids prior to presentation to the small intestine.[1,2]

Solids

Owing to the primary function of the stomach, the ingestion of food delays the gastric emptying rate.[3] In addition, the magnitude of this decrease in GER is dependent on the volume and the type of meal ingested (see Table 2.1). High-fat meals tend to slow the rate of gastric emptying to a greater degree than one rich in carbohydrates or amino acids. The ingestion of food elevates gastric pH and slows the longitudinal motility of the stomach to allow food sequestration in the stomach for processing. Changes in stomach pH that result from food ingestion can produce significant effects on drug absorption for those drugs whose dissolution is dependent on low pH. This topic will be covered in the section on Drug Dissolution.

In some instances, food can alter the rate order of drug absorption. The amount of the vitamin riboflavin absorbed has been studied in fasted and fed subjects.[3] In fasted subjects, riboflavin is absorbed in a zero order fashion. In other words, the amount of drug absorbed as a function of time will not change regardless of the magnitude of the dose. In the presence of food, the presentation of riboflavin to

Table 2.1   Circumstances That Influence Gastric Emptying

Circumstance	Influence on Gastric Emptying
Volume of substance ingested	In general, the slowing of gastric emptying is proportional to the volume of substance ingested
Type of Meal	
Fatty acids	Reduction in the gastric emptying rate is proportional to the amount of fatty acid in the stomach as well as the side chain length
Triglycerides	Unsaturated triglycerides reduce the gastric emptying rate to a greater extent than saturated triglycerides
Carbohydrates	Reduction in the gastric emptying rate is proportional to the amount of carbohydrates in the stomach
Amino acids	Reduction in the gastric emptying rate is proportional to the amount of amino acids in the stomach
Physical properties of stomach contents	Liquids empty faster than solids; the rate of gastric emptying is reduced in proportion to the size of the solid material that must be broken down
Drugs	
Anticholinergics	Reduce gastric emptying rate
Narcotic analgesics	Reduce gastric emptying rate
Ethanol	Reduces gastric emptying rate
Metoclopramide	Increases gastric emptying rate
Miscellaneous	
Body position	Gastric emptying rate is reduced in a patient lying on left side
Emotional states	Stress and aggression increase gastric emptying rate; depression reduces gastric emptying rate
Disease states	Dependent upon the disease
Exercise	Vigorous exercise reduces gastric emptying rate

Source: Adapted from Shargel, L. and Yu, A., *Applied Biopharmaceutics and Pharmacokinetics,* 3rd ed., McGraw-Hill/Appleton & Lange, New York, 1996, 126. With permission.

the absorption site is slowed to the point that absorption occurs at a first order rate. The presentation of riboflavin was sufficiently slow that the transport carriers were not saturated. Thus, the amount of drug absorbed increased as the dose increased (Table 2.2).

Liquids

The ingestion of liquids does not significantly reduce the GER, primarily because liquids need minimal physiological processing before their presentation into the small intestine. Recent studies suggest, however, that liquids can indeed slow the GER as a function of their caloric content.[2–3] This theory is supported by data obtained in various laboratories that investigated whether the use of an acidic beverage, such as Coca-Cola® or grapefruit juice, may lower the pH of the stomach and thus promote the dissolution of the weakly basic drugs (e.g., itraconazole and ketoconazole). In addition, this longer residence time in the stomach may aid in the solvation of poorly

Table 2.2 First Order and Zero Order Absorption as a Function of Food Presence

Dose (mg) of Riboflavin	Percent Absorbed		Amount Absorbed (mg)	
	Fasting	Fed	Fasting	Fed
5	48	62	2.4	3.1
10	30	63	3.0	6.3
15	16	61	2.4	9.15

Source: Adapted from Levy, G. and Jusko, W.J., *J. Pharm. Sci.,* 55, 285, 1966.

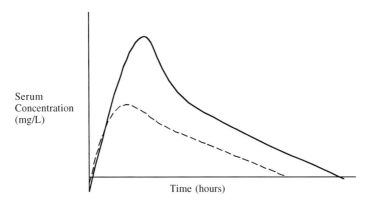

Figure 2.4 Influence of coingestion of water or Coca-Cola® on the blood levels of itraconazole. (Adapted from Jaruratanasirikul, S. and Kleepkaew, A., *Eur. J. Clin. Pharmacol.,* 52, 235–237, 1997. With permission.)

soluble, lipophilic drugs such as itraconazole.[5–8] Figure 2.4 depicts the benefit of a delay in gastric emptying as the C_{MAX} and AUC of itraconazole were dramatically improved by the reduction in gastric emptying rate following ingestion of Coca-Cola®. At pH values that should have promoted prompt drug dissolution and absorption (e.g., pH 1–3), the rates of absorption of these drugs, as reflected in T_{MAX} values, was not enhanced by the acidic beverage.[8] To further emphasize the point, Carver and colleagues lowered the gastric pH using glutamic acid and demonstrated that the T_{MAX} of itraconazole was unchanged.[5] Therefore, the caloric content of the liquid may be the determining factor in the magnitude of GER reductions.

The volume of fluid also plays a role in the rate of absorption. This was demonstrated in studies with several antibiotics taken with a small volume of water (e.g., 20–25 mL) or a large volume of water (e.g., 250–500 mL). Dramatic differences were observed in the drug concentration vs. time profiles for these drugs simply as a function of the volume of fluid ingested (Figure 2.5). Thus, patients who take medications with a large volume of water as opposed to a small volume of water may exhibit considerably different onset, duration, and intensity of drug action. Not all drugs will show these substantial changes in their disposition as a function of the type and volume of fluid ingested, but it is wise to instruct patients to be consistent in their chosen method of ingesting medications.

As previously mentioned, the pH of the stomach may play a role in the rate of absorption of drugs. In general, weakly basic drugs, such as antihistamines and nasal

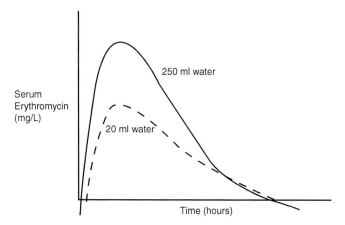

Figure 2.5   Influence of the volume of fluid on the absorption of erythromycin. (Adapted from data
reported in Shargel, L. and Yu, A., *Applied Biopharmaceutics and Pharmacokinetics,*
3rd ed., McGraw-Hill/Appleton & Lange, New York, 1996, 129. With permission.)

decongestants, dissolve rapidly into the low pH environment of the stomach due to
the favorable ionization profile. Conversely, weakly acidic drugs, such as most
nonsteroidal antiinflammatory drugs (NSAIDs), are poorly soluble in the stomach
because acid molecules tend to remain unionized in strongly acidic environments.
One of the fundamental steps in the absorption process is the dissolution (or solvation) of the drug molecules into stomach fluids from the administered dosage form.
If a drug is poorly soluble in the stomach and, as a result, the dissolution of the
drug molecules is slow, then the rate of absorption of the drug will decrease.
Paradoxically, a solubilized drug in an ionized state is considered to be poorly
absorbed. Drugs must be deionized to cross a lipophilic biological membrane, unless
a specific active transport mechanism exists to facilitate its movement across membranes. Ideally, a drug molecule must be ionized to facilitate its dissolution and then
unionized to be absorbed. In reality, even ionized drug molecules are absorbed well
in the small intestine due to its tremendous surface area and lengthy residence time.
Table 2.3 displays the pH values and residence times of various portions of the GIT
during a fasted condition.

**Table 2.3   Physiological Properties of the
GIT in the Fasted State**

Region	pH	Residence Time (h)
Stomach	1.5–2	0–3
Small Intestine		
Duodenum	4.9–6.4	3–4
Jejunum	4.4–6.4	3–4
Ileum	6.5–7.4	3–4
Colon	7.4	Up to 18

Source: From Fleisher, D. et al., *Clin. Pharmacokinet.,* 36(3): 237, 1999. With permission.

Intestinal Transit

Whereas the GER is sensitive to ingested solids and liquids, the intestinal emptying rate is virtually independent of food or liquid ingestion.[9] Numerous drugs, however, can affect intestinal tone and motility. Stimulant laxatives increase the movement of material from the small intestine distally, and this disruption in homeostasis can easily affect the extent of drug absorption. Alternatively, antidiarrheals, such as loperamide as well as narcotic analgesics, significantly slow intestinal motility, and this may alter the extent of drug absorption. Concomitantly administered medications that affect intestinal tone also affect intestinal transit to a greater degree than food ingestion.

Drug Dissolution

The physical and chemical microphenomena that characterize drug dissolution are covered in great detail in several biopharmaceutics textbooks. It is important to mention in this forum a few basic concepts of drug dissolution. The measurement of the rate of drug dissolution is a prime aspect in the Food and Drug Administration (FDA) review of new drug applications. As previously mentioned, weakly basic drugs dissolve well in acidic environments and weakly acidic drugs dissolve well in basic environments. If food (solid or liquid) alters the pH of the stomach fluid, then the dissolution rate of weak acids and bases will be affected.

The dissolution rate of many drugs is slower than the overall rate of drug absorption. For such drugs, the dissolution rate limits their absorption. Tablets, capsules, and other compressed, oral dosage forms typically belong to this category. Circumstances that influence the dissolution rate for these drugs will have a substantial impact on drug absorption. Whereas food and calorie-laden liquids reduce the gastric emptying rate and thereby reduce the rate of absorption of drugs, the effect of food on the dissolution rate of drug molecules is not as clear. The dissolution rate of numerous drugs is unaffected by the ingestion of food; however, this is not the case for all drugs.

In general, the dissolution rate of highly lipophilic drugs is enhanced when the drug is taken with food, especially foods rich in fat. A great example is the original formulation of the antifungal drug, griseofulvin. The dissolution rate and, thus, the rate of absorption of griseofulvin is substantially increased when taken with food. The dissolution rate of highly lipophilic drugs, therefore, may be enhanced when taken with a fatty meal. In the case of griseofulvin, its absorption has been remarkably enhanced by reducing the particle size of the drug aggregates and thus improving its dissolution characteristics.

Complexation and Degradation

In addition to the influence on the GER and dissolution rate, the ingestion of food may endanger the drug molecule. These dangers are manifested in the forms of acidic degradation, food–drug adsorption, and complexation. Any of these may significantly reduce or prevent drug absorption.

Acidic degradation of acid-sensitive drugs is a primary concern when drugs and food are taken together. Classic examples of acid-sensitive drugs include aspirin and the various first-generation penicillins. If the residence time of these drugs in the stomach is increased by the presence of food, then the degradation of these drugs increases. As a result, the extent of drug absorption may be substantially reduced because the active degradation reduces the amount of drug available to be transported across the mucosa and distributed in the circulation.

Drug molecules may adsorb onto food components and, thus, may lead to a reduction in the rate and extent of absorption. Conversely, food particles may interact with drug molecules in the stomach and small intestine. Numerous instances of multivalent cation complexation with the older tetracyclines exist. When these medications are taken with food (or other drug preparations) containing iron, calcium, aluminum, magnesium, and other multivalent cations, insoluble complexes may be formed that render the drug unabsorbable.

The effect of food on the rate and extent of absorption, by any of the above mechanisms, is generally considered to be less critical when drugs are taken 30 min or more before feeding or 2 h postprandial. Although the preceding sections contained several examples of prescription drugs, these types of interactions may easily occur with OTC medications. Indeed, with the recent increasing trend of prescription to OTC movement, these interactions may become more prevalent.

REFERENCES

1. Shargel, L. and Yu, A., *Applied Biopharmaceutics and Pharmacokinetics,* 3rd ed., McGraw-Hill/Appleton & Lange, New York, 1996, 126.
2. Yu, L.X., Crison, J.R., and Amidon, G.L., Compartmental transit and dispersion model analysis of small intestinal transit flow in humans, *Int. J. Pharm.,* 140, 111, 1996.
3. Levy, G. and Jusko, W.J., Factors affecting the absorption of riboflavin in man, *J. Pharm. Sci.,* 55, 285, 1966.
4. Shafer, R.B. et al., Do calories, osmolality or calcium determine gastric emptying? *Am. J. Physiol.,* 248, 479, 1985.
5. Carver, P., Wellace, L., and Kauffman, C., The effect of food and gastric pH on the oral bioavailability of Itraconazole in HIV+ patients. Paper presented at *Pharmacokinetics and Pharmacodynamics,* 36th ICAAC Conference, 1996.
6. Chin, W.W., Loeb, M., and Fong, I.W., Effects of an acidic beverage (Coca-Cola®) on absorption of ketoconazole, *Antimicrob. Agents Chemother.,* 39, 1671, 1995.
7. Lange, D. et al., Effect of a cola beverage on the bioavailability of itraconazole in the presence of H_2 blockers, *J. Clin. Pharmacol.,* 37, 535, 1997.
8. Jaruratanasirikul, S. and Kleepkaew, A., Influence of an acidic beverage (Cola-Cola) in the absorption of itraconazole, *Eur. J. Clin. Pharmacol.,* 52, 235, 1997.
9. Penzak, S.R. et al., Grapefruit juice decreases the systemic availability of itraconazole capsules in healthy volunteers, *Ther. Drug. Monit.,* 21, 304, 1999.
10. Fleisher, D. et al., Drug, meal and formulation interactions influencing drug absorption after oral administration: clinical implications, *Clin. Pharmacokinet.,* 36, 237, 1999.

CHAPTER **3**

Drug Interactions: Basic Concepts

Eric H. Frankel

CONTENTS

OVERVIEW

    Drug–drug interaction refers to an alteration of the effect of one drug caused by the presence of a second drug. Drug–nutrient interactions similarly refer to the alteration of the effect of a drug or nutrient caused by the presence of a second agent. Drug interactions can be beneficial or detrimental. At times we intentionally produce a drug–drug interaction. One example would be administering a drug product like carbidopa/levodopa (Sinemet®). Levodopa is converted to dopamine in the central nervous system (CNS), thereby exerting an effect against symptoms of Parkinson's disease. Carbidopa acts as a chemical decoy, which binds to the enzyme that converts levodopa to domapine outside the CNS. This increases dopamine levels in the CNS while limiting side effects of increased dopamine in peripheral tissues. In combination, the paired drugs produce additive effects. Patients with numerous disease states may require treatment with interacting drugs. Where these interactions

0-8493-1531-X/03/$0.00+$1.50

cannot be avoided, the fact is taken into account when planning therapy. Many times dosing is not altered at all, but usual monitoring is increased.

TYPES AND MECHANISMS OF DRUG–DRUG AND DRUG–NUTRIENT INTERACTIONS

Now that basic information about pharmaceutics, pharmacokinetics, and pharmacodynamics has been presented, drug interactions can be appreciated. The types of interactions that can occur include potentiation, inhibition, alteration of absorption, direct chemical interaction, alteration of metabolism, alteration of distribution, competition at the site of action, and alteration of elimination.

Potentiation can be additive or synergistic and refers to an increase in the effect of one drug as a result of a second drug or nutrient. The increased pain relief experienced when acetaminophen is combined with a narcotic (Tylenol #3®, Vicodin®, Lortabs®) illustrates a positive example of this effect. Adding bananas, potatoes, and other foods rich in potassium to the diet at the same time a patient is taking a prescribed potassium supplement (e.g., Kaon-Cl®) would cause an additive food–nutrient effect with a therapeutic purpose.

Inhibition refers to the decrease of effect when two substances have opposite effects on a process. The decreased anticoagulant effect of warfarin (Coumadin®) seen when vitamin K intake is increased is a negative example of this type of interaction. Warfarin therapy frequently requires adjustment because of such inhibition, especially when patients suddenly increase their intake of green leafy vegetables rich in vitamin K. This is a real hazard for patients who are avid gardeners and whose vitamin K intake can vary drastically from season to season. Caffeine, a nonnutritive food constituent, may oppose the pharmacological effect of tranquilizers.

Decreased absorption of nonheme iron from food is seen when antacids are taken on a chronic basis with iron-containing foods. This may result in iron deficiency anemia with its characteristic microcytic, hypochromic, red blood cells. Grapefruit juice will increase the bioavailability of cyclosporine (Sandimmune®). This will decrease the potential for organ rejection by recipients of organ transplants, but may also increase the potential for cyclosporine toxicity. Deliberate ingestion of grapefruit to decrease cytosporine doses is not advised due to the unpredictable nature of this interaction.

An example of a direct chemical interaction is the reaction between dextrose and amino acids in parenteral nutrition. This is the same reaction seen when meats are cooked and is known as the Maillard reaction. The substrates involved tend to reduce sugars and amino acids, and these factors limit the storage time for parenteral nutrition solutions. The reaction results in a darkening of the solution.

Alterations of metabolism may also occur. This generally occurs in the liver but may also be peripheral. Many enzymes responsible for drug metabolism are part of the cytochrome P-450 family. St. John's Wort induces an increase in the activity of one P-450 isoform termed CYP 3A4. This can result in decreased levels of cyclosporine, indinavir, and oral contraceptives. This drug interaction with St. John's Wort demonstrates the potential for herbal products to participate in significant herb-drug interactions when used in combinations with conventional medications.

Alterations of distribution may occur when drugs are protein-bound. Binding to protein will generally reduce the amount of free drug. Decreased amounts of free drug may decrease the activity of the drug and also decrease the metabolism and elimination of the drug. In this type of interaction, one substance that is bound displaces another bound substance from a binding site. The effect, if any, may be transient because the increased effect of the free drug may be countered by increased metabolism and excretion of the free drug. Some significance is possible if the second agent is taken on an intermittent basis. A nontransient example of this is the need to adjust measured serum total calcium levels based on serum albumin levels. Only ionized Ca++ is physiologically active. Most clinicians do not have rapid access to ionized calcium levels; total serum calcium levels are commonly available. Because each gram of albumin in the bloodstream will bind with approximately 0.8 mg of calcium, serum with a lower than normal albumin concentration will have a lower amount of bound calcium. This will result in a lower total calcium level, even if the ionized (unbound) calcium is normal. Many clinicians calculate the corrected calcium level by subtracting the patient's albumin level from either 4.0 g/dL (mid-point of normal range) or 3.5 g/dL (low normal albumin), then multiplying this by 0.8 mg/g, and adding this factor to the total serum calcium.

An example of competition at the site of action is best illustrated by the effect of naloxone (Narcan®) on narcotics. Naloxone reverses the effects of narcotics at a receptor site. This can be useful after surgery to reverse the effects of intraoperative narcotics. Naloxone is also useful in the treatment of narcotic overdoses. Caution is needed if an individual is dependent on narcotic drugs because naloxone can cause withdrawal symptoms. This interaction is further modified by drug metabolism. Naloxone is eliminated faster than the narcotics that it affects. It is, therefore, necessary to monitor a patient who has received a narcotic overdose even after he appears to have recovered. The naloxone may wear off, and then the narcotic effect will recur.

Renal excretion may also be involved in interactions between drugs and nutrients. The classic example is the effect of most diuretics (e.g., loop diuretics and thiazide diuretics) on potassium. These diuretics result in increased loss of potassium in the urine. This may require pharmacological or nutritional supplementation of potassium intake.

Drug Interaction Risk Factors and the Unknown

By now, the potential for unexpected effects as a result of interactions between a drug and other drugs or foods has been well established. The risk of having drug interactions will be increased as the number of medications taken by an individual increases. This also implies a greater risk for the elderly and the chronically ill, as they will be using more medications than the general population. Risks also increase when a patient's regimen originates from multiple prescribers. Filling all prescriptions in a single pharmacy may decrease the risk of undetected interactions.

The method for getting new drugs approved has increased in efficiency in recent years. Drug studies done to seek approval of a new agent are often done on "ideal" populations, that is, individuals with a single ailment. This highlights the effect of the drug being studied. As a result, few subjects are taking other medications. Once the drug is approved, it is used by a less select group of patients. As a result, the full extent of drug interaction potential may be only recognized after the drug is widely available. In addition, medical practice is highly individualized and managed based on specific patient response. This may delay or prevent recognition of interactions. Taking a thorough medical, drug, and nutritional history from patients when they seek medical attention may help identify drug–drug and drug–nutrient interactions.

UNCLASSIFIED INTERACTIONS

Effects of Nutritional Status on Drugs

The presence of nutritional abnormalities may have an effect on drugs. Drug dosages may need adjustment based on actual body weight for some drugs. Other drugs may need to be dosed differently in obese, normal, and underweight patients, based on actual, ideal, or an adjusted body weight corrected for lean body mass. Somatic protein status may affect the dosing of medications that bind to somatic protein.

Effects of Drugs on Nutritional Status

The converse effect may also be observed. Some drugs will have an effect on a patient's nutritional status. The mechanisms for these effects are varied and are usually due to drug side effects. Medications may have direct effects on the gastrointestinal tract (GIT), which can affect food ingestion. Nonsteroidal antiinflammatory agents, commonly used to treat arthritis, including aspirin, can cause irritation of the upper gastrointestinal mucosa and even cause ulcers. This can depress appetite and produce weight loss. Chemotherapeutic agents used to treat cancer can affect rapidly growing tissues, particularly the lining of the GIT. Nausea is a common side effect and will interfere with eating. Some patients develop oral and esophageal lesions that cause pain upon chewing and swallowing (odynophagia), which limits oral intake. Antibiotics can suppress commensal bacteria, and this may result in overgrowth of other organisms such as *Candida albicans*. Overgrowth in the GIT may produce malabsorption and, subsequently, diarrhea. Overgrowth in the mouth may result in candidiasis or thrush, which can reduce oral intake. Drug-related dysgeusia may result in alteration of taste perceptions and avoidance of certain foods. Many drugs reduce salivation and cause dryness of the mucus membranes. This may also inhibit oral intake. Nausea, vomiting, diarrhea, and constipation are ubiquitous side effects associated with most medications and even with placebo medications. Again, oral intake of food may be reduced due to these effects.

Some drugs have a direct effect on digestion. Orlistat (Xenical®) interferes with the digestion and subsequent absorption of fat intentionally to enhance weight loss.

Pancreatic enzymes enhance digestion for patients with limited amounts of digestive enzymes. Several types of drugs interfere with hydrochloric acid production, but none have demonstrated a significant effect on macronutrient absorption. Increasing the gastric pH may affect absorption of weakly acidic drugs, as well as iron and vitamin B_{12}. Intrinsic factor requires an acidic pH to bind with vitamin B_{12}. Without the acidic pH, B_{12} deficiency can have an irreversible effect on brain function if prolonged without treatment.

Some drugs have a direct effect on appetite. The amphetamines and their derivatives were long used for weight loss. Unfortunately, side effects and transient results for most patients have limited their usefulness. Sibutramine (Meridia®) has both an appetite suppressing effect and a mild antidepressant effect and is approved by the Food and Drug Administration (FDA) for weight loss. These drugs are discussed in more detail in the Chapter 11, Obesity and Appetite Drugs, and Chapter 7, Gastrointestinal and Metabolic Disorders and Drugs.

Dronabinol (Marinol®), also known as THC (from tetrahydracannabinols), the active principle in cannabis, is also used as an appetite stimulant. Oxandrolone (Oxandrin®) is an anabolic steroid approved for weight gain. Megesterol (Megace®), a progestin used to treat certain types of cancer, is also indicated to enhance appetite. Cyproheptadine (Periactin®) has been used to enhance appetite, although this is an off-label use and not an FDA-approved indication.

Besides drugs specifically indicated to effect changes in appetite, some drugs may affect appetite as a side effect. Several antidepressants have been observed to consistently increase or decrease appetite. When these drugs are prescribed, their relative side-effect profiles in relation to weight change may make one or another a preferred agent for an individual who would benefit from an increase or decrease in weight.

REFERENCE MATERIALS

This chapter has presented a brief overview of fundamental ways to categorize and describe drug–drug interactions. Understanding pharmacology is central to the process, for it uses information about drug actions and side effects to identify problematic characteristics in another drug that may be added to a patient's regimen. Interactions are also characterized as clinically significant when they are documented to occur and either interfere with care or pose a danger to the patient. Some interactions are deemed potential. Potential interactions are those that pharmacology predicts are possible, but their significance is as yet not documented. Readers who wish to know more about drug–drug interactions may consult the following references for further information and for in-depth and authoritative information. The list includes several items already noted in Chapter 1, but repeated here for ease of access.

Textbooks and References

Hansten & Horn's Drug Interactions Analysis and Management, Hansten, P.D. and Horn, J.R., Eds. Facts & Comparisons, Inc., St. Louis, MO, updated quarterly.

(This text is the touchstone for learning about drug–drug interactions. It details the mechanism of various drug interactions. It is useful for someone seeking a comprehensive understanding of how drugs interact and a guide to clinically significant interactions.)

Goodman and Gilman's The Pharmacological Basis of Therapeutics, 9th ed., Hardman, J.F. and Limbird, L.E., Eds., McGraw-Hill, New York, 1996. (This is the classic reference for pharmacology. It can guide the reader to an understanding of how particular drugs or classes of drugs exert their pharmacological effects, and what the mechanisms for side effects are.)

Drugs Manuals and References

Drug Interaction Facts, Tatro, D.S, Ed., Facts & Comparisons, Inc., St. Louis, MO, updated quarterly. (Providing extensive information about drug–drug and drug–food interactions, this reference examines mechanisms, clinical significance, timing, and management of interactions. The information is quite clear and accessible. Case and study descriptions are provided, and the information is referenced. It is available in both a hardbound and a computer format. Subscribers are provided with quarterly updates.)

Evaluations of Drug Interactions, Vol. 1, II (EDI), Zucchero, F.J., Hogan, M.J., and Schultz, C.D., Eds., First DataBank, St. Louis, MO, 1999. (This book is a comprehensive reference for both prescription and over-the-counter (OTC) drug conflicts. It covers more than 34,000 drug interactions. Each interaction is outlined in a monograph format. The monographs include severity coding of the interaction, a summary of the overall effect of the interaction, and a synopsis of documented cases. Mechanisms of action and related agents that are chemically similar to the interacting drugs are discussed. Helpful recommendations, when available, for acceptable alternative therapies supported by primary literature are also included. EDI is updated six times a year.)

Drug Facts and Comparisons, Facts & Comparisons, Inc., St. Louis, MO, updated monthly. (This is the drug reference that is most extensively used by pharmacists. It is somewhat more oriented to community practice. A loose-leaf format that is updated monthly, a hardbound format that is updated annually, and a CD-ROM are all marketed. The CD-ROM can be made accessible on a computer network. It covers over 10,000 products and includes comparison charts between similar products. Both OTC and prescription products are covered. Both FDA-approved and non–FDA-approved (off-label) uses of drugs are covered. Information is presented on a large number of, but not all, investigational agents. The monthly updates highlight product changes. Manufacturer addresses, normal lab values, and pharmaceutical abbreviations are included. It includes the information that is commonly required by practitioners about medications. Pharmacology, pharmacokinetics, adverse reactions, drug interactions, and food interactions are all covered. Information about side effects and interactions is presented in tabular form for many classes of drugs at the beginning of each chapter. This reference will answer the great majority of inquiries about possible drug–drug interactions in everyday practice.)

AHFS Drug Information 2003, McEvoy, G.K., Ed., American Society of Health-System Pharmacists, Bethesda, MD, 2003. (This reference provides detailed monographs on most drugs and includes both FDA-approved and non–FDA-approved (off-label) uses and information on the stability and incompatibility of drugs. Monographs cover pharmacology, pharmacokinetics, dosages, contraindications, precautions, adverse effects, and interactions. It is an essential supplement to other commonly available sources of information about drug interactions. Quarterly updates issued but most revision is done annually. This reference is also available in hard and soft cover editions as well as on CD-ROM, Personal Digital Assistant (PDA) compatible format (abridged but personalized format), and online by subscription. The soft cover edition usually gets dog-eared after a year in a busy pharmacy department. It is most commonly found in hospital pharmacy settings because the American Society of Health-System Pharmacists is the publisher. The information on each agent in this reference is more extensive than *Drug Facts and Comparisons*.)

King Guide to Intravenous Admixtures, Catania, P.N., Ed., King Guide Publications, Inc., St. Louis, MO, updated quarterly. (This reference is of concern for caregivers involved with intravenous medications and in parenteral nutrition. It contains authoritative information on the stability and compatibility of parenteral drugs. The book also makes clear that some incompatibilities are significant only for long-term admixtures, which are then to be stored for long times. Other incompatibilities relate immediately to direct mixing of drugs (e.g., when a clinician wishes to draw two drugs into the same syringe). It is in loose-leaf format and is updated quarterly. The information is presented in tabular form.)

Handbook on Injectable Drugs, 10th ed., Trissel, L.A., American Society of Health-System Pharmacists, Bethesda, MD, 1998. (*Handbook on Injectable Drugs* contains stability and compatibility information on roughly 300 drugs that are commercially available as well as investigational drugs, with references. Drug administration via Y-site is also covered. This reference is also essential for caregivers involved with injectable medications and parental nutrition.)

Micromedex [Healthcare series on CD-ROM], Micromedex, Inc., Greenwood, CO. A multiple CD-ROM, PDA, or *Micromedex*-based drug interaction reference. The PDA version is abridged due to electronic data storage constraints. *Micromedex* allows electronic searches of its database. Besides the information available in the printed references, it also provides citations for the primary information sources used to compile the monographs. It can be networked within an institution for availability at multiple workstations. This reference helps the user locate hard to find information without consulting the primary literature. Unapproved but literature-supported uses for medications are well documented in this reference, and the citations are included. The CD-ROM contains multiple references. A user may subscribe to all or only part of the services, as practice requirements dictate. Subscriptions are available for all the modules at additional cost. The available modules are DRUGDEX, POISINDEX, IDENTIDEX, EMERGINDEX, PDR, MARTINDALE, TOMES, and DRUG-REAX. Identidex is a feature of *Micromedex* that can help identify drugs based on the color, shape, and markings on the tablets. It is particularly helpful when trying to identify generic drugs and products of foreign origin.)

Physician's Desk Reference, Medical Economics Inc., Montvale, NJ, 2002. (Known as the PDR, this is reference consists of paid advertisements placed by pharmaceutical companies. The advertisement for each drug is limited to the package labeling (package insert) approved by the Federal Drug and Cosmetic Agency (FDC). The limitations of the information exceed its benefits for health professionals. Literature-supported but unapproved uses of drugs are not covered. The information is current only as of the last time the package insert was changed (possibly when the drug was first introduced for sale in the U.S.). Drugs that are widely marketed in generic versions but no longer marketed by the originator company may not appear at all, even though they are useful and cost effective agents. One helpful feature of the PDR is the drug identification section with color pictures of dosage forms. The best thing about the PDR is that it may be readily available since it is given away to physicians for free and may be available on nursing units, nursing homes, and clinics.)

United States Pharmacopeia, Vol. I, Drug Information for Health Care Professionals (USP-DI, I), U.S. Pharmacopeial Convention, Inc., Rockville, MD, 1995. (This is an excellent source of authoritative drug information. Micromedex has recently become the publisher in collaboration with the U.S. Pharmacopeial Convention. It contains monographs on most brand and generic prescription drugs including side effects, dosing, drug interactions, precautions and storage information, labeled and off-label uses, and patient counseling guidelines. Subscribers also have access to a Web site and online updates as well as online information that can be printed readily.)

United States Pharmacopeia, Vol. II, Drug Information for the Patient (USP-DI, II), U.S. Pharmacopeial Convention, Inc., Rockville, MD, 1995. (This is an excellent source of simplified drug monographs (corresponding to *Drug Information for Health Care Professionals*). This reference is designed to provide direct, reassuring guidance on proper drug use for non–health professionals and may be useful to nonpharmacists as well. Information in this reference can be photocopied for patient distribution.)

Internet-Based Resources

Edmund Hayes Homepage, http://www.edhayes.com/. (Edmund Hayes, Pharm.D., R.Ph. maintains a page with multiple pharmacy, medical, and nutritional links to other Web sites. Check out the site and follow the links.)

RxList, http://www.rxlist.com. (This URL leads to a professionally-oriented source of drug information. This site includes links to other sites and provides a medical dictionary and an abbreviations reference. It is frequently updated and has patient-oriented information as well.)

Intelihealth for the general public, http://www.intelihealth.com/. (A Web site that provides quality medical information for the public, it includes access to three USP resources: USP-DI, II, USP-DI patient education leaflets, and USP-DI medicine charts, which provide summaries of drug treatments.)

Gold Standard Multimedia, http://www.gsm.com/. (This Web site provides access to *Clinical Pharmacology 2000,* Integrated Medical Curriculum, Virtual Human Gallery (three-dimensional anatomy), and Faculty Development Resources. Registration requires payment of an annual fee.)

Intelihealth Drug Interactions Checker (powered by MicroMedex Drug-Reax Software), http://www.intelihealth.com/cgi-bin/drugreax.p1?st=8124&r=WSIHW000. (This site features an application that will check a group of drugs for any interactions.)

Drug Interaction Checker from Cerner, http://www.drugs.com/xq/cfm/pageID_1150/ 9x/index.htm (This is another Web-based, computerized drug interaction checker. You enter the medications that someone is taking one at a time. When you check for interactions, drug–nutrient interactions are displayed as well as the drug–drug interactions.)

CHAPTER 4

Nutrition and Metabolism

Ronni Chernoff

CONTENTS

Nutrients and drugs share many common characteristics in their basic metabolism that may lead to competition between the two and, thus, reduce the benefits derived from either or both of these essential elements of modern health maintenance. Other distinctively different characteristics may create adverse events.

Understanding these basic similarities and differences may contribute to more effective interdisciplinary healthcare. The intent of this chapter is to present an overview of basic concepts in metabolism with a comparison of the similarities and

0-8493-1531-X/03/$0.00+$1.50

differences between nutrition and pharmacy. The basic concepts presented will include ingestion, digestion, metabolism, and elimination.

INGESTION AND ABSORPTION CONCEPTS

Food nutrients are ingested orally, with the exception of those persons who are unable to ingest or digest food through the gastrointestinal tract (GIT) and must be fed through a parenteral route. The vast majority of drugs are taken orally. The first similarity in the metabolism of nutrients and drugs is that both share common routes of ingestion or administration, whichever term is used. "Sip or drip" may apply equally to nutrition and pharmacy. From there, the underlying concepts of therapeutic interventions by dietitians and pharmacists diverge. Dietitians are taught that food is not nutrition until it passes the lips or is consumed. The physiologist and biochemist are more likely to point out that it is truly not nutrition until it passes from the gut lumen into gastrointestinal cells. Thus, the nutritionist operates under the concept that a substance is not nutrition until it is consumed and passes from the gut lumen into the circulation or a cell. The pharmacist, on the other hand, views a drug entity as not being therapeutic until it passes into a system for distribution to the target organ, a mass of cells where its site of action resides.

Whereas the major components of the gastrointestinal tract (e.g., mouth, esophagus, stomach, small intestine, and large intestine) are really the only truly important routes of introducing nutrition into the body, the opposite is true of drugs. Multiple routes (e.g., intramuscular, intravenous, buccal, or sublingual) may provide major sites of introduction for certain drugs. With the exception of alcoholic beverages, the stomach plays only a minor role in direct absorption of food components, while the stomach serves as a major site of absorption for weakly acidic drugs.

ABSORPTION AND DIGESTION

In general, foods require digestion to enable them to be absorbed. Other than simple sugar beverages, food undergoes multiple processes for digestion that allow passage through the gastrointestinal tract in a serial absorptive process with specific areas where different nutrients are absorbed. If damage occurs in a given segment of the gut, adaptation may occur and absorption of one or more nutrients may be taken over by another segment.

Drugs, on the other hand, generally are destroyed by digestion, needing to pass unchanged into the circulation. Transformation may occur (primarily in the liver via first-pass effect) before the active molecule or compound reaches the site of action. (Biotransformation is a term used to refer to chemical alterations that a substance undergoes in the body.)

DIGESTION

Generally speaking, digestion prepares ingested foods for absorption in forms useful to the body. Foods require digestive enzymes and secretions to break down to their constituent parts and become bioavailable. Even food substances that are not absorbed, such as insoluble fiber, may be important to the digestive process of some nutrients. Drugs, on the other hand, almost always are degraded and made either useless or harmful if altered by the digestive process.

Factors Affecting/Regulating Digestion

Digestion of foods depends on the combination of macronutrients present and the digestive compounds released by the presence of specific macronutrients in the gut. Some nutrients are also influenced by the presence or absence of specific micronutrients. Macronutrients are generally categorized as carbohydrates, proteins, and fats, although, from an energy-intake viewpoint, alcohol may also be considered by some as a macronutrient. The influence of each macronutrient is discussed in more detail in the following sections.

Other characteristics of the drug may also influence whether a drug is digested prior to absorption. The dose level of the drug is one such characteristic; if an individual requires that a certain drug be taken with food, the usual dosage may not reach the effective therapeutic level. The physical characteristics of food (e.g., liquid vs. solid) also influence food digestion and absorption. Equally important to the absorption of drugs is the form (e.g., tablet, elixir, syrup).

The presence or absence of digestive secretions or enzymes strongly influences the potential digestion of both food and drugs. For example, the absence of hydrochloric acid in the stomach interferes with the digestion of vitamin B_{12} and may adversely affect the absorption of mildly acidic drugs. Another similarity is that both nutrients and drugs obtain needed hormones or enzymes from the same sources. Inborn errors of metabolism may occur for each of the macronutrients; inborn errors of metabolism may influence the metabolism of selected drugs as well. Some adverse events that occur with a given medicine may be due to the existence of an inborn error of metabolism, which may influence the ability of that individual to metabolize or eliminate certain drugs. Owing to genetic differences, some individuals metabolize drugs slowly while others may metabolize drugs faster. Polymorphorism is a term used to describe some of these genetic differences.

Additionally, the tolerance of some drugs by the digestive system may constitute an issue. For example, a drug with an extremely low pH may have an unacceptable taste or have an adverse effect on food intake by leaving an unpleasant aftertaste (e.g., carbencillin (Geocillin®)).

Carbohydrates

As the name implies, carbohydrates are made up of carbon, hydrogen, and oxygen with the general formula of $C_nH_{2n}O_n$. In general, carbohydrates are divided into two broad categories: sugars and starches. Table 4.1 provides a list of the common dietary carbohydrates, samples of food sources, and the enzymes required for their digestion.[1] All dietary carbohydrates have to be metabolized to their constituent monosaccharides in order to be absorbed across the intestinal wall. After absorption, most of the monosaccharides pass into the portal circulation to the liver, although small quantities are used by the gut wall for its own metabolic processes.

Table 4.1 Common Dietary Carbohydrates, Food Sources, and Primary Digestive Enzymes

Carbohydrate	Food Sources/Example	Digestive Enzymes
A. Free Sugars		
Monosaccharides ($C_6H_{12}O_6$)	Fruits and vegetables	None required
Glucose	Fruit/grapes	
	Vegetables/onions	
Fructose	Fruits, honey/syrups	
Mannose	Manna/lichens	
Galactose	Milk/cheeses	
Sugar alcohols ($CH_2OH)_6$		
Sorbitol	Fruit/cherries	
Mannitol	Mannose	
Dulcitol	Galactose	
Inositol	Cereals	
Disaccharides ($C_6H_{12}O_6)_2$	Fruits, vegetables, dairy	Disaccharidases in the brush border
Sucrose	Table sugar/beets	Sucrase
Lactose	Milk	Lactase
Maltose	Table sugar/beets	Maltase
	Starchy vegetables/cereal	
Oligosaccharides	Short-chain sugars of glucose, galactose, and fructose	
Raffinose	Seeds/legumes/	No endogenous enzymes
Stachyose	Dried beans/peas	Fermented in colon
Verbascose		
Fructans		
B. Dextrins		
($C_6H_{10}O_5)_{11}$	Starch byproducts/liquid glucose	Amylase
C. Polysaccharides		
Starch	Breads, cereals	Salivary or pancreatic:
Amylose	Starchy vegetables	Amylase
Amylopectin		Amylopectinase
Nonstarch (fiber)		Resistant
Cellulose	Wheat bran	
Hemicellulose	Cereals	
Pectins	Fruits/vegetables	
Xylans	Wheat, rye, barley	
Gums	Guar, locust bean	
Mucilages	Seeds, seaweeds	

Source: Adapted from Garrow, J.S. and James, W.P.T., Eds., *Human Nutrition and Dietetics,* 9th ed., Churchill Livingstone, Edinburgh, 1993, 40. With permission.

Overall, the digestion of carbohydrates is actually more complex than commonly taught in most nutrition courses. Fiber content of foods is highly dependent upon the method of analysis and on the definition of fiber. The resistance of starch to digestion in the small intestine is also highly influenced by additional factors, such as individual human variation and food processing variations in heating temperatures and times, pH, freezing, drying, water content, and others.[1] To fully understand the metabolism of starches, a mastery of some basic concepts of food science and technology must exist, but these are beyond the scope of this book.

An overview of digestive enzymes is best seen as occurring along with the progression of food through the GIT. The digestion of carbohydrates begins in the mouth. The salivary glands produce an enzyme classified as salivary α-amylase. This enzyme is responsible for the first step in the change from a starch to its sugars. Adequate chewing of food mechanically breaks down cells, promotes the mixing of starch with salivary amylase, and acts on some of the food before the pH in the stomach deactivates the enzyme. Digestion can be affected both by the quality and quantity of saliva produced. Various therapies such as radiation therapy and drug therapy may modify saliva production (viscosity and volume) and impact on the efficiency of this enzyme.

Mechanical thrashing of starchy food in the stomach may reduce the particle sizes of poorly chewed food and, therefore, better prepare the starch for further digestion in the small intestine. Smaller particles expose more surface area to digestive compounds. The stomach, however, has little influence on carbohydrate digestion in general because the salivary amylase in a starch bolus is deactivated in a relatively short time.

The pancreas secretes amylase and sodium bicarbonate, which promote the digestion and absorption of carbohydrates in the small intestine. The bulk of carbohydrate digestion occurs due to the action of pancreatic amylase in the mildly basic environment of the small intestine. The change in pH in the small intestine from the acid environment of the stomach is accomplished by the release of sodium bicarbonate with the pancreatic enzymes through the sphincter of Oddi. Newborns may not produce adequate amounts of this pancreatic enzyme to digest starch for several months.

When the common bile duct is obstructed by gallstones, problems occur in the digestion of all macronutrients. Pancreatitis may result due to the effects of pancreatic enzymes being blocked from entering the small intestine and being activated in the pancreas.

The small intestine is the main site of carbohydrate digestion and absorption. The rate of absorption depends on the amount of peristalsis and the viscosity of the bolus. Monosaccharides and disaccharides were once thought to be absorbed more quickly than starches, but later findings have suggested that glucose, dextrins, and soluble starch are absorbed at equal rates.[1] The final cleavage of carbohydrate compounds into monosaccharides is accomplished by brush border enzymes (e.g., lactase, maltase, and sucrase). Several mechanisms exist for the transport of monosaccharides across the intestinal mucosa, including diffusion, facilitated diffusion, and active transport.

Passive diffusion, which is the transport mechanism for the sugar alcohols, L-glucose, and L-galactose, serves to prevent large quantities from being absorbed. Water withdrawal, associated with the presence of these compounds in the gut, prevents large quantities of the simple sugars from being transported across the gut wall. About 50 g of these substances can be consumed before symptoms associated with overdoses appear.

The only actively transported monosaccharides in humans are D-glucose and D-galactose; these two compete with each other for absorption sites. Sodium is the key to active transport of glucose. When the sodium/potassium/ATPase system is inhibited, the active transport of sugar is inhibited.

Facilitated diffusion is the third method of absorption. An example of facilitated diffusion is the absorption of fructose, one of the two monosaccharides in sucrose. If more sucrose or fructose is ingested, the level of brush border enzymes will increase. This is not true of increased ingestion of lactose. If large quantities of lactose are ingested, and there is a limited amount of the enzyme lactase, which is not uncommon, gastrointestinal side effects, including cramping, flatulence, bloating, and diarrhea, may occur.

Once the food leaves the small intestine, no more digestive enzymes are available. Further digestion of carbohydrates in the large intestine is accomplished by a complex fermentation process that has been described by Cummings.[2,3]

The colon has no role in the digestion of carbohydrates except through fermentation that converts undigested fiber or resistant starch into short-chain fatty acids (SCFAs). These fatty acids serve as the preferred fuel of the coloncyte, providing over 70% of the energy required by these cells. Resistant starch is, by definition, carbohydrates that escape digestion in the small intestine. Soluble fibers such as pectin are degraded almost completely, while the insoluble fibers such as lignin found in wheat bran are only partially degraded.

Ideally, carbohydrates constitute the major component of the diet. All dietary guidelines recommend that carbohydrates provide the major portion of energy in the total diet. Carbohydrate foods are the primary source of fiber in the diet as well as the primary provider of many micronutrients (e.g., B vitamins, folate, vitamin C, and trace nutrients). The main function of dietary carbohydrate is to provide energy; another role is to serve as the primary sweetening agents in foods and drugs. Other functions include being a source of flavor and texture, contributing to the viscosity of food products and liquids, stabilizing emulsions, and preserving foods.

Carbohydrates play only a minor role as drug products. Most drugs are protein or other more complex organic molecules. The carbohydrate-based drugs are mostly laxative in their effects because they attract water into the lumen of the large intestine. Drugs may have sugar moieties (e.g., in alkaloids) that expose the drugs to the action of the digestive process.

Proteins

Food proteins provide the smallest percentage of total kilocalories, ranging from approximately 10 to 20%. Proteins are composed of smaller subunits termed amino acids; their nomenclature is derived from the presence of an amine group on one end and a carboxyl group on the other end. Amino acids have traditionally been categorized as either essential amino acids (EAAs), meaning that humans must consume these as part of the diet, or as nonessential amino acids (NEAAs), meaning they may be produced in the body by physiologic processes or converted from other amino acids.

Table 4.2 Precursors of Conditionally
Essential Amino Acids

Amino Acid	Precursors
Cysteine	Methionine, serine
Tyrosine	Phenylalanine
Arginine	Glutamine/glutamate
Proline	Glutamate
Histidine	Adenine, glutamine
Glycine	Serine, choline

Source: From Garrow, J.S. and James, W.P.T., Eds., *Human Nutrition and Dietetics*, 9th ed., Churchill Livingstone, Edinburgh, 1993, 72. With permission.

$$H_3N \text{----} \overset{\displaystyle COO^-}{\underset{\displaystyle R}{C}} \text{----} H$$

Figure 4.1 General formula of an amino acid, where *R* can be several different components from a single hydrogen atom or an alkyl, aryl, or heterocyclic group.

Table 4.3 Mnemonic Device for Remembering
Essential Amino Acids, Including
Conditionally Essential Amino Acids

Word	Amino Acid	State of Essentiality
Any	Arginine	Conditionally essential
Help	Histidine	Conditionally essential
Given	Glycine	Conditionally essential
In	Isoleucine	Essential
Learning	Leucine	Essential
These	Tryptophan	Essential
Little	Lysine	Essential
Molecules	Methionine	Essential
Proves	Phenylalanine	Essential
Truly	Threonine	Essential
Valuable	Valine	Essential
To	Tyrosine	Conditionally essential
Physicians	Proline	Conditionally essential
Chemists	Cysteine	Conditionally essential

More recently, a new concept of conditionally essential amino acids has evolved. Table 4.2 provides the precursors of conditionally essential amino acids. This theory states that although an amino acid may be nonessential in a healthy person with no ongoing physiological stress, it becomes an essential amino acid in certain conditions for selected individuals. Figure 4.1 provides the general formula of an amino acid, and Table 4.3 provides a mnemonic device for remembering which amino acids are considered essential. About 20 different amino acids are common in the diet and in the body. Certain amino acids, for example, methionine and tryptophan, are generally present in all proteins, although protein amino acid composition varies greatly.

The distinguishing feature of all protein is nitrogen, generally considered to provide about 16% of the weight of an amino acid. Hence, 6.25 (1/16th) is used as the factor by which grams of nitrogen are converted into grams of protein needed. In general, proteins are more complex and variable than carbohydrates and contain a greater number of elements. This means that protein foods are generally good sources of several minerals. One gram of dietary protein, for example, provides about 1 meq of potassium. Differences in the structure of side chains, normally designated as the "R" group, largely determine the functions of the various proteins.

The general structure of a protein is provided by peptide bonds that tend to link folds of polypeptide chains, which ultimately provide a three-dimensional structure. A major new field (proteomics) is focused on determining why proteins made from the same chromosome genetic code fold differently and, thus, function differently.

Proteins serve many functions in the body: structural tissue, organ tissue, enzymes, blood transport molecules, blood compounds, membrane-imbedded cellular carriers, intracellular matrix, immune bodies, hair, fingernails, and many hormones. Changes in the structure of a protein in which the folds or linkages are broken are termed denaturation. Denaturation can occur by three different mechanisms: acid, mechanical, and enzymatic. The beating of meringue from egg whites is a denaturing process that demonstrates the effects of mechanical (whipping) and acid (cream of tartar) actions.

The mouth, beyond mechanical chewing or breaking food into smaller particles, is not involved in protein digestion. The stomach provides several different digestive processes. The grinding and mixing of protein with hydrochloric acid is an important process that stimulates the release of gastric enzymes, which signal the release of pancreatic enzymes. The stomach, thus, illustrates all three methods of denaturating food protein.

The small intestine is the main site of digestion and absorption for proteins. Several proteolytic enzymes are produced by the pancreas. Table 4.4 provides some common enzymes involved in the digestion of protein and the sources of these enzymes. Some enzymes attack the amine end, while others split off the carboxyl ends, yet others break the protein into smaller amino acids segments, usually into tripeptides and dipeptides. These smaller segments are generally better absorbed than either single amino acids (monopeptides) or complex amino acids (oligopep-

Table 4.4 Main Enzymes Involved in the Digestion of Proteins

Enzyme	Source of Enzyme
Pepsin	Gastric juice
Chymosin (Rennin) (animal)	
Trypsin	Pancreatic juice
Chymotrypsin	
Elastase	
Carboxypeptidase	
Aminopeptidase	Intestinal mucosa
Dipeptidase	

tides) because of greater gut absorption site options. Amino acids consumed in excess of need are not stored as protein but are used as metabolic fuel and ultimately may be modified into fatty acids and stored in adipocytes.

Some drugs are proteins and may be derived from plants, animals, or genetic engineering. As such, some are readily digested if consumed orally and, therefore, must be taken by injection or spray (e.g., insulin, heparin). Traditionally, insulin was derived from the pancreas of pigs (porcine) or cattle (beef); long-term use of these compounds sometimes led to allergy to the foreign protein. Today, human insulin and several human insulin analogues are genetically engineered and manufactured.

Orally administered drugs are absorbed mainly by active processes in the small intestine as intact molecules. The ability to reach the small intestine as intact molecules is preferred for most drug products. The fragility of proteins due to the adverse environment in the gastrointestinal tract is a major problem for drug designers. The designers of functional foods want normal digestion and absorption to occur at appropriate places in the gut, while drug designers work to prevent digestion and delay absorption until the drug reaches an appropriate site.

Fat

Lipid is the term used by chemists to describe a group of hydrophobic substances that contain basically only hydrogen, carbon, and oxygen and are immiscible in water. No precise definition of the word "fat" actually exists. Lipids are the major components of many cell membranes in animals and serve as the primary storage form of energy in the body. Lipids are stored in adipose tissues in the form of triglycerides. A triglyceride or triacylglycerol consists of a molecule of glycerol to which three fatty acids are attached with ester bonds (esterified). In edible fats, the term triacylglycerols is used to distinguish these lipids from industrial hydrocarbons. Among nutritionists, distinction is made by the common use of the word fat to refer to these compounds in foods, while lipids refer to the fats found in the body. In most industrialized countries, fat intake provides about 35–45% of caloric intake.

In foods, the characteristics of the fat are determined by chain length and degree of saturation. Table 4.5 lists some important fatty acids in foods by saturation status and chemical definition. Figure 4.2 provides general structures and nomenclature of fatty acids. Carbon chain length determines their transport after absorption. The most common dietary fats are the long-chain fatty acids that are usually 16–18 carbons in length and the degree of saturation is dependent on the original source. In general, fats from animal sources are saturated (all their binding sites are occupied) with the exception of the polyunsaturated fatty acids in the omega-three classification, commonly referred to as fish oils. Fats from plant origin are predominantly a combination of monounsaturated fatty acids (MUFAs) or polyunsaturated fatty acids (PUFAs) depending on the specific plant source. Certain plants (e.g., safflower, sunflower, corn) have traditionally been regarded as being predominantly polyunsaturated, but newer varieties of plants, particularly safflower, have been developed that are higher in MUFAs and lower in PUFAs. A small number of plant sources yield predominantly saturated fats (SFAs) (e.g., coconut, palm, and date palm oils). In these oils, the ratio of saturated vs. unsaturated fat is higher for the saturated side

Table 4.5 Some Commonly Occurring Fatty Acids in Foods

Saturation State, Common Name	Chemical Name	Shorthand Nomenclature
Saturated		
Short Chain (4–6)		
Butyric	Butanoic	4:0
Caproic	Hexanoic	6:0
Medium Chain (8–10)		
Caprylic	Octanoic	8:0
Capric	Decanoic	10:0
Long Chain (12–18)		
Lauric	Dodecanoic	12:0
Myristic	Tetradecanoic	14:0
Palmitic	Hexadecanoic	16:0
Stearic	Octadecanoic	18:0
Monounsaturated (18–22)		
Oleic	*cis*-9-Octadecenoic	18:1 (*n*-9)
Elaidic	*trans*-9-Octadecenoic	
Erucic	cis-13-Docosemnoic	22:1 (*n*-9)
Polyunsaturated (18–22)		
Linoleic	*cis-cis*-9,12-Octadecadienoic	18:2 (*n*-6)
α-Linolenic	all-*cis*-9,12,15 Octadecatrienoic	18:3 (*n*-3)
Arachidonic	all-*cis*-5,8,11, 14–20:4 Eicosatraenoic	20:4 (*n*-6)
EPA	all-*cis*-5,8,11,14,17-Eicosapentaenoic	20:5 (*n*-3)
DHA	all-*cis*-4,7,10,14,16,19-docasahexaneoic	22:6 (*n*-3)

Source: From Garrow, J.S. and James, W.P.T., Eds., *Human Nutrition and Dietetics*, 9th ed., Churchill Livingstone, Edinburgh, 1993, 77. With permission.

```
        Saturated                Monounsaturated              Polyunsaturated
     H H H H H H                 H H H H H H                 H H H H H H H
     R-C-C-C-C-C-R               R-C-C-C=C-C-C-R             R-C-C=C-C-C=C-C-R
     H H H H H H                 H H    H H                    H   H   H

              Cis-fatty acid                        Trans-fatty acid

            H H H H                                  H H  H
           R-C-C=C-C-R                              R-C-C=C-C-R
            H    H                                   H  H H
```

Figure 4.2   General structures and nomenclature of fatty acids.

effects; this has been of some concern due to the role of saturated fats in atherogenesis.

Debate has arisen about the ratio of monounsaturated to polyunsaturated fats because of the differences in the production of other lipid compounds in the body. The ratio of omega-three and omega-six fatty acids has been of concern due to their roles as precursors for different types of prostaglandins in the body. Because the human body cannot incorporate a carbon chain double bond below carbon 9, two fatty acids, linolenic (n-3) and linoleic (n-6), cannot be synthesized from other fats and are, therefore, termed essential fatty acids. In infants, arachidonic acid may also be considered essential. All other fatty acids can be synthesized from any excess of dietary energy. The rate of fatty acid synthesis is strongly related to the availability of glucose and is suppressed by fasting, dietary fat, and insulin deficiency.

The digestion of triglycerides is very complex and involves interactions among many different lipolytic products, phospholipids, bile salts, proteins, and carbohydrates. Two initial steps in digestion are: (1) to prepare for enzymatic hydrolysis by increasing the surface area of a fat-containing molecule and (2) to make the surface of that molecule accessible to the action of lipase.

While a small amount of lipase is produced sublingually, this enzyme, lingual lipase, plays a minor role in the digestion of fats, with the possible exception of very young infants for whom lingual lipase may be important. Some very small amounts of lipase exist in human milk, meat, cheese, vegetables, salad dressings, and soy sauce. When triglycerides enter the stomach, another enzyme, gastric esterase, breaks down the medium and short-chain fats but does not affect long-chain fatty acids. The combination of an acid pH, the presence of amino acids, fatty acids, and monoglycerides stimulates the release of cholecystokinin, usually abbreviated as CCK, and another enzyme, secretin, from the duodenal mucosa into the circulation. Secretin is the physiologic stimulant for the release of most of the pancreatic electrolytes. CCK stimulates synthesis and release of exocrine pancreatic enzymes and pancreatic bicarbonate; the latter helps to modulate the duodenal pH. CCK also induces sustained gall bladder contraction and synthesis and the release of hepatic bile.

Once the acid chyme (the mixture of food and gastric secretions, e.g., acid, enzymes) has been alkalinated and pancreatic enzymes in excess have been added to the mix, triglycerides are hydrolyzed or broken down. Bile salts and phospholipids displace lipase from the cell surface, and another enzyme, colipase, supplants these enzymes in the cell binding sites. Bile salts and phospholipids, mainly lecithin (phosphatidyl choline), form mixed micelles because of being both hydrophilic and hydrophobic. The micelles contain triglycerides, diglycerides, 2-monoglycerides, and fatty acids. Only the latter two components can pass through the membrane by diffusion. The micelles are in constant motion, allowing lipid monomers to pass into the cell membrane and then refilling from other micelles in a chain reaction.

Long-chain triglycerides, which are the major proportion of fats in the diet, must be broken down in the small intestine by pancreatic lipase to partial glycerides and fatty acids before efficient absorption can occur. Unfortunately for modern sedentary man, absorption of fats is highly effective, with an absorption rate in excess of 90% in moderate amounts (100–250 g/d).

Adults have a great capacity for fat absorption but have a normal, average daily stool excretion of 4–6 g, even in the presence of 100 g of dietary fat. When more fat is ingested, absorption just continues more distally in the small intestine. Newborns, however, do not have a reserve capacity for fat absorption, so the source of fat is important. Breast milk contains a lipase that provides some protection from fat malabsorption, but infants who consume cow's milk formulas may have a certain degree of fat malabsorption. Elderly adults may have a limited capacity for lipid absorption, but this is usually offset by a reduced fat intake. The greater likelihood of achlorhydria in the elderly adult may contribute to a higher pH in the proximal duodenum and, hence, may produce a mild steathorrea.

The liver produces bile salts that are stored in the gallbladder to be released through the common bile duct where it mixes with pancreatic lipase. Bile salts act as emulsifiers and aid in the digestion of fat. Reabsorption of bile acids is necessary to meet the needs of a high-fat diet, and this occurs in the distal ileum. Damage to the ileum or to the ileocecal valve may induce diarrhea and contribute to further malabsorption of dietary fat.

Absorption of fat varies with the type of fat. In general, long-chain fatty acids (LCTs) are transported from the mucosal cell to the circulation via the lymphatic system, entering the blood stream near the thoracic artery. Medium-chain triglycerides (MCTs), on the other hand, enter the circulation directly via the portal vein to the liver. Short-chain fatty acids are fairly rare in foods, but are produced in the colon as an end product of the fermentation of nonstarch polysaccharides such as those found in legumes. MCT oil is generally produced by the fractional distillation of coconut oil. The transformation of an oil into a solid or semisolid margarine or shortening requires a process of hydrogenation. Many of the fatty acids are transformed into *trans* fatty acids, rather than the *cis* form from which they started. In the *cis* form, the two hydrogens would be added on the same side (sisterly fashion) while in the *trans* form, a hydrogen would be added on each side (across from each other). The amount of processing determines the amount of *trans* fatty acids from a practical viewpoint. *Trans* fatty acids do occur naturally in foods but in relatively small amounts. The *trans* form may be less desirable than the *cis* form in cardiovascular disease prevention. If total dietary fat is kept to a modest amount, the presence of *trans* fatty acids in small amounts is unlikely to significantly impact health. The melting point of a triglyceride is determined by the specific types of fatty acids (e.g., carbon chain length) as well as the number, location, and *cis* and *trans* configurations of the double bonds. The melting point of a triglyceride is important in the process of intestinal absorption.

Dietary Fat and Drug Absorption

Few drugs originate from fat, but fat may serve as a carrier for active molecules, especially when introduced through intramuscular injections and for some active molecules (e.g., doxsorubicin microsphere). The few fat-soluble drugs may have a higher absorption rate in the presence of a fatty meal. The intravenous lipid used as a second calorie source and a primary source of essential fatty acid for parenteral nutrition are emulsions because free oils may not be administered intravenously.

METABOLISM

Metabolism is defined as the process of energy production in the adult, with repair and healing as secondary functions. In children, metabolism is generally assessed by the continuation of a good growth pattern when charted over time.

The production of energy is essential because all active absorption of both foods and drugs requires energy. Only passive absorption, where nutrients will cross the cell wall with the usual flow of water across the cell membrane, can take place without energy. Most nutrients require facilitated or active transport that requires energy. The ultimate end products of all energy metabolism, regardless of substrate source, are water and carbon dioxide.

Carbohydrates

Glucose is the most common source of energy, and most cells are able to metabolize glucose to carbon dioxide and water. In this process, glucose is phosphorylated, converted to trioses, and then enters the tricarboxylic cycle. The production of energy is not the only fate of glucose; glucose can also be converted to glycogen or fat for storage. Although glucose can be used by all cells, it is essential for energy in only brain and red blood cells. Under normal circumstances, the adult brain requires approximately 40 g glucose/d and the red blood cells about 40 g glucose/d.

Nevertheless, glucose is not considered an essential nutrient because the body can make glucose in a process called gluconeogenesis. As the name implies, this process means the creation of glucose from new sources (e.g., amino acids) up to 130 g/d. The only form of glucose storage is the glucose polymer, glycogen. This storage process is termed glyconeogenesis. The glycogen stored in the adult liver is about 90 g, and averages about 150 g in the muscles, although this can be increased by training and dietary manipulation. Glycogen is not as energy dense as fat and requires about 2.7 g of bound water for each gram of glycogen deposited. Fat cells (adipocytes) can convert glucose into fatty acid.

The basic pathways of energy metabolism are divided into oxidative (in which oxygen is required) and nonoxidative, sometimes called the anaerobic cycle. The primary oxidative pathway for all macronutrients, including alcohol, is the Krebs or tricarboxylic acid (TCA) cycle. The mitochondria, often termed the powerhouses of the cell, are the sites for the Krebs cycle (energy metabolism) in all mammals. The Krebs cycle produces most of the reduced coenzymes, nicotinamide adenine dinucleotide (NADH), and flavin adenine dinucleotide ($FADH_2$) that drive the electron transport chain and that are essential in oxidative phosphorylation. This cycle serves as the intermediary by which the simple forms of all the macronutrients get converted into energy in the form of adenosine triphosphate (ATP). Prominent TCAs, including citric acid, are important intermediates of the cycle leading to the term TCA cycle or the citric acid cycle. Four major functions of the Krebs cycle are to: (1) be the source for the reduced coenzymes that drive the respiratory chain at the completion of the cycle, (2) produce carbon dioxide for the maintenance of acid–base balance, (3) convert intermediaries to precursors of fatty acids, and (4) provide precursors for the synthesis of proteins and nucleic acids.[4]

An important part of carbohydrate metabolism is glycolysis. Glycolysis is the degradation pathway whereby glucose is oxidized to pyruvate. Pyruvate, in turn, is further metabolized by one of two processes. In the presence of adequate oxygen for complete oxidation, the pyruvate is decarboxylated to acetyl CoA, which then enters the Krebs cycle and is completely broken down to carbon dioxide and water. If oxygen is present in inadequate amounts (a condition known as oxygen debt by athletes), pyruvate is reduced to lactate to maintain the necessary levels of NAD^+. This process is called anaerobic glycolysis. When lactate levels in the blood rise, the pH falls, and symptoms of rapid breathing and exhaustion begin; runners may refer to this as "hitting the wall." When oxygen levels are once again adequate, the lactate will be converted back into pyruvate, which is a pathway known as the Cori cycle.

Protein Metabolism

The metabolism of protein is more complex than that of carbohydrate and may involve many different pathways. Nearly half of the weight of a cell is protein. Proteins are very large molecules because they are polymers of amino acids joined by peptide linkages. A vast variability exists in protein structure and complexity. The specific amino acids that are present, their position in the peptide chain, and the spatial arrangement of the molecule determine the properties and characteristics of the protein. Proteins form the structural component of the cell, antibodies, hormones, and enzymes.

Amino acids are distinguished by their carboxyl and amine groups. This structure allows for three major reactions: transamination, deamination, and decarboxylation. These types of transformations serve different purposes. Amino acids are usually thought of first as building blocks for new substances and are thought to be transiently found in a free amino acid pool. Free amino acids in protein synthesis are thought to be quickly assimilated or else they will be oxidized. Amino acids are the primary building blocks for the creation of new glucose that occurs in the process of gluconeogenesis. Hormonal signals or the existence of low serum glucose (hypoglycemia) will stimulate the process of gluconeogenesis.

Amino acids consumed or infused in amounts that exceed the need for protein synthesis will be used as a metabolic fuel. The alpha amino group is removed, and the remaining carbon skeleton is transformed into acetyl CoA, acetoacetyl CoA, pyruvate, ketoglutarate, succinate, fumarate, or oxaloacetate. The remaining keto acids are, of course, active compounds in the Krebs cycle. Amino acids may enter the Krebs cycle at many different points, not only as acetyl CoA.

Through the action of glutamate hydrogenase, activated by low ATP levels and high ADP levels, glutamate is formed from transamination of amine groups and the amine group combining with ketoglutarate. Deamination of the glutamate leads to the release of ammonia, which will then be converted into urea. Alanine transaminase is an enzyme that catalyzes the transfer of nitrogen to pyruvate from other amino acids, alanine, and the keto acid of the amino acid that has been transaminated. Alanine, in turn, can transfer its nitrogen to ketoglutarate to form glutamate. These two enzymes funnel the nitrogen from excess protein into urea; the remaining carbon skeletons are used for energy. The carbon skeletons are oxidized via the Krebs cycle, eventually leading to excretion as CO_2 or deposition as glycogen and fat. Some free amino acids are used for the synthesis of new nitrogen compounds such as purine bases, creatine, and epinephrine. These are usually degraded without being returned to the free amino acid pool.

Purine bases are degraded to uric acid, creatine to creatinine, and epinephrine to vanillylmandelic acid. A fasting individual will excrete nitrogen at a rate proportional to his or her metabolic rate but clearly less than his or her intake; this is known as negative nitrogen balance. When a fasted person is fed protein, nitrogen excretion does not rise in proportion to intake, contributing to a net gain in body nitrogen or positive nitrogen balance. This positive nitrogen balance in early refeeding is due to accumulation of nitrogen in the liver with smaller amounts being retained by the kidneys. Only a small amount of nitrogen or new protein is retained in muscle tissue. This nitrogen retention is not sustained, however, and the nitrogen retention rate slows after 4–7 d. Rebuilding of lean tissues is a very slow process. Little progress in protein refeeding can be detected by any usual clinical indicators until about 10 d after feeding has restarted.

Dietary glucose and fat will increase the retention of nitrogen by 2–4 mg per extra kilocalorie fed. This process is sometimes called protein sparing. If adequate kilocalories are not provided to stressed persons, protein will become an important source of energy. This is expensive, both financially and physiologically.

Fat Transportation and Metabolism

The metabolism of fat is a more complex process than that of carbohydrate or protein because not only does fat have to be broken into its basic components as do other macronutrients, but these components have to be reassembled before transportation across the intestinal mucosa can occur. Additionally, lipids cannot travel unaided in the water-based environment of the blood vessels, so they are joined to four types of carrier molecules categorized as lipoproteins. These are chylomicrons, very low-density lipoprotein (VLDL), low-density lipoprotein (LDL), and high-density lipoprotein (HDL). The characteristics and functions of each of these are described in Table 4.6.

In the gut lumen, the components are assembled into micelles to begin the process of absorption. In the intestinal cell, long-chain triglycerides are reformed and incorporated into chylomicrons. Chylomicrons consist of 86% triglycerides, 9% phospholipid, 3% cholesterol and cholesteryl esterase, and 2% protein. Intestinal VLDL is a transport protein for exogenous lipids. Chylomicrons and VLDL are the principal vehicles for transport of triglycerides from the gut to tissues via lymph and blood circulation to the liver, fat depots, and muscles. Hepatic VLDL and LDL function primarily as an internal transport mechanism for triglycerides, phospholipids, and cholesterol. HDLs function primarily as a reverse transport system of delivering tissue cholesterol to the hepatocytes.

Alimentary lipemia starts about 1–2 h after ingestion of fat, reaches a maximum level at 3–5 h, and decreases to fasting levels usually by 8–10 h. Hydrolysis of chylomicrons and VLDL triglycerides occurs through the catalytic action of lipoprotein lipase, an enzyme found on the luminal surface of the endothelium but also present in fat cells. Liver also contains a lipase that hydrolyzes lipoprotein trigylcerides into component compounds.

The fatty acids of chylomicrons and VLDL triglycerides are mostly absorbed by extrahepatic tissues and are used: (1) for energy production (particularly by the heart, red muscle fibers, smooth muscle cells, kidney, and platelets); (2) for incorporation into phospholipids in all cellular membranes (the fatty acid composition determines the biomembrane function), as well as in the biosynthesis of prostaglandins, throm-

Table 4.6 Major Classes of Human Lipoproteins

Lipoprotein Class	Composition (%)					Function	Origin
	TG	Cholesterol	Ester	Phospholipid	Protein		
Chylomicrons	86	1	5	7	2	Transport of dietary lipids	Intestine
Very low-density lipoprotein (VLDL)	50	7	13	20	10	Transport of endogenous and exogenous lipids	Liver, intestine
Intermediate-density lipoprotein (IDL)[a]	35	33	—	17	15	LDL precursor	VLDL catabolism
Low-density lipoprotein (LDL)[b]	8	10	30	30	22	Transport of cholesterol; regulation of cholesterol metabolism.	IDL catabolism
High-density lipoprotein (HDL)[c]	8	4	12	24	52	Reverse transport of cholesterol from peripheral tissues to liver	Intestine, liver, surface of CM and VLDL remnants

[a] Also called a VLDL remnant.
[b] Also termed bad cholesterol.
[c] Also termed good cholesterol.

Source: Adapted from Cohn, R.M. and Roth, K.S., *Biochemistry and Disease: Bridging Basic Science and Clinical Practice,* Williams & Wilkins, Baltimore, 1996, 266 and Zeman, F.J., *Clinical Nutrition and Dietetics,* 2nd ed., Macmillan, New York, 1983, 366. With permission.

boxane, and leukotrienes; and (3) as a major source of stored energy through its deposition in adipose tissue as triglyceride.

In the liver, fatty acids are generally incorporated into triglycerides, and some may be stored there for energy production. The major proportion of the fatty acids is incorporated into VLDL and secreted again into the plasma. An increased peripheral lipolysis during prolonged starvation or diabetes will result in greater esterification of fatty acids into triglycerides in the liver, thereby producing a fatty liver. Increased synthesis of VLDL also leads to hypertriglyceridemia.

The properties of the lipoproteins secreted by the liver are partly dependent upon the load of triglycerides requiring transport. High-carbohydrate feeding in humans results in increased production of VLDL with the characteristics of chylomicrons. Diets high in saturated fat and cholesterol are associated with a marked reduction in HDL without apolipoprotein E (sometimes termed good cholesterol). Apparently, the regulating role of HDL in cholesterol metabolism is stressed beyond its capacity. Other lipoproteins may transport this excess lipid to tissues other than the liver and contribute to arterial wall changes. The consequences of these actions are beyond the scope of this chapter, but they have been well described elsewhere.[5-7]

Energy production from fatty acids is also a multiple-step process often pictured as a wheel. Almost all fatty acids endogenously produced by mammals and found in the foods they consume contain an even number of carbons so that their hydrolysis yields two-carbon acetyl CoA, which enters the mitochondrial Krebs cycle. Fatty acids, however, cannot cross the inner mitochondrial membrane without assistance. This assistance is provided by a carrier molecule, carnitine, which is synthesized from lysine and methonine in humans and is found abundantly in muscle. Other transferases activate the fatty acid in preparation for oxidation via a cyclic degradative pathway termed mitochondrial β oxidation. In this pathway, two-carbon units in the form of acetyl CoA are cleaved unit by unit from the carboxyl end. This pathway is illustrated in Figure 4.3.

ELIMINATION/EXCRETION

For both foods and drugs, digestive and metabolic end products are produced following the absorption and metabolism of foodstuffs and drugs. Just as in absorption, foods and drugs often share the same mechanisms, enzymes, and routes of excretion. The route of excretion or elimination may reflect routes unique to dietary sources of food and specific nutrients, as well as endogenous products of metabolism. Indeed, half the bulk of feces may represent wastes from sloughed gastrointestinal cells and dead bacteria. Undigested fiber from foods and nonabsorbable endogenous materials such as bile salts are also eliminated in feces.

The end products of absorbed carbohydrates are stored as glycogen or are fully oxidized to metabolic water and carbon dioxide. Excretion of carbon dioxide may occur either via the kidneys or the lungs. Whereas water is excreted mainly as urine, it may also be excreted as perspiration, through respiration, and in the feces. Soluble fiber that escapes digestion in the small intestine may be fermented and converted to short-chain fatty acids, which are the preferred fuel of colonocytes.

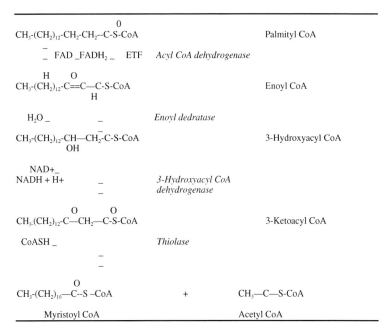

Figure 4.3 The oxidation pathway: an intramitochondrial process. A circular process in which a C-16 fatty acid results in cleavage of the carbon skeleton at the original carbon to form a C-14 fatty acyl CoA compound and acetyl CoA. The process will be repeated until the chain is depleted of two-carbon units. (From Cohn, R.M. and Roth, K.S., *Biochemistry and Disease: Bridging Basic Science and Clinical Practice*, Williams & Wilkins, Baltimore, 1996, 46–47. With permission.)

End products of nitrogen metabolism, mainly coming from the oxidation of amino acids, are potentially toxic and, therefore, must be excreted in a form that will not harm the individual. The by-products of ammonia and urea are processed by the liver. Urea is formed in the liver in a two-step process that leads to the combination of two molecules of ammonia with a carbon dioxide molecule. First, one of two possible enzymatic reactions occurs. Transamination is a reversible reaction that uses the keto acid products of glucose metabolism (e.g., pyruvate, oxaloacetate, and α-ketoglutarate) as nitrogen acceptors. For most of the amino acids, these processes occur in the liver. For the three essential branched-chain amino acids, valine, isoleucine, and leucine, however, transamination occurs predominantly in the peripheral tissues, particularly muscle cells. The second possible enzymatic reaction is deamination. Deamination is the stripping of the amine group from the carbon structure to form ammonia and then combining with carbon dioxide to form urea.

Although absorption of fat is approximately 90% complete, a small amount will be excreted in feces. If fat is incompletely absorbed, steatorrhea (fat in the stool, characteristically producing a grayish, floating stool) may occur. If lipids are incompletely metabolized in liver or muscle cells during fasting, acetoacetate and 3-hydroxybutyrate, known as ketone bodies, are formed. Ketone bodies are water-soluble and are able to cross the blood–brain barrier to help meet energy needs of the brain. Ketone bodies can be oxidized to water and carbon dioxide and, thus, can be excreted by the same routes as carbohydrate metabolism end products: through respiration, perspiration, or urine.

The elimination of micronutrients, vitamins, and minerals is determined largely by their polarities. Most minerals are excreted via the kidneys, as are the metabolites of water-soluble vitamins. Polyuria, or diuresis, will increase the loss of these nutrients. When renal thresholds are reached for reabsorption of water-soluble vitamins that are poorly stored in the body, high doses of these vitamins in supplements will be simply excreted. High doses of fat-soluble vitamins can be stored in excess in the liver. Fat-soluble vitamins are eliminated via feces; increased losses occur in the presence of diarrhea or steatorrhea. To compensate for the effects of new food products made with nonabsorbable fat substitutes, some manufacturers have added extra fat-soluble vitamins to these products.

Drug Elimination/Excretion

Phase II biotransformation is the process through which the functional group of drugs are conjugated to become more polar and, therefore, readied for excretion.[8] The excretion of drugs is dependent on transformation by various metabolic processes at the site of action or at remote sites (e.g., liver, by enzymes, or filtered by the kidneys). Possible routes for the excretion of drugs include all those for foods (i.e., feces, urine, perspiration, respiration) as well as biliary and hepatic pathways. Some drugs may pass unchanged from the body, but usually only if they are nonabsorbable compounds.

SUMMARY

Although different terms may be used to describe the metabolic processes of food and drugs, in reality more similarities than differences exist in the digestion, absorption, metabolism, and excretion or elimination of the waste and end products of these vital elements in health maintenance.

REFERENCES

1. Garrow, J.S. and James, W.P.T., Eds., *Human Nutrition and Dietetics,* 9th ed., Edinburgh, Churchill Livingston, 1993, 42–46.
2. Cummings, J.H., Fermentation in the human large intestine: evidence and implications for health, *Lancet,* I, 1206–1209, 1983.
3. Cummings, J.H. and Englyst, H.N., Fermentation in the large intestine and the available substrate, *Am. J. Clin. Nutr.,* 45, 1243–1255, 1987.
4. Montgomery, R. et al., Eds., *Biochemistry: A Case-Oriented Approach,* 6th ed., St. Louis, MO, Mosby, 1996.
5. Semenkovich, C.F., Nutrition and genetic regulation of lipoprotein metabolism, in Shils, M.E. et al., Eds., *Modern Nutrition in Health and Disease,* 9th ed., Baltimore, Williams & Wilkins, 1999, 1191–1198.
6. Grundy, S.M., Nutrition and diet in the management of hyperlipidemia and athersclerosis, in Shils, M.E. et al., Eds., *Modern Nutrition in Health and Disease,* 9th ed., Baltimore, Williams & Wilkins, 1999, 1199–1216.

7. Groff, J.L. and Gropper, S.S., Eds., *Advanced Nutrition and Human Metabolism,* 3rd ed., Belmont, CA, Wadsworth/Thomson Learning, 1999.
8. Utermohlen, V., Diet, nutrition, and drug interactions, in Shils, M.E. et al., Eds., *Modern Nutrition in Health and Disease,* 9th ed., Baltimore, Williams & Wilkins, 1999, 1625.

CHAPTER 5

Food and Nutrition Update

Beverly J. McCabe

CONTENTS

Dietitians tend to think of nutrition in terms of foods more so than in terms of nutrients. Their roles have traditionally been those of assessing and feeding the hospitalized patient or planning and directing the service of foods in a variety of settings. Food is served in relatively large sizes compared with drugs. Information about the nutrient content of foods is usually given in terms of grams or milligrams per 100 g of food. Food is usually served in a solid or semisolid state. Thus, the dietitian tends to think in terms of grams, ounces, or household cups for solids and in fluid ounces or milliliters for liquid foods. Although he or she is familiar with chemical milliequivalents such as used in electrolyte solutions and formulas, the dietitian converts diet prescriptions, often written in milliequivalents, into milligrams in order to plan a food pattern or a menu to meet the prescription. Analysis of nutrient content is generally reported in metric units (gram, milligram, or microgram) per 100 g, readily converted then into amount per 1 g of food calculating content per various serving portions in grams. Appendix A contains the formulas for these conversions.

Food composition data are largely determined by the Agriculture Research Service of the U.S. Department of Agriculture (USDA) in its Food and Nutrition Information Center (FNIC). Traditionally, the data have been placed in government print publications. Two examples, commonly referred to as *Handbook No. 8* and *House and Garden Bulletin No. 72,* are periodically updated and expanded.[1–2] *Handbook No. 8,* formally titled *Composition of Foods … Raw, Processed, Prepared,* now contains 21 volumes, although some are no longer in print. Presently, the most current data analysis is first made available online through the FNIC Web site, www.nal.usda.gov/fnic/foodcomp/. Nutrient values for a food can be readily assessed one food at a time from the online Standard Reference Release No. 15.[3] This Web site also contains provisional tables of Vitamin K and selenium. Additional data on a limited number of foods are available for selected five classes of flavonoids and will soon be available for *trans* fatty acids and choline.[4] The Nutrient Data Laboratory has a cooperative research and development agreement with Healthtech to develop PALM OS and PC versions of USDA's search program for nutrient data.[4]

NUTRIENT RECOMMENDATIONS

Interest in diet and nutrition has grown steadily as epidemiological studies and clinical trials continue to produce more evidence of the relationships between nutrition and chronic diseases. The focus of nutrition has changed from the prevention of nutrient deficiency states to the prevention or delay of degenerative diseases such as cardiovascular disease, osteoporosis, hypertension, obesity, and cancer.[5] Most health professionals today were trained in nutrition guidelines that emphasized meeting the recommended dietary allowances (RDAs). The RDAs were intended to ensure an intake of macronutrients and micronutrients that would be adequate to prevent deficiency states, to maintain growth in children, and to maintain and repair the body in adults.[5,6]

During the 1960s, questions were raised about the possible role of macronutrients, such as fat, in the development of cardiovascular diseases.[7] In the 1980s, micronutrients such as minerals were being examined for their possible roles in the development of hypertension and osteoporosis. By the 1990s, research began to look more at other micronutrients, such as the folate, B_6, and B_{12} vitamins, in the prevention of neural tube defects, cardiovascular disease, and dementia.[8] At the end of the 20th century, attention was directed toward food constituents not defined as nutrients per se but as protectants against diseases such as cancer and perhaps even against the consequences of aging.[6]

The RDAs were designed to plan an adequate intake, but not to provide guidance for an optimal diet for chronic disease prevention.[5,6] The scientific debate over where to set the RDA for calcium for the prevention or delay of osteoporosis serves to illustrate the need for a new method of making dietary recommendations. The release of the first set of dietary reference intakes (DRIs) in 1997 enlarged the concept of

Table 5.1   Definitions of Terms Used in the 1997–2001 Dietary Reference Intakes (DRIs)[6,9–13]

Requirement:	The lowest continuing intake level of a nutrient that, for a specified indicator of adequacy, will maintain a defined level of nutriture in an individual
Basal requirement:	The level of intake needed to prevent pathologically relevant and clinically detectable signs of a dietary inadequacy
Estimated average requirement (EAR):	The daily intake estimated to meet the requirement, as defined by the specific indicator of adequacy, in 50% of the individuals in a life stage or gender group; the EAR is used to determine the RDA
Recommended dietary allowance (RDA):	The daily intake that is sufficient to meet the daily nutrient requirements of most individuals in a specific life stage and gender group; if the variation in requirements is well defined, the RDA is set at 2 standard deviations (SD) above the EAR

$$RDA = EAR + 2SD_{EAR}$$

If the variation is not known, a standard estimate of variance is applied; a coefficient of variation of 10% and equal to one standard deviation is assumed for most nutrients

$$RDA = 1.2 \times EAR$$

If the coefficient of variation is greater than 10% (example, niacin = 15%), then the RDA formula would be adjusted accordingly

$$\text{Niacin } RDA = 1.3 \times EAR$$

Adequate intake (AI):	The recommended daily intake based on observed or experimentally determined approximations of the average nutrient intake by a defined population or subgroup that appears to sustain a defined nutritional state; the AI is used when scientific data are insufficient to determine an EAR and subsequently the RDA
Tolerable upper limit (UL):	The highest daily intake level that is unlikely to pose a risk of adverse health effects in almost all individuals in the specified life stage and gender group; the UL is used to examine the potential fortification of foods and the use of dietary supplements; the UL is not intended as a recommended level of intake; the UL is based on a risk assessment model developed specifically for nutrients from careful literature review with systematic scientific considerations and judgments; the model is based upon the lowest levels at which no observed adverse effects (NOAE) are found; lack of data on adverse effects has limited the number of nutrients for which ULs have been set

Source: From The Institute of Medicine, Food and Nutrition Board, *Dietary Reference Intakes: Calcium, Phosphorus, Magnesium, Vitamin D, and Fluoride, 1997* and Yates, A.A. et al., *J. Am. Diet. Assoc.,* 98, 699–707, 1998. With permission.

the single-value RDAs to a range of values designed to go beyond the prevention of deficiency diseases and to include current concepts of the role of nutrients and food components in long-term health. [6,9–13] While the RDA is still present, its purpose is to serve as a goal for individuals. [6,9] For all other purposes, the three other reference values should be selected: the adequate intake (AI), the tolerable upper limits (UL), and the estimated average requirement (EAR).[11] Table 5.1 provides the definitions of the DRIs.[4,6,9–13] Despite many studies, the National Research Council DRI committee did not judge the evidence as strong enough to name an RDA for calcium, but left the calcium recommendation as an AI (adequate intake) and provided a UL (tolerable upper limit).[9]

USES OF THE DRIs

The uses and preferred values for the DRIs include four primary areas: (1) assessing intakes of individuals for which the EAR would be used to examine potential for inadequacy and for which the UL would be used to examine for overconsumption; (2) assessing intakes of population groups for which the EAR would be used to examine prevalence of inadequate intakes within a group; (3) planning diets for individuals for which the RDA would be the target value if available, otherwise, the AI would be the target value[9–14]—the UL would be used as a guide to limit intake of individuals on a chronic basis but not as a target intake;[6,9,14] and (4) planning diets for groups for which the EAR would be used to set goals for the mean intake of a specified population. Note that an estimate of the variability of the group's intake would be required to set realistic goals. Thus, the appropriate use of the DRIs requires the dietetic and other health professionals to invest time and effort in understanding how to use the DRIs as well as in collecting baseline data (e.g., a group's intake of nutrients with which to use these tools most effectively).[14]

The DRIs have been set for most of the essential vitamins and minerals in four volumes, and the DRIs for the macronutrients were scheduled for release late in 2002.[14] The first volume presents the minerals and vitamins related to bone health.[9] The second volume presents most of the B vitamins including those related to energy metabolism.[10] The third volume presents the vitamins and minerals related to anti-oxidant activity.[15] The fourth volume establishes micronutrient DRIs including vita-mins A and K, and 12 trace elements.[16] A fifth volume released in 2002 provides a proposed new definition of dietary fiber.[17] A sixth publication provides development background and recommendations on uses and interpretation of the new DRIs.[18] For example, a probability approach to assessing the adequacy of an individual's diet allows a calculation of the confidence that an individual's intake meets his or her requirement for a nutrient. A seventh volume provides a risk assessment model for establishing tolerable upper limits for nutrients.[19] With the release of the DRIs for macronutrients, additional attention will be focused on better data on various types of dietary fats, including changing fatty acid profiles of dietary fats and *trans* fatty acids.[20] The fatty acid composition of oils that are expected to change include canola oil, sunflower oil, and safflower oil. New varieties of soybeans have been developed to reduce the omega-three fatty acid levels to improve cooking stability and increase shelf life.[20] The results of work to develop DRIs for fluid and electrolytes could be found in a prepublication copy available in late 2002.[14] If DRIs are not available for a nutrient, the 1989 RDAs remain the best available guidelines for assessing and planning diets.[4,6,14]

DIETARY GUIDELINES FOR PLANNING

Food Pyramids

While recommended intakes guide dietitians in planning specific diets, the DRIs do not readily allow other health professionals or consumers to plan menus or select

Table 5.2   Dietary Guidelines for Americans: 2000: Your ABCs of Good Health[21]

ABCs of Good Health

Aim for fitness
  Build for a healthy base
    Choose sensibly

Ten Guidelines for Good Health

Aim for fitness
  Aim for a healthy weight
  Be physically active each day
Build for a healthy base
  Let the pyramid guide your food choices
  Choose a variety of grains daily, especially whole grains
  Choose a variety of fruits and vegetables daily
  Keep food safe to eat
Choose sensibly
  Choose a diet that is low in saturated fat and cholesterol and moderate in total fat
  Choose beverages and foods that limit your intake of sugar
  Choose and prepare foods with less salt
  If you drink alcoholic beverages, do so in moderation

Source: From the U.S. Departments of Agriculture and Health and Human Services, *The ABCs for Your Health: Dietary Guidelines 2000,* http://www.usda.gov/cnpp/dietgd.pdf.

specific foods. Tools available to translate these recommendations given in scientific units of individual nutrients include food pyramids, dietary guidelines, cancer guidelines, exercise pyramids, and nutrition labeling. The USDA has released the new *Dietary Guidelines 2000* with three basic messages termed "the ABCs for your health ..." as outlined in Table 5.2.[21] The first message is "aim for fitness" and encourages the maintenance of a healthy weight and physical activity. The first guideline defines a healthy weight and includes exercise recommendations. The second message, "build a healthy base," urges the use of the food pyramid and adds a new emphasis on keeping food safe. Food safety is defined as avoiding foodborne illnesses and keeping food temperatures in a safe range as shown in Table 5.3. The third message, "choose sensibly," emphasizes food selection to lower risk of heart disease, obesity, and hypertension and to control sugar and alcohol intakes.[21] The addition of exercise and the reordering of the guidelines reflect attempts to address the increasing problem of obesity and its sequela, especially among children and young adults.

Another attempt to address obesity has been the development of food pyramids and exercise pyramids specific to special groups in the population. The food pyramid, first released in 1990, is an attempt to translate dietary guidelines into food servings for ease of menu planning and food selection [22] The USDA released a set of food and exercise pyramids for children in 1999 (see Figure 5.1).[23] The food and nutrition for older Americans campaign of the American Dietetic Association introduced a senior's pyramid with fluid as its base, reflecting the special attention needed for fluid intake in this population (see Figure 5.2).[24] An exercise pyramid was also developed to reflect the benefits of exercise in this population.[24]

Table 5.3   Safe Time and Temperatures for Control of Bacteria in Food

Temperature		
(°C)	(°F)	Time
100	212	Boiling Point of water at sea level
80	180	Cooking temperatures
60–83	140–181	Pasteurizing temperature, less time at higher temperature
60	140	Some bacteria growth, many bacteria survive, keep only short time at these temperatures
!!! Danger zone !!!		
51.5	125	Rapid growth of bacteria and production of toxins
!!! Discard food kept in this zone for 2–3 hours !!!		
Important Temperature Points		
4–60	40–140	Allows bacteria and mold growth
4	40	Optimum refrigerator temperature
0	32	Freezing temperature stops bacteria growth but does not kill bacteria
18	0	Optimum freezer temperature

Source: From American Home Economics Association, *Handbook of Food Preparation,* 9th ed., Kendall/Hunt Publishing Company, Dubuque, IA, 1993, 49. With permission.

Cancer Guidelines

Another approach to promote a healthier diet in Americans has been the five-a-day program sponsored by the National Cancer Institute (NCI). This program encourages the consumption of a minimum of five servings of vegetables and fruits a day as protection against the development of cancer and to meet the food pyramid recommendation.

An advisory committee on food, nutrition, and cancer prevention of the American Cancer Society has published a set of diet guidelines to protect against the development of cancer.[25]

These 1996 guidelines recommend the following:

1. Choose most of the foods you eat from plant sources. Eat five or more servings of fruits and vegetables each day. Choose green and dark yellow or cabbage-family vegetables. Use soy products and legumes. Eat other plant source foods including breads, cereals, grain products, rice, pasta, and beans several times each day. Choose whole grains in preference to refined grains. Choose beans as a replacement for meats.
2. Limit the intake of high-fat foods, particularly from animal sources. Choose foods low in fat. Prepare foods with little or no fat. Bake or broil meats and vegetables rather than fry foods. Choose nonfat and low-fat milk and dairy products. Eat smaller portions of high-fat dishes.
3. Select low-fat food items when snacking or eating in restaurants. Limit meat intake, especially high-fat meats. Use lean meat more as a condiment and less as an entree. Choose seafood, poultry, or beans over beef, pork, and lamb.

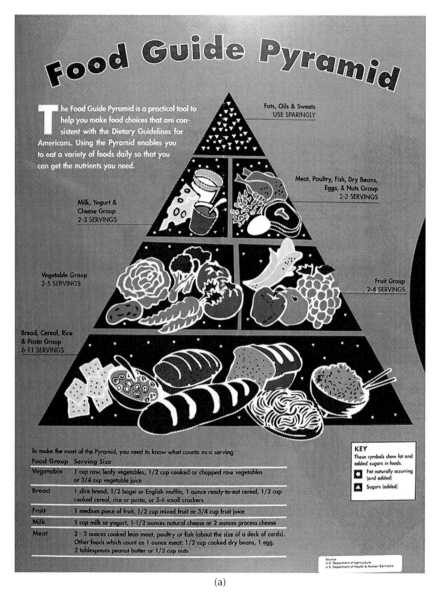

The Food Guide Pyramid is a practical tool to help you make food choices that are consistent with the Dietary Guidelines for Americans. Using the Pyramid enables you to eat a variety of foods daily so that you can get the nutrients you need.

Fats, Oils & Sweets
USE SPARINGLY

Milk, Yogurt & Cheese Group
2-3 SERVINGS

Meat, Poultry, Fish, Dry Beans, Eggs, & Nuts Group
2-3 SERVINGS

Vegetable Group
3-5 SERVINGS

Fruit Group
2-4 SERVINGS

Bread, Cereal, Rice & Pasta Group
6-11 SERVINGS

To make the most of the Pyramid, you need to know what counts as a serving:

Food Group	Serving Size
Vegetable	1 cup raw, leafy vegetables, 1/2 cup cooked or chopped raw vegetables or 3/4 cup vegetable juice
Bread	1 slice bread, 1/2 bagel or English muffin, 1 ounce ready-to-eat cereal, 1/2 cup cooked cereal, rice or pasta, or 5-6 small crackers
Fruit	1 medium piece of fruit, 1/2 cup mixed fruit or 3/4 cup fruit juice
Milk	1 cup milk or yogurt, 1-1/2 ounces natural cheese or 2 ounces process cheese
Meat	2 - 3 ounces cooked lean meat, poultry or fish (about the size of a deck of cards). Other foods which count as 1 ounce meat: 1/2 cup cooked dry beans, 1 egg, 2 tablespoons peanut butter or 1/3 cup nuts

KEY
These symbols show fat and added sugars in foods.
■ Fat naturally occurring (and added)
▲ Sugars (added)

Source:
U.S. Department of Agriculture
U.S. Department of Health & Human Services

(a)

Figure 5.1 Food and exercise pyramids for (a) adults and (b) children. (From the U.S. Department of Agriculture and the U.S. Department of Health and Human Services.)

4. Be physically active: achieve and maintain a healthy weight. Be active for at least 30 minutes several times a week. Control caloric intake. Be within your healthy weight range.

5. Limit consumption of alcoholic beverages, if you drink at all. Limit alcoholic beverages to two or less drinks a day. Do not combine the use of tobacco and alcohol.[25]

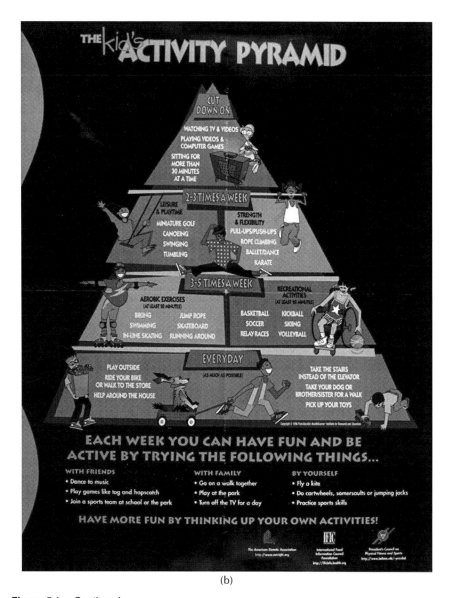

(b)

Figure 5.1 *Continued.*

In a review of 206 human epidemiologic studies and 22 animal studies on diet and cancer prevention, the consumption of vegetables and fruit was most favorable toward cancer prevention.[26] The evidence is particularly strong for cancers of the gastrointestinal and respiratory tracts but less strong for prevention of cancers related to hormones such as breast cancer and prostate cancer.[26] The types of vegetables and fruits most often cited as protective are raw vegetables, allium vegetables (onion and garlic), carrots, green vegetables, cruciferous (cabbage family) vegetables, tomatoes, soy protein, and legumes.[25–27] This protective effect is not limited to the value

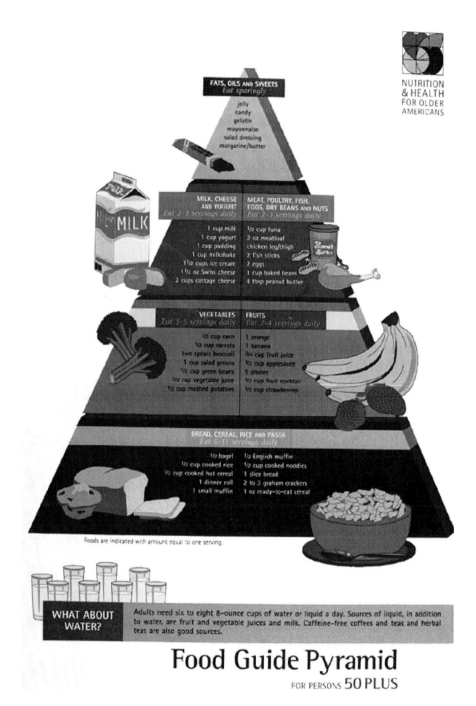

Figure 5.2   Food pyramid for older Americans. (From the American Dietetic Association Foundation © 1998. With permission.)

of vitamins such as beta carotene and minerals such as selenium[28] but appears to include many other food constituents that are not classified as nutrients.[25–27,29] Examples of potential protective substances are fiber, phytochemicals such as flavonoids, terpenes, sterols, indoles, and phenols that are of plant origin.[25,27]

Foods not previously noted for antioxidant activity are being considered as additives to functional foods. Whereas oats and barley have been evaluated for antioxidant activity, buckwheat or groats, commonly used in traditional dishes such as kasha, have only recently been evaluated for antioxidant activity.[30] Buckwheat honey and other types of commercial honeys, royal jelly, and propolis were recently analyzed for antioxidative activities.[31] Although Americans may use honey as a sweetening agents, other countries also use it as a food preservative, a quality attributed to its antioxidative effects.[31]

ASSESSMENT OF DIET QUALITY

To assess overall diet quality better and to monitor the compliance of Americans to the food pyramid and the dietary guidelines, the healthy eating index (HEI) was first computed using 1989 data from the continuing survey of food intakes by individuals (CSFII).[32–33] The CSFII survey is a nationally representative survey containing information on people's consumption of foods and nutrients.[32] The healthy eating index is the sum of 10 components, each representing different aspects of a healthful diet. Figure 5.3 illustrates the distribution of these components into a score of 100.[32] The first five components measure the degree to which a person's diet complies with the recommendations for the five major food groups of the pyramid: grains, vegetables, fruits, meats, and milk. The percentage of total kilocalories from fat is the sixth component, while percentage from saturated fat is the seventh, and total cholesterol intake is the eighth component. Total sodium intake is the ninth component, while variety in the diet is the tenth component. An HEI score over 80

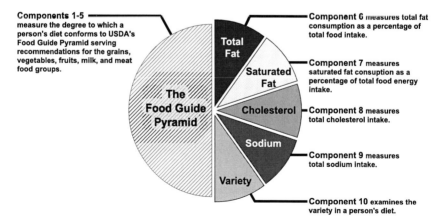

Figure 5.3   Healthy eating index. (From the U.S. Department of Agriculture for Nutrition Policy and Promotion, CNPP-5, 1998.)

is considered a good diet; a HEI score between 51 and 80 indicates a diet that needs improvement; and a HEI score below 51 is considered a poor diet.[32-33]

NUTRITION LABELING AND HEALTH CLAIMS

Another important development was the 1990 Nutrition Labeling and Education Act (NLEA), which simplified the nutrition information provided on a label and required only those nutrients associated with chronic disease risks.[7-8] This act also allowed food manufacturers to petition the Food and Drug Administration (FDA) for approval of health claims by providing data to demonstrate the validity of the claim. The approved health claims are listed in Table 5.4. This significant change in food policy enabled food manufacturers to provide messages about the role of nutrients and food constituents in health promotion and disease prevention.[7-8] One of the latest health claims, approved in 1999, recognized soy as being protective against heart disease.[21] It is important that consumers may see soy protein as being protective against other diseases, but the current evidence is insufficient to allow claims for other diseases such as cancer. The use of health claims as a marketing strategy has had two positive effects. The health claims encouraged the development of new products, and the new products were advertised widely in print and mass

Table 5.4   FDA-Approved Health Claims

Specific Health Claim	Citation from Federal Register
Calcium and osteoporosis	21 CFR 101.72
Dietary lipids (fats) and cancer	21 CFR 101.73
Sodium and hypertension	21 CFR 101.74
Dietary saturated fat, cholesterol, and risk of coronary heart disease	21 CFR 101.75
Fiber-containing grain products, fruits and vegetables, and cancer	21 CFR 101.76
Fruits, vegetables, and grain products that contain fiber, particularly soluble fiber and risk of coronary heart disease	21 CFR 101.77
Fruits and vegetables and cancer	21 CFR 101.78
Folic acid and neural tube birth defects	21 CFR 101.79
Dietary sugar alcohol and dental caries (cavities)	21 CFR 101.80
Soluble fiber from certain foods and risk of coronary heart disease, whole oats, and psyllium seeds	21 CFR 101.81
Soy protein and risk of coronary heart disease	21 CFR 101.82
Stanols/sterols and risk of coronary heart disease	21 CFR 101.83

FDAMA Health and Nutrient Content Claim Based on Authoritative Statement of a Scientific Body

Choline: nutrient content claim	August 30, 2001
Potassium and the risk of high blood pressure and stroke: health claim	October 31, 2000
Whole grain foods and the risk of heart disease and certain cancer: health claim	July 8, 1999

Source: Compiled from the Center for Food Safety and Applied Nutrition Web site: cfsan.fda.gov/list.html, July 7, 2001.

media. The advertisement also managed to increase the awareness of many hard-to-reach Americans regarding the protective benefits of some foods.[7–8] More traditional nutrition messages generated by government and private health organizations have failed to effectively reach limited-resource populations, the lesser educated, and minority groups. The use of mass media to deliver very short nutrition messages has increased awareness, but left many without sufficient information on how to implement sufficient changes in food intake.[7]

The Nutrition Education Labeling Act (NLEA) states that label formation must be conspicuously displayed and written in terms that the ordinary consumer is likely to read and understand under ordinary conditions of purchase and use.[34] Details concerning type sizes, location, etc. of required label information are contained in FDA regulations (21 CFR 101) and are available online through the FDA Web site, http://csfan.fda.gov/list.html.[34] The NLEA updated the nutrition label with a box design resembling a bar code with the title "Nutrition Facts." The label must contain a serving size in both a household measure and gram weight. Only five core foods listed in bold print are required on the label if the other nutrients are present in "insignificant" amounts. An amount is considered insignificant is it provides less than 2% of the U.S. RDA for micronutrients and less than 0.5 g for macronutrients. The five required nutrients must be listed even if the amount is zero. Required nutrients are calories, total fat, sodium, total carbohydrates, and protein. Special regulations apply to nutrition facts labeling on foods designed primarily for children or for foods that are insignificant sources of seven nutrients, in which simplified nutrition labels are acceptable. The amounts of calories from fat, cholesterol, dietary fiber, and sugars are commonly listed. The percent of the RDAs for vitamin C, vitamin A, calcium, and iron are listed or included in a statement "not a significant source of …"[35] The manufacturer may voluntarily include other nutrients such as monounsaturated and polyunsaturated fats. The mandatory listing of *trans*-fatty acids is under consideration.

The values listed on nutrition labels must be regarded as estimates. All analyzed and computer-generated values are rounded under very specific rules. For example, the following rounding rules apply to fats:

Below 0.5 g fat per serving: use the declaration "0 g" for total fat.
Above 0.5 g and below 5.0 g: round to the nearest 0.5 g (e.g., 1.5, 2.0, 2.5)
Above 5 g per serving: Use 1 g increments rounded to the nearest 1 g

For vitamins and minerals, the percent of the RDAs for those nutrients are rounded to the nearest 2%.[34–35]

For example, a serving labeled as containing 16% of the RDA for vitamin C might actually contain between 15 and 17.4%. A set of reference serving sizes are available on the FDA Web site.[35] For example, a reference serving size for cookies is 28 g. The manufacturer will list the number of whole cookies nearest to 28 g, usually 4–6 for smaller cookies or 2–3 for larger cookies.

In an effort to make the label user-friendly, the precision of nutrient values, even if initially available, is lost in the preparation of the label. The FDA still holds the manufacturer responsible for accuracy in label information with the 20/80 rule. This rule requires that no more than 120% of the amount listed for a nutrient such as saturated fat be present and no less than 80% of the amount listed for a nutrient such as protein should the FDA pull the product from a grocery shelf and run an independent analysis of the product.[34–35]

FUNCTIONAL FOODS

The onset of health claims fostered the development of specially modified foods, generally termed functional foods. Functional foods may be modified in several different ways. The term enriched refers to the replacement of a nutrient removed or lessened by food processing. The addition of B vitamins to white rice is an example of enrichment. If the amount of a nutrient added to the product exceeds the original content of the food, the food is referred to as a fortified food. To be labeled as an excellent source of a nutrient, the food must provide 20% of the DRI or RDA. To be labeled as a good source, the food must contain 10% of the DRI or RDA.[35] A popular functional food is the calcium-fortified orange juice developed to provide calcium to those individuals who cannot or will not consume dairy products. Orange juice contains some calcium naturally, but the amount added is far beyond the original amount. Another functional food is a chocolate candy fortified with 500 mg calcium. A new group of products to lower serum cholesterol comes from the modification of plant sterols. These products are consumed as margarine spreads or salad dressings. These products are designed to be less well absorbed and to induce a mild fat malabsorption for which extra fat-soluble vitamins have been added. These products are examples of the blurring between food and drugs. For older individuals at the 90th percentile of calcium intake (955 mg for women and 1240 mg for men ages 55–60), three calcium-fortified products a day would be well below the tolerable upper limits of 2500 mg calcium.[36] Nevertheless, foods fortified with calcium could play a significant role in assisting elderly people to obtain these new recommended intakes of calcium. Table 5.4 presents the FDA-approved claims.

Even with hormone replacement therapy (HRT), an adequate intake of calcium remains essential.[37] The use of HRT reduces the recommended daily calcium intake from 1500 mg back to 1000 mg per day.[37] The good news is that the latest CSFII data suggest that the elderly are increasing their intakes of calcium; and many elderly persons are using calcium supplements.[34–39]

An emerging functional food group is termed symbiotic and consists of probiotics and prebiotics. Probiotics modulate the indigenous intestinal flora by live microbial adjuncts and now comprise about 65% of the functional food world market with estimated sales of $75 million.[40] Prebiotics are indigestible yet fermentable dietary carbohydrates that may selectively stimulate certain bacterial groups usually found in the colon. Some examples of the bacterial groups are bifidobacteria, lactobacilli, and cubacteria, all of which are generally regarded as beneficial for the human host.[40–41] Some resistant short-chain carbohydrates or low-digestible carbohydrates are also termed prebiotics. Some dose-related undesirable effects may result when both prebiotics and probiotics are together in very large amounts.[40] The amounts found in usual amounts in foods such as fermented milk products (e.g., yogurt) present few side effects. Many fermented foods have become potential probiotics with the introduction into the U.S. of a host of fermented vegetables beyond the traditional sauerkraut, fermented meat products, and a variety of fermented milk products such as kir.

Several beneficial effects have been suggested, from nutritional benefits (e.g., vitamin production, increasing bioavailability of minerals and trace elements, production of important digestive enzymes) to treatment benefits as either a barrier or restorative (e.g., infectious diarrhea, antibiotic-associated diarrhea, cholesterol-lowering, immune system stimulant, enhancement of bowel motility, and maintenance of mucosal integrity). Direct health-related claims for foods are not allowed in the European Union or the U.S.[40] Since the 1960s, folic acid deficiencies have been increasingly recognized in the presence of disease, polypharmacy, and poverty.[42–45] From 11 to 28% of the elderly have been estimated as having folic acid deficiency, largely from poor dietary intake.[44] A low red cell folate suggests a long-term dietary inadequacy.[43] Dietary folate varies greatly in bioavailability and may also be destroyed in prolonged food preparation. When increased food folate intake did not lead to significant increases in folate status, attention turned to food fortification.[45] Ready-to-eat cereals were fortified with folate, and then it was mandated that flour be fortified with folate, mostly to provide additional folate to women of child-bearing age as a prevention of neural tube defects.[44–45] Cereals and breads, however, are consumed in limited amounts by many women and by some elderly who are also at increased risk of folate deficiency. Institutionalized elderly are more likely to have low serum folate.[44] Milk was selected as a vehicle for folic acid supplementation in a prospective clinical trial. Forty-nine subjects received the fortified milk for at least 6 months and 40 controls received unfortified milk. The experimental group had a mean serum folate of 5.81 μg/L compared with 2.16 μg/L for the control ($p < 0.0001$); thus, fortified milk appears to be a potential vehicle for fortification in some populations.[29] In recognition of the limited bioavailability of food folate and the increased fortification with folic acid with near perfect bioavailability, the DRIs are now using dietary folate equivalents (DFEs) rather than metric units for folate content of food.[46]

Although functional foods may provide a wonderful benefit to one population group, such as the elderly or women of child-bearing age, the question must be raised whether it could be detrimental to another population group, such as young children.[47–50] For example, young children who use dry cereals not only as breakfast foods but also as snacks throughout the day might exceed the upper limits for folate. Widespread iron fortification of foods or dietary supplements might lead to problems of iron overloading in individuals with hemochromatosis or in the elderly.[47–50] Thus, functional foods must be carefully examined both in their design states and subsequent recommendation for individuals of various ages, gender, and conditions.

FOOD SAFETY

Although not a new topic, interest has risen dramatically in food safety. As Americans eat less foods at home and more in restaurants, more takeout foods, more vended foods, and other convenience food sources, the possibility of foodborne

Table 5.5   Contaminants and Microorganisms of Current Concern in American Food Supplies

Contaminants and Microorganisms Traditionally Considered as Important Food-Borne Pathogens and Toxicants

Salmonella
Staphylococcus
Clostridium perfringens
Clostridium botulinum
Giardia

Contaminants and Microorganisms Recently Considered as Important Food-Borne Pathogens and Toxicants

Aspergillus (Aflatoxins)
Campylobacter jejuni
Ciguatera toxins
Cryptosporidium parvum (Cryptosporiasis)
Dinoflagellates (e.g., red tide)
Escherichia coli 0157:H7
Listeria monocytogenes
Norwalk virus
Toxoplasma gondii
Yersinia

illness has grown.[51–56] Food supplies have become global.[52] Organisms and toxicants, other than those commonly associated with foodborne illness, such as salmonella, have been identified as the culprits in serious and sometimes fatal episodes.[51–55] A detailed list of common contaminants and microorganisms found in foods is presented in Table 5.5. Children, pregnant women, and the elderly are particularly prone to suffer serious illnesses from foodborne organisms or toxins.[51,56] Certain drugs also increase the potential for serious reactions to food that is slightly spoiled.[57–58] Biogenic amines form in contaminated foods during spoilage and pose particular threats to those taking certain medications such as isonizaid and monoamine oxidase inhibitors (MAOIs).[57–58] These issues are discussed in more detail in Chapter 14.

The federal government has established several programs to promote food safety not only to homemakers but also to school children, educators, food service establishments, food manufacturers, and the general public. Four main federal agencies are involved in food safety: the Center for Disease Control (CDC, a division of the Department of Health and Human Services), the Center for Food Safety and Applied Nutrition (a division of the FDA), the Environmental Protective Agency (EPA), and the Food Safety Inspection Service (a division of the USDA). These agencies are part of a food safety initiative launched in July 1999. Fight Bac™ is the title of the food safety materials aimed at educating school children about the prevention of foodborne illness. Another new program is Thermy™, designed to encourage the use of thermometers to test for safe temperatures in food in both cooking and storage. Several Internet sites focus on food safety, including the USDA site for educators and consumers (www.foodsafety.gov)[58] and a collaboration of agricultural academics, government, and industry called the Council for Agricultural Science and Technology (CAST) at www.cast-science.org.[51] The goal of the National Food Safety

Database project is to develop an efficient management system of U.S. food safety databases, which are used by the Cooperative Extension Service (CES), consumers, industry, and other public health organizations, intended to be a one-stop shopping source for food safety information on the Internet.[59] This is available at a new URL at the University of Florida, foodsafety.ifas.ufl.edu.[59]

CONSUMER HEALTH INFORMATION (CHI)

The Internet has become an increasingly popular source of health information for the consumer. Consumers without computers frequently access the Internet at public libraries, or they ask librarians to conduct Internet searches. In recognition of this, the National Library of Medicine has begun a Consumer Health Information Index (CHI) to encourage and assist local libraries in this endeavor.[61] Grants have been awarded to some medical libraries to provide leadership within their states to conduct local workshops and establish Web sites for each state (e.g., www.arhealth-link.org).[61]

FUTURE TRENDS

As mentioned earlier, the FDA's Center for Food Safety and Applied Nutrition (CFSAN) is considering several new areas of regulation and rules: *trans*-fatty acids on nutrition labeling, restaurant menu claims for health, meat irradiation, and allergenic ingredients declaration.[4,62–64] The guidelines for *trans*-fatty acids and menu claims for restaurants have been proposed and are in the review process.[4,62–64] Meat irradiation is being developed commercially, and regulations will likely be completed in the near future. An international effort is under way to address concerns about allergenic ingredients. Voluntary declarations of allergens or other food substances that are potentially dangerous to selected individuals (such as phenylalanine) have begun. The intent is to provide ingredient lists that allow these individuals to identify potential problems for themselves. The more difficult problem lies in inadvertent addition of tiny amounts of allergenic constituents, such as peanut dust, from the manufacture of products in the same plant. No simple solutions to this complex problem or to the issues surrounding genetically modified foods have evolved. The government will likely review much scientific data before establishing final rules, while trying to keep nutrition labels simple and understandable to the average consumer. Over 150 studies were evaluated by the FDA before the approval of the first synthetic fat-based fat substitute by the FDA scientific staff.[63] Industry and consumers push for timely approval of modified foods and health claims they believe will assist the pursuit of health by consumers. A shorter approval time for health claims and new food products appears likely as technology advances knowledge and product development.

In summary, new and revised nutrition recommendations are likely to continue to evolve as more scientific data provide more evidence on which health professionals will base future practice. The food industry, from the farmer to processor to food service operators, will strive to meet consumer demands for healthy yet convenient foods.

REFERENCES

1. Consumer and Food Economics Institute, Composition of Foods: Raw, Processed, Prepared. Agricultural Handbook No. 8–1 to 8–15, U.S. Department of Agriculture, Washington, D.C., 1989–1991.
2. Nutritive Value of Foods, USDA Home and Garden Bulletin No. 72, U.S. Department of Agriculture, Washington, D.C., 1986.
3. Food and Nutrition Information Center, Standard Reference Database, Release No. 15, U.S. Department of Agriculture, Washington, D.C., 2002, http://www.nal.usda.gov/fnic/foodcomp.
4. Holden, J.M., Progress in Food Composition, paper presented at the 26th National Nutrient Databank Conference, Food Composition Databases: Important Tools for Improving National Health, Baton Rouge, 2002.
5. National Research Council Subcommittee on the 10th Edition of the RDAs, Food and Nutrition Board, Commission on Life Sciences, *Recommended Dietary Allowance,* 10th ed., National Academy Press, Washington, D.C., 1994.
6. Yates, A.A., Schlicker, S.A., and Suitor, C.W., Dietary reference intakes: the new bases for recommendations for calcium and related nutrients, B vitamins, and choline, *J. Am. Diet. Assoc.,* 98, 699–707, 1998.
7. Ippolito, P.M. and Mathios, A.D., Information and Advertising Policy: A Study of Fat and Cholesterol Consumption in the United States, 1977–1990, Bureau of Economics Staff Report, Federal Trade Commission, Washington, D.C., 1996.
8. Mackey, M.A. and Hill, B.P., Health claims regulations and new food concepts, in *Nutrition in the 90s: Current Controversies and Analysis,* Vol. 2, Kotsonis, F.N. and Mackey, M.A., Eds., Marcel Dekker, New York, 1994.
9. Institute of Medicine, Food and Nutrition Board, *Dietary Reference Intakes for Calcium, Phosphorus, Magnesium, Vitamin D, and Fluoride,* National Academy Press, Washington, D.C., 1997.
10. Institute of Medicine, Food and Nutrition Board, *Dietary Reference Intakes for Thiamin, Riboflavin, Niacin, Vitamin B-6, Folate, Vitamin B-12, Pantothenic Acid, Biotin, and Choline,* National Academy Press, Washington, D.C., 1998.
11. Sims, L.S., Uses of the recommended dietary allowances: a commentary, *J. Am. Diet. Assoc.,* 96, 659–662, 1996.
12. Most frequently asked questions … about the 1997 dietary reference intakes (DRIs), *Nutr. Today,* 32, 189–190, 1997.
13. Yates, A.A., Process and development of dietary reference intakes: basis, need, and application of recommended dietary allowances, *Nutr. Rev.,* 56, S5–S9, 1996.
14. Murphy, S.P., Overview of New Dietary Recommendations and Impact on Nutrient Calculation Programs, paper presented at the 26th National Nutrient Databank Conference, Food composition databases: important tool for improving national health, Baton Rouge, 2002.
15. Institute of Medicine, Food and Nutrition Board, *Dietary Reference Intakes for Vitamin C, Vitamin E, Selenium, and Carotenouids,* National Academy Press, Washington, D.C., 2000.

16. Institute of Medicine, Food and Nutrition Board, *Dietary Reference Intakes for Vitamin A, Vitamin K, Arsenic, Boron, Chromium, Copper, Iodine, Iron, Manganese, Molybdenum, Nickel, Silicon, Vanadium, and Zinc,* National Academy Press, Washington, D.C., 2001.
17. Institute of Medicine, Food and Nutrition Board, *Proposed Definition of Fiber,* National Academy Press, Washington, D.C., 2002.
18. Institute of Medicine, Food and Nutrition Board, *Dietary Reference Intakes: Applications for Dietary Assessment,* National Academy Press, Washington, D.C., 2000.
19. Institute of Medicine, Food and Nutrition Board, *Dietary Reference Intakes: A Risk Assessment Model for Establishing Upper Intake Levels for Nutrients,* National Academy Press, Washington, D.C., 1998.
20. Kris-Etherton, P.M., Impact of the Changing Fatty Acid Profiles of Fats, paper presented at the 26th National Nutrient Database Conference: Food Composition Databases: Important Tools for Improving National Health, Baton Rouge, 2002.
21. U.S. Department of Agriculture and U.S. Department of Health and Human Services, *The ABCs for Your Health: Dietary Guidelines 2000,* http://www.health.gov/dietary guidelines/dga2000/document/content.htm.
22. U.S. Department of Agriculture and U.S. Department of Health and Human Services, *Nutrition and Your Health: Dietary Guidelines for Americans,* 4th ed., Home and Garden Bulletin No. 232. U.S. Government Printing Office, Washington, D.C. 1995.
23. U.S. Department of Agriculture and U.S. Department of Health and Human Services, *Food and Exercise Pyramid for Children,* Washington, D.C., 1999.
24. Expert Committee of Nutrition and Health for Older Americans, Nutrition and Health for Older Americans—A Campaign of the American Dietetic Association, *Food Guide for Older Adults,* The American Dietetic Association, Chicago, 1998.
25. American Cancer Society Advisory Committee on Diet, Nutrition and Cancer Prevention, Reducing the risk of cancer with healthy food choices and physical activities, *CA Cancer J. Clin.,* 46, 325–341, 1996.
26. Steinmetz, K.A. and Potter, J.D., Vegetables, fruits and cancer prevention: a review, *J. Am. Diet. Assoc.,* 96, 1027–1039, 1996.
27. Tong, Y.M., Tomlinson, B., and Benzie, I.F.F., Total antioxidant and ascorbic acid content of fresh fruits and vegetables: implications for dietary planning and food preservation, *Brit. J. Nutr.,* 87, 55–59, 2002.
28. Murphy, J. and Cashman, K.D., Selenium content of a range of Irish foods, *Food Chem.,* 74, 493–498, 2001.
29. Brouns, F., Soya isoflavones: a new and promising ingredient for the health foods sector, *Food Res. Int.,* 35, 187–193, 2002.
30. Holasova, M. et al., Buckwheat—the source of antioxidant activity in functional foods, *Food Res. Int.,* 35, 207–211, 2002.
31. Nagai, T. et al., Antioxidative activities of some commercially honeys, royal jelly, and propolis, *Food Chem.,* 75, 237–240, 2001.
32. Kennedy, E.T. et al., The healthy eating index, 1994–96, U.S. Department of Agriculture for Nutrition Policy and Promotion, *CNPP-5,* 1998.
33. U.S. Department of Agriculture Center for Nutrition Policy and Promotion, *CNPP-1,* The Healthy Eating Index, 1995.
34. Food and Drug Administration, FDA approves new health claim for soy proteins and coronary heart disease, *Federal Register,* October 26, 1999.
35. United States Code of Federal Regulations, *CFR Title 21 (Food and Drugs),* U.S. Government Printing Office, Washington, D.C., Updated 1998.

36. McCabe, B.J., Champagne, C.M., and Allen, H.R., Calcium intake of selected age and gender groups from CSFII 1994–96, Abstract, *Exp. Biol.,* April, 1999, Washington, D.C.; Addendum to *J. Fed. Amer. Soc. Exper. Biol.,* 1999.

37. N.I.H. Consensus Development Panel on Optimal Intake, N.I.H. consensus: optimal calcium intake, *J. Am. Med. Assoc.,* 272, 1942–1948, 1994.

38. Mares-Perlman, J.A. et al., Nutrient supplements contribute to the dietary intake of middle- and older-aged adult residents of Beaver Dam, Wisconsin, *J. Nutr.,* 123, 176–188, 1993.

39. Food and Drug Administration, Center for Food Safety and Applied Nutrition, www.cfsan.fda.gov/list.html, April 6, 2000.

40. Holzapfel, W.H. and Schillinger, U., Introduction to pre- and probiotics, *Food Res. Int.,* 35, 109–116, 2002.

41. Reuter, G., Klein, G., and Goldberg, M., Identification of probiotics cultures in food samples, *Food Res. Int.,* 35, 119–124, 2002.

42. Ebly, E.M. et al., Folate status, vascular disease, and cognition in elderly Canadians, *Age and Aging,* 27, 485–491, 1998.

43. Bogden, J.B. and Louria, D.B., Micronutrients and immunity in older people, in *Preventive Nutrition: The Comprehensive Guide for Health Professionals,* Bendich, A. and Deckelbaum, R.J., Eds., Humana Press, Totowa, NJ, 1998.

44. Keane, E.M. et al., Use of folic acid-fortified milk in the elderly population, *Gerontology,* 44, 336–339, 1998.

45. Cuskelly, G.J., McNulty, H., and Scott, J.M., Effect of increasing dietary folate on red cell folate: implications for prevention of neural tube defects, *Lancet,* 349, 657–659, 1996.

46. Trumbo, P., Schlicker, S., and Yates, A.A., Impact of the DRIs on food composition databases, paper presented at the 26th National Nutrient Databank Conference, Food Composition Databases: Important Tools for Improving National Health, Baton Rouge, 2002.

47. Omenn, G.S., An assessment of the scientific basis for attempting to define the Dietary Reference Intakes for beta carotene, *J. Am. Diet. Assoc.,* 98, 1406–1409, 1998.

48. Mertz, W., Food fortification in the United States. *Nutr. Rev.,* 55, 44–49, 1997.

49. Connor, J.R. and Beard, J.L., Dietary iron supplements in the elderly: to use or not to use, *Nutr. Today,* 32, 102–109, 1997.

50. Russell, R.M., The impact of disease states as a modifying factor for nutrition toxicity, *Nutr. Rev.,* 55, 50–53, 1997; Council for Agricultural Science and Technology (CAST), Foodborne Pathogens: Review of Recommendations, Ames, IA, 1998, www.cast-science.org, 1999.

51. Caceres, V.M. et al., A foodborne outbreak of cyclosporiasis caused by imported raspberries, *J. Fam. Pract.,* 47, 231–234, 1998.

52. Quinn, K. et al., Foodborne outbreak of cryptosporodiosis—Spokane WA, 1997, *Morbidity Mortality Wkly. Rep.,* 47, 565–567, 1998.

53. Millard, P.S. et al., An outbreak of cryptosporidiosis from fresh-pressed apple cider, *J. Am. Med. Assoc.,* 272, 1592–1596, 1994.

54. Center for Disease Control, Outbreaks of Escherichia coli 0157:H7 infection and cryptosporidiosis associated with drinking unpasteurized apple cider—Connecticut and New York, October 1996, *Morbidity Mortality Wkly. Rep.,* 46, 4–8, 1997.

55. Klontz, K.C., Adler, W.H., and Potter, M., Age-dependent resistance factors in the pathogenesis of foodborne infectious disease, *Aging Clin. Exp. Res.,* 9, 320–326, 1997.

56. Shalaby, A.R., Significance of biogenic amines to food safety and human health, *Food Res. Int.,* 29, 675–690, 1996.

57. Stratton, E.J., Hutkins, W.R., and Taylor, L.S., Biogenic amines in cheese and other fermented foods. A review, *J. Food Prot.,* 54, 640–670, 1991.

58. Center for Disease Control, Food and Drug Administration, and FSIS Educators Network for Food Safety, http://www.foodsafety.gov.

59. The National Food Safety Database, http://www.foodsafety.ifas.ufl.edu, 2000.

60. Bougard, R., CHI Activities on a National Level, paper presented at Regional Technology Awareness Conference, Dissemination of Consumer Health Information: Technology, Services and Resources, Little Rock, 2000.

61. Food and Drug Administration, Federal Register notice: food labeling, nutrient content claims, and health claims. Proposed rule, *Federal Register,* November 17, 1999.

62. Food and Drug Administration, *Food Labeling Questions and Answers, Volume II—A guide for restaurants and other retail establishments,* Superintendent of Documents, U.S. Government Printing Office, Washington, D.C., 1999.

63. Food and Drug Administration, *Food Labeling Questions and Answers,* Vol. I, Booklet, August, 1993, www.cfsan.fda.gov/list.html.

64. Food and Nutrition Section. American Home Economics Association. *Handbook of Food Preparation,* 9th ed., Kendall-Hunt Publishing Company, Dubuque, IA, 1993, p. 49.

CHAPTER 6

Monitoring Nutritional Status in Drug Regimens

Beverly J. McCabe, Eric H. Frankel, and Jonathan J. Wolfe

CONTENTS

Drug–nutrient interactions have been categorized by Trovato into three categories: drugs affecting nutritional status, drug–food incompatibilities, and drug–alcohol interactions.[1] Three other categories, however, might well be considered by the nutrition professional. One is the case of nutrients becoming drugs, as can occur with megadose ingestion in the place of ordinary supplementation.[2] In this case, a product not known to be toxic at customary intake levels can become harmful based solely on dose. The second category to supplement Trovato's three is interaction of alcohol, food, and drug together to produce adverse events that can lead to a multinutrient state termed nutritional polyneuropathy of alcoholism.[3] Another category is the increasing potential interactions of foods and nutrients with herbal medicines discussed in Chapter 13 of this volume. This chapter discusses nutrition monitoring needed to prevent or minimize these five sorts of interactions. Other chapters present greater detail about mechanisms and specific drugs involved in interactions. Chapter 10 on nutritional assessment in the elderly provides detailed information that may apply to other age groups.

Although many nutrient–drug interaction references provide extensive lists of drugs involved in reactions with food, this chapter focuses on those reactions with the greatest potential for severity or occurrence. Other chapters discuss some of these in more depth. Some less commonly encountered interactions are also discussed briefly because the dietitian or the pharmacist is perhaps better situated to spot them than the nurse or physician. The intent is not to attempt to provide an exhaustive list of interactions, but rather to provide guidance to the nutrition professionals most likely to encounter them in practice.

Most drug–nutrient interactions involve food interfering with drugs, rather than drugs interfering with nutrient status.[4] The pharmacist is most often involved in acute effects of drug–nutrient interactions. A common example would be noting that warfarin has lessened effectiveness in a patient due to unusually high dietary intake of foods rich in Vitamin K. The phylloquinone from foods and the exogenous phytonadione from supplements may require a careful adjustment to a higher dose of warfarin.[5] The pharmacist may recognize the problem very quickly. The dietitian, on the other hand, is most often involved with managing chronic diseases and the long-term health effects of drug–nutrient interactions. An example of this is the dietitian's monitoring of long-term use of anticonvulsants, especially in children on high dosages. Children with refractory seizure disorders may even come to suffer from rickets, secondary to drug interference with vitamin D and calcium status. Another example might be B vitamin deficiencies (including vitamin B_6, B_{12}, or riboflavin deficiencies) that may not become evident for months or even years.[6,7] Symptoms of drug interference with nutrient status may be very slow and gradual—even to the point of having imperceptible onsets.

Diet interference with drug absorption and metabolism is more likely to be readily identified than the converse. Food interference with drug effectiveness is more obvious.[8] It is, therefore, more likely to be recognized quickly, studied clinically, and characterized more fully. If a drug known to be effective in a given condition and at a given dose fails to achieve expected results, caregivers are likely to start investigating the cause quickly. On the other hand, drugs may slowly, subtly interfere with nutrient status. The occurrence may prove important, but may not be detected or studied early. Indeed, negative influences on nutrient status may well occur more frequently than thought, but may not be recognized for what they are.[7]

Drug influences on nutrient status are less obvious because the nutrient deficiency symptoms are not specific and may be attributed to primary disease effects. Although nutrient adequacy is extremely important for quality of life, overt symptoms that are readily recognized may not appear until months or even years of inadequate intake.[4,6] These slow-appearing nutrient deficiencies are more likely to occur in individuals who had marginal intakes prior to starting the interfering drug regimen. The drug did not so much create the problem as it drove it toward more serious levels as nutrient status deteriorated.[3,4,8,9] Some drug metabolism requires micronutrients; and therapy with these drugs places a greater demand for adequate intake. Without adequate nutrition, drug clearance may also be slowed.[9,10] In these days of short-term stays or outpatient diagnosis and treatment, dietary assessment for marginal or submarginal intakes may simply not be done. It may indeed be objectively impossible in some cases.

Clinical drug trial studies for the efficacy and safety of a drug are usually done only on a short-term basis with a small number of subjects (e.g., 20–80) and often in a fasting state.[9] Assessments of beginning and ending nutritional status are not customarily part of drug studies, unless the experimental drug or drug combination is considered a nutrient per se, such as vitamin E and selenium supplements as a combination in cancer treatment. With no baseline nutritional assessment, small and gradual changes in status are unlikely to be detected. Hence, any nutritional inadequacies that result from the drug regimen are not likely to be detected until the drug is on the market for an extended period of time. Premarketing clinical drug trials are classified into one of four phases. Appendix C.2 contains a general description of the four phases of clinical trials of drugs.

In the past, when drugs were tested in a metabolic unit, subjects were often placed on formula feedings for the test duration. The formula diet was easier to control, plan, and monitor than diverse diets. Whether drug effects during formula feedings bore any close relationship to the effects of drugs upon regular diets was seldom questioned or studied. Recently, healthy subjects have often been studied short term in the fasting state.[9] This mandates little consideration of the potential effect of foods on the drug or the drug on nutritional status.[6] With the expansion of outpatient settings for drug studies, initial assessment and monitoring of nutritional status in drug trials has received minor attention, unless a potential mechanism was identified early. Another change is that clinical trials of drugs are being done increasingly in community hospital settings, rather than research university settings with full research staff. Potential mechanisms by which drugs can influence nutritional status are outlined in Table 6.1.

Table 6.1   Mechanisms by Which Drug Groups Can Induce Nutrient Depletion Metabolically and Physiologically

Mechanism	Nutrient	Drug Groups
Malabsorption	Folate	Anticonvulsants Antiinflammatories (Sulfasalzine, Azufidine®)
	B_{12}	Bile acid sequestrants Biguanides
	A Beta carotene	Antihyperlipidemics (Clofibrate®, Colestipol®)
Competitive binding	Folate Thiamin Antacids	Salicylates
	Potassium Magnesium Phosphates	Aluminum preparations
Inhibition of coenzyme	Folate	B_6 antagonists (INH)
Biosynthesis	B_6	Antituberculars (Pyrimethamine), antineoplastics (Cytarabine), folate antagonists
	B_{12}	Methotrexate, nitrous oxide
Selective effect on apoenzyme or holoenzyme	B_6	Contraceptive steroids, hypotensives (hydralazine, Apresoline®, Serpasil®)
Hyperexcretion by kidneys	Ascorbic acid Potassium Amino Acids Magnesium Zinc	Glucocorticoids Antiarthritics (Indomethacin) Diuretics (furosemide, Lasix®)
	Folate B_6	B_6 and folate antagonists
Increased turnover, especially in children	D K	Anticonvulsants (phenytoin, phenobarbital, primidone)
Changes pH in gastrointestinal tract	Iron (nonheme) B_{12}	H_2 inhibitors (Tagamet®, Cimetidine®)

Source: Adapted from Roe, D. A., *Drug-Induced Nutritional Deficiencies*, 2nd ed., AVI Publishing, Westport, CT, 1985 and White, J.V., Ed., *The Role of Nutrition in Chronic Disease Care: Executive Summary,* National Nutrition Screening Initiative, Washington, D.C., 1997. With permission.

MAJOR DRUG-INDUCED MALNUTRITION

Roe[11] noted that drugs may induce nutrient deficiencies in several unusual circumstances:

1. Deficiencies that are rarely seen due to inadequate diets (e.g., pyridoxine deficiency)[12]
2. Slow and gradual storage deficiencies
3. Unusual and complex nutrient deficiencies, such as vitamin D and folate in anticonvulsant therapy[13]
4. Either single or multivitamin deficiencies
5. Mineral imbalances secondary to increased urinary excretion[14]

Underlying causes of drug-induced malnutrition are often multifactorial in origin, including such elements as marginal intake or marginal synthesis, physiological stress, increased nutrient requirements secondary to a particular disease state, and (lastly but certainly not least) decreased absorption of nutrient(s).[4] The picture can be further confused by the use of several drugs at one time. Polypharmacy within a study may cloud the issues because drug–drug interactions can occur simultaneously with drug–nutrient interactions.[1,2,4] When a potential nutritional complication is commonly recognized—such as diarrhea with an enteral feeding—the rate or concentration of enteral feeding may be blamed for placing a hyperosmolar load on a malnourished gut. The hyperosmolar load from exogenous potassium chloride supplements administered by the same route, the use of a liquid medication containing sorbitol, or the impact of antibiotics taken simultaneously may, thereby, pass unnoticed in the shadow of the assumed cause of the problem.

NUTRIENTS COMMONLY AFFECTED BY DRUGS

Some nutrients are more widely recognized as being affected by drugs than others. Traditionally, the nutrients most often cited in drug-induced malnutrition were summarized by Roe and seconded by Williams,[7,9] as follows:

1. Vitamin B_{12} because its digestion, absorption, and utilization can be impacted at several points and by multiple drugs and conditions
2. B vitamins, in general, secondary to initial low body stores leading to early depletion
3. Iron and other nutrients important in red blood cell production
4. Calcium and vitamin D important to maintenance of healthy bones in adults and avoidance of rickets in children

More attention has recently been placed on drug-induced deficiencies of folate, thiamin, and protein.[3,4,14–16] Increased numbers of these reactions have occurred as a result of drugs having greater potency and specificity.[4,11] Special attention has been paid to the numerous drugs that negatively influence folate status.[11–15,17–19] The multiple mechanisms by which folate status can be impacted are summarized in

Table 6.2 Folate and Pyrodoxine Antagonists: Drugs That Work by Interfering with Metabolic Pathways Dependent on Folate and B_6 as Coenzymes

General Classification	Generic Name	Product Name
Folate Antagonists: May Require Supplementation or Special Fortified Foods		
Antineoplastics	methotrexate	Mexate®
Antipsoriatrics	acitretin	Soriataine®
Antiarthritic		Rheumatrex®
Antiinflammatories/(ulcerative colitis, Crohn's)	sulfasalzine	Azulfidine®
Antiprotozoals/(HIV/AIDS)	pentamidine	Pentam®
Diuretic (potassium-sparing)/Hypotensive	triamterene	Dyrenium®, Diazide®
Antituberculars	pyrimethamine	Daraprim®, Fansidar®
Anticonvulsants	phenytoin	Dilantin®
	primidone	Mysoline®
Alcohol	ethyl alcohol	
Immunosuppressants	azathioprine	Imuran®
Pyridoxine Antagonists: May Require B_6 Supplementation or Rich Food Sources		
Antiarthritics	penicillamine[a]	Cuprimine®
Antineoplastics	cytarabine	Cytosar®
Antituberlins	isoniazid	INH®
Hypotensives	hydralazine	Apresazide®, Apresoline®, Ser-Ap-Es®, Serpasil®
Antiparkinsonism	levodopa[a]	Larodopa®, Sinemet®

[a] Use food rather than oral supplements.

Table 6.2. The widespread use of certain drugs in cardiovascular disease has led to a much greater appreciation of the potential dangers of poor thiamin status because that syndrome may be perceived as simply another symptom of the underlying cardiac disease itself.[16] Another example is the real influence of drugs on the many disease states that may be misdiagnosed as dementia or Alzheimer's disease. Such masqueraders may include vitamin deficiency, drug–drug interactions, or water and sodium imbalances.[17–22] When checking vitamin B_{12} status by biochemical methods, the most commonly used test is the Schilling's test. Although this is a valid and valuable test for identifying malabsorption secondary to lack of intrinsic factor, it does little to identify other causes of poor B_{12} status.[17] Lack of dietary folate or drugs interfering with folate both can lower vitamin B_{12} status.[17–18] Among patients with marginal folate status, the requirement for vitamin B_{12} increases as different pathways are used.[19]

In the total picture, the most common symptoms associated with drug influences on nutritional status may well be commonly occurring symptoms, such as dry mouth, nausea and vomiting, constipation, or diarrhea, that discourage adequate intake of food. These are indirect influences of drug, which may exacerbate the disease state. They are not necessarily side effects of the drug(s).

Monitoring the influence of drugs on nutrient status must begin with a general recognition of the importance of nutrition in total health and in disease management.

History of clinical diseases, drug intakes, and physical examination are the starting point of nutritional monitoring in drug regimens.[7]

CLINICAL OR MEDICAL HISTORY

In a review of systems, the gastrointestinal system has the most direct influence on nutrient status. As such, past medical history for gastrointestinal surgeries and diseases is especially important to clinicians seeking to guard against risk for malnutrition. From a clinical viewpoint, recent weight changes can be extremely important in screening for protein–calorie malnutrition and fluid retention. Assessment of body mass index (BMI) has sometimes been used in population studies as the sole criterion for judging dietary adequacy. Changes in body weight and use of various weight indices are the most common starting points for nutritional assessment employed by American dietitians. Pharmacists and physicians use actual body weight, ideal body weight, adjusted lean body mass, or body surface area as starting points for calculating appropriate drug dosage.

Any significant change in weight, either loss or gain, must be recognized and the cause identified. The dietitian needs to assess whether dietary intake, including enteral feeding, has changed and can explain weight change. If intake remains the same, other potential causes need to be evaluated. Weight gain in the face of no change in caloric intake or exercise patterns suggests fluid retention. A sudden gain in body weight may be an early warning of pending sepsis in trauma patients, such as those severely burned. If fluid retention occurs, the dietitian must assess protein status. Edema occurs in the presence of a lowered protein status, as indicated by a drop in serum albumin below 3.5 g/dL. A significant drop in serum albumin may be indicative of increased urinary losses of protein or of gluconeogenesis. The drop may occur slowly over many months and even years. For those on long-term drug therapy, especially children and the elderly, regular monitoring of serum albumin is advisable. For those drugs that may negatively impact renal or liver functions, monitoring serum albumin is especially critical. Dietary protein exerts a major influence on serum albumin level, on drug-metabolizing enzymes such as P_{450} cytochrome families, and intestinal flora.[2]

Evaluation of mental status may also constitute an important index for nutrition risk. Indeed, Benton has suggested that changes in cognition may well be the first sign of a subclinical deficiency of the B vitamins.[20] Patients in whom depression, mania, or mental confusion exist are frequently found to be malnourished. This is especially the case when deficiency proves to be secondary to decreased dietary intake, or to treatment with drugs that may increase the need for riboflavin. This is especially likely when little or no milk products, the leading dietary sources of riboflavin, are consumed. When folate status was clinically evaluated in psychiatric admissions in England, the majority of patients were found to have either submarginal or deficient levels of red blood cell folate.[21] Dementia may occur secondarily to vitamin B_{12} deficiency. It may not be diagnosed from a positive Schilling test, for that determination is really more a test for B_{12} absorption than a measure of B_{12}

status.[17] Part of the nurse's role is to monitor for another potential cause of confusion: dehydration. Dehydration occurs much more readily in the elderly due to a decreased effectiveness of the normal thirst mechanism. People with a poor food intake are also likely to have a poor fluid intake because foods are a major source of fluid in the American diet. When energy intake is low, glycogen stores may be burned, and this means a loss of 2–4 g of body water for each gram of glycogen metabolized.[23] Such body water waste produces the rapid weight loss seen early in fasting and severe dieting. Characteristically, most of this weight loss is rapidly regained when fluid, protein, and carbohydrate intake improve. Thus, poor food intake may mean a lower intake of water and an increased loss of metabolic water.[23]

DRUG HISTORY

It is important to identify the use of drugs (both prescription and nonprescription) that may interfere with nutrient status when monitoring nutrient status.[24–26] The simple identification of each drug a patient uses does not constitute a history of drug intake. The potential for a drug–nutrient interaction is not solely based on drugs in use and adequacy of diet prior to and during drug use. It also includes the dosage level and duration of the drug regimen. True risk for a drug–nutrient interaction is multifactorial and must be viewed in the complete picture of disease state, dietary adequacy, dosage level, and duration of the drug regimen. Figure 6.1 features a drug history form suggested by Roe[27] that includes the current and previous health problems, proprietary and generic drug names, duration of intake, frequency of intake, and dose. It also allows for the recording of complaints for which the patient has self-prescribed. Today, the clinician also needs to specifically ask the same set of questions for the use of herbal and other dietary supplements.[28–30] The dietitian might well adopt the "brown bag approach" used by many pharmacists to assess drug intake by requesting that the patient bring in all current medications, including herbal or dietary supplements packaging. Brand names, herbal mixtures, and production aspects of these supplements change frequently, making a precise herbal databank almost impossible to compile and maintain. More detailed discussion of these issues appears in Chapter 13.

Drugs used to treat gastrointestinal disorders and diseases are especially important to identify and review with the patient.[1–6,31–33] These drugs are discussed in detail in Chapter 7. With the movement of histamine-H2 receptors from prescription to nonprescription status, both dietitians and pharmacists need to inquire about frequent or long-term use of drugs such as cimetidine (Tagamet®), famotidine (Pepcid®), and ranitidine (Zantac®) as self-prescribed medications that may impact on iron and B_{12} status.

DIET HISTORY

A diet history that identifies marginal diets can lead to improved nutrient intake prior to the development of overt nutrient deficiency states. Whereas a complete nutrient intake analysis requires a typical or usual day's diet history conducted by a

Drug		Duration of Intake	Frequency	Dose	Health Problem
Proprietary Name	Generic Name				
	`				

Self-Prescribed for Complaints

Complaint	Yes	No	Some-times	Drug	Duration	Frequency	Dose
Constipation							
Indigestion							
Headache							
Nervousness							
Insomnia							
Pain							
Menstrual cramps							
Cold and sinus trouble							
Diarrhea							
Depression							
Other (state)							

Dietary Supplements

Supplement	Recommended by		Purpose	Brand	Duration	Frequency	Dose
	Self	Other					

Figure 6.1 Sample drug intake form. (Adapted from Roe, D.A., *Drug-Induced Nutritional Deficiencies,* 2nd ed., AVI Publishing, Westport, CT, 1985, 129–131. With permission.)

dietitian, other types of dietary intake screening can be done by other health professionals. If the patient has the prerequisite characteristics needed to complete a 3-day food record, the adequacy of the usual diet can be better assessed. Although a 24-h dietary recall for the previous day is frequently done in research studies for assessing the mean intake of a group, this method is inappropriate for assessing the adequacy of any individual's intake.[34] A dietary screen that can identify the most likely nutrient(s) to be low, secondary to inadequate intake of key foods, is featured in Table 6.3.

The amount, type, and frequency of alcoholic beverage consumption forms an essential part of any diet history. Such an inventory bears particular importance in dietary counseling for drug regimens.[35] Acute and chronic alcohol intake may lead to: (1) lower or elevated drug levels; (2) lower or elevated plasma levels of glucose, and (3) depletion of vitamins and minerals.[36–40] Alcohol exhibits many effects usually associated with drugs. It also is a potent depressant substance. For these reasons, it

Table 6.3   Key Foods in Global Screening for Dietary Adequacy

Key Foods	Primary Food Sources of Nutrients
Dairy products:	
Milk, cheese, yogurt	Riboflavin, calcium, protein
Meat, poultry	Protein, iron, B vitamins
Citrus fruits, tomatoes, melons, potatoes	Vitamin C
Deep yellow or leafy green vegetables	Vitamin A, folate
Whole grain cereals and breads	Fiber, B-complex vitamins

acquires an extraordinary importance in dietary counseling. More details of the mechanism involved in these effects are provided in Chapter 9.

PHYSICAL EXAMINATION FOR DRUG-INDUCED MALNUTRITION

Physical examination should pinpoint clinical and biochemical signs of several disease states including gastrointestinal diseases, symptoms, and conditions that may be related to malnutrition. Many of the symptoms may be nonspecific for malnutrition, but together with dietary and medical history can identify potentially modifiable nutritional risks.[34]

MALABSORPTION

Maldigestion may arise from many drug-related factors. Such factors certainly include use and abuse of laxatives and gastric antacid products. The former markedly decrease gastrointestinal transit time (e.g., bisacodyl [Dulcolax®]), mineral oil). The latter change the pH to decrease adsorption of dietary folate (aluminum and magnesium hydroxides [Maalox®], sodium bicarbonate).[1–3]

Drugs used specifically to treat gastrointestinal disorders (such as ulcerative colitis and Crohn's disease) may have the undesirable side effect of contributing to folate deficiency by decreasing hydrolysis of dietary folate polyglutamate.[2] This can be counterbalanced by use of folate supplementation either with vitamin tablets or folate-fortified foods that require less hydrolysis. Another positive step is not to take drugs such as sulfasalazine with meals because the drug is thought to interfere with folate absorption.[2] Patients with celiac disease or with hemolytic anemia may be particularly vulnerable to drug–folate malnutrition.

Vitamin B_{12} is another vitamin particularly vulnerable to gastrointestinal drugs.[17–18] The preparation of vitamin B_{12} for absorption and the amount absorbed are dependent on several factors. Dietary B_{12} is found only in foods of animal origins; thus, vegan vegetarians are particularly vulnerable to depletion. Dietary B_{12} must be bound to intrinsic factor that is produced in the stomach. The vitamin also requires an acid environment for the binding to occur. Potassium chloride supplements, particularly the slow-release form, may yield an abnormal Schilling test suggestive of vitamin B_{12} impairment. Secondary malabsorption can occur with the chronic use of H_2 histamine receptor antagonists. Various formulations of H_2 antagonists and proton pump inhibitors, including nonprescription strengths, prevent intrinsic factor (IF) binding. Later on, the absorption of the B_{12}-IF complex requires the basic environment found in healthy mucosa near the ileocecal valve to complete its cycle. Maximum B_{12} absorption occurs at pH 6.6 and has been said to be absent below a pH of 5.5.[40] The last step in the absorption of B_{12} occurs in the lower small intestine proximal to the ileocecal valve. Gastrointestinal disease and especially surgery in this area of the small intestine can greatly reduce the absorption of B_{12} and the reabsorption of bile acids. Thus, fat malabsorption may also occur, thus lowering absorption of the fat-soluble vitamins as well as B_{12}.

ANEMIAS

Vitamin B_{12} deficiency that arises from the lack of intrinsic factor has been termed pernicious anemia, a fatal disease where the original treatment was the feeding of desiccated liver. Once the process of vitamin B_{12} absorption was understood, intramuscular injections of B_{12} provided relief from this megaloblastic anemia. With the low cost of injections, physicians no longer need to order laboratory tests to confirm the diagnosis of pernicious anemia; they can simply treat patients with monthly injections. B_{12} deficiency may occur as part of achlorhydric anemia, a form of microcytic anemia secondary to a lack of gastric acid. This form of anemia is more likely to occur in the elderly or in adults who heavily use over-the-counter (OTC) antacids. Other drugs that are antagonists of folate may lead to a secondary B_{12} deficiency. This occurs because a lack of folate drives metabolic pathways that require B_{12}, producing a consequent increase in the need for B_{12} at a time when intake is level or declining and stores are depleted. Heavy alcohol use may further complicate these interactions because it constitutes another mechanism by which B vitamin requirements are increased.[42]

Anemia may also arise from a little-recognized side effect of taking vitamin C supplements in amounts greater than 1 g daily, or as a constituent of multivitamin–mineral supplements, according to Herbert.[17] The actions of the vitamin C, iron, and other antioxidant nutrients in high-dose supplements may convert vitamin B_{12} into analogues that are useless to humans. Supplemental vitamin B_{12} may not be sufficient protection. Herbert recommends that persons taking megadoses of vitamin C be checked regularly for vitamin B_{12} deficiency or stop taking high-dose supplements.[17] Others disagree that excess vitamin C destroys vitamin B_{12}, but the upper limit of daily vitamin C intake is set at 1 g to avoid other adverse events.[24]

Multiple forms and causes of anemia may exist, but exact diagnosis may not be attempted. The busy practitioner who sees a low hemoglobin value may simply prescribe iron supplements, especially in the elderly. In reality, iron supplementation may provide no positive effect on the anemia but may instead pose a risk of iron overload in the elderly patient.[42,43] In addition, iron supplements, as well as supplements of other divalent ion minerals, may complex with other drugs the patient takes, reducing effectiveness of those agents through decreased absorption. Appendices D.3, D.5, D.6, and D.10 list foods high in calcium, iron, magnesium, and zinc.

The assessment of anemia should begin with a simple finger prick and microscopic blood smear examination to distinguish between microcytic and macrocytic anemia, as well as hypochromic or normochromic erythrocytes. If the erythrocytes are judged microcytic, the question of occult bleeding secondary to drugs or lack of dietary protein should be raised. Another potential form of microcytic, hypochromic anemia is the "anemia of chronic disease" associated with some other major disease states such as rheumatoid arthritis, inflammatory bowel disease, cancer, and some vascular disorders.[42,43] The hypochromic cell appears pale due to lack of iron. If the erythrocyte is judged to be macrocytic, distinction needs to be made as to the potential for folate, B_{12}, and B_6 deficiency, as well as copper deficiency. A dietary and drug history can be used to judge likely causes, and corrective action can be taken that will resolve the anemia.

Drugs that interfere with folate or pyridoxine status can create a deficiency of B_{12} as well. A lack of one vitamin may shift metabolism to an alternate pathway, which increases the need for other vitamins. This is especially true for the six B vitamins found in many important pathways, including the Krebs cycle.

Anemia may also develop from the use of a single-mineral supplement that creates an unbalanced competition for other minerals, thereby creating a relative deficiency. For example, use of zinc supplements may induce a copper deficiency. Drugs that chelate minerals, such as penicillamine (Cuprimine®) used in Wilson's disease to reduce serum copper, may also chelate other minerals.

NEUROPATHIES

Neuropathies may occur as a result of vitamin deficiency or toxicity. Until recently, water-soluble vitamins were thought to be incapable of producing toxicity. A number of neurologic diseases such as premenstrual syndrome, carpal tunnel disease, foot drop, and others were treated with megadoses of various B vitamins including pyridoxine. Physicians prescribing B_6 in 2-g doses began to recognize a neuropathy that largely but slowly resolved after cessation of the B_6 regimen.[44]

Drug-induced imbalances of vitamin B_6 or vitamin B_{12} can lead to the development of a neuropathy.[7,44] Common to both are the slow development of paresthesias, numbness, and the development of pareses of the lower limbs. Vibration sense may be reduced, especially in vitamin B_{12} deficiency. Vitamin B_{12} deficiency has often been spotted by the "burning feet" syndrome, muscle soreness in the legs, and atrophy of the peroneal muscles.[7,17] It is often difficult to diagnose drug-induced B_6 deficiency by biochemical means because the B_6 antagonists may well produce the deficiency by inducing hyperexcretion of the vitamin in the urine. Urinary measures are commonly used to screen for water-soluble vitamin deficiency, but are not particularly helpful in drug-induced deficiency states if the drug's action is to increase urinary excretion. Vitamin B_6 deficiency does not commonly occur in isolation.[45] Other B-vitamin deficiencies, most notably riboflavin deficiency, also affect B_6 status and share clinical signs such as stomatitis, cheilosis, glossitis, irritability, depression, and confusion.[45–48] Riboflavin is needed in the metabolism of vitamin B_6.[44]

Paradoxically, the drug-induced toxicity of B_6 megadoses also presents a neuropathy with similar characteristics to those of deficiency neuropathy. The most commonly described symptoms of the toxic neuropathy were the "white glove/sock" feel of the hands and feet.[44] Affected patients describe touch sensations as being similar to touching objects while wearing cotton gloves or socks over the hands.

DERMATITIS

Although drug-induced dermatitis is seldom of nutritional origin, important nutrient deficiencies have been first identified by dermatitis, especially in early days of total parenteral and enteral nutrition. Vitamin B_6 antagonists, such as levodopa in large doses, can produce a seborrheic dermatitis and pellagra (a dermatitis of light-exposed areas of the body such as collarbone, neck, arms, hands, feet, and legs).[7] Pellagra may be caused by a lack of several B vitamins, but most notable is the lack of niacin.[46] Pellagra is still found in the U.S. today, usually in those patients with poor diets and other conditions, such as alcoholism, that may further aggravate a poor intake. In dermatitis that not only involves the outer skin, but also alters the oral mucosa, the tongue becomes a bright red color. Thus, the tongue and other gastrointestinal symptoms should be checked for causation by impaired niacin status.[46] If accompanied by neurological symptoms of depression, apathy, headache, fatigue, and loss of memory, dermatitis may well arise from nutrient deficiencies of one or more B vitamins.[7]

Riboflavin deficiency may develop with long-term use of several psychotherapeutic drugs, including some of the newer generation of tricyclic antidepressants and antipsychotic drugs (e.g., thiothiexene/Navane®). See Table 6.4 for details. Tricyclic antidepressants (e.g., amitriptyline/Elavil®) have chemical structures very similar to riboflavin.[47] The classic phenothiazines (imipramine/Tofranil®, chlorpro-

Table 6.4 Drugs and Conditions That May Interfere with Riboflavin Absorption or Metabolism; Encourage Milk Products or Supplement Use

Drug Class/Condition	Generic Name	Brand Name
Anticonvulsants[a]	Phenobarbital (long term)	Barbital, Luminal
Antimalarial[a]	Quinacrine	
Antineoplastic[b]	Adriamycin	
Bile acid sequestrants[c]	Cholestryamine (severe diarrhea)	Questran
Psychotrophic[b]	Chlorpromazine	Thorazine
	Imipramine	Tofranil
	Amitriptyline	Elavil
Adrenal insufficiency[a]		
Diarrheal diseases[a]		
Thyroid disorder[a]		

[a] McCormick, D.B., Riboflavin, in *Modern Nutrition in Health and Disease,* 9th ed., Shils, M.E. et al., Eds., Williams & Wilkins, Baltimore, 1999, 391–399.
[b] Rivlin, R.S., Riboflavin, in *Present Knowledge in Nutrition*, 7th ed., Ziegler, E.E. and Filer, L.J., Jr., Eds., ILSI Press, Washington, D.C., 1996, 170–171.
[c] Roe, D.A., *Drug-Induced Malnutrition,* 2nd ed., AVI Press, Westport, CT, 1985.

mazine/Thorazine®) increase the need for riboflavin. Patients requiring such drugs frequently present with limited dietary intake for several weeks prior to hospital admission. The elderly or substance abusers, especially those recently dieting, stand at greater risk for lack of dietary riboflavin. Riboflavin is a vitamin with a limited number of rich food choices. The absence of or limited intake of milk products should serve as a red flag to monitor riboflavin status. Clinical symptoms associated with riboflavin deficiency are not specific and may represent other causes including submarginal intakes of several other vitamins. Thus, screening for milk and meat intake becomes a primary means of identifying the readily corrected dermatitis induced by these drug–nutrient interactions. Antitubercular (isoniazid [INH®]/Isotamine®) and antimalarial drugs (pyrimethamine/Daraprim®) may also induce dermatitis secondary to nutrient deficiencies of B vitamins.[46]

BONE DISEASES

A number of drugs can induce such bone diseases as osteomalacia in adults and rickets in children. The causation derives from secondary interference with uptake of vitamin D, calcium, and other vitamins only recently recognized as involved in bone metabolism (e.g., Vitamin K).[48] Other disease states, most notably end-stage renal disease, can make people much more vulnerable to the nutritional problems inherent with these drugs. The absence of dairy products in the diet should serve as a red flag to monitor vitamin D and calcium status in drug regimens such as the antituberculars (rifampin/Rifamate®), anticonvulsants (phenobarbital, primidone/Mysoline®), and antilipidemics (cholestyramine/Questran®). End-stage renal disease and liver disease diminish a number of hormones that are produced either in lower amounts or not in an activated form. This deficiency may require the use of several nutrient supplements, especially in activated form. For example, cholecalciferol (D_3), the active form of vitamin D (calcitriol/Rocaltrol®), is often given during dialysis, combined with administration of intraluminal phosphate binders.[48] Care must be taken not to give excess vitamin D (D_2) or magnesium supplements with this regimen because impaired renal function may lead to toxicity.[49,50]

GASTROINTESTINAL DISEASES

The impact of gastrointestinal diseases and the drugs to treat them can create major nutritional problems. As aging may bring more or worsening of gastrointestinal diseases, these are discussed in greater detail in the separate chapters on drugs in the elderly and gastrointestinal diseases. The major impact of drugs on nutritional status may, however, be more commonly induced by generic side effects of anorexia, dry mouth, nausea, and vomiting—all of which may reduce food intake. The majority of drugs carry some risks for these side effects as well as risks for stomach pain, diarrhea, or constipation that may serve as negative reinforcers for food intake. These and more specific nutritional problems are addressed by general drug categories later in this chapter.

CHRONIC DISEASES

Several chronic diseases may lead to long-term malnutrition known as marasmus or cachexia. Most notable among these are cardiac cachexia, cancer cachexia, chronic obstructive pulmonary disease (COPD), HIV/AIDS, and frailty due to a number of disease states in the elderly. The term sarcopenia has been coined to describe the slow, steady loss of lean muscle mass secondary to severe inactivity, disease states, and aging.[51] In many of these states, aggressive nutrition support is inadequate to produce regain of lean muscle mass. The addition of appropriate exercise prescription to a well-designed nutritional care plan should be considered. If these therapies prove inadequate, another potential therapeutic approach is the use of appetite-stimulating drugs, including prednisone/Orasone®, dronabinol/Marinol®, oxandrolone/Oxandrin®, and megestrol acetate/Megace®. These drugs bring both benefits and risks to the nutritional care plans. Prednisone has been in use longer and has proved effective for short-term (4 weeks or less) stimulation. Cost is modest. Prednisone, however, carries risks of hypokalemia, muscle weakness, cushingnoid features, hyperglycemia, immune suppression, and other pathologies. These risks make prednisone a poor choice for stimulating appetite in patients with diabetes mellitus or HIV/AIDS.

Dronabinol, a derivative of marijuana, has been shown to improve appetite, but does not appear to bring any significant weight gain. Taken before meals, appetite may be improved, but avoidance of alcohol is recommended. Nausea and vomiting are side effects. Other risks include mental changes such as euphoria, somnolence, dizziness, and confusion. Monthly costs are high. Another new appetite stimulant is megestrol acetate sold under the brand name Megace®, which has been shown to improve appetite, body weight, well-being, and quality of life when combined with exercise and nutrition support. Risks include impotence, vaginal bleeding, and deep-vein thrombosis. The costs can also run to several hundred dollars per month when taken in higher doses (400 mg/d).

SIDE EFFECTS AND IMPACT ON DIETARY INTAKE BY DRUG CATEGORY

In general, adequate intakes of kilocalories and protein are necessary for the optimal use of many drugs. All drug metabolism requires energy. Without adequate dietary intake or appropriate nutrition support, medications cannot have desired results at reasonable dose levels. Adequate protein is essential for the immune response and for healing in general to occur. Although correction of nutrient deficiencies cannot cure diseases or extend life in chronic disease states such as cancer, adequate intake and correction of nutrient imbalances can improve the quality of life. Therapeutic drugs essential to the treatment of these diseases may create nutrient deficiency states that must be corrected or minimized. Another general guideline is to take medications with appropriate fluid to prevent or minimize side effects, including damage to mucosal linings of the gastrointestinal tract.

Absorption of the majority of drugs taken orally is profoundly reduced or delayed by the presence of food, therefore, most drugs should not be taken with food.[3,14,15] Two exceptions require mentioning. First, when a drug is identified as a likely cause of gastric upset, a small amount of food or milk may be desirable. Second, a very few drugs (e.g., metronidazole/Flagyl®) are best absorbed in the presence of a fatty meal.

Analgesics

Among OTC drugs, analgesics account for a large portion of the market and are found in almost every American home. Regular and long-term use, however, is appropriate mostly for patients suffering chronic pain such as that of arthritis. Salicylates, including aspirin, have long been recognized to induce gastric distress. This may progress to anemia secondary to occult blood loss in patients who take large doses over an extended period of time. If taken with meals or milk, the potential for gastric distress is reduced. Aspirin is absorbed faster in the presence of a higher pH, so antacids may produce quicker onset and higher blood levels. If taken with alcohol, gastric damage and distress from nonsteroidal antiinflammatory drugs (NSAIDs) becomes far more likely. Besides salicylates and NSAIDs, acetaminophen (APAP) is the one major remaining OTC medication for analgesia and it, too, has interactions. The ingestion of acetaminophen (Tylenol®) and alcohol may cause liver toxicity and is not recommended.

Hyperexcretion of some nutrients is also a possibility in long-term use of high NSAID doses, most notably ascorbic acid, folate, and potassium.[1] Protein and vitamin K status may also become marginal. Iron deficiency anemia secondary to microhemorrhages may necessitate consumption of foods high in iron and vitamin C.[1] Chronic use of acetaminophen (APAP/Tylenol®), another commonly used OTC analgesic, may increase the risk of renal disease, especially in the presence of chronic alcohol intake. APAP use may also increase the need for folate.

Opioids are the drugs of choice for pain control involving both chronic pain of cancer and severe acute pain. With these drugs (e.g., morphine/Duramorph®, Astramorph®), there is no toxicity because they have no peripheral target organ, but act on the central nervous system (CNS). As such, appetite may be suppressed due the development of dysgeusia (i.e., foods may taste differently). Constipation will present a continuing and significant problem, particularly when opioids are taken orally. Patients on these drugs must regularly take stimulant laxatives such as bisacodyl or senna. They must never take mineral oil by mouth. They must minimize any use of milk of magnesia or other saline cathartics. Opioid-related constipation stems from direct opioid action on inhibitory receptors in the bowel. This is the mechanism by which opioids (e.g., diphenoxylate with atropine/Lomotil®) control diarrhea. Use of oral mineral oil exposes the patient to the risk of lipoid aspiration pneumonia, but does not stimulate the intestine to expel the lubricated feces. Administration of saline cathartics exposes the patient to risks of CNS depression (e.g., from hypermagnesemia), but also does not stimulate the musculature of the bowel to expel a fecal mass. Bulk-forming laxatives (psyllium/Metamucil®) have no stimulant powers, but instead place the patient at risk for impaction with a fecalith.

As a general rule, alcohol and analgesics do not mix well. Analgesics such as propoxyphene/Darvon® and propoxyphene with APAP/Darvocet®, or oxycodone/APAP/Lorcet®, produce abdominal discomfort and CNS symptoms if mixed with alcohol.[1] The combination of depressant analgesics related to opioids and alcohol (also a CNS depressant) can place life itself at hazard.

Nonsteroidal antiinflammatory drugs are frequently used for chronic pain. Hence, their doses can be properly used long term. The need to suppress inflammatory processes properly dictates high doses in many cases. Sodium and water retention may occur as a consequence. Examples of this classification of drugs are ibuprofen (Motrin IB®, Advil®) and naproxen (Anaprox®, Naprosyn®, and the OTC product Aleve®). All these drugs are similar in molecular structure to aspirin. They can produce similar toxicities, although the side-effect profile varies from one NSAID to another. They are not benign drugs. At prescription strengths and doses, they require regular monitoring for toxicities. If purchased OTC for self-medication, they are safe only so long as used according to package instructions. This means that their use by lay persons (patients) may only be at lower doses and for strictly limited periods of time. If a patient exceeds either the maximum dose or the maximum length of time for use stated in the packaging, that use must be under the direction of a physician. In every case, caregivers will monitor for gastric distress, occult bleeding, tarry stools, renal changes, and electrolyte disturbances (edema).

Antibiotics

In general, broad-spectrum antibiotics related to penicillin (including cephalosporins) need to be taken under two important considerations:

1. Some should be taken 1 h before or 2 h after meals for best effects. Check for specific information on each agent.
2. Take with an adequate amount of fluid.

If significant gastrointestinal distress occurs, these drugs can be taken with food, although that will alter the pharmacokinetics of the dose. Avoid coadministration with milk products that are rich sources of divalent ions, such as calcium and magnesium, that complex with some antibiotics and prevent their absorption. The intake of dairy products, however, needs to be monitored and encouraged with appropriate consideration of the specific antibiotics involved. Milk products are among the few rich sources of riboflavin, as well as an easily consumed and inexpensive protein source. This monitoring is needed especially when antibiotics are used long term by adolescents and young adults who are maximizing bone density. Advice to limit milk products when taking antibiotics may lead to elimination of milk products from the diet and greatly increase the long-term risk of osteoporosis. The patient requires encouragement to continue appropriate dietary intake of dairy products, but only at times that minimize interference with antibiotic regimens.

If significant gastric distress necessitates combining the drug with food, the intake of vitamins C and K and riboflavin needs to be monitored more closely. With some antibiotics such as cephalosporins, watch for hypokalemia and vitamin K deficiency when taken with food. Not all antibiotics are affected in amount or rate of absorption by food intake. Some tetracycline products (minocycline/Minocin® and doxycycline/Vibramycin®) are not affected by dairy product intakes. Among the penicillins, amoxicillin/Amoxil® and bacampicillin/Spectrobid® appear to be unaffected by food intake.

Take all antibiotics, as indeed most drugs, with sufficient fluid to reduce or minimize side effects. Fluid intake is especially important with urinary tract antibacterial drugs (nitrofurantoin/Macrodantin®). Absorption of these may be increased with milk or food. With some antibiotics, especially those taken long term (clindamycin, tetracyclines), inadequate fluid intake with oral capsules may lead to esophageal irritation.[52] Counsel adolescents and young women on acne regimens to take at least 8 oz (240 mL) of fluid with each capsule. With erythromycin, fluids other than acidic juices or carbonated beverages are advised. With sulfonamides (Bactrim®, Gantrisin®, Septra®, Thiosulfil®), advise a minimum fluid intake of 1500 mL/d. Remember that food is an important source of fluid in most American diets. If food intake is limited, monitoring and encouragement of fluid intake becomes even more crucial. Anorexia is common in stress states secondary to hormonal influences as well as a common side effect of the actual drugs.

Second- and third-generation cephalosporins (cefoperazone/Cefobid®, ceftriaxone/Rocephin®) have been implicated in several cases of hypoprothrombinemia. These cases appear to occur in patients with low vitamin K status.[53] Vitamin K supplementation of those on long-term total parenteral nutrition and with biliary obstruction is advised, especially when placed on antibiotics. The new vitamin formulation for intravenous use contains vitamin K, while the prior standard did not. A significant decline in prothrombin time is a late sign of vitamin K deficiency in long-term regimens. As methodology improves, the monitoring of milder forms of vitamin K deficiency may allow detection prior to a large decrease in vitamin K–dependent clotting.[53]

In infections and stress states, iron status may appear to be poor, especially in infants and in elderly patients with chronic diseases.[54–56] Prescribing iron supplements, however, may not be helpful and may indeed be counterproductive. Part of the body's immune response appears to be sequestration of iron. As infection abates, iron status appears to normalize without iron therapy. Provision of additional iron supplements may not be effective, especially in the elderly who are at risk of iron overload in the absence of blood loss.[42] Finally, bear in mind that most antibiotic regimens last a relatively short time (typically from single doses to 2 weeks). Even when antibiotic/nutrient interactions occur, the long-term effect is likely to be minimal. High levels of concern are appropriate mainly for patients who stand at obvious risk of inadequate nutrition. Regardless of the reason for prescription, iron supplementation should be monitored for effectiveness in the short and long term, especially in the elderly.

Antituberculars

For many years, antituberculars ranked among the leading producers of drug-induced malnutrition. As such, they were regularly monitored by dietitians until the number of tuberculosis cases fell. That decline also greatly diminished interest in this facet of counseling. Today, the rise in tuberculosis, especially among elderly persons in institutionalized and group housing, warrants renewed attention to the potential for negative influence on nutritional status. The increase of cases among patients suffering from HIV/AIDS and persons with substance abuse problems only increases the challenge of adequate surveillance.

INH is a B_6 antagonist, as well as a weak monoamine oxidase inhibitor (MAOI). Rifampin (Rifamate®) may induce a vitamin D deficiency, especially if given in tandem with isoniazid to elderly subjects with limited sunshine exposure. Monitor dairy products for enrichment with vitamin D, as well as calcium intake levels. For example, while made from milk, frozen yogurt is made from milk that has not been fortified with vitamin D.[56] Check label information before assuming that all dairy products are rich sources of vitamin D. Pyrimethamine (Daraprim® and Fansidar®) antagonizes folate and indirectly may lead to low vitamin B_{12} levels. If platelets or white blood cell count are low, folate supplementation may be required to normalize both vitamin levels.[58] Advise patients to take these drugs on an empty stomach, if tolerated.

Cycloserine is a bacteriostatic antitubercular agent used in combination with other drugs to treat resistant tuberculosis.[59] Effects of other drugs, such as antacids, or high-fat meals that decrease serum concentrations of antitubercular drugs can lead to incomplete eradication of the bacteria. Avoidance of high-fat meals with cycloserine is necessary, but orange juice and antacids are not problematic.[59]

Antiprotozoals

Folate supplementation may also be necessary during use of pentamidine (Pentam 300®).[58] Monitor this drug for hypoglycemia and hypocalcemia, as well as for folate deficiency.

Alcohol intake may be especially troublesome for patients taking this class of drugs, given the interference alcohol has on folate absorption as well as the need for folate in alcohol metabolism.

Anticonvulsants

The anticonvulsant drugs have long been recognized as posing a significant risk for drug-induced malnutrition, partly because of their long-term use and partly because of their use in children. Drug regimens tend to be more carefully monitored in children. These drugs require careful attention to protein intake because low protein intake may lead to toxicity secondary to delayed drug clearance. Bone density changes are a risk with phenobarbital, phenytoin (Dilantin®), and primidone (Mysoline®), especially in children, due to an increased turnover of vitamins D and K, and, consequently, decreased calcium absorption. Megaloblastic anemia may develop secondary to low serum folate, vitamin B_{12}, and vitamin B_6.[47] If megaloblastic anemia occurs, then folate supplementation may become necessary. Folate supplements may, however, act as drug antagonists. Counsel for adequate dietary intakes of folate, vitamins D and K, calcium, protein, fiber, and fluid before encouraging supplement usage.

With newer anticonvulsants in the carbamazepine group (Tegretol®, Carbatol®), serum iron and sodium need to be monitored. Advise users not to drink grapefruit juice within 1–2 h of taking these anticonvulsants. Children and the elderly are most likely to need vitamin D and folate supplementation.[58] Weight changes in the face of adequate kilocalories and protein need to be assessed because possible renal or hepatic changes in long-term, high-dose use may result in anemia and hyperammonemia in newer drugs such as valproate (Depacon®, Depakene®).[58]

Antineoplastics

As a single category, antineoplastics present the greatest challenge to maintenance of good nutritional status. A major reason is that almost all antineoplastics cause some degree of gastrointestinal distress. This is to be expected because antineoplastic drugs typically affect rapidly dividing cells. The healthy cells most likely to be stricken by drugs intended for malignant cells are the mucosal cells lining the mouth, genital tract, and the gastrointestinal tract. It is no surprise that cancer treatment directly leads to the anorexia, nausea, and vomiting that decrease food intake and produce weight loss and fatigue. Individualization of nutritional care plans cannot be overemphasized, including use of aggressive nutrition support in meal supplementation by favorite foods, high-calorie beverages, fortified puddings, enteral feedings, and parenteral feeding when indicated.

The first folate antagonist recognized was methotrexate (Mexate®), which may also lower absorption of vitamins (B_{12} and carotene), fat, lactose, and calcium.[7] Avoidance of milk products at the time of taking methotrexate is also advised. Mercaptopurine (Purinethol®) may serve as an antagonist of purines (bases for RNA and DNA) and pantothenic acid, an essential component of Coenzyme A. Procarbazine (Matulane®) is a weak MAOI and requires avoidance of high tyramine foods. See Chapter 14 for more discussion of MAOI drugs interactions with food.

Hypoglycemic Agents

Oral antidiabetic agents are designed to prevent or lower elevated blood glucose levels, some by stimulating the release of more insulin.[60] They also may act by increasing the effect of endogenous insulin within the cells.[61] Regular monitoring of these agents is needed to assure that serum levels do not fall to dangerously low levels. Three factors are most likely to lead to hypoglycemia: (1) inadequate food intake, (2) prolonged exercise without increased food intake, or (3) significant alcohol intake.

Alcohol intake in conjunction with these oral agents may cause gastrointestinal symptoms (e.g., nausea and vomiting), especially in early administration of chlorpropamide (Diabinese®) and in higher doses. Side effects may be mild or may diminish within 1–2 months. Limited alcohol intake is advised as well as avoidance of high intakes of nicotinic acid (niacin).

Treatment with the second generation of sulfonylureas (glimepiride/Amaryl®, glyburide, and glipizide/Glucotrol®) needs to be carefully monitored for hypoglycemia if the patient has hypoalbuminemia or other signs of debility. Avoidance of alcohol and high doses of niacin/nicotinic acid are essential. These agents are not adequate to maintain good glucose control in pregnancy.[58]

Among the biguanides (metformin hydrochloride/Glucophage®), additional monitoring of vitamin B_{12} status every 1–2 yr is recommended because malabsorption may occur.[58] This is especially important when these drugs are being used by elderly diabetic patients. Lactic acidosis may occur, therefore, the clinician needs to monitor for signs including diarrhea, severe muscle cramps, shallow and fast breathing, increased tiredness, and increased sleepiness.[58] Advise taking with food and avoiding alcohol. Although hypoglycemia is of little risk in monotherapy, a combination regimen with insulin may increase insulin effectiveness and reduce the amount of insulin required. Dietary counseling with these drugs, especially with therapy that combines them with insulin, is needed for sick days associated with diminished oral intake to prevent potential hypoglycemic effects. A list of carbohydrate replacements for sick days is given in Appendix C.6.

Dietary counseling to maintain an adequate and balanced food intake will improve maintenance of appropriate serum glucose levels. Watch for changes in appetite because either hyperphagia or anorexia may occur with several of these drugs. Serum monitoring of glucose, sodium, and glycosylated hemoglobin is good practice.

Cardiovascular Agents

These disease-grouped drugs are frequently used for the elderly and in persons of any age suffering from chronic disease. Drug usage may accordingly be long term. Therapy may be made more difficult to manage by use of polypharmacy among high-risk individuals. These drugs will be discussed in five subgroups: diuretics, anticoagulants, antihyperlipidemics, antihypertensives (including beta blockers, calcium channel blockers, and ACE inhibitors), and antiarrhymthmics. In general, four basic precautions are commonly appropriate with many of these drugs: (1) restriction of fluid, (2) restriction of electrolytes, (3) weight loss recommendations, and (4) avoidance of alcohol. All four promote better cardiac health while limiting influences that may make drug–nutrient or drug–drug interactions extremely hazardous.

Diuretics

Diuretics can produce vexing adverse effects even while playing a significant role in treating cardiovascular disease, especially congestive heart disease.[37] As a general rule, diuretics may cause some degree of glucose intolerance, especially when taken in high doses and in the face of poor dietary intake of potassium. The use of diuretics by the elderly has been considered the most common cause of mineral imbalances and a major factor in the development of thiamin deficiency.[7,16] Thiamin deficiency in patients with congestive heart failure can greatly exacerbate the clinical picture. Poor thiamin status produces a loss of appetite that, in turn, decreases food intake and may induce wet beriberi, which is a form of deficiency characterized by peripheral vasodilation. This outcome further overloads the strained cardiovascular system. A small study of congestive heart failure patients on loop diuretics found that approximately 20% had biochemical evidence of thiamin deficiency, but the majority of these appeared to have an adequate dietary intake of thiamin.[16] Given that clinical signs of thiamin deficiency may be difficult to distinguish from symptoms of congestive heart failure, thiamin supplementation with its low cost and low toxicity risk appears to be a prudent step in long-term loop diuretic regimens. The dry mouth and anorexia associated with diuretics may also play a role in reducing food intake.

Loop diuretics (furosemide/Lasix®, bumetanide/Bumex®) also increase the excretion of potassium, calcium, sodium, chloride, and magnesium. It is, therefore, appropriate to encourage patients receiving loop diuretics to maintain a reasonable dietary intake of potassium-rich foods. A number of common, inexpensive foods provide rich sources of potassium (e.g., potatoes, citrus fruits, and coffee). These offer options beyond the usual "banana-a-day" advice. See Appendix D for a more extensive list of potassium sources. If serum potassium levels are low, even in the presence of high dietary intake or potassium supplements, it is important to check serum magnesium levels. Another potential cause of hypokalemia is the consumption of natural licorice. Most licorice-flavored foods in the U.S. contain an artificial licorice flavoring, but imported candies and dietary supplements may well contain natural licorice.

Patients taking potassium-sparing diuretics (spironolactone/Aldactazide®, triamterene/hydrochlorothiazide/Dyazide®, Maxzide®) should be monitored for high intakes of dietary potassium or use of potassium supplements. Use of potassium-containing salt substitutes or any other sources of supplemental potassium must be avoided with potassium-sparing diuretics. Patients can easily reach toxic hyperkalemia by taking potassium supplements and potassium-sparing diuretics. These same drugs may also cause hyperglycemia.

Thiazide diuretics, such as chlorothiazide/Aldoclor®, Diuriland® hydrochlorothiazide/Aldoril®, and Hydrodiuril®, are potassium-wasting drugs. Others, such as triamterene-hydrodiuril/Dyazide® and spironolactone-hydrodiuril/Aldactazide®, combine thiazides with potassium-sparing diuretics with a view toward avoiding electrolyte disturbances. Minimal doses of thiazide diuretics may support good blood pressure control without causing either significant glucose or mineral metabolic changes.[58] Alterations are, however, sufficiently likely that monitoring glucose and electrolyte, especially potassium and magnesium, levels on higher doses is important with appropriate dietary counseling provided.

Antiarrhythmics

In general, antiarrhythmics are given to patients at high risk for life-threatening disturbances of the cardiac rhythm. The patients' poor cardiac statuses may be rooted in prior limitations of food intake and exercise during the progression of cardiovascular disease. In addition, these patients may have previously been subject to strict dietary restrictions of sodium and fluids. Good practice indicates a careful evaluation of prior dietary intake, dietary restrictions, weight changes, gastrointestinal difficulties, and exercise. Inactivity, especially if combined with low protein intake, may result in loss of lean muscle tissue.

Digoxin/Lanoxin®, although not a true antiarrhythmic, constitutes a common treatment for cardiac failure and offers protection against certain complications of rhythm disturbance. The drug may be taken with a small amount of food if gastric distress occurs, but high-fiber foods and fruit juices need to be withheld for 2 h after the daily dose because they may interfere with drug absorption. If body potassium levels fall, as may occur with fasting, prolonged poor food intake, or potassium-wasting diuretics, digoxin toxicity may occur. Indeed, hypokalemia is a well-established cofactor in digoxin toxicity. Consumption of more dietary potassium or use of potassium supplements may be needed. Other forms of antiarrhythmics (e.g., procainamide/Procan®, Pronestyl®) may cause less gastric upset than digoxin, but may still lower appetite. Others, such as quinidine/Cardioquin®, Duraquin®, may produce toxicity if taken with citrus juice or high-dose vitamin C supplements. The need for vitamin K may also be increased.

Nonselective beta-adrenergic blockers (propranolol/Inderal®, Inderide®) may cause these and other side effects. Elevation of triglycerides with lowering of high-density lipoprotein (HDL) levels may occur. In diabetic patients with cardiac rhythm disorders, special precautions are needed because beta blockers can mask symptoms of hypoglycemia.

Anticoagulants

This group of drugs is among the top 50 of the 200 most commonly prescribed medications, as listed in Appendix A.4. Owing to the frequency of its use and its critical interactions with vitamin K, warfarin/Coumadin® has top priority for nutrition monitoring and counseling by pharmacists, dietitians, and other nutrition professionals.

Historically, patients taking warfarin were advised to avoid foods with vitamin K because that nutrient directly antagonized the anticoagulant effect. A provisional table for vitamin K content of foods was not available until the early 1990s, making careful assessment of dietary vitamin K intake difficult at best. Although analysis of phylloquinone can be done in the laboratory, technology has not advanced to the point of making this easy or feasible to do as part of clinical assessment. The prothrombin time (PTT), a measure of clotting time, is used clinically to judge changes in vitamin K status. The measure is now reported as international normalized ratio (INR), a score that allows for normalizing clotting time values against a known standard. Use of this process has made warfarin therapy both more effective and safer. Changes detected by INR, however, occur late in the depletion of vitamin K stores. For this reason, advice to avoid all foods containing vitamin K is not appropriate.

Whereas excess vitamin K may undo drug efficacy, too low a vitamin K dietary intake may lead to submarginal deficiency state. The best practice is to identify an approximate intake of vitamin K and work proactively with the patient to maintain that intake. Warfarin is dosed to clinical effect, with dosage varying considerably among the patient population. The individual's warfarin dose is, therefore, titrated in the face of that person's customary diet. Weight loss and taking a vacation are events that place patients at risk for overanticoagulation, although habitual alcohol consumption, even high habitual intake, was not.[5] The hazard from significant increases or decreases in vitamin K intake (lowered vs. increased drug effect) occur in the face of departures from normal dietary or lifestyle practices. Once an effective drug dosage is established at a patient's usual diet, monitoring for changes in the INR or in the diet needs to be done on a regular basis. Early in therapy, patients customarily have the INR checked at least monthly. Some clinicians will move to a longer interval, such as every 3 or 6 months, after the patient exhibits a stable INR.

Dietary intake of vitamin K is most likely to increase when locally grown green leafy vegetables become available. Another less recognized problem may be the consumption of warfarin antagonists in the diet. Avocado and other foods eaten in large quantities have been suggested as antagonistic to warfarin secondary to high fat content.[62] Megadoses of the fat-soluble vitamins A and E antagonize vitamin K in animals.[63] In humans, a case of bleeding was reported by Corrigan and Marcus in a middle-aged man taking both warfarin and megadoses of vitamin E.[64] Cessation of the vitamin E supplement resulted in correction of the bleeding and normalization of the PTT. It would appear prudent to advise against megadoses of fat-soluble vitamins during warfarin regimens.[64]

A recent presurgery survey found that 38% of 24 patients on warfarin were also taking vitamin E supplements.[65] Over 40% of the patients using an anticoagulant were concomitantly taking dietary supplements that contain naturally occurring couramins or that inhibit platelet aggregation. These supplements included garlic, ginkgo, ginseng, herbal teas, and fish oils.[65]

Antihypertensives

As a general rule, patients placed on antihypertensive drugs will benefit from concurrent moderate sodium-restricted diets.[38] A notable exception is the caution to avoid beginning a sodium-restricted diet when a patient is initially placed on captopril/Capoten®. Starting both antihypertensive therapies together may result in a precipitous drop in blood pressure. This proves particularly confounding because symptomatic hypotension (particularly orthostatic hypotension) frequently occurs during the induction period of antihypertensive therapy. Food intake may initially be reduced because of short-term loss of taste that should resolve in a few months. Another exception is the blunting of the efficacy of calcium channel blockers by sodium-restricted diets.[38]

Although high sodium intakes may not have caused hypertension, implementation of a modest or lower sodium intake may reduce the drug dosage needed to normalize blood pressure. In addition, weight loss of even 10 pounds may prove beneficial in obese hypertensives in reducing blood pressure.[66] Another general rule is that lower dose levels produce fewer, milder side effects and lower costs.

Sulfonamide-based diuretics (e.g., medapamide/Lozol®) may cause potassium depletion and require monitoring of electrolytes, especially magnesium, and of glucose. Glucose intolerance may develop and weight loss may occur.[37] Other antihypertensives, such as clonidine/Catapres®, may induce hyperglycemia.

Hydralazine products, such as Apresazide® and Apresoline®, are vitamin B_6 antagonists and may require supplemental B vitamins, especially if the diet history suggests a marginal intake of B vitamins. A poor dietary intake of one B vitamin, such as B_6, is seldom found in isolation. Particularly in the presence of polypharmacy, a modest level of multiple B vitamin supplementation may be prudent. Gastric distress may occur and food intake may be advisable when taking these drugs.

Antihypertensives containing methyldopa (e.g., Aldomet® and Aldoril®) are greatly influenced by high protein intake. The recommendation has been made to take these with a high-carbohydrate meal at least 3 h before or after a high-protein meal. This is not as critical if the patient is also being given a combination of levadopa and carbidopa.[67]

Newer drugs used as antihypertensives include cardioselective beta blockers, calcium channel blockers, and angiotensin-converting enzyme (ACE) inhibitors. If individuals have been on diuretics or have a restricted sodium intake, monitoring blood chemistries is important when any of these drugs is introduced into the regimen.[38] Selective beta blockers (e.g., metoprolol/Lopressor®, Toprol®) need to be used with caution among diabetic patients. Calcium channel blockers (such as amlodipine/Norvasc®, nicardipine/Cardene®, nifedipine/Adalat®, Procardia®, dilt-iazem/Cardizem®, Dilacor®, Tiamate®, and felodipine/Plendil®) may be used as antihypertensive or antianginal drug therapy. In either case, caution should be used if the patient's diet includes grapefruit juice, licorice, or is considered low in sodium.[38,68,69] These drugs should not be taken within 3 h of consuming grapefruit juice.[70] The first recognized grapefruit juice–drug interaction was reported with felodipine.[71] Since then, many reports of other drugs interacting with grapefruit have been published, but the majority of these have not identified clinically significant interactions. See Appendix C.3 for drug–grapefruit juice interactions and their clinical significance. Although it is prudent not to use grapefruit juice as a medication beverage, elimination of grapefruit juice from commercial or home menus does not appear warranted based on the literature, except for a limited number of drugs.[68] Some drugs associated with serious adverse events from grapefruit juice interactions have been withdrawn from the American market, particularly terfenadine/Seldane® and cisapride/Propulsid®.[71] Natural licorice and dietary supplements containing natural licorice (glycyrrhizin) should be avoided with the ACE inhibitors.[70,71]

ACE inhibitors include altace/Ramipril®, fosinopril/Monopril®, benazepril/Lotensin®, and quinapril/Accupril®. The use of potassium supplements (including salt substitutes containing potassium) needs to be avoided. Monitor potassium status carefully during ACE inhibitor therapy. Once again, it is important also to avoid intake of natural licorice.[70] Natural licorice is not currently allowed in American foods, but natural licorice is found in a number of herbal supplements, as discussed in Chapter 13. A high-fat meal (50 g) may lower drug absorption by 25–30%, with a significant effect on blood pressure control.[70] Many restaurant meals easily contain 50 g of fat. An 8 oz steak dinner with either French fries or baked potato loaded with butter or sour cream will easily reach this level, especially if combined with a buttered roll and dessert. Patients require careful teaching, so that they will not unknowingly select menu items directly antagonistic to important drug treatment.

Antihyperlipidemics

Drugs that bind bile salts within the intestinal lumen have long constituted the mainstay for treatment of hyperlipidemia. They work by reducing reabsorption of bile salts into the circulation. The drugs typically will induce at least a mild diarrhea or loose stools, especially when used long term or in higher doses. The bound bile salts then pass out in the feces, lowering the pool of bile acids available for uptake by the blood. Examples of this type of drug include cholestyramine/Questran® and colestipol/Colestid®.[71]

Interference with enterohepatic circulation of bile acids is also likely to impair absorption of fat-soluble vitamins A, D, E, and K. Dietary counseling is advisable to guide restrictions of total fat, saturated fat, and cholesterol, as well as to encourage adequate fluid and fiber intake. Vitamin supplementation of the fat-soluble vitamins in water-miscible form may be needed in long-term use. Recommend that supplement administration occur 1 h before or 4 h after any dose of bile acid sequestrants in order to minimize interference with nutrient absorption. Monitoring of calcium, electrolytes, and iron status needs to be done periodically.[38] Fibric acid derivatives, such as clofibrate/Atromid-S® and gemfibrozil/Lopid®, are thought to act by increasing the activity of lipoprotein lipase and may also lead to loose stools and gastric distress.

The HMG-CoA reductase inhibitors, also commonly called "statins" for convenience, make up another class of antilipidemic agents. Gastric symptoms are likely to be milder with these drugs than with bile acid sequestrants. The statins, however, may lower some gastrointestinal enzymes. Examples of these include lovastatin/Mevacor®, fluvastatin/Lescol®, pravastatin/Pravachol®, and simvastatin/Zocor®. High-fiber diets may lower the efficacy of these drugs.[71] Until recently, none of these drugs were recommended in combination with high doses of niacin. Currently, none should be taken concurrently with grapefruit juice. See Appendix C.3 for specific recommendations pertaining to drugs and CYP3A4 enzyme inhibition.

Niacin or Nicotinic Acid

Before bile acid sequestrants, niacin offered the sole pharmacologic approach to reducing serum lipids. The drug proved troublesome to most patients for two reasons. First, the effective dose is quite high and may only be reached by initiating therapy at a lower dose and working up. Second, niacin in pharmacologic doses often causes severe itching, as well as severe episodes of hypotension. Its use is challenging, and it is clearly now a second-line agent. Nevertheless, this inexpensive B vitamin in high doses is sometimes effective as a drug to lower serum lipids, particularly when dosed along with bile acid sequestrants. Recently, a combination product, lovastatin/niacin (Advicor®), was introduced, which contains immediate release lovastatin and extended release niacin. In general, niacin/Nicolar® should not be combined, however, with the statins. In large drug doses, niacin-induced hyperglycemia may occur. Thus, use of niacin may be difficult and is often not desirable for use with diabetic patients.

DIGESTIVE DISEASES

Drugs used in the treatment of digestive diseases are discussed in detail in Chapter 7. In these disease states, some general monitoring of severity of symptoms is important from a nutritional viewpoint. Diarrhea, if severe or prolonged, can have negative effects on several nutrients, especially water-soluble vitamins and minerals involved in fluid equilibrium. Occult blood loss, whatever the origin, increases the need for nutrients involved in hemopoiesis (e.g., iron, folate, vitamin B_{12}). Steatorrhea, whatever the cause, places fat-soluble vitamin status at risk and may produce anorexia and weight loss.

Antacids, especially if used frequently and for extended periods of time, can raise the stomach pH to a level that lowers the ability to digest and absorb nutrients, most notably vitamin B_{12} and nonheme iron. The histamine-H_2 receptor inhibitors, (e.g., cimetidine/Tagamet®) are particularly effective in reducing acid secretion. Proton pump inhibitors (e.g., omeprazole/Prilosec®), a newer type of medication that directly stops acid secretion, are even more effective in raising the pH of the stomach. Proton pump inhibitors suppress daytime gastric acidity more when taken before breakfast.[32] Thus, long-term usage warrants monitoring of B_{12} status.

RESPIRATORY AGENTS

Drugs used to treat pulmonary and respiratory tract disorders are not usually considered to any great extent in a discussion of drug–nutrient interactions. These patients, however, frequently present at great nutritional risk, sometimes at the point of gauntness in late stages of chronic obstructive pulmonary disease (COPD). Chronic difficulty in breathing almost always leads to reduced food intake and eventually to marginal nutritional status. Swallowing food may result in decreased air entry to the lungs because it does require holding one's breath. Patients may feel as though they need to choose between eating or breathing, and breathing takes precedence. Poor protein status related to dietary insufficiency (usually assessed by a serum albumin below 3.5 g/dL) may alter drug metabolism.[9] On the other hand, severe obesity that produces the Pickwickian syndrome or other forms of apnea may also lead to potentially lethal respiratory difficulties as well. Drugs used to treat respiratory illnesses may well induce a number of problems for which nutritional supplementation may be beneficial.[72] Patients who receive anticoagulants for deep-vein thrombosis and pulmonary embolic disease require monitoring of vitamin K status.

Bronchodilators

Some bronchodilators used to relax bronchial and pulmonary blood vessels also act to increase gastric acid secretion and to decrease the lower esophageal sphincter (LES) pressure. Both effects can lead directly to gastric disturbances. Xanthine derivatives (e.g., theophylline/Elixophyllin® and diyphylline/Difor®, Lufyllin®) may cause gastric discomfort, including gastroesophageal reflux. Overdosage may lead to nausea and vomiting. Food may induce a sudden release (dose dumping) of sustained-release one-a-day preparations. The sudden increase in drug absorption can result in toxicity. Caffeine, a chemical cousin to theophylline, may further enhance the pharmacologic effects of theophylline and other drugs that are substrates of P_{450} CYP1A2.[9,73] In a recent review, Durrant identified over 80 prescription drugs with caffeine and over 80 nonprescription drugs, mainly analgesics and stimulants, with added caffeine.[73] Although not required to list caffeine as an ingredient on the label, many herbal/dietary supplements contain caffeine, especially South American *mate* beverage products.

Monitoring caffeine intake and advice to limit coffee or other caffeine-containing foods to less than six servings a day may be prudent.[72] Vitamin B_6 supplementation has been suggested to reduce the CNS effects of theophylline.[74] See Appendix D.1 and Appendix D.2 for tables with content of methylxanthines in foods and drugs.

Corticosteroids

Corticosteroids in both systemic and inhalant therapy can create nutritional challenges. Systemic corticosteroids (e.g., prednisolone/Predalone®, Predcor®) commonly used in respiratory diseases have similar adverse effects when used as immunosuppressant or chemotherapeutic agents. These effects include glucose intolerance, sodium retention, nitrogen loss secondary to gluconeogenesis, hyperphagia, and weight gain.[72] These, in turn, increase the workload on respiratory muscles. When used long term for childhood asthma, cushingoid features and growth suppression may occur. Inhaled corticosteroids (e.g., triamcinolone/Azmacort®) that are not administered properly may lead to oropharyngeal fungal overgrowth and pain, leading to less food intake.

IMMUNOSUPPRESSANTS

Glucocorticoids may be ordered for systemic, ophthalmic, or inhalant administration as therapy for a variety of disorders in which immunosuppression or antiinflammatory effects are needed.[71] Immunosuppressive agents reduce the rate of protein synthesis and depress the migration of cells involved in inflammation. As in the acute stress response, anorexia, hyperglycemia, and sodium and water retention may occur. Sodium retention can induce potassium wasting and ascorbic acid excretion. Dietary advice should encourage a modest reduction in sodium intake (e.g., eliminate use of a salt shaker and highly salted processed foods) and to increase consumption of foods rich in potassium and vitamin C (e.g., citrus fruits, tomatoes, potatoes). See Appendix D for additional foods rich in minerals. In long-term use, these drugs can lead to growth retardation, muscle wasting, decreased bone density, hypercholesterolemia, and development of cushingoid symptoms. Cushingoid symptoms include moon face, truncal fat deposits, glucose intolerance, weight gain, and appetite increase.

The development of cyclosporine/Neoral®, Sandimmune® led to a great improvement in the success of organ transplants and relief from many side effects of the glucocorticoids.[38] Certain dietary cautions need to be observed. Potassium supplements, including salt substitutes containing potassium, should be avoided. Sodium depletion may increase the risk of toxicity.[38] Grapefruit juice may increase the serum concentration to toxic levels.[69] Coadministration of grapefruit juice is inappropriate and hazardous as a possible means to lower doses. Any advice to intentionally create this interaction for intended therapeutic effect is entirely premature, based on current data.[9,14,15]

Another class of immunosuppressant is azathioprine/Imuran®.[3] The drug works by suppressing purine synthesis. It is used widely in bone marrow transplantation, renal transplantation, or refractory rheumatoid arthritis. If macrocytic anemia occurs, supplementation with folate is likely needed secondary to folate antagonism and inadequate dietary folate intake. Esophagitis, stomatitis, and gastric upset may lead to reduced food intake. If pancreatitis occurs, steatorrhea and muscle wasting may result. Special counseling may be needed to maintain adequate food intake.

A fourth type of immunosuppressant is mycophenolate/CellCept®, a potent inhibitor of guanosine nucleotide synthesis.[71] This drug may be used concurrently with cyclosporine to lower costs and toxicology risks. Although it is less likely to severely depress bone marrow functions, anemia is still a possible side effect. Hypertension, fever, and diarrhea are common and may require appropriate medical nutrition therapy.

Sirolimus/Rapamycin® is a recently approved immunosuppressant for kidney transplant patients.[75] A high-fat meal causes a small increase in whole blood concentration.[75] Thus, it is advisable for individuals to consistently take this medication with or without meals.

Tacrolimus (Prograf®), another immunosuppressant used for organ transplant recipients, has multiple food interactions, including decreased rate and extent of absorption when taken with food.[72] High-fat meals have the most pronounced effect, resulting in a 35% decrease in overall bioavailability and a 77% decrease in maximal concentration. Grapefruit juice, a CYP3A3/4 inhibitor, may increase the serum level and risk for toxicity of tacrolimus as noted in Appendix C.3. St. John's Wort, a common herbal supplement, may reduce tacrolimus serum concentrations; therefore, avoid concurrent use.

PSYCHOTROPIC AGENTS

This classification of drugs includes a wide variety of medications with several chemical classes and different mechanisms. Weight gain has been a clinically reported side effect in almost every class and is likely multifactorial in origin. Appetite stimulation, restricted physical activity, organized group activities with food, increased sleep patterns, and regain of previously lost weight are just a few possible contributing factors related to psychiatric hospitalization. Nutritional professionals need to monitor weight and offer assistance in preventing excessive weight gain. Smoking is extremely prevalent among mental health patients, bringing increased requirements for certain nutrients (e.g., vitamin C) and lower intakes of other nutrients (e.g., folate and vitamin B_{12}).[47,73]

In general, patients requiring pyschotropic medications should be carefully assessed for nutritional status upon admission to a clinic or hospital. Depression or mania may mean that poor food intake has led to anorexia and marginal B-vitamin status (e.g., folate depletion). Apathy and lethargy may have led to poor food choices, even if energy intake has been maintained. Snacking may have replaced meals for an extended period of time. Increased intake of alcohol and increased smoking may also be factors in impaired dietary status. Diet history, biochemical assessment, and physical examination, including anthropometric measures and clinical signs of malnutrition, are needed to fully assess nutritional status.[10–13]

Some antianxiety drugs (e.g., alprazolam/Xanax®) depress the CNS and are usually used for only a short time (less than 3 months). The short usage, therefore, may not affect nutritional status. Patients, however, need to be counseled to limit intake of methylxanthines/caffeine, theobromine, and theophylline-containing foods to avoid counteracting the medications.[76–78] Other antianxiety drugs (e.g., chlordiazepoxide/Librium® and diazepam/Valium®, which are both benzodiazepines) may be taken long term and require monitoring of weight as either gain or loss may occur. In general, appetite and thirst may be increased. If a patient presents with hypoalbuminemia, drug effects may be increased. Grapefruit presents clinically significant interactions with buspirone/BuSpar®.

Phenothiazines comprise a large group of drugs including chlorpromazine/Thorazine®, Prochlorperazine/Compazine®, thioridazine/Mellaril®, and fluphenazine/Prolixin®. Individuals taking these drugs need to be monitored for appetite and weight changes.[46] Glucose homeostasis may be altered, leading to weight changes.[46,77] Because these drugs are similar in chemical structure to riboflavin, an adequate intake of riboflavin either in dairy products or in supplements is important. Salivary changes signal the need for dental monitoring.

Tricyclics constitute another group of antidepressants that have been widely used. Some (e.g., amitriptyline/Elavil® and imipramine/Tofranil®) also closely resemble the structure of riboflavin and require either an adequate intake of dairy products or use of a riboflavin supplement in lactose intolerant individuals.[46,77] Although it has been suggested that herbals such as St. John's Wort should be avoided when taking tricyclic antidepressants, the Commission E monographs lists no other drug interactions.[77] As with other antidepressants, alcohol should be avoided.[77] Appetite may be increased, especially for sweets if taste acuity drops. One should monitor sodium, potassium, and uric acid status in patients taking clomipramine/Anafranil®. Individuals taking some tricyclics (e.g., clomipramine/Anafranil®) should avoid grapefruit juice.

MAOIs are drugs used to treat depression mixed with anxiety and are implicated in one of the earliest recognized and serious food–drug interactions. Counseling on these drugs is discussed in detail in Chapter 14. Tables to update previous reviews by McCabe[76] of tyramine and histamine content of foods are in Appendix D.1 and Appendix D.2.

Newer, but among the most widely used of all prescription drugs, are the selective serotonin reuptake inhibitors (SSRIs). Prozac®, a brand name for fluoxetine, is part of every American's vocabulary, and doctors may be asked to prescribe it as a means of weight loss. Glycemic control may be altered. Although short-term anorexia and weight loss are common, prolonged use may result in weight gain. Riboflavin supplements should not be taken with Prozac®. As with other psychotropic agents, alcohol should be avoided. Other SSRIs (e.g., sertraline/Zoloft®) may also decrease appetite, while citalopram/Celexa® may cause increased appetite, weight gain, or weight loss.[71] Caffeine intake and smoking may also alter the metabolism of these drugs. In general, SSRIs should not be taken concurrently with MAOIs, and a 2-week interval after stopping MAOIs before starting a SSRI regimen is prudent.

Other antipsychotic agents such as the butyrophenones (e.g., haloperidol/Haldol®, resperidone/Resperdal®, and thiothixene/Navane®) may increase the appetite and cause weight gain. Thiothixene/Navane® also increases the need for riboflavin.[77] Hypoalbuminemia may increase the drug effects of Clozapine (Clozaril®), a potent dibenzodiazepine antipsychotic agent.

Drugs used specially to treat mania or bipolar depression (e.g., lithium/Eskalith®, Lithane®) alter sodium transport in nerve and muscle. Large shifts in dietary sodium can significantly modify the drug's absorption and may result in a toxic serum level. [1,2,5,77] Dehydration is a risk for toxicity. Consistent intake of sodium in foods allows for effective and safe use of the drug.[77] Encourage a fluid intake of at least 2–3 L a day. Monitor for signs of vomiting and diarrhea that may reflect a toxic serum level. Appetite stimulation may be another side effect.[77]

FOOD AND SUPPLEMENT PRECAUTIONS

In reviewing these various drug categories, certain foods and beverages appear frequently: alcohol, grapefruit juice, citrus juice, and licorice. These items share one commonality. Each is processed by the same family of hepatic enzymes: the P_{450} cytochrome series. These potential interactions should not lead to total elimination of indicated foodstuffs from menus, partly because not everyone has the same risk of experiencing adverse events and because risk is related to genotype. A large number of drugs are metabolized by these enzymes, but actual clinical events are rare. For simplicity, if a food is not highly popular it may be prudent for acute care health institutions to eliminate foods such as grapefruit juice and fava beans from their limited menus. Thus, the potential for a negative event to occur even in a small fraction of patients admitted is avoided.

For clinical reactions to occur, several conditions may need to exist: coadministration of the drug and the food/beverage; presence of large amounts of one or the other; and use in a person whose phenotype creates a risk.[14,15] When chronic and heavy use of alcohol is involved, the risks increase considerably.[41,78,79] Chronic abusers of alcohol have altered their enzymatic systems, often making drug metabolism and nutrient requirements quite different from the patterns found in persons not addicted to alcohol.[79]

Certain vitamin supplements may actually become hazardous, most notably vitamin A supplements in alcoholic liver disease or potential candidates for the disease.[78,80]

Certainly upper limits of nutrients must be carefully considered in giving nutrients as treatment.[73,80] Recommendations as to the use of grapefruit, citrus fruits, and other indole-containing foods need to be considered on an individual drug basis.[14]

In general, medications are best not taken concurrently with acidic beverages, caffeine-containing beverages, or alcohol. Unless specifically prescribed, vitamin

Table 6.5   Chronic Drug Therapy and Nutrient Supplementation
in the Elderly

Drug	Supplement(s)
Antacids	Folic acid, B_{12} (if needed)
Aspirin	Folic acid, iron, vitamin C
Chloretetracycline	Calcium, vitamin C, riboflavin
Cholestyramine resin	Vitamins A, D, E, K, folic acid, calcium
Colestipol	Vitamins A, D, E, K, folic acid, calcium
Estrogens/progestin	Vitamin B_6, folic acid
Hydralazine hydrochloride	Vitamin B_6
Phenothiazines	Riboflavin
Phenytoin	Folic acid, vitamin D, vitamin K, calcium
Primidone	Vitamin D
Rifampin	Vitamin B_6, niacin, vitamin D
Sulfasalzine	Folic acid
Tetracycline	Calcium, riboflavin, vitamin D
Triamterene	Folic acid

Source: From Blumberg, J. and Couris, R., in *Geriatric Nutrition: The Health Professional's Handbook,* 2nd ed., Chernoff, R., Ed., Aspen Publishers, Gaithersburg, MD, 1999, 359. With permission.

and mineral supplements need to be used carefully below the upper limits and ideally near the estimated average requirement (EAR) level. If an EAR is not available, the adequate intake (AI) is generally considered the next best guideline.[47,48,73,80]

Certain chronic drug regimens are more likely to require consideration of supplements, either in the form of fortified foods or medications. Blumberg and Couris have compiled a summary list of drugs for which nutrient supplementation in older adults might be considered.[81] This list, presented in Table 6.5, can serve as a starting checklist for chronic drug therapy in general.

In the future, more functional foods are likely to appear that may need to be encouraged or discouraged in certain drug regimens. Testing of all possible reactions is not feasible if new drugs or new foods are to be made available to improve health and treat diseases. Diet histories may well need to include specific questions about the use of functional foods or highly fortified foods as well as dietary supplements. Clinicians from all disciplines must step forth and take responsibility for monitoring their patients for drug–nutrient interactions.

REFERENCES

1. Trovato, A., Nuhlicek., D.N., and Midtling, J.E., Drug–nutrient interactions, *Am. Fam. Physician,* 44, 1651–1658, 1992.
2. Knapp, H.R., Nutrient–drug interactions, in *Present Knowledge in Nutrition,* 7th ed., Ziegler, E.E. and Filer, L.J., Jr., Eds., ILSI Press, Washington, D.C., 1996, chap. 54.
3. Jeffery, D.R., Nutrition and diseases of the nervous system, in *Modern Nutrition in Health and Disease*, 9th ed., Shils, M.E. et al., Eds., Williams & Wilkins, Baltimore, 1999, 1545.
4. Thomas, J.A., Drug–nutrient interactions, *Nutr. Rev.,* 3, 271–282, 1995.

5. Penning-van Beest, F.J.A. et al., Lifestyle and diet as risk factors for overanticoagulation, *J. Clin. Epidemiol.,* 55, 411–417, 2002.

6. Force, R.W. and Nahata, C., Effect of histamine H2-receptor antagonists on vitamin B$_{12}$ absorption, *Ann. Pharm.,* 26, 1283–1286, 1992.

7. Roe, D.A., *Drug-Induced Malnutrition,* AVI Publishing, Westport, CT, 1985.

8. Murray, J.J. and Healy, M.D., Drug–mineral interactions: a new responsibility for the hospital dietitian, *J. Am. Diet. Assoc.,* 91, 66–70, 1991.

9. Williams, L., Davis, J.A., and Lowenthal, D.T., The influence of food on the absorption and metabolism of drugs, *Med. Clin. N. Am.,* 77, 815–829, 1993.

10. Silkroski, M., Collaborative care to improve nutrition outcomes, *Consultant Pharmacist,* 17, 567–578, 2002.

11. Roe, D.A., *Drug-Induced Malnutrition,* AVI Publishing, Westport, CT, 1985, pp. 125–127.

12. Leklem, J.E., Vitamin B$_6$, in *Present Knowledge in Nutrition,* 7th ed., Ziegler, E.E. and Filer, L.J., Jr., ILSI Press, Washington, D.C., 1996, 174–183.

13. Jeffery, D.R., Nutrition and diseases of the nervous system, in *Modern Nutrition in Health and Disease,* 9th ed., Shils, M.E. et al., Eds., Williams & Wilkins, Baltimore, 1999, 1552–1553.

14. Fleisher, D. et al., Drug, meal and formulation: interactions influencing drug absorption after oral administration: clinical implications, *Clin. Pharmacokinet.,* 36, 233–254, 1999.

15. Quinn, D.I. and Day, R.O., Drug interactions of clinical importance: an updated guide, *Drug Safety,* 12, 393–452, 1995.

16. Brady, J.A., Rock, C.L., and Horneffer, M.R., Thiamin status, diuretic medications, and the management of congestive heart failure, *J. Am. Diet. Assoc.,* 95, 541–544, 1995.

17. Herbert, V., Vitamin B$_{12}$, in *Present Knowledge in Nutrition,* 7th Ed., Ziegler, E.E. and Filer, L.J., Jr., Eds., ILSI Press, Washington, D.C., 1996, pp. 191–205.

18. Weir, D.G. and Scott, J.M., Vitamin B$_{12}$ and cobalamin, in *Modern Nutrition in Health and Disease,* 9th Ed., Shils, M.E. et al., Eds., Williams & Wilkins, Baltimore, 1999, pp. 447–458.

19. Herbert, V., Folic acid, in *Modern Nutrition in Health and Disease,* 9th Ed., Shils, M.E. et al., Eds., Williams & Wilkins, Baltimore, 1999, pp. 433–446.

20. Benton, D., Fordy, J., and Haller, J., The impact of long-term vitamin supplementation on cognitive functioning, *Psychopharmacology,* 117, 298–305, 1995.

21. Carney, M.W. et al., Red cell folate concentrations in psychiatric patients, *J. Affect. Disord.,* 19, 207–213, 1990.

22. Bottiglieri, T., Folate, vitamin B$_{12}$, and neuropsychiatric disorders, *Nutr. Rev.,* 54, 382–390, 1996.

23. Hoffer, L.J., Metabolic consequences of starvation, in *Modern Nutrition in Health and Disease,* 9th ed., Shils, M.E. et al., Eds., Williams & Wilkins, Baltimore, 1999, pp. 645–665.

24. Levine, M. et al., Criteria and recommendations for vitamin C intake, *J. Am. Med. Assoc.,* 281, 1415–1423, 1999.

25. Gore, M.J., Common pain relievers may pose hidden dangers, *Dig. Health Nutr.,* 11, 14, 1999.

26. Blumberg, J. and Couris, R., Pharmacology, nutrition, and the elderly: interactions and implications, in *Geriatrics Nutrition: Handbook for Health Professionals,* 2nd ed., Chernoff, R., Ed., Aspen Publishers, Gaithersburg, MD, 1999, p. 359.

27. Roe, D.A., *Drug-Induced Malnutrition,* AVI Publishers, Westport, CT, 1985, pp. 129–131.

28. Tyler, V.E., *Herbs of Choice: The Therapeutic Use of Phytomedicinals,* Pharmaceutical Products Press, an imprint of Haworth Press, Binghamton, NY, 1994.

29. Miller, C.A., Drug, food, food supplements interactions, *Geriatric Nursing,* 20, 164–168, 1999.

30. Smeeding, S.J.W., Nutrition, supplements, and aging, *Geriatric Nursing,* 22, 219–224, 2001.

31. Medhus, A.W. et al., Low dose intravenous erythromycin: effects on postprandial and fasting motility of the small bowel, *Aliment. Pharmacol. Ther.,* 14, 233–240, 2000.

32. Hatlebakk, J.G. et al., Proton pump inhibitors: better acid suppression when taken before a meal than without a meal, *Aliment. Pharmacol. Ther.,* 12, 1267–1272, 2000.

33. Lowe, N.K. and Ryan-Wenger, N.M., Over-the-counter medications and self-care, *Nurse Pract.,* 24, 34–44, 1999.

34. Gibson, R.S., *Principles of Nutritional Assessment,* Oxford University Press, New York, 1990, p. 37.

35. Ramchandani, V.A., Kwo, P.Y., and Li, T.-K., Effect of food and food composition on alcohol elimination rates in healthy men and women, *J. Clin. Pharmacol.,* 41, 1345–1350, 2001.

36. Ginsberg, E.S. et al., Estrogens in postmenopausal women, *J. Am. Med. Assoc.,* 276, 1747–1751, 1996.

37. Pandit, M.K. et al., Drug-induced disorders of glucose tolerance, *Ann. Intern. Med.,* 118, 529–539, 1993.

38. Bennett, W.M., Drug interactions and consequences of sodium restriction, *Am. J. Clin. Nutr.,* 65, 678S–681S, 1997.

39. Roe, D.A., *Alcohol and the Diet,* AVI Publishing, Westport, CT, 1979.

40. Carmel, R. et al., Vitamin B_{12} uptake by human small bowel homogenate and its enhancement by intrinsic factor, *Gastroenterology,* 56, 548–555, 1969.

41. Halstead, C.H., Alcohol: medical and nutritional effects, in *Present Knowledge in Nutrition,* 7th ed., Ziegler, E.E. and Filer, L.J., Jr., ILSI Press, Washington, D.C., pp. 547–556, 1996.

42. Mansouri, A. and Lipschitz, D.A., Anemia in the elderly patient, *Med. Clin. N. Am.,* 76, 619–630, 1992.

43. Sears, D.A., Anemia of chronic disease, *Med. Clin. N. Am.,* 76, 567–579, 1992.

44. Schaumburg, H. et al., Sensory neuropathy from pyridoxine abuse: a new megavitamin syndrome, *New Engl. J. Med.,* 309, 445–448, 1983.

45. Jacob, R.A. and Swenseid, M.E., Niacin, in *Present Knowledge in Nutrition,* 7th Ed., Ziegler, E.E. and Filer, L.J., Jr., Eds., ILSI Press, Washington, D.C., 1996, 184–190.

46. Rivlin, R.S., Riboflavin, in *Present Knowledge in Nutrition,* 7th ed., Ziegler, E.E. and Filer, L.J., Jr., ILSI Press, Washington, D.C., 1996, pp. 167–173.

47. Food and Nutrition Board, Institute of Medicine, Dietary reference intakes for thiamin, riboflavin, niacin, vitamin B_6, folate, vitamin B_{12}, pantothenic acid, biotin, and choline, National Academy Press, Washington, D.C., 1998.

48. Food and Nutrition Board, Institute of Medicine, Dietary reference intakes for calcium, phosphorus, magnesium, vitamin D, and fluoride, National Academy Press, Washington, D.C., 1997, p 38.

49. Kopple, J.D., Renal disorders and nutrients, in *Modern Nutrition in Health and Disease,* 9th ed., Shils, M.E. et al., Eds., Williams & Wilkins, Baltimore, 1999, p. 1479.

50. Food and Nutrition Board, Institute of Medicine, Dietary reference intakes for vitamin C, vitamin E, selenium, and cartenoids, National Academy Press, Washington, D.C., 2000.

51. Campbell, W.W. et al., Increased protein requirements in the elderly: new data and retrospective reassessments, *Am. J. Clin. Nutr.,* 60, 501–509, 1994.
52. Smilack, J.D., The tetracyclines, *Mayo Clin. Proc.,* 74, 727–72, 1999.
53. Suttie, J.W., Vitamin K, in *Present Knowledge in Nutrition,* 7th ed., Ziegler, E.E. and Filer, L.J., Jr., Eds., ILSI Press, Washington, D.C., 1996, chap. 14.
54. Yip, R., Iron status defined, in *Dietary Iron: Birth to Two Years,* Filer, L.J., Jr., Ed., New York, Raven Press, 1989, pp. 19–36.
55. Yip, R., and Dallman, P.R., Iron, in *Present Knowledge in Nutrition,* Ziegler, E.E. and Filer, L.J., Jr., Eds., ILSI Press, Washington, D.C., 1996, chap. 28.
56. Chanarin, I., Nutritional aspects of hematologic disorders, in *Modern Nutrition in Health and Disease,* 9th ed., Shils, M.E. et al., Eds., Williams & Wilkins, Baltimore, 1999, chap. 88.
57. McCabe, B.J., Champagne, C.M., and Allen, H.R., Estimated impact of calcium fortification of frozen yogurt bars on calcium intake of women, Addendum to FASEB Proceedings, Federation of American Societies of Experimental Biology, Bethesda, MD, 1999.
58. Ellsworth, A.J. et al., Eds., *Mosby's Medical Drug Reference, 1999–2000*, Mosby and Co., St. Louis, 2000, pp. 918–919.
59. Zhu, M. et al., Pharmacokinetics of cycloserine under fasting conditions and with high-fat meal, orange juice, and antacids, *Pharmacotherapy,* 21, 891–897, 2001.
60. Marathe, P.H. et al., Pharmacokinetics and bioavailability of a metformin/glyburide tablet administered alone or with food, *J. Clin. Pharmacol.,* 40, 1494–1502, 2000.
61. Karara, A.H., Dunning, B.E., and McLeod, J.F., The effect of food on the oral bioavailability and the pharmacodynamic actions of the insulinotrophic agent nateglinide in healthy subjects, *J. Clin. Pharmacol.,* 39, 172–179, 1999.
62. Blickstein, D., Shaklai, M., and Inba, A., Warfarin antagonism by avocado, *Lancet,* 337, 914–915, 1991.
63. Olson, R.A., Vitamin K, in *Modern Nutrition in Health and Disease,* 9th ed., Shils, M.E. et al., Williams & Wilkins, Baltimore, 1999, chap. 20.
64. Corrigan, J.J. and Marcus, F.L., Coagulopathy associated with vitamin E ingestion, *J. Am. Med. Assoc.,* 230, 1300–1301, 1994.
65. Collins, S.C. and Dufresne, R.G., Dietary supplements in the setting of Mohs surgery, *Am. Soc. Dermatol. Surg.,* 28, 447–452, 2002.
66. White, J., Ed., The Role of Nutrition in Chronic Disease Care, Executive Summary, Nutrition Screening Initiative, Washington, D.C., 1997.
67. Karstaedt, P.J. and Pincus, J.H., Protein redistribution diet remains effective in patients with fluctuating Parkinsonism, *Arch. Neurol.,* 49, 149–152, 1992.
68. Ameer, B. and Weintraub, R.A., Drug interactions with grapefruit juice, *Clin. Pharmacokinet.,* 32, 103–121, 1997.
69. Bailey, D.G. et al., Grapefruit juice and drugs: how significant is the interaction? *Clin. Pharmacokinet.,* 26, 91–98, 1991.
70. Yamreudeewong, W. et al., Drug–food interactions in clinical practice, *J. Fam. Practice,* 40, 376–384, 1995.
71. *Drug Facts and Comparisons,* Facts and Comparisons, Inc., St. Louis, MO, 2001.
72. Johnson, M.M., Chin, R., Jr., and Haponik, E.F., Nutrition, respiratory function and disease, in *Modern Nutrition in Health and Disease,* 9th ed., Shils, M.E. et al., Eds., Williams & Wilkins, Baltimore, 1999, pp. 363–380.
73. Durrant, K.L., Known and hidden sources of caffeine in drug, food, and natural products, *J. Am. Pharmacol. Assoc.,* 42, 625–637, 2002.

74. Bartel, P.R. et al., Vitamin B_6 supplementation and theophylline-related effects in humans, *Am. J. Clin. Nutr.*, 60, 93–99, 1994.

75. Zimmerman, J.J. et al., The effect of a high-fat meal on the oral bioavailability of the immunosuppressant sirolimus (Rapamycin), *J. Clin. Pharmacol.*, 39, 1155–1161, 1999.

76. McCabe, B.J., Dietary tyramine and other pressor amines: a review, *J. Am. Diet. Assoc.*, 86, 1059–1064, 1986.

77. Blumenthal, M. et al., Eds., *The Complete German Commission E Monographs: Therapeutic Guide to Herbal Medicine,* American Botanical Council, Boston Integrative Medicine Communications, Austin, TX, 1998, pp. 214–215.

78. Utermohlen, V., Diet, nutrition, and drug interactions, in *Modern Nutrition in Health and Disease,* 9th ed., Shils, M.E. et al., Williams & Wilkins, Baltimore, 1999, chap. 99.

79. Lieber, C.S., Mechanisms of ethanol–drug–nutrition interactions, *Clin. Toxicol.*, 32, 631–681, 1994.

80. Food and Nutrition Board, Institute of Medicine, *Dietary Reference Intakes for Vitamin A, Vitamin K, Arsenic, Boron, Chromium, Copper, Iodine, Iron, Manganese, Molybdenum, Nickel, Silicon, Vanadium, and Zinc,* National Academy Press, Washington, D.C., 2001.

81. Blumberg, J. and Couris, R., Pharmacology, nutrition, and the elderly: interactions and implications, in *Geriatric Nutrition: The Health Professional's Handbook,* 2nd ed., Chernoff, R., Ed., Aspen Publishers, Gaithersburg, MD, 1999, 359.

82. McCormick, D.B., Riboflavin, in *Modern Nutrition in Health and Disease,* 9th ed., Shils, M.E. et al., Eds., Williams & Wilkins, Baltimore, 1999, pp. 391–399.

CHAPTER 7

Gastrointestinal and Metabolic Disorders and Drugs

Fantahun Yimam and Razia Malik

CONTENTS

The body can be characterized as a tube inside a tube. The gastrointestinal (GI) tract is the inner tube, which extends from the mouth to the anus. It is contiguous with the outside environment at both ends. Substances, both food and drug, passing through this channel may gain passage to the interior of the body. The GI tract serves as the highway for delivery of raw materials and energy needed for life support. The health and well-being of the GI tract is of paramount concern to practitioners who focus on the nutrition of the organism.

Disorders and diseases of the GI tract will interfere with nutrient intake and absorption. A thorough understanding of gastrointestinal disorders, therefore, is an essential part of nutritional training. An in-depth review of GI pathophysiology is not within the scope of this text. This chapter focuses on drugs used to treat GI and metabolic disorders and diseases. This material would not have been covered in pathophysiology courses, many of which are not specifically designed for nutritional professionals and do not focus on the GI tract. Some programs may provide instruction in pharmacology, but unless the instructor specializes in nutritional support, these drugs may not be a focus.

This chapter traverses the GI tract and, while doing so, presents the diseases and disorders that affect each segment, while at the same time highlighting the classes of drugs and individual agents used to treat such problems. The name of each agent, both generic and brand (brand names are capitalized and followed by the ® symbol) is presented along with the mechanism of action (MOA) of the drug, the accepted dosages, and the common side effects seen with each agent. Finally, a tabular summary of the information is also provided. These tables and figures are intended to be a valuable reference for practitioners of nutritional support.

MEDICATIONS USED TO TREAT DISORDERS OF THE MOUTH AND THROAT

The mouth is the entranceway to the GI tract. Disorders affecting the mouth may interfere with adequate nutrient acceptance. These disorders include dental problems ranging from inadequately fitting dentures to abscesses involving the teeth and gums. It is also important to remember that patients at nutritional risk may also have a greater risk of contracting oral candidiasis. Interestingly, medications such as inhaled steroids can contribute to yeast infections. A common complaint of patients with this type of infection is that food tastes different, thereby increasing the risk that the patient will not eat. Cold sores, fever blisters, and canker sores are also common and can make ingestion of food uncomfortable. In addition, hyposalivation or xerostomia may cause dry mouth and throat, making ingestion uncomfortable.

The main causes of hyposalivation are surgery, radiation near to salivary glands, infection, dysfunction or obstruction of the salivary glands, inflammation of the mouth, and emotional factors such as fear and anxiety. If left untreated, hyposalivation may put an individual at higher risk for malnutrition. Patients should receive saliva substitute therapy (Salivart®, Mouthkote®, Xerostoma®, etc.), and candies, especially lemon flavored, may help. See Table 7.1 for a more complete description of specific drugs, indications for use, mechanism of action, dose, and side effects.

Cold sores, oral candidiasis, inflammation, and gingivitis can also interfere with oral intake.

GASTROINTESTINAL DISEASE STATES

Gastroesophageal Reflux Disease (GERD)

The lower esophageal sphincter (LES) is the major physiologic barrier to reflux of gastric contents into the esophagus. Abnormally low LES pressure may lead to pathologic reflux manifested by esophageal inflammation, ulceration, and heartburn. Complications include Barrett's esophagus, esophageal stricture, pulmonary aspiration, and bleeding. The treatment options include nonpharmacological measures such

Table 7.1　Medications for Oral Disorders

Drug	Indication	Mechanism of Action	Dose	Side Effects
Nystatin (Mycostatin®)	Oral candidiasis	Binds to sterols in fungal cell membrane, changing cell wall permeability	Adult and children: Oral suspension 400,000 to 600,000 units 4 times daily Infants: 200,000 to 400,000 units 4 times daily	Nausea, vomiting, GI distress, and diarrhea
Tannic Acid (Zilactin®)	For temporary relief of pain, burning, and itching caused by cold sores, fever blisters, and canker sores	Forms a thin, pliable film over sores and blisters	Apply every 4 h for the first 3 d and then as needed	Stinging sensation, infection
Amphotericin B (Fungizone®)	Oral candidiasis	Binds to ergosterol altering cell membrane permeability in susceptible fungi and causing leakage of cell components with subsequent cell death	1 mL (100 mg) 4 times daily; administer between meals to permit prolonged contact with the oral lesions × 2 weeks	Cardiac arrest, arrhythmias, hypokalemia, hypomagnesemia, thrombocytopenia, increased serum creatinine and azotemia, etc.
Chlorhexidine gluconate (Peridex®)	Gingivitis	Provide bactericidal effect by binding to the bacterial cell walls and extramicrobial complexes during oral rinsing	Swish undiluted oral rinse around in mouth for 30 sec, and then expectorate; avoid eating for 2–3 h after treatment	Skin and tongue irritation, increased tartar on teeth, staining of oral surfaces
Carbamide peroxide (Proxigel®, Gly-Oxide®, Orajel®, Perioseptic®)	Oral inflammation	Release oxygen on contact with mouth tissues to provide cleansing effects; help reduce inflammation, relieve pain, and inhibit odor-forming bacteria	Apply several drops undiluted to affected area of the mouth 4 times/d and at bed time up to 7 d	Dizziness, rash, tenderness, pain, and redness
Clotrimazole (Mycelex®)	Prophylaxis of oropharyngeal candidiasis	Inhibit yeast growth by altering cell membrane permeability	Treatment: Administer 1 troche 5 times a day for 14 d Prophylaxis: Administer 1 troche 3 times a day for duration of chemotherapy or until steroid are reduced to maintenance levels	Erythema, pruritus, abnormal liver function test, stinging of skin, nausea, and vomiting

Note:　Other mouth and throat products are also available. For more information, refer to Riley, M.R. et al., *Drug Facts and Comparisons*, Kluwer, St. Louis, 1999.

as using 4- to 6-inch bed blocks under the head of the bed; avoiding alcohol, peppermint, and chocolate because these substances can lower LES pressure; avoiding food or drink before retiring; and avoiding cigarette smoking and medications that increase acid reflux.

Pharmacological management includes the use of histamine 2 (H_2)-receptor antagonists, antacids, proton pump inhibitors, and motility agents. Histamine 2 (H_2)-receptor antagonists are highly effective in improving symptoms and healing esophageal inflammation. Antacids may be used by patients with mild or intermittent symptoms, two tablespoons of high-potency liquid antacid nightly or when needed for heartburn works quickly, is most economical, and may be sufficient. Proton pump inhibitors are highly effective and decrease gastric acid secretion by blocking parietal cell release of hydrochloric acid. Metoclopramide improves gastric emptying and increases LES pressure. Surgery should be considered in patients with strictures, bleeding, aspiration, or intractable esophagitis despite aggressive medical therapy. Infectious esophagitis usually presents with odynophagia and dysphagia. It is most common in patients with malignancy, diabetes, or impaired immunity resulting from other causes. One of two organisms is usually responsible for causing this disorder: *Candida albicans* or *Herpes simplex*. Viscous lidocaine 2% may be given to relieve the discomfort. The usual dose is 15 mL swished around in the mouth and then swallowed. This may be repeated every 3 to 4 h as needed. Nystatin (Mycostatin®) oral suspension (500,000 units in water taken orally four times a day) and nystatin oral lozenges (one lozenge taken five times daily for 2 weeks) are effective treatments for *Candida albicans*. Herpes simplex should be treated with acyclovir (Zovirax®) 5 mg/kg administered intravenously every 8 h for 7 d.

Esophageal motility disorders may cause noncardiac chest pain or intermittent dysphagia to both liquids and solids. Optimal treatment is not defined. A gastroenterology consultation is recommended for advice regarding diagnosis and therapy.

Peptic Ulcer Disease

Peptic ulcer disease (PUD) is a group of disorders characterized by sharply circumscribed loss of mucous membrane of the stomach, duodenum, or any other part of the GI system exposed to gastric juices containing acid and pepsin. It can occur anywhere in the GI tract. Normally, a layer of mucus covers the GI tract and protects the GI endothelium from being acted on by gastric acid and digestive enzymes. In the absence of this protection, the acid and enzymes will attempt to digest the endothelial layer of the GI as they would any other collection of animal-derived cells organized into proteins (meat).

There is growing evidence from research that a bacterium present in the gut may be responsible for PUD. *Helicobacter pylori* (formerly *Campylobacter pylori*), a gram-negative bacterium that resides in the human stomach and duodenum, is strongly associated with antral gastritis and PUD. If *H. pylori* are present, a two-drug, three-drug, or four-drug regimen may be given for 2 weeks as shown in Table 7.2. Surgery is required in patients with perforation, obstruction, or bleeding.

Table 7.2   Drug Regimens Used to Treat H. pylori

Two-Drug Regimens	Three-Drug Regimens	Four-Drug Regimens
Clarithromycin + PPI Clarithromycin + RBC Amoxicillin + PPI	Clarithromycin + Amoxicillin + PPI Clarithromycin + Metronidazole + PPI Clarithromycin + Metronidazole + RBC Amoxicillin + Metronidazole + PPI Tetracycline + Metronidazole + Sucralfate	Tetracycline or Amoxicillin + Metronidazole + PPI + BSS Tetracycline or Amoxicillin + Metronidazole + H_2RAs + BSS PPI + Metronidazole + BSS + Clarithromycin

Note: H_2RAs = H_2 receptor antagonist (e.g., ranitidine), BSS = bismuth subsalicylate (Pepto-Bismol®). PPI = proton pump inhibitor (e.g., omeprazole), RBC = ranitidine bismuth citrate (Tritec™).

PUD Manifestations

Gastric ulcers form most commonly in the antrum or at the antral–fundal junction, and duodenal ulcers almost always develop in the duodenal bulb (the first few centimeters of the duodenum). A few ulcers, however, arise between the duodenal bulb and the ampulla of Vater.

Less common forms of PUD also develop. Drug-induced ulcers occur in patients who chronically ingest substances that damage the mucosa, such as nonsteroidal antiinflammatory drugs (NSAIDs). Stress ulcer result from serious trauma or illness, major burns, or ongoing sepsis. The most common site of ulcer formation is the proximal portion of the stomach. Zollinger–Ellison syndrome is a severe form of peptic ulcer disease in which intractable ulcers are accompanied by extreme gastric hyperacidity and at least one gastrinoma (a non–beta islet cell tumor of the pancreas or another site).

Treatment of PUD

The goals of treatment of PUD, regardless of origin, are to relieve pain, to enhance ulcer healing, to prevent complications such as GI bleeding or perforation, and to prevent recurrence of the ulcer. Table 7.3 summarizes the types of drugs used in the treatment of PUD.

Antacids

Antacids neutralize gastric acidity, resulting in an increase in the pH of the stomach and duodenal bulb. In addition, they inhibit the proteolytic activity of pepsin and increase the lower esophageal sphincter tone. Aluminum ions inhibit smooth muscle contraction, thus inhibiting gastric emptying. Use aluminum-containing antacids with caution in patients with gastric outlet obstruction. Also use these antacids with caution for patients in renal failure, for this may increase the potential for aluminum toxicity.

Table 7.3 Medications in the Treatment of Peptic Ulcer Disease (PUD)

Drug	Mechanism of Action	Dose	Side effects
Antacids	Neutralize gastric acid; mucosal protection; bind bile acid and pepsin	Give amounts sufficient to neutralize	Constipation or diarrhea, hypermagnesemia, hypophosphatemia and milk-alkali syndrome; may interfere with the absorption of tetracyclines, quinolones, and Azoles
H₂ Antagonists	Selectively antagonizes histamine (H₂) receptors (H₂ blocker)		Confusion, neurological dysfunction, elevated serum creatinine, thrombocytopenia and antiandrogenic effect (gynecomastia, impotence); most prevalent with cimetidine
Cimetidine (Tagamet®)		Oral: Short-term treatment of active ulcers: 300 mg QID or 800 mg Q HS or 400 mg BID × 8 weeks DU prophylaxis: 400–800 mg q HS Gastric hypersecretory conditions: Oral, IM or IV 300–600 mg q 6 h, and dosage not to exceed 2.4 g/d IM OR IV: 300 mg every 6 h Children: Oral IM or IV 20–40 mg in divided doses every 4 h	Decrease absorption of Azoles, Digoxin and increase plasma levels of Fluorouracil and opioid analgesics, etc.
Famotidine (Pepcid®)		Oral: GERD: 20 mg BID × 6 weeks; duodenal or gastric ulcer: 40 mg Q HS × 4–8 weeks Hypersecretory conditions: 20 mg q 6 h, then increase up to 160 mg q 6 h IV: 20 mg every 12 h Children: Oral, IV 1–2 mg/kg/d Max: 40 mg/d	

Table 7.3 Medications in the Treatment of Peptic Ulcer Disease (PUD) (*Continued*)

Drug	Mechanism of Action	Dose	Side effects
Nizatidine (Axid®)		Active duodenal ulcer: Treatment: 150 mg BID or 300 mg Q HS Maintenance: 150 mg/d Meal induced heartburn, acid digestion, and sour stomach: OTC: 75 mg twice daily	
Ranitidine (Zantac®)		Oral: Short-term treatment of ulceration: 150 mg BID or 300 mg Q HS Prophylaxis of recurrent DU: 150 mg Q HS Gastric hypersecretory: 150 mg BID, up to 6 g/d IM or IV: 50 mg every 6–8 h Max: 400 mg/d Children: Oral: 1.25–2.5 mg/kg every 12 h Max: 300 mg/d IM or IV: 0.75–1.5 mg/kg every 6–8 h Max: 400 mg/d	
Proton pump inhibitors	Block gastric acid secretion by binding to H+/K+ ATPase Competitive Inhibitor of histamine at H_2 receptors of the gastric parietal cells, which inhibits gastric acid secretion		Constipation, nausea, abdominal pain, vomiting, headache, and regurgitation; inhibits cytochrome P450; may increase concentration of phenytoin, warfarin, diazepam, etc.
Omeprazole (Prilosec®)		20 mg QD For ZE Syndrome: 60 mg QD (Max: 120 mg TID)	Headache

Drug	Action	Dose	Side effects
Lansoprazole (Prevacid®)		30 mg QD (Max: 180 mg)	
Rabeprazole (Aciphex®)		20 mg QD For hypersecretory conditions including Zollinger–Ellison (EZ) syndrome: 60 mg QD (Max: 100 mg QD or 60 mg BID)	
Pantoprazole (Protonix®)		Oral: 40–80 mg PO QD IV: 40 mg QD times 7 d through in-line filter; 80 mg IV q12 h for the treatment of EZ	
Cytoprotective agents A. Sucralfate (Carafate®)	Bind to protein at GI lesion, forming protective barrier	1 g tab 30 min Pc and HS or 2 g BID; 200 mg QID	Constipation, fullness, and rash; interferes with absorption of quinolones, theophylline, and phenytoin; diarrhea
B. Misoprostol (Cytotec®)	Stimulates mucous secretion (replaces the protective prostaglandins); used for prevention of NSAID-induced gastric ulcers	200 µg PO QID with food	Diarrhea, abdominal pain, constipation, flatulence, uterine stimulation, and vaginal bleeding
Anticholinergic agents Propantheline (ProBanthine®)	Block gastric acid secretion by inhibiting the action of acetylcholine	30 mg q HS	Dry mouth, blurred vision, tachycardia, and gastric and urinary retention

H_2 Antagonists

H_2 antagonists are reversible competitive blockers of histamine at the H_2 receptors, particularly in the parietal cells. They are effective in alleviating symptoms and in preventing complications of PUD. The drugs have similar adverse reaction profiles. Cimetidine appears to have the greatest degree of antiandrogenic (e.g., gynecomastia, impotence) and central nervous system (CNS) (e.g., mental confusion) effects. Cimetidine also is involved in more drug interactions because it inhibits the cytochrome P_{450} oxidase system that affects metabolism of other drugs (e.g., warfarin, theophylline.). In addition, cimetidine causes rare hematological adverse effects, as compared to other H_2 antagonists. Ranitidine, on the other hand, may cause reversible thrombocytopenia.

Proton Pump Inhibitors

Proton pump inhibitors suppress gastric acid secretion by specific inhibition of the H^+/K^+ ATPase enzyme system at the secretory surface of the gastric parietal cell. They block the final step of acid production. This effect is dose-related and leads to inhibition of both basal and stimulated gastric acid secretion regardless of the stimulus.

Nausea and Vomiting

Nausea and vomiting are symptoms that may result from systemic illness, CNS disorders, and primary GI disease, as well as side effects of medications. The most common cause of these symptoms for the healthy individual is viral illness. Pregnancy, in women of childbearing age, should be ruled out before treatment is initiated. Intestinal obstruction can cause nausea and vomiting and can be diagnosed radiographically. Once an etiology is established, specific therapy can often be initiated.

Nausea and vomiting are common side effects of many antineoplastic agents and radiation therapy. Uncontrolled nausea and vomiting can result in dehydration, metabolic disturbance, weight loss, malnutrition, aspiration pneumonia and decrease quality of life. It can have a significant impact on a patient's overall therapy and response to treatment.

The frequency of chemotherapy and radiation induced emesis depends primarily on the emetogenic potential of the specific chemotherapeutic agents used and the area receiving radiation. The onset, duration, and intensity of acute and delay nausea and vomiting secondary to chemotherapy are dependent on many factors. You should be aware of the relative emetic potential of all antineoplastic agents, as well as the relationship of dose, onset, duration, and mechanism of emetic activity.

Treatment of Nausea and Vomiting

The treatment of nausea and vomiting beyond establishment of a firm etiology falls into two categories: supportive measures and pharmacology. As supportive measures, the patient should be nothing by mouth (nihil per orem, npo) or on clear liquid diet, if tolerated. Nasogastric decompression may be beneficial for patients with protracted nausea and vomiting. Parenteral fluid resuscitation is necessary for patients with significant intravascular volume depletion or electrolyte derangement.

Pharmacotherapy

Drugs that are effective as antiemetics are the anti-dopaminergic agents (phenothiazines and metoclopramide) which are effective for drug-induced emesis. Anticholenergic agents (antihistamines, trimethobenzamide, and scopolamine) may be more appropriate in motion sickness, labyrinthine disorders, etc. Selective 5-HT3 receptor antagonist agents (Dolasetron, Granisetron, and Ondansetron) are used for prevention and treatment of nausea and vomiting associated with chemo and radiation therapy. Owing to the nature of the malady, the use of other than orally administered dosage forms, such as suppositories or intravenous or intramuscular injections, is sometimes necessary. Chewable oral doses may be better tolerated than dosage forms that need to be swallowed whole with water.

Antidopaminergic, anticholenergic and selective $5HT_3$ receptor antagonists are presented in more detail in Table 7.4.

Diarrhea

Diarrhea is characterized by the abnormal frequency and liquidity of fecal discharge compared with the normal stools. It results in an imbalance in the absorption and secretion of water and electrolytes. Frequency and consistency are variable within and between individuals. Diarrhea may result from systemic illness, gastrointestinal disease, toxins, or poisons and as a side effect of medications. It can be a major health hazard if left untreated, especially in children, elderly, and already debilitated patients. Diarrhea can lead to fluid and electrolyte imbalances, acid–base disturbances, and even cardiovascular collapse. In general, diarrhea can be the result of osmotic abnormalities or secretory abnormalities. Diarrhea can be divided into three classifications: (1) Acute diarrhea (less than 3 d), (2) chronic diarrhea (greater than 14 d), and (3) diarrhea in patients with AIDS. Table 7.5 summarizes the diagnostic and general therapeutic strategies for diarrheal conditions.

Causes of Diarrhea

Antimicrobial agents may produce diarrhea by causing nonspecific alteration of the enteric flora or by causing pseudomembranous colitis, which is associated with overgrowth of *Clostridium difficile* and requires specific therapy. Antibiotic-associated diarrhea without evidence of pseudomembranous colitis usually responds to cessation of the offending agent.

Bile-induced diarrhea is caused by excessive production of bile or poor bile reabsorption in the intestine. Ileal resection can deplete the bile salt pool, owing to inadequate reabsorption and recirculation. Bile salt malabsorption induces diarrhea after bile salts are converted into bile acids, which stimulate secretion and evacuation,

Table 7.4 Treatment of Nausea and Vomiting

Drug	MOA	Dose	Side Effects
Prochlorperazine (Compazine®)	Blocks postsynaptic mesolimbic dopaminergic receptors in the brain, including the medullary chemoreceptor trigger zone; exhibits a strong alpha-adrenergic blocking effect	5–10 mg PO TID or QID; 10 mg IM q 4 h (maximum IM dose = 40 mg/d); 25 mg PR BID	Orthostatic hypotension, dystonias
Promethazine (Phenergan®)	Blocks postsynaptic mesolimbic dopaminergic receptors in the brain; exhibits a strong alpha-adrenergic blocking effect, etc.	12.5–25 mg PO, IM, or PR q 4–6 h	Thrombocytopenia, jaundice, drowsiness
Trimethobenzamide (Tigan®)	Acts centrally to inhibit the medullary chemoreceptor trigger zone	250 mg PO TID or QID; 200 IM TID or QID or 200 mg PR TID or QID	Drowsiness, hypotension, seizures; injection contraindicated in children, especially if fever is present
Thiethylperazine (Torecan®)	Blocks postsynaptic mesolimbic dopaminergic receptors in the brain; exhibits a strong alpha-adrenergic blocking effect, etc.	10 mg PO, IM, or PR QID or TID is effective	Drowsiness, hypotension
Metoclopramide (Reglan®)	Blocks dopamine receptors in chemoreceptor trigger zone of the CNS	10 mg PO 30 min ac and hs	Drowsiness, diarrhea, weakness
Diphenhydramine (Benadryl®)	Competes with histamine for H1-receptor sites on effective cells in the gastrointestinal tract, blood vessels, and respiratory tract	IV: 10–50 mg every 2–4 h, not to exceed 400 mg/d; PO: 25–50 mg every 6–8 h	Drowsiness, thickening of bronchial secretion, headache, appetite increase etc.
Meclizine (Antivert®)	Has central anticholinergic action by blocking chemoreceptor trigger zone; decrease excitability of the middle ear labyrinth and blocks conduction in the middle ear vestibular-cerebellar pathways	PO: 12.5–25 mg one hour before travel, repeat dose every 12–24 h if needed; dose up to 50 mg may be needed	Drowsiness, thickening of bronchial secretion, headache, appetite increase, etc.

Table 7.4   Treatment of Nausea and Vomiting *(Continued)*

Drug	MOA	Dose	Side Effects
Scopolamine (Isopto® Hyoscine)	Blocks the action of acetylcholine at parasympathetic sites in smooth muscle, secretory glands and the CNS; increase cardiac output, dries secretions, antagonizes histamine and serotonin	IV, IM, SC: 0.3–0.65 mg; may be repeated every 4–6 h Transdermal: apply one disc behind the ear at least 4 h prior to exposure and every 3 d as needed	Blurred vision, photophobia, local irritation, increase intraocular pressure, respiratory congestion, etc.
Dolasetron (Anzemet®)	Selective 5-HT$_3$ receptor antagonist, blocking both serotonin, both peripherally on vagal nerve terminals and centrally on the chemoreceptor trigger zone.	IV: 100 mg or 1.8 mg/kg; PO: 100 mg	Headache, diarrhea, fever, etc.
Granisetron (Kytril®)		IV: 1 mg or 0.01 mg/kg; PO: 2 mg	Headache, diarrhea, constipation, etc.
Ondansetron (Zofran®)		IV: 8 mg or 0.15 mg/kg; PO: 12–24 mg/d	Headache, diarrhea, fever, constipation, etc.

Table 7.5   Diagnostic and Therapeutic Strategies for Diarrhea

Diarrhea Work-Up Diagnosis/Treatment Protocol

Special Tests

Stool examination for parasite and ova, mucus, fat, or blood
Stool osmolality, pH, and electrolytes
Direct endoscopic visualization and biopsy: can be used to diagnose conditions such as colitis
Radiographic studies: help in diagnosing neoplastic and inflammatory conditions

Therapeutic Strategies of Diarrhea Treatment

Identification and treatment of the specific disease
Correction of electrolyte, fluid, and acid–base disturbance
Occasional use of nonspecific antidiarrheal agents

in the colon. Bile-acid-induced diarrhea can be treated with small amounts of cholestyramine (Questran®, Questran Lite®), which binds to bile salts and prevents their conversion to bile acids.

Agents to Treat Diarrhea

Drugs or agents used in the treatment of diarrhea fall into four general categories: (1) antimotility, (2) adsorbents, (3) antisecretory, and (4) bulk-forming agents (used for constipation as well as diarrhea).

Antimotility

Opioid agents have a potential for abuse that should be recognized. These agents are listed in order of potency and potential for narcotic side effects, weakest first:

1. Loperamide (Imodium®): 2–4 mg by mouth (PO) after each loose stool until diarrhea is controlled (Max: 16 mg/d).
2. Diphenoxylate and atropine (Lomotil®): 1 tablet PO 4 times daily (QID) until control of diarrhea is achieved. Each tablet or 5 mL of liquid contains 2.5 mg of diphenoxylate hydrochloride and 0.025 mg of atropine sulfate.
3. Codeine: 30–60 mg PO twice daily (BID)-QID
4. Paregoric (camphorated tincture of opium) (morphine equivalent): 4–8 mL QID or after each liquid stool, not to exceed 32 mL/d.
5. Tincture of opium (morphine equivalent): 0.3–1.0 mL PO QID (Max: 6 mL/d).

Caution: It is vitally important not to confuse paregoric and tincture of opium. Inadvertent administration of tincture of opium in a volume appropriate to paregoric will result in a potentially severe overdose of morphine.

6. Atropine: 0.4–0.6 mg Q 4–6 h (nonnarcotic used synergistically at times).

Adsorbents

Atapulgite (Kaopectate®) 600 mg/15 mL: Use 60–120 mL of regular strength or 45–90 mL of concentrate PO after each loose stool.

Antisecretory

A. Bismuth subsalicylate (Pepto-Bismol®): Use two tablets or 30 mL every 30 min to 1 h as needed, up to 8 doses/24 h.
B. Octreotode (Sandostatin®): 50–100 μg IV Q8H; increase by 100 μg/dose at 48 h intervals; maximum dose: 500 μg Q 8 h.

Bulk-Forming Agents

These agents promote bowel regularity and may be used for both diarrhea and constipation. See Table 7.2 for details about drugs used in constipation and in diarrhea.

Specific Agents of Choice

Octreotide blocks the release of serotonin and other active peptides, and is effective in controlling diarrhea and flushing. It is also used for the symptomatic treatment of carcinoid tumors and vasoactive intestinal peptide-secreting tumors (VIpomas). Dose: Carcinoid: 100–600 μg/d in 2–4 divided doses subcutaneously. VIpomas: 200–300 μg/d in 2–4 divided doses subcutaneously.

Metronidazole is the drug of choice for treating pseudomembranous colitis (PMC), which results from toxins produced by *Clostridium difficile*. It has been associated most often with broad-spectrum antibiotics, such as ampicillin, clinda-mycin, and cephalosporins. Dose: 250–500 mg four times daily orally. Orally administered vancomycin is effective, but should be reserved for patients not responding to metronidazole, patients who are pregnant, or patients under 10 years of age.

Note: It is administered for its intraluminal effect, not for systemic effect. Intravenous administration of vancomycin produces no effect on pseudomembranous colitis. Dose: 125–500 mg four times daily orally.

Cholestyramine (Questran®, Questran® Light) is used for diarrhea associated with excess fecal bile acids. MOA: Forms a nonabsorbable complex with bile acids in the intestine, inhibits enterohepatic reuptake of bile salts, and thereby increases the fecal loss of bile salt–bound, low-density lipoprotein cholesterol. Dose: 4 g 1–6 times daily; maximum dose: 16–32 g/d.

Probiotic agents (lactobacillus, acidophilus, live culture yogurt) are used for antibiotic-associated diarrhea. It is intended to replace colon microflora. This supposedly restores intestinal functions and suppresses the growth of pathogenic microorganisms.

Constipation

Constipation is defined as the difficulty of passing stools, incomplete passage, or infrequent passage of hard stools. It can be further defined as having less than three stools per week for women and five for men despite a high residual diet, or a period greater than 3 d without a bowel movement. It can be caused by gastrointestinal disorders, metabolic and endocrine disorders, pregnancy, neurogenic and psychogenic problems, or it could be drug induced.

Treatment of Constipation

Laxative Mechanisms of Action

Laxatives promote bowel evacuation by decreasing water and electrolyte absorption, increasing intraluminal osmolarity, or increasing hydrostatic pressure in the gut. Chronic use of laxatives, particularly stimulants, may lead to laxative dependency. Laxative dependency, in turn, may result in fluid and electrolyte imbalances, steatorrhea, osteomalacia, and vitamin and mineral deficiencies. Known as laxative abuse syndrome (LAS), it is difficult to diagnose. LAS is often seen in women with anorexia nervosa, depression, and personality disorders and also in elderly patients with quasimedical concerns about their bowel movements. Table 7.6 outlines important properties of six types of laxatives.

Bulk-Forming Agents

Bulk-forming agents are used to promote regularity and are equally indicated for both constipation and diarrhea. The mechanism of action (MOA) is to provide fiber that is not digested or absorbed. This adds bulk to the stool and retains some water in the lumen of the GI tract.

Side effects can include fluid and electrolyte imbalance. Specific drugs and usual dosages are as follows:

1. Methylcellulose (Citrucel®): 4–6 g/d
2. Polycarbophil (FiberCon®, Mitrolan®): 4–6 g/d
3. Psyllium (Fiberall®, Metamucil®, Konsyl®, etc.): Dose varies with product

Table 7.6   Properties of Laxatives

Laxatives	Onset of Action (h)	Site of Action
Bulk-forming Methylcellulose Polycarbophil Psyllium	12–24 (up to 72)	Small and large intestine
Stool softeners/surfactants Docusate sodium Docusate calcium Docusate potassium	24–72	Small and large intestine
Saline cathartics Magnesium citrate Magnesium hydroxide Magnesium Sulfate	0.5–3	Small and large intestine
Lubricant Mineral oil	6–8	Colon
Stimulants/irritant Bisacodyl Senna Casanthranol	6–10	Colon
Evacuant Glycerin suppository	0.25–0.5	Local irritation, hyperosmotic action

Stool Softeners/Surfactants

These agents provide detergent activity and facilitate admixture of fat and water to soften stool. They also will retain water in the lumen of the GI tract. They do not add volume to the stool, but they do prevent hardening of the stool and may prevent pain on defecation. They may be used postoperatively to decrease discomfort caused by defecation and for patients with heart disease to prevent Valsalva's maneuver efforts upon defecation, which can produce cardiac arrhythmias. Commonly used stool softeners and surfactants include docusate sodium (Colace®, Doxinate®), 50–360 mg/d; docusate calcium (Surfak®), 50–360 mg/d; and docusate potassium (Dialose®, Diocto-K®, Kasof®, etc.), 100–300 m/d.

Saline Cathartics

These agents attract and retain water in intestinal lumen, increasing intraluminal pressure and cholecystokinin release. These drugs contain an anion or cation that is poorly absorbed and remains in the lumen of the GI tract. In an effort to maintain equal osmotic pressure on both sides of the cell membranes of the GI tract, water will be secreted and not resorbed within the lumen. Agents and their dosages include magnesium citrate (Citrate of Magnesia®, Citroma®), 4 oz to 1 full bottle 120–300 mL; magnesium hydroxide (Phillips'™ Milk of Magnesia), 5–15 mL or 650 mg to 1.3 g tablets up to 4 times/d as needed; magnesium sulfate (Epsom salts®), 10 to 15 g in a glass of water; and sodium phosphate (Fleet®), 20–30 mL as a single dose.

Lubricant Cathartics/Emollients

These agents act to ease passage of stool by decreasing water absorption and lubricating the intestine. One agent is mineral oil (Kondremul®). Dosage for adults and children ≥12 years of age is 15 to 45 mL once daily or divided dose. For children 6 to ≤12 years of age, dosage is 5 to 15 mL once daily or divided dose.

Note: All use of mineral oil, especially chronically, poses a significant nutritional problem, since mineral oil reduces absorption of the lipid-soluble vitamins (e.g., vitamins A, D, E, and K). Use in elderly patients, particularly those who exhibit high risk for aspiration, is not appropriate. Orally administered mineral oil can produce lipid pneumonia in these patients, a fatal complication. Prolonged, frequent, or excessive use may result in dependence or decrease absorption of fat-soluble vitamins.

Intestinal Stimulants/Irritants

These agents directly act on intestinal mucosa, stimulate myenteric plexus, and alter water and electrolyte secretion. Specific agents and usual dosages are bisacodyl (Dulcolax®), 5 to 15 mg (usually 10 mg) as a single dose daily; senna, dose varies with formulation; and casanthranol (Dialose Plus®, Peri-colace®), dose varies with formulation.

Hyperosmotic

Local irritation and hyperosmotic action are produced by these agents. Examples and usual dosage include two types of agents. The first type is glycerin, adults and children ≤12 years of age, one suppository high in the rectum and retained 15 to 30 minutes; it need not melt to produce laxative action. A second type is lactulose (Cephulac®, Chronulac®), adults and children ≤12 years of age, 15 to 30 mL (10 to 20 g) daily, increased to 60 mL/d if necessary.

A third agent is the sugar alcohol, sorbitol 70%, 30–50 g/d. See bowel-cleansing (also called bowel preparation) agents for a discussion of GoLytely® (polyethylene glycol-electrolyte solution). Combination products include docusate and casanthranol (Peri-Colace®), one or two at bedtime with a full glass of water.

Bowel Preparation Agents for Surgery or GI Procedures

Bowel cleansing is done prior to GI surgery to reduce the bacterial load and thereby decrease the risk of peritoneal contamination by fecal material and subsequent infection. Similar treatment with the laxative component may be performed prior to endoscopic colonoscopy in order to provide better visualization of the bowel surface. The oral component of these treatments is administered the day before surgery. Sometimes, enemas may also be given prior to colonoscopy.

Polyethylene Glycol Electrolyte Solution

Polyethylene glycol electrolyte solution (PEG ES) (GoLytely®, CoLyte®, NuLytely®), 4 liters, can be administered orally prior to GI examination. It can be given via a nasogastric tube to patients who are unwilling or unable to drink the preparation. The patient is instructed to drink 240 mL every 10 min until 4 L are consumed or until the rectal effluent is clear. Tap water may be used to reconstitute the solution. The first bowel movement should occur in about 1 h. Side effects include nausea, abdominal cramps, fullness and bloating, vomiting, and anal irritation. These adverse reactions are transient and subside rapidly.

Erythromycin

Another set of agents used in bowel preparation include: 1 g erythromycin base at 1, 2, and 11 p.m. on the day before surgery, combined with mechanical cleansing of the large intestine and oral neomycin (90 mg/kg/d), divided every 4 h for 2 d or 25 mg/kg at 1, 2, and 11 p.m. preoperatively.

Oral Electrolyte Replacements

Oral fluid and electrolyte replacements include Pedialyte®, Rehydralyte®, Ricelyte®, Infalyte®, Lytren®, and Gatorade®. These agents are used to replace electrolytes lost with incessant diarrhea. They are particularly necessary in infants and small children whose electrolyte reserves are much less than that of adults. The elderly are also more susceptible to disastrous results from electrolyte imbalances and may be candidates for oral electrolyte replacement therapy.

These solutions contain varying amounts of glucose, sodium, and potassium and some form of buffer. Some are, however, poor choices for fluid replacement in prolonged or severe diarrhea because of high glucose and low electrolyte concentrations.

Pancreatitis

Acute pancreatitis is an inflammatory disorder of the pancreas resulting from premature activation of proteolytic enzymes within the pancreas. This acute condition resolves both clinically and histologically. Chronic pancreatitis results in functional and structural damage to the pancreas that persists after the causative factor is eliminated. Histological changes persist even after the clinical condition resolves.

The most frequent causes of pancreatitis are gallstones that block the pancreatic duct and alcoholism that leads to blockage of the pancreatic ductules. Endoscopic retrograde cholangiopancreatography (ERCP), trauma, drugs, infection, hypercalcemia, anatomical abnormalities of the pancreas, recent surgery, cancer, hypertriglyceridemia, chemical exposure, and biliary tract cysts may cause pancreatitis. In addition, some cases are idiopathic. The most common symptoms are nausea, vomiting, fever, ascites, swelling of the upper abdomen, pain radiating to the back, and hypotension. Abdominal x-ray, ultrasound, CT scan, and ERCP diagnose the disorder. Calcium, potassium, triglycerides, and glucose levels should be monitored closely.

Treatment of Pancreatitis

Initial treatment is aimed at relieving pain, replacing fluid, minimizing complications, and preventing pancreatic necrosis and infection. Any medication that can cause or exacerbate pancreatitis (e.g., furosemide, metronidazole, tetracycline, thiazide diuretics, valproic acid, sulfonamides, mercaptopurine) should be discontinued. Alcohol also needs be avoided. For pain management, many clinicians favor meperidine (Demerol®), 50–100 mg, intramuscularly (IM) q 3–4 h for analgesia because it may cause less spasm of the sphincter of Oddi than other opioids (morphine). Meperidine's usefulness is limited because its metabolite normeperidine is associated with seizures, particularly in the setting of decreased renal function.

Stimulation of the pancreas should be minimized as much as possible. The patient must take nothing by mouth and continue to receive intravenous fluids. Current practice recommends the use of tube feedings of an elemental or semielemental nature because this will result in less stimulation of the pancreas than oral feedings. The tube feeding should be administered distal to the Treitz's muscle (ligament) to minimize pancreatic stimulation. Bowel sounds may be hypoactive or absent if inflammation is severe. In the seriously ill patient, total parenteral nutrition (TPN) may be needed for 4–6 weeks. A nasogastric (NG) tube may be used to decompress the intestine until the acute inflammation subsided. The NG tube will be needed only if ileus or emesis was present and medications were of little help in resolving the disease.

Intravenous (IV) fluid may be required to maintain intravascular volume and blood pressure in severe pancreatitis. Potassium, magnesium, and calcium should be checked and corrected. The endocrine function of the pancreas and insulin production may also be affected. Insulin may be needed to treat hyperglycemia with glucose above 250 mg/dL. Histamine$_2$ blockers (e.g., famotidine, cimetidine) are added intravenously to reduce secretin, a hormone that increases the flow of pancreatic juices.

Oral pancreatic enzyme supplementation can be used to treat chronic pancreatitis. The most important determinant of the effectiveness of pancreatic enzyme replacement therapy is the quantity of active lipase delivered to the duodenum rather than actual dosage forms (tablet vs. capsule, enteric coated vs. non–enteric coated). The use of antibiotics is controversial and should be reserved for specific infections. If a pancreatic infection is suspected, a CT-guided needle aspiration of the pancreas can be done.

Inflammatory Bowel Disease

Inflammatory bowel disease is a generic term used to refer to two chronic diseases that cause inflammation to the intestines, Crohn's disease and ulcerative colitis. There are differences in the histology between these diseases. Many similarities, however, exist, such as symptoms and age of onset, and severity ranges from mild to severe. Inflammatory bowel disease symptoms can include continuous or intermittent flare-ups. The diagnosis of the disease is made by the symptoms and the exclusion of other diseases by endoscopy examination. Flexible sigmoidoscopy and colonoscopy are endoscopic procedures that allow the physician to see the large intestine. Table 7.7 presents the agents used to treat inflammatory diseases.

Crohn's disease is a transmural (mucosal, submucosal, and deeper layers) inflammation. The terminal ileum is the most common site of involvement but can occur in any part of the GI tract (mouth to anus). The inflammation may also appear in

Table 7.7 Agents to Treat Inflammatory Bowel Disease

Drug	MOA (Mechanism of Action)	Indication	Dose	Side Effects
Mesalamine, (Asacol®, Pentasa®, Rowasa®)	Unknown	Ulcerative colitis, Crohn's disease	Asacol®: 800 mg 3 times daily a total dose of 2.4 g/d for 6 weeks Pentasa®: 1 g 4 times daily for a total of 4 g for up to 8 weeks Rowasa®: One suppository (500 mg) 2 times daily; 60 mL units (4 g) enema once a day	Headache, fever, dizziness
Olsalazine (Dipentum®)	Unknown, but appears to be local rather than systemic	Ulcerative colitis	1 g per day in two divided doses	Headache, watery diarrhea, abdominal pain/cramps
Sulfasalazine (Azulfidine®)	Acts locally in the colon to decrease the inflammatory response and interfere with secretion by binding prostaglandin synthesis	Ulcerative colitis, Crohn's disease	3 to 4 g daily in divided doses; may need to take up to 6 g/d	Nausea, heartburn, headache, dizziness, anemia, skin rashes, reduced sperm counts
Infliximab (Remicade®)	Neutralizes biological activity of TNF and inhibits TNF receptor binding	Crohn's disease	5 mg/kg gives as a single IV infusion; may use additional 5 mg/kg doses at 2 and 6 weeks after the first infusion	Nausea, vomiting, abdominal pain, upper respiratory infection
Mercaptopurine (Purinethol®)	Metabolites of the drug interfere with metabolic reactions necessary for nucleic acid biosynthesis	Ulcerative colitis, Crohn's disease	50 mg/d, titrate to response and tolerance	Pancreatitis, bone marrow suppression, immune suppression, nausea, vomiting, anorexia, rash
Azathioprine (Imuran®)	Affects purine nucleotide synthesis and metabolism, alters the reactions necessary for nucleic acid biosynthesis, suppresses cell-mediated type hypersensitivity, and has antiinflammatory properties	Ulcerative colitis, Crohn's disease	2–3 mg/kg/d, benefits not achieved until at least 3 months of continuous treatment	Bone marrow suppression, nausea, vomiting, pancreatitis, hepatotoxicity
Cyclosporine (Neora®, Sandimmune®, Sang Cya®)	Inhibits the antigenic response of helper T cells, decreases the production of interleukin-2 and interferon gamma, and inhibits the production of the receptor site for interleukin-2 on T cells	Ulcerative colitis, Crohn's disease	8–10 mg/kg/d, treatment not to exceed 4–6 months	Bone marrow suppression, hypertension, tremor, seizures, neurotoxicity, paresthesia, hyperlipidemia, nausea, vomiting, gingival hyperplasia, nephrotoxicity, hepatotoxicity
Methotrexate (Methotrex®, Trexall®)	Folic antagonist, thus interferes with the synthesis of DNA and cell reproduction	Crohn's disease	25 mg IM weekly	Alopecia, fatigue, headache, hyperuricemia, nausea, vomiting, stomatitis, anemia, myelosuppression, hepatotoxicity

more than one part of the gastrointestinal tract while skipping other parts. No cure exists for the disease; unless necrosis occurs, surgery has not proved helpful. Continuous monitoring of nutritional status is needed in order to replete any deficiencies that may develop during acute episodes.

Ulcerative colitis is confined to the colon and rectum and primarily affects the mucosa and the submucosa. In some cases, small segments of the terminal ileum may be inflamed, which is referred to as backwash ileitis. It can be accompanied by complications that may be local (involving the colon) or systemic (not directly associated with colon). Surgical treatment is a curative treatment in severe cases. Monitoring of nutritional status is important to prevent the development of anemia secondary to occult blood losses. Table 7.7 presents the agents used to treat ulcerative colitis.

Motility Agents

These agents act to stimulate motility of the upper GI tract without stimulating gastric, biliary, or pancreatic secretions. Usual manifestations of delayed gastric emptying (i.e., nausea, vomiting, heartburn, persistent fullness after meals, anorexia) respond within different time intervals. Significant relief of nausea occurs early and improves over 3 weeks. Relief of vomiting and anorexia may precede the relief of abdominal fullness by ≥ 1 week. Table 7.8 outlines the motility agents used to treat delayed gastric emptying.

Miscellaneous GI Tract Agents

Emetics

Emetic agents are substances that induce vomiting and can be critical in early treatment of the ingestion of some toxic substances, including some common household chemicals. A call to a poison control center may direct the caller to immediately use an emetic. Other emetics are invaluable in treating accidental or intentional overdoses of other drugs and are commonly administered in the hospital emergency room.

Ipecac syrup should be kept in every home with children. The recommended dose is 15 mL (one tablespoonful) followed by two full glasses of water. Repeat once if unsuccessful. Abuse potential exists in patients with bulimia nervosa. Ipecac syrup is used to treat drug overdosage and in certain poisonings. The poison control center needs to be called to see if Ipecac use is possible with the ingested poison.

Nonspecific Antidote

Other agents are used as nonspecific antidotes. Activated charcoal (SuperChar®) works by adsorbing toxic substances from the GI tract and inhibiting GI absorption. Its use is in emergency treatment of poisoning by drugs and chemicals with administration via tube.

The usual dose is 30–100 g or 1 g/kg PO

Table 7.8 Motility Agents

Drug	Indications	Mechanism of Action	Dose	Side Effects
Metoclopramide (Reglan®)	Increases gastric emptying Diabetic gastroparesis Antiemetic for patients receiving chemotherapy Helps pass feeding tubes into the duodenum and jejunum	Stimulate motility of upper GI tract without stimulating gastric, biliary or pancreatic secretions	Diabetic gastroparesis: 10 mg 30 min before meal and at bedtime × 2–8 weeks Symptomatic GERD: 10 to 15 mg PO 4 times daily 30 min before meal and at bedtime Prevention of postoperative nausea and vomiting: 10–20 mg IM near the end of surgery Prevention of chemotherapy-induced emesis: 2 mg/kg slow IV infusion for high emetogenic drugs 1 mg/kg slow IV infusion for low emetogenic drugs	Extrapyramidal symptoms (EPS) including motor restlessness (akathesia), tardive dyskinesia (involuntary movement of the tongue, mouth, face, or jaw)
Cisapride (Propulsid®), restricted access in USA, no longer commercially available	Nocturnal heartburn due to gastroesophageal reflux disease (GERD), heartburn, diabetic gastroparesis and other GI motility problems	Enhance release of acetylcholine at the myenteric plexus	LESP: 20 mg QD GERD: 10 mg four times daily Gastric emptying: 10 mg doses IV or oral (PO) 10 mg orally 3 times daily up to 6 weeks	Headache, diarrhea, abdominal pain, ventricular tachycardia, ventricular fibrillation, torsades de pointes (very rapid ventricular tachycardia) and qt prolongation (heart wave transmission prolongation)
Erythromycin	Improves gastric emptying time and intestinal mobility (used for its side-effect profile) This use has never been submitted for approval to the FDA and is therefore considered outside of the approved indications or off label.	Inhibit bacterial RNA dependent protein synthesis at the chain elongation step (antibiotic)	Initial: 200 mg IV followed by 250 mg orally three times daily, 30 min before meals	Abdominal pain, diarrhea, ventricular arrhythmias, torsades de pointes, qt prolongation, elevated liver transaminases, and cholestatic hepatitis
Dextro-pentothenyl alcohol (Dexpanthenol®)		Unknown	250–500 mg IM repeat in 2 h, followed by doses every 6 h	

Anorectal Preparations

Anorectal preparations are used for the symptomatic relief of the discomfort associated with hemorrhoids and perianal itching or irritation. Maintenance of normal bowel function by proper diet (fiber), adequate fluid intake, and regular exercise are important. In addition, it is important to avoid excessive laxative use. Stool softeners or bulk laxative may be useful adjunctive therapy. A softer stool can reduce mechanical trauma that exacerbates local discomfort. Examples of anorectal preparation agents include but are not limited to the following:

1. Hydrocortisone (Hydrocortisone, Anusol-HC®) will reduce inflammation, itching, and swelling. Apply as directed, usually 10–100 mg 1–2 times/d to affected area.
2. Local anesthetics (Pramoxine HCl® Anusol®) will relieve pain, itching, and irritation. Apply as directed, usually every 3–4 h to affected area; maximum adult dose is 200 mg.
3. Vasoconstrictors (Ephedrine/PazoHemorroid®) act to reduce swelling and congestion of anorectal tissues.
4. Astringents (witch hazel/Tucks®) act by coagulating the protein in skin cells, protecting the underlying tissue, and decreasing the cell volume.

APPETITE ENHANCERS

Numerous disease states can affect the patient's appetite and, therefore, cause already debilitated patients to suffer nutritional compromise. Some common disease states that can affect appetite are cancer and AIDS. These patients, in addition to nutritional advice, may need drug therapy to help them eat. Five different types of appetite enhancers are available: anabolic steroids, antihistamine (off-label use), cannabinoid, progestin derivative, and recombinant human hormone.

Anabolic Steroids (FDA Label Indicated)

Oxandrolone (Oxandrin®) is a synthetic derivative of testosterone. It is used as an adjunctive therapy to promote weight gain in a variety of patient conditions, such as extensive surgery, chronic infection, long-term steroid use, and trauma. This agent has an orphan drug status for HIV-wasting syndrome. The usual dose to promote weight gain is one 2.5-mg tablet two to four times daily, up to 20 mg/d. The typical duration is 2–4 weeks, with repeated courses as needed. Potentially important adverse effects occur with this agent, such as virilization, hepatic dysfunction, lipid abnormalities, edema, weight gain, and psychotic-like symptoms. The patient will need to be monitored closely for any of these adverse effects, with the possibility of dosage reduction or discontinuation as indicated.

Nandrolone-decanoate (Deca-durabolin®) (non–FDA label indicated) is another testosterone derivative used extensively in renal failure patients prior to erythropoietin availability. This agent has been studied in this population and has been associated with improvements in lean body mass and quality of life. It is given intramuscularly at a dose of 100 mg IM weekly.

Cyproheptadine (Periactin®) (non–FDA label indicated) is an antihistamine that is sometimes used to increase patient's appetite. The dose is 4 mg three times to four times daily. A side effect of the medication is appetite stimulation. Other common side effects are drowsiness, headache, nervousness, abdominal pain, and xerostomia. This agent should be used with caution in patients consuming alcohol or depressant medications because these combinations can cause added drowsiness. The patient needs to be educated regarding this before use.

Dronabinol (Marinol®) (FDA label indicated) is a cannabinoid and is useful in increasing the appetite in AIDS patients. Usual dose is 2.5 mg BID (before lunch and dinner) titrated to a maximum of 20 mg/d. Most common side effects are related to the central nervous system (e.g., drowsiness, dizziness, mood changes). This agent should be used cautiously in patients consuming alcohol or depressant medications as combination can cause added drowsiness. Educate the patient prior to use.

Megesterol (Megace®) (FDA label indicated) is a progestin derivative that is used to stimulate patient's appetite in HIV-related cachexia. It is also used as palliative treatment of breast cancer and endometrial carcinomas. The most common side effects are edema, breakthrough bleeding, spotting or changes in menstrual flow, and weakness. The usual dosage is 800 mg/d in divided doses (480–1600 mg/d).

Somatotropin, rh-GH (Serostim®) (FDA label indicated), a recombinant human growth hormone, has been successfully used for the treatment of HIV-associated failure to thrive in children and for AIDS wasting or cachexia in adults. It should be given subcutaneously, and injection sites should be rotated.

Subcutaneous (SC) dosage (Serostim™ only) is another administration form of somatropin. For adults over 55 kg body weight, the recommended dose is 6 mg SC once daily at bedtime. For adults weighing between 45 and 55 kg, the recommended dose is 5 mg SC once daily at bedtime. For adults between 35 and 45 kg, the recommended dose is 4 mg SC once daily at bedtime. For adults less than 35 kg, the recommended dose is 0.1 mg/kg SC once daily at bedtime. The manufacturer reports that, in two small studies, 11 children with HIV-associated failure to thrive received human growth hormone. In one study, a dose of 0.04 mg/kg/d SC for 26 weeks was used in five children ranging in age from 6 to 17 years. A second study used a dose of 0.07 mg/kg/d SC for 4 weeks in six children ages 8 to 14 years. Treatment was reported to be well tolerated and consistent with safety observations in growth hormone treated adults with AIDS wasting.

ENZYME REPLACEMENTS

Digestive enzymes hydrolyze fats, protein, and starch as described in Table 7.9. Administration reduces the fat and nitrogen content in the stool if malabsorption exists. Digestive enzymes exert their primary effects in the duodenum and upper jejunum. They are indicated for enzyme replacement therapy in patients with deficient exocrine pancreatic secretions, cystic fibrosis, chronic pancreatitis, postpancreatec-tomy, ductal obstructions caused by cancer of the pancreas or common bile duct, pancreatic insufficiency, steatorrhea of malabsorption syndrome, and postgastrec-tomy (Billroth II and total) or post-GI surgery (e.g., Billroth II gastroenterostomy).

Table 7.9   Enzyme Replacements and Probiotics for Treatment of Malabsorption

Drug	Indication	Mechanism of Action (MOA)	Major Side Effects
Pancreatic enzymes Cotazym-S® Pancrease MT® Ultrase MT®	Deficient exocrine pancreatic secretions, cystic fibrosis, postgastrectomy, etc.	Increases the digestion of fat, carbohydrate, and fats in the gastrointestinal tract	Diarrhea, nausea, stomach cramps
Levocarnitine (Carnitor®)	Carnitine deficiency	This enzyme is required for the transport of long chain fatty acids into the mitochondria	Gastrointestinal complaints (nausea, vomiting, cramps, diarrhea), drug-related body odor
Lactobacillus (Bacid®, Lactinex®)	Dietary supplement, antibiotic-associated diarrhea (non–FDA label indicated)	Maintain the homeostasis of normal fecal flora during antibiotic administration	

Table 7.9 also presents probiotics used to treat malabsorption as well as digestive enzymes.

Drugs to Treat Metabolic Disorders

Diabetes mellitus (DM) refers to a group of disorders manifested by hyperglycemia. Patients with DM ultimately demonstrate an inability to produce insulin in amounts necessary to meet their metabolic needs. Type 1 diabetes is thought to be secondary to an autoimmune process that causes pancreatic beta cell destruction leading to an inability to produce insulin. In contrast, significant insulin resistance and the inability of beta cells to hypersecrete insulin sufficiently to overcome this resistance characterize type 2 diabetes. Diet, drug therapy, exercise, glucose monitoring, patient education, and self-care are all crucial in the management of DM. All diabetic patients must eat a consistent amount of carbohydrates to support drug therapy and to regulate blood glucose. Dietary modification is important in all types of DM and may also be beneficial to patients with impaired glucose tolerance. Simple avoidance of refined sugars and sweets is not adequate treatment or even necessary. In type 2, even small weight loss can be highly beneficial in obese patients. Gestational diabetes is a secondary form of type 2 diabetes present during pregnancy in women at risk of later development of full-blown type 2. Another form of secondary diabetes may be a result of chronic steroid dosing or of postoperative stress. Impaired glucose tolerance (IGT) may be seen with high glucose intake such as when patients receive total parenteral nutrition. This, too, usually resolves once the causative factor is no longer present.

Insulin

Exogenous insulin replacement therapy is indicated for all type 1 diabetes patients and for type 2 diabetes patients whose hyperglycemia does not respond to

Table 7.10 Pharmacokinetics of Insulin Preparations in Subcutaneous Dosing

Type	Onset of Action (h)	Peak Effect (h)	Duration (h)
Fast Acting			
Insulin lispro (Humalog®)	0.25	1	2–3
Insulin aspart (Novolog®)	0.25	0.75–1.5	3–5
Regular	0.5–1	2–3	4–6
Semilente	0.5–1	3–10	8–18
Intermediate Acting			
NPH (isophane)	2–3	6–9	10–14
Lente (zinc suspension)	2–3	6–12	10–18
Long Acting			
PZI	3–8	14–26	24–40
Ultralente (extended zinc suspension)	6–10	No peak	18–24
Insulin glargine (Lantus®)	6–10	No peak	24+

Note: Major side effects are weight gain and hypoglycemia.

diet or to oral hypoglycemic agents. Many different types of human insulin are used, with varying characteristics in terms of onset of action, time to peak effect, and duration of action. The pharmacokinetics of these various forms of insulin are presented in Table 7.10.

Fast-acting insulin products include regular, insulin lispro (Humalog®), insulin aspart (NovoLog®), and insulin zinc suspension (Semi-lente insulin®). Only regular insulin is appropriate for intravenous use. All insulins, including regular, can be given subcutaneously. Please note that administering regular insulin intravenously results in a considerably shorter duration of action as compared with the same medication given subcutaneously.

Intermediate-acting insulin products include lente and NPH (isophane insulin suspension). Long-acting insulin products include PZI (protamine zinc insulin), ultralente (extended insulin suspension), and insulin glargine (Lantus®). These can be administered to provide a nearly constant level of circulating insulin when given in daily or twice-daily injections.

Insulin mixture therapy using two different insulin types is employed to meet needs for variable insulin delivery while providing a convenient dosing regimen. When two different insulin types are drawn into the same syringe, care must be taken to avoid cross-contamination of the bottle. When regular insulin is used, it should be drawn first. Regular insulin, insulin lispro, insulin aspart, and insulin glargine are clear liquids. All others are white suspensions. Every patient and caregiver who prepares insulin mixtures must keep in mind the simple rule "always cloudy into clear." This will ensure that the solution, regular human insulin, is drawn into the syringe prior to the suspension. The modified insulin suspension will always be drawn second. PZI should not be mixed with other types.

Table 7.11 Dosages and Characteristics of Oral Hypoglycemic Agents

Agents	Onset of Action (h)	Duration of Action (h)	Usual Daily Dose (mg)	Major Side Effects
Sulfonylureas				
Chlorpropamide (Diabinese®)	1	24–60	250–500	Hypoglycemia, weight gain, diarrhea
Glyburide (Diabeta®, Micronase®)	1–2	16–24	5–10	
Glyburide (micronized) (Glynase®)		16–24	3–6	
Glimepiride (Amaryl®)		16–24	4–8	
Biguanides				
Metformin (Glucophage®)		6–12	500–2000	Diarrhea, lactic acidosis, bloating, cramps
Meglitinides				
Repaglinide (Prandin®)	Short	Short	3–6	Low risk of hypoglycemia, weight gain
Nateglinide (Starlix®)	Short	Short	360	
Alpha-Glucosidase Inhibitors				
Acarbose (Precose®)	<30 min	4–6	150–300	Flatus, bloating
Miglitol (Glyset®)	Short	Short	150–300	
Thiazolidinediones				
Rosiglitazone (Avandia®)	Short	Short	2–8	Weight gain, edema
Pioglitazone (Actos®)	Short	Short	2–8 15–45	

Oral Hypoglycemic Agents

Until the 1990s, only one class of oral agents, the sulfonylureas, was available for type 2 diabetes. These agents are now divided into first- and second-generation types. Three other classes of oral agents with differing methods of action are now available to be used alone or in combination with the sulfonylureas. The dosage and characteristics of the oral hypoglycemic agents are presented in Table 7.11.

Sulfonylureas

First-generation sulfonylureas include acetohexamide (Dymelor®), chlorpropamide (Diabinese®), tolazamide (Tolinase®), and tolbutamide (Orinase®).

Second-generation sulfonylureas include glipizide (Glucotrol®), glyburide (Diabeta®, Micronase®), glyburide (micronized) (Glynase®), and glimepiride (Amaryl®).

In general, these agents are well tolerated. The most common side effect is hypoglycemia. Sulfonylureas should be avoided with alcohol because of a possible disulfiram-like reaction (flushing, throbbing pain in the neck and head, shortness of breath, nausea, vomiting, chest pain, palpitations, sweating, anxiety). Also, a combination of some alternative herbal agents with these agents can increase the risk of hypoglycemia (ginseng, garlic, fenugreek, coriander, celery). Glipzide (Glucotrol®) is the only sulfonylurea that needs to be taken 30 min before eating, due to the impaired absorption when taken concomitantly with food.

Biguanides: Metformin (Glucophage®)

This class of drugs, unlike any other class of oral drugs discussed here, is not a hypoglycemic agent, but rather an agent to increase insulin sensitivity in the muscle. The patient needs functioning pancreatic islet cells for this drug to work. The common side effects are gastric disturbances, such as anorexia, nausea, and vomiting. Lactic acidosis is the most serious, yet rare, adverse effect. If this effect occurs, electrolyte disturbances, elevated blood lactic acid levels, an increased anion gap, and decreased blood pH will occur. Another interesting adverse effect is asymptomatic vitamin B_{12} deficiency.

Alpha-Glucosidase Inhibitors

Alpha-glucosidase inhibitors include acarbose (Precose®) and miglitol (Glyset®). These agents delay the absorption of ingested carbohydrates and, thus, are taken with the first bite of each meal. The most common side effect is gastric distress, such as abdominal pain, diarrhea, and flatulence. A very serious side effect is elevated liver function enzymes and hyperbilirubinemia.

Meglitinides include repaglinide (Prandin®) and nateglinide (Starlix®). This is a new class of agents that are similar to sulfonylureas, although the side effect of hypoglycemia is rare. Also, these agents have a very rapid elimination so insulin levels return to normal baseline ranges before the next meal. These agents need to be taken with the first bite of each main meal.

Thiazolidinediones

These agents include troglitazone (Rezulin®), rosiglitazone (Avandia®), and pioglitazone (Actos®). Troglitazone has been withdrawn from the market due to its association with hepatotoxicity, which resulted in some cases of hepatic failure and death. Neither rosiglitazone nor pioglitazone was associated with significant rises in hepatic enzymes. At present, there does not appear to be an increased risk of severe hepatotoxicity with either drug. Thiazolidinediones should not be used in patients with known hepatic dysfunction. The serum alanine aminotransferase (ALT) level should be checked every 2 months during the first year of treatment and every 3 months thereafter. Patients with ALT levels higher than three times the upper limit of normal should not be given this class of drugs.

Lipid Control Agents

Although coronary artery disease (CAD) is not generally regarded as a disease of the GI system, several of the agents used to lower the risks for CAD act on the

Table 7.12 Adult Treatment Panel III Goals for LDL, HDL, and Total Cholesterol

LDL Cholesterol (mg/dl)

<100	Optimal
100–129	Near optimal
130–159	Borderline high
160–189	High
≥190	Very high

Total Cholesterol (mg/dl)

<200	Desirable
200–239	Borderline high
≥240	High

HDL Cholesterol (mg/dl)

<40	Low
≥60	High

GI tract. These drugs may interfere with nutritional status, or diet modification may be necessary to allow effective use of the drugs. Awareness of both the benefits and risks involved with these agents is essential for a good standard of practice.

CAD can lead to one of the most serious health threats to Americans today — myocardial infarction. Numerous studies have shown that lowering serum cholesterol, triglycerides (TG), low-density lipoprotein (LDL), and increasing high density lipoprotein (HDL) can slow or reverse the progression of coronary artery disease and associated complications. The National Heart, Lung, and Blood Institute's adult treatment panel (ATP) III report has recently been published and has further defined cholesterol levels and drug and diet management. The report also has added information on assessing risk for cardiovascular disease. The ATP III classifies LDL, total, and HDL cholesterol based on a patient's 9–12 h fast according to Table 7.12.

Once the physician has obtained the patient's fasting cholesterol levels, the risk factors need to be identified. The guidelines for LDL cholesterol goals and cutoff points for therapeutic lifestyle changes (TLC) and drug therapy for the different categories are stated in Table 7.13.

Agents to Treat Lipid Disorders

The agents used in lipid treatment are in the different categories because of different mechanism of actions and different effects on the lipid panel. The patient should have the lipid panel checked periodically to assess individual response to medication, diet, and exercise.

Although drug therapy is important, a low-fat diet and increased exercise need to be emphasized to the patient. If the LDL is above goal, more stringent dietary guidelines are implemented. The National Cholesterol Education Program (NCEP)

Table 7.13 Guidelines for LDL Goals and Cutoff points for Beginning of Drug
          Therapy

Risk Category	LDL Goal (mg/dl)	LDL at Which to Initiate TLC (mg/dl)	LDL at Which to Consider Drug Therapy (mg/dl)
Coronary heart disease (CHD) or CHD risk equivalents (10-yr risk >20%)	<100	≥100	≥130 (100–129: drug optional)
2+ risk factors	<130	≥130	10-yr risk 10–20% 10-yr risk <10%: ≥160
0–1 risk factor	<160	≥160	≥190 (160–189: LDL-lowering drug optional)

has a set of dietary guidelines for what is usually called the NCEP step two diet, which consists of the patient eating saturated fat <7% of calories and cholesterol <200 mg/d. Increased soluble fiber of 10–25 g/d and plant stanols/sterols to 2 g/d are options to the above dietary changes. Also, weight management and increased physical activity need to be emphasized to the patient. The dietitian is the most appropriate professional to educate the patient about dietary changes, which should be implemented along with the drug therapy.

It is important to note that lipid-lowering agents from different classes are sometimes combined to enhance lipid-lowering effects, the exception being that HMG-CoA reductase inhibitors (statins), which should not be combined with fibric acid derivatives and nicotinic acid agents due to the risk that the patient may develop myositis and rhabdomyolysis. Drug therapy classes include bile acid sequestrants, HMG-CoA reductase inhibitors (statins), nicotinic acid, and fibric acid. With all these agents, liver function tests need to be done periodically or as recommended by the pharmaceutical manufacturer or physician.

Table 7.14 outlines the approximate benefit from the lipid-lowering agents. The physician will assess the patient's lipid panel and decide on a drug product based on many factors, including the relative success for each agent in lowering cholesterol, LDL, and TG and increasing HDL. Table 7.15 describes the classes of lipid-lowering agents, mechanisms of action, and major side effects. The dietitian will need to check for these potential side effects if the patient has gastrointestinal complaints.

Table 7.14 Benefits from Different Drug Classes of Lipid-Lowering
          Agents on the Lipoprotein Profile

Drug Class	Total Cholesterol (%)	LDL (%)	TG (%)	HDL (%)
Bile acid sequestrants	↓20–25	↓20–35	↑5–20	No change
Fibric acid derivatives	↓10	↑ or ↓10	↓40–55	↑10–25
Statins	↓15–35	↓20–40	↓7–25	↑2–15
Nicotinic acid	↓25	↓20	↓40	↑20

Table 7.15 Mechanism of Action (MOA) and Major Side Effects of Lipid-Lowering Agents

Bile Acid Sequestrants	Mechanism of Action (MOA)	Major Side Effects
Colestipol (Colestid®) Colesevelam® Cholestyramine (Questran®)	Binds bile acids in intestine, interrupting enterohepatic circulation of acids	Constipation, bloating, flatulence, unpalatability

The bile acid sequestrants are gritty powders that must be mixed with a beverage (juice, water, milk, or carbonated beverage) (except Questran); Colestid (Colestipol) may have better palatability because it is tasteless and odorless; it is important that the bile acid sequestrants are taken 1 h before or 4 h after ingesting certain medications in order to decrease the possibility that these agents bind and reduce absorption of the other medications.

Fibric Acid Derivatives	Mechanism of Action (MOA)	Major Side Effects
Gemfibrozil (Lopid®) Clofibrate (Atromid-S®) Fenofibrate (Tricor®)	Increase activity of lipoprotein lipase	Nausea, diarrhea, rash, dizziness, gallstones, myopathy

HMG-CoA Reductase Inhibitors (Statins)	Mechanism of Action (MOA)	Major Side Effects
Atorvastatin (Lipitor®) Cerivstatin (Baycol®) removed from market 8/2001 Fluvastatin (Lescol®) Lovastatin (Mevacor®) Pravastatin (Pravachol®) Simvastatin (Zocor®)	Inhibit the early stage of cholesterol synthesis	Constipation, flatulence, dyspepsia, headache, elevations in liver function tests, myopathy, muscle aches, and weakness

These agents are to be taken in the evening, except for atorvastatin due to its long half-life, because cholesterol synthesis occurs at night; lovastatin is the only statin that needs to be taken with food, otherwise administration on an empty stomach will decrease the absorption by 30%.

Nicotinic Acid Derivatives	Mechanism of Action (MOA)	Major Side Effects
Niacin	Inhibit lipolysis and hepatic triglycerides production	Generalized flushing, itching, GI distress, hyperglycemia, hyperuricemia (gout), hepatotoxicity

Alcoholic drinks should be avoided in conjunction with nicotinic acid due to the possible magnification of flushing and itching.

Table 7.16 Common Disease States Producing Fluid
Retention or Fluid Depletion

Conditions That Can Cause Fluid Depletion	Condition That Can Cause Fluid Retention or Overload
Diarrhea	Congestive heart failure
Diabetes mellitus	Edema
Diabetes insipidus	Renal disease
Vomiting	Hepatic cirrhosis
Adrenal disease	Reduced albumin synthesis (malnutrition, liver disease)
Bartter's syndrome	Adult respiratory distress syndrome

DRUGS AFFECTING FLUID BALANCE

Many drugs and disease states can alter fluid balance. When fluid balance is altered, nutritional consequences may arise. Given the frequent use of these drugs, especially in the elderly, the potential impact of these drugs is important to recognize. Some of the more commonly used drugs and disease states encountered in everyday clinical practice are described next. See Table 7.16 for more details.

Diuretics

Diuretics as a class can cause fluid depletion due to different mechanisms of action on sections of the kidney. The diuretics are indicated to enhance the elimination of fluid in patients with certain disease states, including congestive heart failure (CHF), hypertension, edema, and urinary retention. The carbonic anhydrase inhibitors are used primarily to treat glaucoma, refractory seizures, acute altitude sickness, and (non–FDA label indicated) metabolic alkalosis.

The different classes of diuretics cause different electrolyte abnormalities. It is important to know that if the patient is on a diuretic, he or she may also be on an electrolyte replacement. Many combination products are available that are formulated to minimize electrolyte imbalances.

The four classes of diuretics include loop, thiazide and thiazide-like, carbonic anhydrase, and potassium sparing; the possible electrolyte imbalances they can cause are discussed next.

Loop Diuretics

Electrolyte changes that may be produced by loop diuretics are hypokalemia, hyponatremia, hypochloremia, hypercalciuria, and hyperuricemia. Drugs in this class include furosemide (Lasix®), ethacrynic acid (Edecrin®), bumetanide (Bumex®), and torsemide (Demadix®)

Thiazide and Related Diuretics

These agents can cause the same electrolyte problems as for loop diuretics, except for hypercalcemia. Specific agents are chlorothiazide (Diuril®), hydrochlorothiazide (HydroDIURIL®), metolazone (Zaroxolyn ®, Mykrox®), and indapamide (Lozol®).

Potassium-Sparing Diuretics

Electrolyte changes in this class are the opposite of the hypokalemia of the first two classes. Hyperkalemia is the electrolyte disorder more likely to occur. Specific agents in this class are amiloride (Midamor®), spironolactone (Aldactone®), and triameterene (Dyrenium®).

Carbonic Anhydrase Inhibitors

Although used for different disorders, similar electrolyte changes may occur including hyperchloremic metabolic acidosis and hypokalemia. The current agent in this class is acetazolamide (Diamox®).

Corticosteroids

Corticosteroids can cause fluid retention. Corticosteroids are used in a variety of medical disorders such as arthritis, asthma, and dermatological and connective tissue disorders. Corticosteroids with the most pronounced mineralocorticoid properties are more likely to cause fluid retention. Common corticosteroids that can cause fluid retention are cortisone (Cortone®), hydrocortisone (Cortef®), prednisone (Orasone®), and prednisolone (Prelone®).

Nonsteroidal Antiinflammatory Drugs (NSAIDs)

These agents are used to treat inflammatory conditions and pain. NSAIDs are used quite often by patients, since they are available both over the counter (OTC) and through prescription. These agents can cause sodium retention and, thus, fluid retention. Some of the more commonly used NSAIDs are ibuprofen (Motrin®, Advil®), naproxen (Naprosyn®, Aleve®), and indomethacin (Indocin®)

Caution: Because of its propensity to cause serious bleeding in the GI tract and at other sites, this drug must be used with extreme caution—if at all—in older patients and in any patient who has shown a bleeding diathesis. It is also not appropriate for combination therapy with any drug known to inhibit coagulation.

Antihypertensive Agents

The three classes of antihypertensives that can cause fluid retention and thus, at times, increase blood pressure are $alpha_2$ agonists, $alpha_1$ adrenergic blockers, and vasodilators. The patient needs to be monitored closely for the side effect of fluid retention, especially with agents that can affect the patient's medical status. The following agents are the ones most likely to cause fluid retention: methyldopa (Aldomet®), prazosin (Minipress®), terazosin (Hytrin®), and doxazosin (Cardura®).

High Sodium Content Medications and Dietary Supplements

Numerous classes of prescription and OTC drugs may cause fluid retention, secondary to the high sodium content of the product. Dietitians need to look for these agents when reviewing a patient's chart if fluid retention and/or increasing sodium blood levels are seen. At times, the dietitian may need to alter the patient's diet due to the necessity to continue medications that cause fluid retention. A list of the more common agents to cause fluid retention, either due to the active or inactive ingredients, include ticarcillin (Ticar®) and some other penicillin derivatives, citric acid/sodium bicarbonate/potassium bicarbonate (Alka-Seltzer®), sodium polystyrene sulfonate (Kayexalate®), and sodium phosphate/sodium biphosphate (Fleet Enema®, Phospho-Soda®).

Table 7.16 provides a list of the more common disease states that can cause either fluid retention or fluid depletion. The patient's disease state will need to be considered when planning a patient's diet. For example, patients with CHF may have a fluid restriction and may need calorically dense foods (e.g., fortified puddings and sauces) rather than nutritional supplements (Boost®, Ensure®) with a caloric density of approximately 1 kcal/mL.

DIABETES INSIPIDUS

This is a hypothalamic-pituitary disorder in which a deficiency in vasopressin (antidiuretic hormone, ADH) causes excretion of copious and very dilute urine. The cause of diabetes insipidus is a neurological disease process affecting the hypothalamus, posterior pituitary gland, or the supraoptic and paraventricular nuclei. The patient ingests large amounts of water (polydipsia) and urinates large amounts of fluid (polyuria). Other characteristics of this disorder are very dilute urine (specific gravity <1.005) and osmolality (<200 mOsm/L.)

Treatment

The patient will need fluid replacement, otherwise dehydration and hypovolemia can ensue rapidly. The initial treatment is to give the patient water by mouth, or, in cases where the patient is unable to drink, intravenous hydration. The patient may also need administration of an antidiuretic hormone in order to slow the renal water losses. Depending on the severity of the patient's condition, the dose and route of administration differ.

Desmopressin acetate (DDAVP®) is given intranasally in children 3 months to 12 years, usually 5 µg/d in one administration, but a range of 5–30 µg/d may be used. Intravenously, children may receive 0.3 µg/kg by slow infusion over 15–30 min. For adults, IV or SC administration of 2–4 µg/d may be given in two doses or 1/10 of the maintenance intranasal dose with a range of 5–40 µg/d 1–3 times/d.

Vasopressin (Pitressin®) is usually given to children as 2.5–10 units vasopressin IM or SC 2–4 times/d as needed. For adults, 5–10 units vasopressin IM or SC 2–4 times/d (dosage range 5–60 units/d). Another form of administration is continuous

IV infusion at a rate of 0.5 milliunits/kg/h (0.0005 units/kg/h), and double dose as needed every 30 min to maximum of 0.01 unit/kg/h.

The therapeutic effect of vasopressin is decreased urine output and increased urine osmolarity. Side effects may include pounding sensation in the head, dizziness, chest pain, myocardial infarction, abdominal cramps, nausea, vomiting, paleness, perioral blanching of the skin, and trembling.

Nonhormonal therapy may also be effective in reducing polyuria. Thiazide diuretics and ADH-releasing drugs, such as clofibrate, carbamazepine, and chlorpropamide, are the most common agents. The ADH-releasing drugs are effective in patients with partial diabetes insipidus.

Syndrome of Inappropriate Antidiuretic Hormone Secretion (SIADH)

The syndrome of inappropriate antidiuretic hormone secretion (SIADH) is characterized by inappropriately elevated urinary osmolarity (usually >200 mOsm/L) relative to plasmaosmolarity and hypotonic hyponatremia elevated urinary sodium (typically >20 mEq/L), while other indices remain normal including normal renal, adrenal, and thyroid function; normal acid–base balance; euvolemia; and normal potassium level.

Clinical conditions associated with SIADH include malignant tumors, pulmonary disease, and CNS disorders. Acute treatment of SIADH should be reserved for the patients with severe, symptomatic hyponatremia (serum sodium <110–115 meq/L). This may be accomplished by initiating and maintaining a rapid diuresis with IV diuretics followed by IV replacement of urinary sodium and potassium losses.

Chronic Treatment of SIADH

Water restriction to 500–1000 mL daily is the mainstay of chronic management. Demeclocycline (Declomycin®) (300–600 mg PO, BID) may be effective when restriction alone is unsuccessful; its onset of action for diuresis may be delayed for several days. This drug should be administered 1 h before or 2 h after food or milk with plenty of fluid. The mechanism of action is to reduce the renal response to vasopressin. Side effects include photosensitivity, nausea, and diarrhea.

PRINT RESOURCES

The following references are excellent sources of additional information on the drugs discussed.

1. Riley, M.R., et al., *Drugs Facts and Comparisons,* Kluwer, St. Louis, 1999.
2. Lacy, C., et al., *Drug Information Handbook,* 6th ed., Lexi-Comp, Hudson, OH, 1999.
3. Woodley, M. and Whelan, A., *The Washington Manual,* 30th ed., Department of Medicine, Washington University, 1998.
4. Dipiro, J.T., et al., *Pharmacotherapy Handbook,* 2nd ed., Appleton and Lange, Stamford, CT, 2000.

5. Dipiro, J.T., et al., *Pharmacotherapy: A Pathophysiologic Approach,* 2nd ed., Norwalk, CT, 1993.
6. Beers, M.H. and Berkow, R., *The Merck Manual of Diagnosis and Therapy,* 17th ed., Merck & Co., Inc., Whitehouse Station, NJ, 1999.
7. Micromedex®, online version, 2002.

INTERNET RESOURCES

http://www.pharminfo.com
http://www.vh.org
http://www.aoa.dhhs.gov
http://www.diabetes.org
http://www.powerpak.com
http://www.pharmacytimes.com
http://www.eatright.org
http://www.drugtopic.com
http://www.nutritioncare.org
http://www.asns.org
http://www.am-coll-nutr.org
http://www.micromedex.com
http://www.rxlist.com
http://www.emedicine.com

CHAPTER 8

Drug Interactions in Nutrition Support

Kathleen M. Strausburg

CONTENTS

Nutrition support refers to the provision of nutrients via the intravenous route (parenteral nutrition) or through a tube that accesses the gastrointestinal tract and delivers nutrients distally to the mouth (enteral nutrition).[1] These methods of feeding are indicated in a select group of patients who suffer either partial or total dysfunction of the gastrointestinal tract.[2] Examples are given in Table 8.1. Parenteral nutrition entails providing a completely synthetic diet in which the amount of each nutrient is specifically prescribed and can be adjusted based on individual nutrient needs.[3] Enteral nutrition is provided using formulations with nutrients in fixed amounts that

Table 8.1   Examples of Indications for Nutrition Support

Enteral Nutrition

Cancer/bone marrow transplant
Critical illness (trauma, burn injury, sepsis)
HIV infection
Inflammatory bowel disease
Neurologic impairment (traumatic brain injury)
Organ failure (kidney, liver, lungs, pancreas)

Parenteral Nutrition

Cancer/bone marrow transplant
Enterocutaneous fistulae
Gastrointestinal ischemia
Inflammatory bowel disease
Intestinal obstruction
Necrotizing enterocolitis
Organ failure (kidney, liver, lungs, pancreas)
Short bowel syndrome

Note: HIV = human immunodeficiency virus.

are product specific. The amount of each nutrient in enteral feeding formulas may be supplemented, but may not otherwise be altered.[4]

Patients requiring nutrition support frequently have underlying alterations in their nutrition status including protein–calorie malnutrition and specific nutrient deficiencies. One goal of nutrition support is to replete these deficiencies. Achieving this goal may be complicated by coexisting diseases that affect nutrient requirements and nutrient tolerance (e.g., renal failure, hepatic failure, pancreatitis, or short bowel syndrome). Supervening acute illness, such as infection accompanied by hypermetabolism, may also complicate the provision of adequate nutrients. Furthermore, this patient population commonly receives numerous medications as part of the management of their acute and chronic illnesses. Schneider determined that the concomitant use of medications for patients receiving parenteral nutrition averaged 4.2 medications per patient. It was also noted that 77% of these medications had potential side effects that could affect the parenteral nutrition therapy.[5] Driscoll has also observed a high usage of medications with a high likelihood for drug-induced metabolic disorders in critically ill patients receiving parenteral nutrition.[6] In a study of clinical nutrition patients that included patients receiving enteral and parenteral nutrition, a 30% incidence of drug-related problems has been described.[7]

Patients receiving nutrition support are at increased risk for the occurrence of drug-induced abnormalities in nutrition status and nutrient balance. Several factors contributing to this increased risk have been discussed and are summarized in Table 8.2.[7,8] These drug interactions are likely to result in a clinically significant event requiring adjustments either in the offending medication or in nutrient intake. This chapter reviews those drug interactions that are most likely to occur in patients receiving nutrition support and provides strategies to prevent as well as recognize and manage them.

Table 8.2   Risk Factors for Drug Interactions in Patients Receiving Nutrition Support

Acute illness with hypermetabolic stress
Chronic illness
Inability to take medications via the oral route
Multiple medications
Preexisting specific nutrient deficiencies (e.g., vitamins, trace minerals, electrolytes)
Protein–calorie malnutrition

DRUG-INDUCED METABOLIC ALTERATIONS IN NUTRITION SUPPORT PATIENTS

Alterations in macronutrient metabolism, fluid and electrolyte balance, and micronutrient balance are known side effects of nutrition support therapy.[9,10] These side effects may either be caused by or exacerbated by the medications the patient concurrently receives. Monitoring nutrition support therapy requires frequent evaluation for clinical signs and symptoms associated with such metabolic alterations, appropriate laboratory assessment, and a thorough investigation to identify the cause. In the case of medications, numerous possible causes exist.[8,11–27] See Tables 8.3, 8.4, and 8.5 for more details. These drug-induced metabolic alterations may occur in both enterally and parenterally fed patients.

Table 8.3   Alterations in Macronutrient Metabolism Associated with Drug Therapy*

Hyperglycemia	Hypertriglyceridemia
Chlorpromazine (Thorazine®)	Cyclosporine (Sandimmune®)
Corticosteroids	Dexamethasone (Decadron®)
Cyclosporine (Sandimmune®)	Propranolol (Inderal®)
Dopamine (Intropin®)	Propofol (Diprivan®)
Furosemide (Lasix®)	Tacrolimus (Prograf®)
Indomethacin (Indocin®)	
Meperidine (Demerol®)	**Increased Urinary Nitrogen Excretion**
Norepinephrine/pressors	
Octreotide (Sandostatin®)	Antineoplastic agents
Pentamidine (Pentam®)	Corticosteroids
Phenytoin (Dilantin®)	
Propranolol (Inderal®)	**Decreased Urinary Nitrogen Excretion**
Protease inhibitors	
Tacrolimus (Prograf®)	Pentobarbital (Nembutal®)
Thiazide diuretics	
Thyroid preparations	**Decreased Metabolic Rate**
	Morphine (Duramorph®)
Hypoglycemia	Pentobarbital (Nembutal®)
Disopyramide (Dipyridamole®)	
Haloperidol (Haldol®)	
Octreotide (Sandostatin®)	

* The trade names are examples and may be only one of many products.

Table 8.4   Alterations in Electrolyte Balance Associated with Drug Therapy*

Potassium

Hypokalemia

Amphotericin B (Fungizone®)	Laxatives
Carbamazepine (Tegretol®)	Loop diuretics
Corticosteroids	Metoclopramide (Reglan®)
Digoxin (Lanoxin®)	Salicylates
Inhaled beta agonists	Theophylline (Theo-Dur®)
Insulin	Thiazide diuretics
Lactulose (Chronulac®)	Trimethoprim (Trimpex®)

Hyperkalemia

ACE inhibitors	NSAIDs
Amiloride (Midamor®)	Procainamide (Procan-SR®)
Cyclosporine (Sandimmune®)	Propranolol (Inderal®)
Enalapril (Vasotec®)	Spironolactone (Aldactone®)
Heparin	Succinylcholine

Sodium

Hyponatremia

Cisplatin (Platinol-AQ®)	Mannitol
Clofibrate (Atromid-S®)	Salicylates
Cyclophosphamide (Cytoxan®)	Spironolactone (Aldactone®)
Heparin	Vasopressin (Pitressin®)
Laxatives	Vincristine (Oncovin®)

Hypernatremia

Clonidine (Catapres®)	Lactulose (Chronulac®)
Methyldopa (Dopar®)	Ticarcillin (Ticar®)

Calcium

Hypocalcemia

Cisplatin (Platinol-AQ®)	Laxatives
Corticosteroids	Loop diuretics
Foscarnet (Foscavir®)	Phenobarbital (Luminal®)
Gentamicin (Garamycin®)	

Hypercalcemia

Thiazide diuretics

Magnesium

Hypomagnesemia

Aminoglycosides	Lactulose (Chronulac®)
Amphotericin B (Fungizone®)	Laxatives
Cisplatin (Platinol-AQ®)	Loop diuretics
Cyclosporine (Sandimmune®)	Thiazide diuretics

Table 8.4   Alterations in Electrolyte Balance Associated with Drug Therapy* *(Continued)*

Hypermagnesemia

Lithium (Lithobid®)

Phosphorus

Hypophosphatemia

Aluminum-containing antacids	Corticosteroids
Sucralfate (Carafate®)	Theophylline (Theo-Dur®)

Hyperphosphatemia

Clindamycin (Cleocin®)
Propofol (Diprivan®)
Phosphate enemas (Fleet's Phospho-Soda®)

Note: ACE = angiotensin-converting enzyme; NSAIDs = nonsteroidal antiin-flammatory drugs.

* The trade names are examples and may be only one of many products.

Hyperglycemia is the most common metabolic complication associated with parenteral nutrition.[9] Several factors predispose nutrition support patients to this adverse effect, including critical illness and excess dextrose administration. Several of the listed drugs in Table 8.3, however, may contribute to hyperglycemia, most frequently corticosteroids. Other offending drugs that are administered to patients receiving nutrition support include thiazide diuretics (e.g., hydrochlorthiazide HydroDiuril®) and loop diuretics (e.g., furosemide, Lasix®), cyclosporine (Sandimmune®), tacrolimus (Prograf®),[23–25] and octreotide (Sandostatin®).[16,17] The mechanism by which drug-induced hyperglycemia occurs varies, but frequently includes decreased insulin production, decreased insulin release, increased insulin resistance, or increased insulin clearance. Hyperglycemia may also occur as a result of excess dextrose administration in nutrition support patients whose calorie requirements have been overestimated.[9] Excess dextrose administration, however, may inadvertently occur when intravenous fluids, other than the parenteral nutrition admixtures, are administered in quantities sufficient to contribute significant kilocalories (intravenous 5% dextrose solutions provide 340 kcal per liter). This may occur when patients have large fluid requirements that are met by intravenous fluids or when numerous intravenous medications are delivered via a dextrose-containing solution. These hidden dextrose kilocalories may prove especially significant in neonates and infants, and in any patient with severe impairment of glucose metabolism. They should be counted as part of the daily caloric intake. Provision of hidden dextrose kilocalories will also occur when patients are receiving peritoneal dialysis using large volumes of intraperitoneally infused dextrose-based solutions that can be absorbed via the blood vessels in the omentum.

It has also been demonstrated that corticosteroids have a deleterious effect on protein metabolism in patients receiving nutrition support. Dexamethasone (Decadron®) use for patients with major head injuries resulted in increased urinary nitrogen losses.[20] Similarly, prednisone (Deltasone®) and methylprednisolone (Medrol®) use in kidney transplant patients was correlated with a significant increase in protein catabolic rate that decreased coincidentally with decreasing the corticosteroid dose.[14] Conversely, pentobarbital (Nembutal®) has been shown to decrease urinary nitrogen excretion in critically ill patients.[26]

Lipid metabolism, as measured by serum triglyceride concentrations, is affected by several medications. Hypertriglyceridemia has been shown to occur in transplant patients treated with cyclosporine and tacrolimus.[23,24] This alteration in lipid metabolism is thought to reflect drug-induced posttransplant diabetes mellitus. In extremely low-birth-weight infants receiving parenteral nutrition with intravenous lipids, increased serum triglyceride concentrations occurred in patients receiving Dexamethasone (Decadron®), but not in the placebo group.[18] Proposed causative mechanisms included increased synthesis of lipid-rich lipoproteins, reduced lipoprotein lipase activity, or altered insulin secretion. Propofol (Diprivan®), an anesthetic and sedative agent, has been shown to produce hypertriglyceridemia when given in large, continuous doses that result in the concurrent intake of lipid from the vehicle in which the drug is delivered.[19] Propofol is frequently used in the critical care setting to sedate intubated patients. It is a lipophilic drug solubilized in a 10% soybean oil emulsion.[22] The soybean oil provides 1.1 kcal/mL which, at usual adult doses of propofol for sedation in an intensive care unit, can easily result in a provision of 500 kcal or more per day. These sedative doses may be continued for several days and, when given in conjunction with enteral or parenteral nutrition, have resulted in overfeeding and hypertriglyceridemia.[19,28]

Macronutrient metabolism in nutrition support patients may also be altered by sedative drugs that decrease metabolic rate. Pentobarbital (Nembutal®) is best known for this effect in neurosurgical patients.[15] Pentobarbital is used for patients with traumatic brain injury or with Reye's Syndrome to reduce intracranial pressure. These patients tend to be hypermetabolic and hypercatabolic, and this response is blunted by the continuous infusion of pentobarbital, which induces a pharmacologic coma.

Many drugs are implicated in clinically significant electrolyte imbalance (see Table 8.4). Several drugs stand out, however, as being the most frequent culprits in nutrition support patients. These drugs include aluminum-containing antacids, amphotericin B (Fungizone®), aminoglycosides, carbamazepine (Tegretol®), cisplatin (Platinol-AQ®), cyclosporine (Sandimmune®), thiazide and loop diuretics, lactulose (Chronulac®), sorbitol, and sucralfate (Carafate®). Total body sodium depletion with resultant hyponatremia may occur from renal wasting of sodium secondary to cisplatin and thiazide and loop diuretics. Lactulose-induced diarrhea may result in a loss of water in excess of sodium with resultant hypernatremia. Lactulose (Chronulac®), amphotericin B (Fungizone®), carbamazepine (Tegretol®), thiazide, and loop diuretics may all cause hypokalemia. Loop diuretics also may cause hypocalcemia via urinary wasting, whereas thiazide diuretics may cause hypercalcemia via renal retention. Hypophosphatemia, to which malnourished patients are predisposed especially during refeeding,[29] may be precipitated by sucralfate (Carafate®) and aluminum-containing antacids.[30] These drugs bind phosphorus in the stomach and prevent its absorption and reabsorption. Magnesium balance is primarily affected by drugs that enhance renal excretion of this mineral. Aminoglycosides, amphotericin B

Table 8.5 Alterations in Micronutrient Balance Associated with Drug Therapy*

Micronutrient Imbalance	Offending Drug(s)
Copper deficiency	Penicillamine (Cuprimine®)
Cyanocobalamin	Lansoprazole (Prevacid®)
	Omeprazole (Prilosec®)
Folic acid deficiency	Anticonvulsants [e.g., Phenobarbital (Luminal®), phenytoin (Dilantin®)]
	Antineoplastics [e.g., methotrexate (Mexate®)]
	Sulfasalazine (Azulfidine®)
Pyridoxine deficiency	Cathartics
	Isoniazid (INH®)
Thiamine deficiency	Antacids
	Furosemide (Lasix®)
Vitamin C deficiency	Cathartics
Vitamin D deficiency	Anticonvulsants
	Cathartics
Vitamin K deficiency	Antibiotics
	Warfarin (Coumadin®)
Zinc deficiency	Amphotericin B (Fungizone®)
	Cisplatin (Platinol-AQ®)
	Loop diuretics
	Penicillamine (Cuprimine®)
	Thiazide diuretics

* The trade names are examples and may be only one of many products.

(Fungizone®), cisplatin, loop and thiazide diuretics, and cyclosporine (Sandimmune®) can all cause urinary magnesium wasting.

The micronutrients listed in Table 8.5 may be affected similarly to electrolytes, especially by drugs that enhance renal excretion. For example, amphotericin B (Fungizone®), cisplatin (Platinol-AQ®), and loop and thiazide diuretics all cause increased urinary zinc losses. Furosemide (Lasix®) has been found to increase the urinary excretion of thiamin. Its chronic administration can produce thiamin deficiency.[31] However, most drug-induced alterations result from interference with absorption or metabolism of the micronutrient. Chronic use of omeprazole (Prilosec®) or lansoprazole (Prevacid®) results in decreased absorption of cyanocobalamin.[32] Sulfasalazine (Azulfidine®) a staple treatment of inflammatory bowel disease, impairs the absorption of folic acid. Folic acid supplementation should be routinely given when sulfasalazine (Azulfidine®) is used. Isoniazid (INH®) acts as a pyridoxine antagonist by competing with enzyme systems that are important to that vitamin's role in neurologic function. This effect can be prevented by providing supplemental pyridoxine coincident with isoniazid. Whereas many other drug-induced micronutrient alterations are theoretically possible, most are usually not clinically significant. The exception to this may be the malnourished patient with preexisting, subclinical deficiencies who subsequently requires nutrition support. Drug interactions that would be insignificant in a healthy, well-nourished individual may be important in this setting and, therefore, should be considered as part of the assessment and monitoring of each patient.

DRUG INTERACTIONS SPECIFIC TO PATIENTS RECEIVING PARENTERAL NUTRITION

Parenteral nutrition is a highly technical form of nutrition therapy. Preparation of a sterile, stable nutrient admixture requires adherence to strict compounding guidelines.[33] Although standardized formulas exist for parenteral nutrition, the advent of automated compounding has facilitated the use of more individualized parenteral nutrient admixtures.[3] Knowledge of nutrient compatibility (e.g., calcium and phosphorus; dextrose and lipid) has defined the limits for these individualized formulas.

In addition to nutrient compatibility, the compatibility of intravenous medications added directly to the parenteral nutrient admixture may be of interest. The advantages of admixing medications with the parenteral nutrient admixture include conservation of fluids in fluid-restricted patients, fewer violations of the intravenous catheter, and reduced drug preparation and administration time. These advantages are, in most cases, largely outweighed by the primary disadvantage that limited information exists about the compatibility of each individualized parenteral nutrient admixture with each potential drug additive in these complex nutrient systems. Several reference sources exist that provide a comprehensive overview of existing intravenous drug–nutrient compatibility and stability data.[34,35] When applying these data to an individual patient situation, seldom is there an exact match among the test parenteral nutrient admixture, the desired drug dosage and delivery schedule, and the patient's needs. It becomes necessary to extrapolate from the test circumstances to the clinical circumstances where both represent highly complex physiochemical systems. Therefore, as a general guideline, the parenteral nutrient admixture should not be used as a drug delivery vehicle. There are two notable exceptions—regular human insulin and histamine$_2$-receptor antagonists [i.e., cimetidine (Tagamet®), ranitidine (Zantac®), and famotidine (Pepcid®)]. These drugs have been shown to be compatible with dextrose–amino acid–based and dextrose–amino acid–lipid–based parenteral nutrient admixtures.[36,37] Also, both the histamine$_2$-receptor antagonists and insulin can be appropriately administered via either a continuous or cyclic infusion schedule. In the case of all other drugs, the original drug-specific data need to be carefully evaluated to compare the test conditions to the clinical conditions before extrapolating to an individual patient.

Many drugs that are not compatible or stable for the duration of the parenteral nutrient admixture infusion (usually 24 h per day for a continuous infusion and 10–14 h per day for a cyclic infusion) may be stable for a limited time exposure. When a medication is coinfused with the parenteral nutrient admixture (i.e., given as an intravenous piggyback [IVPB]), the required duration of compatibility and stability decreases to minutes rather than hours. Many drugs have been shown to be compatible with parenteral nutrient admixtures of varying compositions delivered via IVPB.[34–37] As in the case of admixing drugs directly into the parenteral nutrient admixture, however, the original drug-specific data need to be evaluated and the test conditions compared to the clinical conditions before extrapolating to an individual patient. Delivering drugs via IVPB with the parenteral nutrient admixture is most often beneficial in patients with limited intravenous access, such as critically ill pediatric and neonatal patients.[38] In addition to the potential compatibility and stability issues, the IVPB method of drug administration also carries an increased risk of catheter contamination due to frequent violations of the sterile catheter and intravenous delivery system.

DRUG INTERACTIONS SPECIFIC TO PATIENTS RECEIVING ENTERAL NUTRITION

The enterally fed patient will benefit in several circumstances from having medications delivered via the feeding tube. These circumstances include the patient who is intubated, comatose, or otherwise unable to voluntarily swallow oral medications and has no or limited intravenous access. Guidelines for safe and effective administration of medications via a feeding tube need to be general because of the vast number of enteral feeding formula–medication combinations and the frequent introduction of new or reformulated enteral feeding formulas and new medications into the healthcare market. Understanding the factors that contribute to problems with medications, tube feeding formulas, and the feeding tube are essential to interpreting specific formula–medication data and extrapolating these findings to an individual patient.

Drug Absorption and Feeding Tube Position Issues

Several technical aspects of enteral feeding are important to drug administration. The anatomical placement of the feeding tube can dictate which medications can be administered. The distal end of the feeding tube may be in the stomach, duodenum, or jejunum. Medications that are dependent on the acid environment of the stomach, such as ketoconazole, may have impaired absorption if they are given via a duodenal or jejunal feeding tube. Both antacids and sucralfate (Carafate®) act locally within the stomach to prevent or treat gastric ulcers.[22] Thus, they are only effective when given by mouth or via a tube where the tip is in the stomach. Alterations in drug absorption may also occur when drugs are administered beyond the usual site of absorption. This may result in subtherapeutic serum drug concentrations and, in some cases, treatment failure.

One example of this is ciprofloxacin. Ciprofloxacin (Cipro®) is a fluoroquinolone antibiotic that is effective in the treatment of severe systemic infections. It is available for intravenous administration as well as in tablet form for oral administration. The oral form of ciprofloxacin has excellent bioavailability when given by mouth. Ciprofloxacin has been studied extensively in enterally fed patients.[39,40] The clinical circumstances under which it has been studied include administration via gastrostomy; duodenal and jejunostomy tubes; delivery of enteral feeding via continuous, intermittent, and bolus infusion; mixed with the enteral feeding formula; or mixed in water and given directly via the feeding tube and with a variety of enteral feeding products. Administration via jejunostomy tube produced the most profound effects with a 33% decrease in bioavailability and a 59% decrease in peak serum concentration.[41] Furthermore, a 25% decrease in absorption occurs when ciprofloxacin is given via continuous feeding with a significant decrease in peak serum concentrations. Therefore, ciprofloxacin should be given via the feeding tube only after an initial course (i.e., 5 to 6 d) of intravenously administered ciprofloxacin. The enteral feeding formula needs to be discontinued for 1–2 h before and after ciprofloxacin administration.[22,39] Ciprofloxacin should not be given via jejunostomy tube. It is thought that these same guidelines should be applied to the other fluoroquinolone antibiotics such as ofloxacin (Floxin®) and levofloxacin (Levaquin®).[39]

Phenytoin (Dilantin®) is another drug where absorption is affected by enteral feeding, and, therefore, its efficacy is dependent on timing of administration. Phenytoin has been studied extensively under a variety of enteral feeding circumstances.[42–46] The absorption of phenytoin is decreased in the presence of enteral feeding formula by 60–70%, with a resultant decrease in serum drug concentrations of 50–75%. Thus, the enteral feeding infusion needs to be held for 1–2 h before and after phenytoin administration. Also, phenytoin should not be given via a jejunostomy tube.[45]

There are other medications that typically should be taken on an empty stomach for optimal absorption [e.g., ampicillin (Polycillin®), verapamil (Calan®), captopril (Capoten®), theophylline (various), tetracycline (Sumycin®), and rifampin (Rifadin®)]. This may require interruption of continuously infused gastric enteral feeding. The gastric tube feeding should be held 30–60 min before and after the medication is administered.[47] In all cases that require interruption of the continuously infused enteral feeding, the rate of feeding administration needs to be adjusted to assure that the desired 24-h volume of feeding is delivered. Continuously infused small bowel feedings do not need to be held (except with phenytoin and fluoroquinolone antibiotics as previously discussed) because there is no reservoir in which enteral feeding formula can collect. The feeding may be discontinued just prior to medication administration in this setting.

Warfarin (Coumadin®) efficacy may be decreased when this drug is administered via tube in continuously fed patients.[12,48] It is unclear whether this is primarily due to interference with the absorption of warfarin in the presence of enteral feeding formula or due to vitamin K antagonism of warfarin activity. A sufficient amount of vitamin K (e.g., 140–150 µg per day) needs to be delivered via the enteral feeding formula for there to be antagonism of warfarin activity, and most commercial formulas fall below this dose. Warfarin efficacy should be monitored via the international normalized ratio (INR), and the dosage of warfarin adjusted as needed to attain the desired INR. When the patient is transitioned from enteral feeding to an oral diet, the dosage of warfarin may need readjustment.

MEDICATION DOSAGE FORM ISSUES

Drugs are available in numerous oral dosage forms as presented in Tables 8.6 and 8.7.[40,47–53] Each oral dosage form possesses unique pharmaceutical characteristics that define the manner in which the drug is released and where and how it is absorbed. Alterations in dosage form may interfere with a drug's efficacy, potency, or tolerance. Numerous factors specific to each available dosage form must be

Table 8.6 Guidelines for Medication Dosage Forms That Can Be Administered via an Enteral Feeding Tube*

Dosage Form	Guidelines for Administration Via Enteral Feeding Tube	Example Medications
Oral liquids: elixir, solution, suspension	This dosage form is usually the best choice for drug administration via the feeding tube; if liquid is thick or has a high osmolality (>300 mOsm/kg), dilute with water before administering.	Dexamethasone elixir (Decadron®), aminophylline liquid (Theon®), diphenhydramine elixir (Benadryl®), methyldopa suspension (Dopar®)
Compressed tablets	Crush to a fine powder and mix into a suspension with 10–15 mL water.	Ciprofloxacin (Cipro®), captopril (Capoten®)
Hard gelatin capsules filled with a fine powder	Open capsule and mix contents with 10–15 mL water.	Doxycycline (Vibramycin®), ampicillin (Polycillin®)
Hard gelatin capsules filled with microencapsulated contents	Open capsule and pour contents down feeding tube; do not crush pellets; flush tube with water; in the case of omeprazole (Prilosec®) and lansoprazole (Prevacid®) via gastric tube, tube should be flushed with an acidic juice (e.g., apple, orange, tomato); in the case of omeprazole and lansoprazole via a small bowel tube, tube should be flushed with an alkaline liquid (e.g., water, milk, or saline).	Diltiazem (Cardizem®), ferrous gluconate (Fergon®), fluoxetine (Prozac®), verapamil (Calan®)
Soft gelatin capsules	Poke a pinhole in one end of the capsule and squeeze out the contents; mix contents with 10–15 mL water; alternatively, capsule contents may be aspirated with a needle and syringe and then mixed with water; or capsule may be dissolved in 10–30 mL warm water (may take up to 1 h; remove undissolved gelatin prior to administering medication via the feeding tube).	Nifedipine (Procardia®), chloral hydrate (Noctec®), acetazolamide (Diamox Sequels®)
Granular-type medications[a]	Dilute in a sufficient quantity of water (e.g., 80 mL of water with Metamucil®) and quickly administer via feeding tube in ≤5 min; rinse tube thoroughly with water following medication administration.	Methylcellulose, psyllium hydrophilic mucilloid (Metamucil®) cholestyramine resin (Questran®)
Intravenous solution	Dilute in water to reduce osmolarity.	Zinc sulfate

* The trade names are examples and may be only one of many products.
[a] The administration of this dosage form via feeding tubes is controversial due to the high potential for clogging the feeding tube, especially small, bore feeding tubes.

considered prior to administering any medication via an enteral feeding tube. Dosage forms can be divided into two categories: those that can be administered via an enteral feeding tube (see Table 8.6) and those that cannot be administered via an enteral feeding tube (see Table 8.7).

Table 8.7   Medication Dosage Forms that *Cannot* Be Administered via an Enteral Feeding Tube

Dosage Form	Mechanism of Incompatibility Via Enteral Feeding Tube	Example Medications[a]
Buccal or sublingual products	Optimal drug absorption occurs when the drug is absorbed under the tongue or between the gum and cheek; poorly absorbed when given directly in to the stomach or small bowel.	Ergoloid mesylate (Hydergine Sublingual®), nitroglycerine (Nitrostat®)
Enteric-coated products	Enteric coating protects medication from destruction by gastric juices which render the dosage form inactive; enteric coating prevents stomach irritation by allowing irritant drug to pass into the intestine before being released; crushing the medication destroys the enteric coating.	Bisacodyl (Dulcolax®), pancrelipase (Cotazym®), divalproex sodium (Depakote®), erythromycin stearate (E'Mycin®)
Extended-release products	Medication is released over an extended period of time following ingestion by various mechanisms (e.g., layered tablet, wax-matrix tablet, special membranes or capsules containing beads); crushing the dosage form results in immediate release of the entire amount of drug with subsequent increased risk of side effects and toxicities.	Diltiazem (Cardizem®), acetazolamide capsules (Diamox Sequel®), lithium (Lithobid®)
Oral liquids: syrups	Syrups tend to be acidic (pH ≤ 4), which, when in contact with the enteral feeding formula, causes clumping, increased formula viscosity, and subsequent clogging of the enteral feeding tube.	Metoclopramide syrup (Reglan®), pseudoephedrine syrup (Sudafed®)

[a] Not all brands of all medications are in the specified dosage form.

Oral liquid dosage forms are, in general, the preferred forms in which to administer medications via an enteral feeding tube. The exception to this is oral liquid syrups that tend to have a low pH (<4). When syrups are administered via the feeding tube, an interaction may occur between the enteral feeding formula and the medication (even when the medication is not mixed into the feeding formula and is given directly via the tube after flushing with water). The formula tends to clump, increase in viscosity, and cause clogging of the feeding tube. Other liquid dosage forms, such as suspensions, solutions, and elixirs, usually do not react with the enteral feeding formula. However, they may require dilution with 15–30 mL of water if they are viscous liquids or liquids with a high osmolality. Liquid medications with a high osmolality (>300 mOsm/kg) may cause the influx of fluid into the gastrointestinal tract. If the amount of fluid exceeds the absorptive capacity of the gastrointestinal tract, diarrhea may occur. These medications, therefore, should be diluted in water to reduce the osmolality. In a sampling of liquid medications, the osmolality ranged from 450 to 8800 mOsm/kg.[47] This information is typically available in the product literature or from the manufacturer. Intravenous solutions of medications may occasionally be administered via the enteral feeding tube. These medications also tend to have a high osmolality. Their relatively greater expense also renders them typically less desirable alternatives.

Many oral dosage forms can be crushed or otherwise altered in order to deliver them via the enteral feeding tube. Each specific dosage form requires a different preparation technique to optimize drug delivery as well as drug efficacy, as outlined in Table 8.6. Although the various techniques may be tedious or time-consuming, they can result in cost-effective alternatives to administration of the same drug in its parenteral form. In some cases, a parenteral form of the drug is not even commercially available. Also, with some drugs, a pharmacist can extemporaneously prepare a liquid dosage form from a solid dosage form [e.g., omeprazole (Prilosec®),[54] lansoprazole (Prevacid®)[55]]. In all cases, when a medication is administered via the enteral feeding tube, the feeding tube should be flushed with an appropriate amount of water (e.g., 15–30 mL in adults, 5–10 mL in children) before and after the medication is given to prevent incompatibilities and avoid clogging.

An extensive list of solid oral dosage forms that cannot be crushed is published on a biannual basis.[53] Although the list fluctuates as new products enter the market and old products are discontinued, several generalizations can be made regarding which specific dosage forms should never be crushed prior to attempted administration (see Table 8.7). These dosage forms include sublingual and buccal tablets, enteric-coated products, and extended-release products. Sublingual and buccal tablets are designed to be rapidly dissolved and absorbed into the systemic circulation via the highly vascular environment of the mouth. They are intended to avoid the first-pass effect of circulation through the liver. When these tablets are crushed and administered via a gastric or small bowel feeding tube, the absorption of the drug is impaired, and its metabolism is enhanced via the first-pass effect through the liver. The end result is a significant or complete reduction in drug efficacy.

The purpose of enteric coating is twofold. The enteric coating provides a protective barrier against the acid environment of the stomach for acid-labile drugs. The drug is delivered intact to the alkaline environment of the small intestine where it dissolves and is then available for absorption. Destruction of the enteric coating via crushing allows the active drug to be exposed to the gastric acids. Enteric coatings are also used for the purpose of protecting the lining of the stomach from drugs that are gastric irritants [e.g., aspirin and indomethacin (Indocin®)]. Destruction of the enteric coating allows the active drug to come in contact with the lining of the stomach and may result in nausea or even hemorrhage. Delivery of crushed enteric-coated medications into the small bowel via a feeding duodenostomy (or nasoduodenal tube) or jejunostomy, thereby bypassing the stomach, has not been studied. In theory, it may prove an effective option.

Extended-release products are primarily designed to reduce dosing frequency and side effects while sustaining the desired therapeutic effect. Therefore, multiple doses are contained in one capsule, wax-matrix tablet, or layered tablet. When this type of dosage form is crushed and delivered via an enteral feeding tube, the entire amount of drug is immediately available for absorption. There is a high likelihood of adverse or toxic effects from this large bolus of drug, and the overall duration of the therapeutic effect may be reduced.[56] When an immediate-release form (e.g., a compatible liquid or crushable tablet) of the same drug is available, the patient should be switched to this form with an appropriate adjustment in the drug dosage and frequency of administration.

ADMIXING DRUGS WITH THE ENTERAL FEEDING FORMULA

Using the enteral feeding formula as a drug delivery vehicle is undesirable most, if not all, of the time.[47,49] This practice should be avoided for several reasons. First, there is a high likelihood for physical incompatibility between the medication and the enteral feeding formula. Syrups have already been described as one dosage form that may cause curdling or thickening of the enteral feeding formula. Other manifestations of physical incompatibility include granulation, altered flow characteristics, phase separation, and tackiness.[57] These changes in the integrity of the enteral feeding formula may result in altered availability of nutrients and clogging of the feeding tube. Although several studies[57–61] have attempted to define the compatibility of selected drugs and enteral feeding formulas, far more drugs and enteral feeding products exist that have not been tested. Extrapolating the study results to other formulas or other drugs is not recommended. In addition to changes in the enteral feeding formula, there may be changes in the drug's efficacy [e.g., ciprofloxacin (Cipro®)] when it is combined with the formula. Lastly, addition of medications may cause contamination of the enteral feeding formula and subsequent diarrhea or infection if aseptic technique is not strictly followed.[62–65]

MEDICATIONS CLOGGING THE FEEDING TUBE

Several factors influence enteral feeding tube patency when using the tube as a route for medication administration. Proper preparation of acceptable dosage forms as shown in Table 8.6, not using unacceptable dosage forms as shown in Table 8.7, and not admixing medications directly into the enteral feeding formula are all important factors that have been discussed. The ease with which tube patency is maintained is also determined by the inner diameter of the tube—the smaller the inner diameter, the more likely the tube will become clogged. The tube diameter is expressed as the French (F) unit of measure. Each French unit equals 0.33 mm and reflects the outer diameter of the tube. The material from which the tube is made dictates the inner diameter. Thicker materials will have a smaller inner diameter. Most enteral feeding tubes are made from silicone (e.g., gastrostomy tubes) or polyurethane (e.g., nasoenteric tubes). Silicone tubing is a softer, more flexible material, but it is thicker than polyurethane of equal strength; therefore, silicone tubes have a smaller inner diameter than polyurethane tubes of the same outer diameter. Enteral feeding tubes range in size from 6 to 12 F and are from 16 to 60 inches in length accommodating a wide range of adult and pediatric needs. Other characteristics of specific tubes, such as size, number, shape, and position of outflow

Table 8.8   Guidelines for Administration of Medications via an Enteral Feeding Tube

1. Ensure medication is in a dosage form acceptable for administration via the enteral feeding tube (Table 8.6 and Table 8.7).
2. Know the location of the tip of the feeding tube (i.e., in the stomach or small bowel) and determine whether this affects the medication to be administered.
3. Timing:
   a. Intermittent gastric feeding—time medication administration based on need for a full or empty stomach
   b. Continuous gastric feeding—stop feeding for 30–60 min (exceptions are phenytoin and fluoroquinolone antibiotics which require 1–2 h) if medication is to be administered on an empty stomach
   c. Continuous small bowel feedings—stop feeding just prior to administration of medication (exceptions are phenytoin and fluoroquinolone antibiotics which require stopping the feeding 1–2 h prior to administration)
4. Prepare dosage form for administration via the enteral feeding tube (Table 8.6).
5. Flush enteral feeding tube with water (15–30 mL in adults; 5–10 mL in pediatrics) before and after medication administration.
6. Administer each medication separately and flush feeding tube with at least 3–5 mL water in between medications.
7. Allow medications to flow through tube by gravity.
8. Document amount of water used on the patient's fluid intake record (for hospitalized patients only).
9. Monitor patient's response to the medication for therapeutic efficacy.

ports at the distal tip of the enteral feeding tube, may also affect the likelihood of the tube becoming clogged. With this many factors in mind, it is important to adhere to guidelines for administration of medications via the enteral feeding tube, as described in Table 8.8, which are developed to optimize the likelihood of maintaining tube patency.[48,49,52,66] Key points to be emphasized are flushing the tube before and after each medication with an appropriate amount of water and administering only one medication at a time.

ENTERAL TUBE FEEDING INTOLERANCE: MEDICATION CULPRITS

In addition to the concerns for safely administering medications via the enteral feeding tube, there are concerns regarding complications of concomitant drug therapy that may affect enteral feeding tolerance. The most common adverse effect of enteral tube feeding is diarrhea, with an incidence of 2 to 70%.[67–70] Medications are thought to be the most frequent causative factor for diarrhea, with a 61% incidence reported in one study.[71] Antibiotics, sorbitol-containing oral liquids, magnesium-containing antacids, and oral liquids with a high osmolality (discussed previously) are medications frequently involved. Other medications that may cause diarrhea include histamine$_2$-receptor antagonists [e.g., cimetidine (Tagamet®), ranitidine (Zantac®), famotidine (Pepcid®)], antineoplastics, oral potassium, magnesium and phosphorus supplements, prokinetic agents [e.g., metoclopramide (Reglan®), erythromycin (E'Mycin®), and quinidine (Quinaglute®)].[69] Antibiotics prescribed to treat a specific infecting organism may also alter normal intestinal flora, producing a subsequent overgrowth of undesirable flora and concomitant diarrhea. In some instances of antibiotic-associated diarrhea, the offending organism is *Clostridium difficile*. *C. difficile* produces toxins that cause pseudomembranous colitis, an enteric infection characterized by voluminous diarrhea.

Sorbitol-containing oral liquids are often difficult to identify. Sorbitol is considered an inactive ingredient and is, therefore, not always listed as part of the labeled contents of a liquid medication. Sorbitol is a sweetener and may improve solution stability, but it is also an osmotically acting compound that, when ingested in sufficient quantities (≥10 g per day), has been associated with diarrhea.[72,73] Several authors have compiled lists of medications that contain sorbitol and the specific amount of sorbitol per daily dose.[72-74] Product formulations, however, may change over time and without notice. The manufacturer should be contacted for the most current information.

The management of medication-induced diarrhea depends somewhat on the specific medication involved.[53,67,69,70] In all cases, the first step, when possible, is to discontinue the offending medication. When antibiotics have been used and stool cultures are positive for *C. difficile*, treatment is with metronidazole (Flagyl®), the drug of choice, or with oral vancomycin (Vancocin®). When stool cultures are negative, the gut flora may be reestablished using a culture of *Lactobacillus acidophilus* and *L. bulgaricus*. In cases where other medications have caused diarrhea, an antidiarrheal agent, such as loperamide (Imodium®) or diphenoxylate with atropine (Lomotil®), may be prescribed to slow gut motility.

Pulmonary aspiration of enteral feeding formula is another common complication of enteral tube feeding, particularly in patients fed via a nasogastric or gastrostomy tube.[75] Risk factors include altered mental status, impaired gag or cough reflex, and mechanical ventilation. Medications are seldom considered as risk factors, but they should be considered in the case of selected medications. Two categories of medications may increase the risk of pulmonary aspiration: medications that delay gastric emptying and medications that decrease lower esophageal sphincter (LES) pressure. In both cases, gastric contents have an increased likelihood of refluxing into the esophagus and being aspirated into the lungs. Medications that delay gastric emptying include aluminum-containing antacids and narcotics.[47] Medications that decrease LES pressure include phenobarbital (Luminal®), diazepam (Valium®), nifedipine (Procardia®), levodopa (Dopar®), theophylline (Theo-Dur®), and nitroglycerin (Nitrostat®).[76]

MONITORING AND MANAGEMENT STRATEGIES FOR DRUG INTERACTIONS IN NUTRITION SUPPORT PATIENTS

Clearly, numerous possibilities exist for clinically significant drug interactions in nutrition support patients. The first step in the monitoring and management of drug interactions in this population is to review all medications the patient is receiving coincident with a thorough evaluation of the nutrition support regimen. The review should be done daily in hospitalized patients and at each clinic or home visit in home nutrition support patients. Ideally, potential issues can be identified before they incite a problem. For intravenous medications, the vehicle in which the medication is delivered should be identified, and it should be determined whether the vehicle is a significant calorie source (e.g., dextrose or lipid emulsion). When laboratory values are abnormal, medications should be considered in addition to pathophysiologic causes. For example, hyperglycemia may indicate acute infection but may also be due to prednisone or cyclosporine in a transplant patient. In a critically ill patient, hyperlipidemia may be due to hypermetabolism or excessive lipid ingestion with propofol plus a dextrose–lipid–amino acid–based parenteral nutrition formula. Several simple guidelines must be followed once a drug interaction is identified (or suspected):

- Discontinue the offending medication if possible.
- If needed, substitute a therapeutically equivalent alternative if it exists.
- In the case of administering medications via the feeding tube, substitute an acceptable dosage form of the same medication if it exists; if not, substitute a therapeutically equivalent alternative medication that is available in an acceptable dosage form.
- Manage drug-induced metabolic alterations according to standards of practice (e.g., replace electrolytes when electrolyte depletion occurs; use insulin, if appropriate, for hyperglycemia).
- Manage medication-induced diarrhea based on the specific offending agent (see previous discussion).
- Establish parameters by which to evaluate the success of interventions made to manage the drug interaction (e.g., cessation of diarrhea within 3 d of discontinuing the offending medication and instituting antidiarrheal therapy).

Two patient groups that receive nutrition support require special consideration for monitoring: pediatric patients and elderly patients. Both groups have additional age-related factors that may further increase their risk of drug interactions while receiving nutrition support. Pediatric patients, especially neonates, may exhibit an exaggerated response to adverse effects of medications. For example, if diarrhea occurs, infants and young children are more susceptible to dehydration. Neonates have immature organ function during the first few months of life and have limited nutrient stores. Drugs with metabolic effects, therefore, may be more problematic. Infants and young children often have limited intravenous access that may challenge the preference to keep separate intravenous lines for parenteral nutrition and for medications. Finally, there is a bigger impact of intravenous drug diluents (e.g., 5% dextrose in water) on overall calorie and fluid intake, such that the calories and fluids from this source should be included in the daily assessment.

Elderly patients exhibit issues similar to pediatric patients, but for different reasons. These patients may have limited nutrient stores or preexisting deficiencies because of ingesting a restricted diet either by choice or by prescription. Elderly patients have declining organ function particularly affecting the liver, kidney, gastrointestinal tract, and endocrine system. As a result, they are more susceptible to metabolic alterations from both the nutrition support and from medications. They may also have limited accessible veins to establish separate intravenous lines for nutrition and for medications. Finally, and most important, elderly patients typically are receiving numerous medications for several chronic disease states. When reviewing the risk factors for drug interactions in patients receiving nutrition support, as listed in Table 8.2, most elderly patients will have at least two, and potentially all, of the risk factors listed.

CONCLUSION

Patients receiving nutrition support represent a special population when considering drug interactions. The nutrition support itself is a medical therapy that complements but may also negatively impact concomitant medication therapies and vice versa. Nutrition support therapy requires close monitoring to assure nutrition goals are attained with a minimum of adverse effects. This close monitoring includes the regular review of all concomitant medications and an understanding of how medications may affect the outcome of the nutrition support.

REFERENCES

1. ASPEN, Board of Directors, Standards of practice: definition of terms used in ASPEN guidelines and standards, *Nutr. Clin. Pract.,* 10, 1–3, 1995.
2. ASPEN, Board of Directors and the Clinical Guidelines Taskforce, Guidelines for the use of parenteral and enteral nutrition in adult and pediatric patients, *J. Parental Enteral Nutr.,* 26, 185A–215A, 2002.
3. Strausburg, K.M., Parenteral nutrition admixture, in *The A.S.P.E.N. Nutrition Support Manual,* Souba, W.W. et al., Eds., A.S.P.E.N., Kansas City, MO, 8-1–8-12, 1998.
4. Olree, K. et al., Enteral formulations, in *The A.S.P.E.N. Nutrition Support Manual,* Souba, W.W. et al., Eds. A.S.P.E.N., Kansas City, MO, 4-1–4-9, 1998.
5. Schneider, P.J. and Mirtallo, J.M., Medication profiles in TPN patients, *Nutr. Suppl. Serv.,* 3, 40–48, 1983.
6. Driscoll, D.F., Drug-induced metabolic disorders and parenteral nutrition in the intensive care unit: a pharmaceutical and metabolic perspective, DICP, *Ann. Pharmacother.,* 23, 363–371, 1989.
7. Cerulli, J. and Malone, M., Assessment of drug-related problems in clinical nutrition patients, *J. Parental Enteral Nutr.,* 23, 218–221, 1999.
8. Hatton, J., Pharmacotherapy and nutrition, in *Pharmacotherapy Self-Assessment Program, Module 8 Gastroenterology Nutrition,* 3rd ed., Carter, B.L. et al., Eds., American College of Clinical Pharmacy, Kansas City, MO, 1999, pp. 157–183.
9. Rosmarin, D.K., Wardlaw, G.M., and Mirtallo, J., Hyperglycemia associated with high, continuous infusion rates of total parenteral nutrition, *Nutr. Clin. Pract.,* 11, 151–156, 1996.
10. Teasley-Strausburg, K.M., Metabolic and gastrointestinal complications, in *Nutrition Support Handbook—A Compendium of Products with Guidelines for Usage,* Teasley-Strausburg, K.M., Ed., Harvey Whitney Books Company, Cincinnati, OH, 1992, pp. 295–303.
11. Klang, M.G., Hayes, E.M., and Bloss, C.S., Drug-nutrient considerations—parenteral nutrition, in *The A.S.P.E.N. Nutrition Support Manual,* Souba, W.W. et al., Eds., A.S.P.E.N., Kansas City, MO, 10-1–10-11, 1998.
12. Brown, R.O. and Dickerson, R.N., Drug-nutrient interactions, *Am. J. Managed Care,* 5, 345–352, 1999.
13. Pandit, M.K. et al., Drug-induced disorders of glucose tolerance, *Ann. Intern. Med.,* 118, 529–539, 1993.
14. Seagraves, A. et al., Net protein catabolic rate after kidney transplantation: impact of corticosteroid immunosuppression, *J. Parental Enteral Nutr.,* 10, 453–455, 1986.

15. Magnuson, B. et al., Tolerance and efficacy of enteral nutrition neurosurgical patients in pentobarbital coma, *Nutr. Clin. Pract.,* 14, 131–134, 1999.

16. Seidner, D.L. and Speerhas, R., Yes, Octreotide can be added to parenteral nutrition solutions, *Nutr. Clin. Pract.,* 13, 84–87, 1998.

17. Lamberts, S.W.J. et al., Octreotide, *N. Engl. J. Med.,* 334, 246–254, 1996.

18. Sentipal-Walerius, J. et al., Effect of pulsed dexamethasone therapy on tolerance of intravenously administered lipids in extremely low birth weight infants, *J. Pediatr.,* 134, 229–232, 1999.

19. Lowrey, T.S. et al., Pharmacologic influence on nutrition support therapy: use of propofol in a patient receiving combined enteral and parenteral nutrition support, *Nutr. Clin. Pract.,* 11, 147–149, 1996.

20. Greenblatt, S.H. et al., Catabolic effect of dexamethasone in patients with major head injury, *J. Parental Enteral Nutr.,* 13, 372–376, 1989.

21. Teasley-Strausburg, K.M. and Anderson, J.D., Assessment of nutrition status and nutrition requirements, in *Pharmacotherapy—A Pathophysiologic Approach,* 4th ed., DiPiro, J.T. et al., Eds., Appleton-Lange, Stamford, CT, 1999, pp. 2221–2236.

22. Lacy, C.F. et al., Eds., *Drug Information Handbook,* 7th ed., Lexi-Comp, Cleveland, 1999.

23. Fernandez, L.A. et al., The effects of maintenance doses of FK506 versus cyclosporin A on glucose and lipid metabolism after orthotopic liver transplantation, *Transplantation,* 68, 1532–1541, 1999.

24. Carreras, E. et al., Hypertriglyceridemia in bone marrow transplant recipients: another side effect of cyclosporine A, *Bone Marrow Transpl.,* 4, 385–388, 1989.

25. Dresner, L.S. et al., Effects of cyclosporine on glucose metabolism, *Surgery,* 106, 163–169, 1989.

26. Dickerson, R.N. et al., Pentobarbital improves nitrogen retention in sepsis, *J. Parental Enteral Nutr.,* 13, 359–361, 1989.

27. Sacks, G.S. and Brown, R.O., Drug-nutrient interactions in patients receiving nutritional support, *Drug Ther.,* March 25, 1994, 41.

28. Roth, M.S., Martin, A.B., and Katz, J.A., Nutritional implications of prolonged propofol use, *Am. J. Health Syst. Pharm.,* 54, 694–695, 1997.

29. Solomon, S.M. and Kirby, D.F., The refeeding syndrome: a review, *J. Parental Enteral Nutr.,* 14, 90–97, 1990.

30. Miller, J.S. and Simpson, J., Medication-nutrient interactions: hypophosphatemia associated with sucralfate in the intensive care unit, *Nutr. Clin. Pract.,* 6, 199–201, 1991.

31. Brady, J.A., Rock, C.L., and Horneffer, M.R., Thiamin status, diuretic medications, and the management of congestive heart failure, *J. Am. Diet. Assoc.,* 95, 541–544, 1995.

32. Marcuard, S.P., Albernaz, L., and Khazanie, P.G., Omeprazole therapy causes malabsorption of cyanocobalamin, *Ann. Intern. Med.,* 120, 211–215, 1994.

33. National Advisory Group on Standards and Practice Guidelines for Parenteral Nutrition, Safe practices for parenteral nutrition formulations, *J. Parental Enteral Nutr.,* 22, 49–66, 1998.

34. Trissel, L.A., *Handbook on Injectable Drugs,* 12th ed., American Society of Health-System Pharmacists, Bethesda, MD, 2002.

35. King, J.C. and Catania, P.N., ed., *King Guide to Parenteral Admixtures,* King Guide Publications, Inc., Napa, CA, 2002.

36. Trissel, L.A., Gilbert, D.L., and Martinez, J.F., Compatibility of parenteral nutrient solutions with selected drugs during simulated Y-site administration, *Am. J. Health Syst. Pharm.,* 54, 1295–1300, 1997.

37. Trissel, L.A. et al., Compatibility of medications with 3-in-1 parenteral nutrition admixtures, *J. Parental Enteral Nutr.,* 23, 67–74, 1999.
38. Moshfeghi, M. and Ciuffo, J.D., Visual compatibility of fentanyl citrate with parenteral nutrient solutions, *Am. J. Health Syst. Pharm.,* 55, 1194–1197, 1998.
39. Nyffeler, M.S., Ciprofloxacin use in the enterally fed patient, *Nutr. Clin. Pract.,* 14, 73–77, 1999.
40. Wright, D.H. et al., Decreased *in vitro* fluoroquinolone concentrations after admixture with an enteral feeding formulation, *J. Parental Enteral Nutr.,* 24, 42–48, 2000.
41. Healy, D.P., Brodbeck, M.C., and Dlendening, C.E., Ciprofloxacin absorption is impaired in patients given enteral feedings orally and via gastrostomy and jejunostomy tubes, *Antimicrob. Agents Chemother.,* 40, 6–10, 1996.
42. Bauer, L.A., Interference of oral phenytoin absorption by continuous nasogastric feedings, *Neurology,* 32, 570–572, 1982.
43. Yeung, A. and Ensom, M.H., Phenytoin and enteral feedings: does evidence support an interaction? *Ann. Pharmacother.,* 34, 896–905, 2000.
44. Fleisher, D., Sheth, N., and Kou, J.H., Phenytoin interaction with enteral feedings administered through nasogastric tubes, *J. Parental Enteral Nutr.,* 14, 513–516, 1990.
45. Rodman, D.P., Stevenson, T.L., and Ray, T.R., Phenytoin malabsorption after jejunostomy tube delivery, *Pharmacotherapy,* 15, 801–805, 1995.
46. Doak, K.K. et al., Bioavailability of phenytoin acid and phenytoin sodium with enteral feeding, *Pharmacotherapy,* 18, 637–645, 1998.
47. Johnson, D.R. and Nyffeler, M.S., Drug-nutrient considerations for enteral nutrition, in *The A.S.P.E.N. Nutrition Support Manual,* Souba, W.W. et al., Eds., A.S.P.E.N., Kansas City, MO, 1998, 6-1–6-20.
48. Beckwith, M.C., Barton, R.G., and Graves, C., A guide to drug therapy in patients with enteral feeding tubes: dosage form selection and administration methods, *Hospital Pharm.,* 32, 57–64, 1997.
49. Gora, M.L., Tschampel, M.M., and Visconti, J.A., Considerations of drug therapy in patients receiving enteral nutrition, *Nutr. Clin. Pract.,* 4, 105–110, 1989.
51. Dunn, A. et al., Delivery of omeprazole and lansoprazole granules through a nasogastric tube *in vitro, Am. J. Health Syst. Pharm.,* 56, 2327–2330, 1999.
52. Lehmann, S., Medication administration via feeding tubes, in *Nutrition Support Handbook—A Compendium of Products with Guidelines for Usage,* Teasley-Strausburg, K.M., ed., Harvey Whitney Book Company, Cincinnati, OH, 1992, 305–320.
53. Mitchell, J.F., Oral dosage forms that should not be crushed: 2000 update, *Hosp. Pharm.,* 35, 553–567, 2000.
54. Quercia, R.A. et al., Stability of omeprazole in an extemporaneously prepared liquid, *Am. J. Health Syst. Pharm.,* 54, 1833–1836, 1997.
55. Phillips, J.O., Metzler, M.H., and Olsen, K., The stability of simplified lansoprazole suspension (SLS), *Gastroenterology,* 116, A89, 1999.
56. Cleary, J.D. et al., Administration of crushed extended-release pentoxifylline tablets: bioavailability and adverse effects, *Am. J. Health Syst. Pharm.,* 56, 1529–1534, 1999.
57. Cutie, A.J., Altman, E., and Lenkel, L., Compatibility of enteral products with commonly employed drug additives, *J. Parental Enteral Nutr.,* 7, 186–191, 1983.
58. Holtz, L., Milton, J., and Sturek, J.K., Compatibility of medications with enteral feedings, *J. Parental Enteral Nutr.,* 11, 183–186, 1987.
59. Strom, J.G. and Miller, S.W., Stability of drugs with enteral nutrient formulas, DICP, *Ann. Pharmacother.,* 24, 130–134, 1990.
60. Udeani, G.O., Bass, J., and Johnston, T.P., Compatibility of oral morphine sulfate solution with enteral feeding products, *Ann. Pharmacother.,* 28, 451–455, 1994.

61. Crowther, R.S., Bellanger, R., and Szauter, K.E.M., *In vitro* stability of ranitidine hydrochloride in enteral nutrient formulas, *Ann. Pharmacother.,* 29, 859–862, 1995.
62. Bussy, V., Marechal, F., and Nasca, S., Microbial contamination of enteral feeding tubes occurring during nutritional treatment, *J. Parental Enteral Nutr.,* 16, 552–557, 1992.
63. Anderson, K.R. et al., Bacterial contamination of tube-feeding formulas, *J. Parental Enteral Nutr.,* 8, 673–678, 1984.
64. Levy, J. et al., Contaminated enteral nutrition solutions as a cause of nosocomial bloodstream infections: a study using plasmid finger printing, *J. Parental Enteral Nutr.,* 13, 228–234, 1989.
65. Navajas, M. et al., Bacterial contamination of enteral feeds as a possible risk of nosocomial infection, *J. Hosp. Infect.,* 21, 111–121, 1992.
66. Engle, K.K. and Hannawa, T.E., Techniques for administering oral medications to critical care patients receiving continuous enteral nutrition, *Am. J. Health Syst. Pharm.,* 56, 1441–1444, 1999.
67. Bowling, T.E. and Silk, D.B.A., Diarrhea and enteral nutrition, in *Clinical Nutrition—Enteral and Tube Feeding,* Rombeau, J.L. and Rolandelli, R.H., Eds., W.B. Saunders Co., Philadelphia, 1997, pp. 540–553.
68. Guenter, P.A. et al., Tube feeding-related diarrhea in acutely ill patients, *J. Parental Enteral Nutr.,* 15, 277–280, 1991.
69. Fuhrman, P.M., Diarrhea and tube feeding, *Nutr. Clin. Pract.,* 14, 83–84, 1999.
70. Williams, M.S. et al., Diarrhea management in enterally fed patients, *Nutr. Clin. Pract.,* 13, 225–229, 1998.
71. Edes, T.F., Walk, B.E., and Austin, J.L., Diarrhea in tube-fed patients: feeding formula not necessarily the cause, *Am. J. Med.,* 88, 91–93, 1990.
72. Miller, S.J. and Oliver, A.D., Sorbitol content of selected sugar-free liquid medications, *Hosp. Pharm.,* 28, 741–744, 1993.
73. Lutomski, D.M. et al., Sorbitol content of selected oral liquids, *Ann. Pharmacother.,* 27, 269–274, 1993.
74. Thomson, C.A. and Rollins, C.J., Nutrient-drug interactions, in *Clinical Nutrition, Enteral and Tube Feeding,* 3rd ed., Rombeau, J.L. and Rolandelli, R.H., Eds., W.B. Saunders Co., Philadelphia, 1997, pp. 523–539.
75. Hamaoui, E. and Kodsi, R., Complications of enteral feeding and their prevention, in, *Clinical Nutrition—Enteral and Tube Feeding,* 3rd ed., Rombeau, J.L. and Rolandelli, R.H., Eds., W.B. Saunders Co., Philadelphia, 1997, 554–574.
76. Brandt, N., Medications and dysphagia: how do they impact each other?, *Nutr. Clin. Pract.,* 14, 527–530, 1999.

CHAPTER 9

Alcohol and Nutrition

Kim E. Light and Reza Hakkak

CONTENTS

0-8493-1531-X/03/$0.00+$1.50
© 2003 by CRC Press LLC

Without a doubt, ethyl alcohol is the most pervasively used, and abused, drug in the world.[1,2] As a result, ethyl alcohol consumption has the potential to impact individual nutritional status and concurrent pharmacotherapy by alteration of several different biological processes. Because alcohol metabolism results in the availability of kilocalories, the most obvious impact on nutrition stems from an alteration in dietary composition or total caloric intake. As alcohol-derived kilocalories are used for the production of energy, there is a concurrent potential for decreased intake of kilocalories from other sources. Thus, not only is the total caloric intake potentially altered by alcohol consumption, but the decreased intake of nutritional factors important in the multienzymatic conversion of calories to energy can also result in severe consequences.

Alcohol–nutrient or alcohol–medication interactions are evident in two primary areas: the kinetic and dynamic realms. Alterations in the kinetic realm involve changes in absorption, distribution, biotransformation, or elimination.[3] These processes govern the concentration of active ingredient (alcohol, nutrient, or medication) at their particular sites of action. Changes in the dynamic realm (commonly referred to as pharmacodynamics) involve alterations in the ability of an agent (again alcohol, nutrient, or medication) to produce the cellular alterations involved in its particular actions.

This chapter is designed to present a general overview on the consumption of alcohol, its impact on the biochemical machinery of the organism, and its interaction with nutritional substances and pharmacotherapeutic agents. Finally, a brief discussion of the other side of the coin is presented wherein the coassociation is made between individuals whose nutritional selectivity or preferences may have concurrent effects on the intake of alcohol.

KINETICS

Bioavailability

By far, the most common arena for interactions of nutrients and medications with alcohol involves alterations in pharmacokinetic parameters. A common term used in describing alterations in the absorptive aspects of bioactive compounds is bioavailability. This term refers to the ability of the compound to gain access to the circulatory system. Once compounds are absorbed (or delivered directly) into the circulatory system, the absorptive processes are completed.

Alcohol is absorbed primarily in the upper small intestinal segment called the duodenum. Classically, the rate-limiting factor in alcohol absorption is gastric emptying time, and alcohol is one of several factors involved in determination of gastric emptying.[4-24]

The potential impact of alterations to gastric emptying by alcohol, nutrients, or medications on the absorption of each is multifactorial and bidirectional. Thus, nutrients or medications that delay alcohol absorption may result in the consumption of greater than usual amounts of alcohol, leading to even greater consequences. Likewise, the acceleration of gastric emptying will enhance the absorption of alcohol and lead to an earlier and possibly more intense impairment. These reciprocal alterations of bioavailability can clearly lead to multiple levels of problems involving nutritional status, medication effectiveness, and alcohol consumption.

Aside from the alterations of gastric emptying, alcohol has been shown to result in alterations in the absorption of nutrients across the mucosal surfaces of the intestine.[25] Clinical studies have shown that malabsorption is frequent in heavy alcohol drinkers.[26] In addition, the impact of acute or chronic alcohol consumption has been explored in regard to the absorption of selected nutrients.[27-30] It is well known that absorption of water-soluble nutrients, such as B vitamins, glucose, and some amino acids that require active transport processes for their absorption, is severely altered with acute and chronic alcohol intake.[31]

Alcohol consumption, both on an acute and chronic basis, has been shown to alter nutrient intake, so it is reasonable to assume that the bioavailability of a variety of medications will also be altered. For example, alcohol consumption in an acute setting will impair first-pass metabolism resulting in an increased bioavailability for drugs undergoing significant first-pass biotransformation. Additionally, the effect of alcohol to delay gastric emptying will generally delay the rate and extent of drug absorption, which may result in undermedication.[3,32-34]

Distribution

The primary consideration in the distribution of drugs, nutrients, or alcohol is whether, and to what extent, these substances are bound to plasma proteins. Those drugs or nutrients that are highly bound to plasma proteins (e.g., benzodiazepines, phenytoin, tolbutamide, and warfarin) will be most impacted by chronic alcohol consumption. Decreased plasma proteins are comorbid with liver damage or impaired liver function, which is a common result of chronic alcohol consumption over time, especially heavy consumption patterns. Another possibility within a drinking session involving heavy consumption would result from the extent of dehydration that might occur because alcohol inhibits release of antidiuretic hormone, resulting in depletion of body water.

Biotransformation

Perhaps the major interaction among alcohol, nutrients, and medications occurs in the realm of biotransformation. Drugs undergo biotransformation for excretion and even, in some cases, for activation. Biotransformation is usually described in drug literature as either phase I biotransformation or phase II biotransformation. Phase I biotransformation is carried out primarily in the liver by the cytochrome P_{450} system of enzyme families.[35] Differences in individual responses to drugs can largely be attributed to genetic polymorphisms of these 12 genetically determined P_{450} families. This means some individuals metabolize certain drugs faster and other individuals metabolize certain drugs more slowly. Alcohol metabolism also involves P_{450} enzymes.[36] Phase II biotransformation is the conjugation of a parent compound's functional group with a polar group and is the major step in inactivation of most drugs.[35] Individuals vary in this process, and many studies have accessed differences between slow acetylators and fast acetylators. Slow acetylators usually clear drugs at a slower rate and need lower dosages, while fast acetylators clear the same drugs at a faster rate and may need higher dosages for the same effect. The clinical implications of biotransformation in food and drug interactions are not fully delineated.[35]

ALCOHOL CONSUMPTION PATTERNS

In 1997, alcohol consumption in the U.S., on a per capita basis (all individuals over 14 years), was 2.21 gallons of ethanol (http://www.niaaa.nih.gov/publications/). This figure has declined 14% since 1970. Figuring these data on a per drinker basis and by state reveals that ethanol consumption ranged from a high of 4.07 gallons per drinker in New Hampshire to a low of 1.76 gallons per drinker in Kentucky. Utah had the highest percentage of abstainers in its population (70.3%) while only 28.9% of the population of Wisconsin were abstainers. As a result, the prevalence of interactions between alcohol and nutrients and/or medications is undoubtedly significant and likely to account for frequent and unreported problems.

The patterns and extent of alcohol consumption have been investigated and characterized by gender, race, age, occupation, marital status, etc. These data, based on figures obtained in 1992, are quite revealing and are available from the National Institutes on Alcohol Abuse and Alcoholism through the Internet Web site (http://www.niaaa.nih.gov). Looking at the total population, roughly one-third of the population are lifetime abstainers; one-fifth are former or light drinkers; 17% are moderate drinkers, and 7.5% are heavy drinkers. For this study, lifetime abstainers never had 12 or more drinks in any single year of life; former drinkers had more than 12 drinks in a single year but not in the past year; light drinkers had 12 or more drinks in the past year but fewer than 3 drinks per week on average; moderate drinkers had between 3 and 14 drinks per week on average; and heavy drinkers had 2 or more drinks per day on average.[36]

In general, males report higher consumption than females based on the total number of drinks or dosage units of alcohol. This can be deceiving because on a per drink basis, females experience higher blood alcohol concentrations than males.[37] Approximately 14% of men are heavy drinkers and, remarkably, the percentage of heavy drinkers shows little difference across race, income level, education, employment status, or region of the country. Approximately 3% of women report heavy drinking with greater variation with age, education, and income level. (http://silk.nih.gov/silk/niaaa).

Type of Alcohol Consumed

Greater than 50% of alcohol consumed in the U.S. is in the form of beer. Slightly less than one-third is in the form of distilled spirits, and about 14% is in the form of wine. From the perspective of the potential for interactions with nutrients and medications, the composition of the alcoholic beverage and the availability of nutritional factors within the alcoholic drink are necessary considerations. Distilled spirits are higher in their percentage of alcohol and are consumed in smaller volumes (per drink), resulting in a marked reduction in the potential for additional nutrients within the drink. On the other hand, the lower alcohol drinks (on a volume percent basis), such as beer, result in larger volumes being consumed per drink and allow for the inclusion of other nutrients. Nevertheless, little research has been conducted to provide guidance and direction toward an understanding of the impact of the nutritional value of the alcohol drink itself on the overall nutritional status of the individual and on potential interactions with other nutritional sources or medications.

Alcoholism

Although commonly misunderstood, the definition of alcoholism does not rest on the absolute quantity of alcohol consumed, but rather on the control an individual is able to exert over the consumption of alcohol. Alcoholism is considered by addiction professionals to be a disease of impaired control.[38,39] As a result, the existence of interactions among alcohol, nutrients, and medications will be associated with the quantities of alcohol consumed and not primarily among those individuals with the disease of alcoholism.

Ethnic Difference

Studies have shown that the rates of problem drinking are higher among black and Hispanic men than white men.[2] Among women, Native Americans were significantly more likely than Caucasians or African-Americans to receive formal alcohol treatment services.[40]

A common and well-characterized feature of the metabolism of alcohol is the flushing response experienced primarily by a large percentage of Asians, as opposed to other groups. This flushing response is the result of a diminished ability to rapidly metabolize the initial breakdown product of alcohol metabolism—acetaldehyde. The flushing and associated physiological responses are a result of the build up of serum acetaldehyde concentrations. In a study of students in Japan, those with the flushing response reported drinking significantly less than nonflushers with respect to both frequency and amount.[41]

The frequency and number of alcohol-related problems, including dependence-related problems and social consequences from drinking, were greater among Latino compared with Caucasian men.[1] Dependence-related problems showed greater severity among African-Americans as opposed to Caucasians. In contrast, among women the frequency and severity of adverse social consequences attributable to drinking is higher among African-Americans than Caucasians, and highest among Latino women.[2]

The prevalence of a number of alcohol-related problems, the stability and incidence of dependence-related problems, and the incidence of social consequences from drinking are higher in Latino men compared with Caucasian men. Dependence-related problems are more stable among African-American than among Caucasian men. Among women, the reported incidence of dependence-related problems and social consequences from drinking is higher among African-Americans, followed next by Latinos, and then Caucasians. Finally, Irish populations appear to show the highest alcohol-related causes of death among the ethnic populations.[42]

Possible Cooccurrence of Alcohol and Sweet Preference

One of the more interesting observations resulting from studies of alcoholism is the increased evidence of and association between alcoholism and high sweet preference.[43–45] In this regard, selected studies have demonstrated that alcoholics show a greater sweet preference than nonalcoholics. Similar studies have also appeared using animal models of alcoholism and demonstrating that those animals showing specific preference for alcohol also demonstrated a much stronger preference for sweets, compared with controls.[45] It remains unknown as of yet how the neurobiology of alcoholism or sweet preference overlap or interact with each other. However, it is not surprising that drugs and nutrients stimulate a reward pathway and reinforce their consumption. It would not be surprising to identify additional areas of crossover in preference between nutrition and drug intake.

Age and Gender Differences

Although it has been suggested that older adults have a lower tolerance for alcohol, studies of the rate of metabolism have not identified a difference in the rate of absorption or elimination of alcohol by older adults.[46] Nevertheless, individuals frequently describe a lowered tolerance for alcohol as they age. This appears to relate to a gain of body fat and a loss of lean body mass. Thus, a lower amount of total body water means a greater sensitivity to alcohol as a consequence.[46] There appears to be little doubt that women have a lowered tolerance and greater damage from equivalent amounts of alcohol per unit of body weight.[47] Other metabolic differences based on gender appear to exist.[48] Another interesting gender difference is that men tend to reduce other sources of kilocalories in their diets with high alcohol intakes, while women tend to add the alcohol calories on the top of other dietary kilocalories.[47,49–50] Men and most animals appear to substitute the alcohol kilocalorie for other kilocalories from carbohydrate, protein, and fat. Men also have a tendency to consume a higher percentage of kilocalories from meat; they also have a higher caloric intake. It remains unclear whether or not these observed dietary differences account for part of the reason that women have more liver damage. Animal studies suggest that this may well be another influence in a very complex situation.

EFFECTS OF ALCOHOL CONSUMPTION ON NUTRITION

Alcohol consumption, if it includes either binge drinking or chronic intake of more than moderate amounts, clearly can exercise a negative impact on nutritional status.[51] The degree of tissue damage varies and depends on the level and type of alcohol consumption. Studies of the influence of alcohol intake on the development of disease and malnutrition also vary, with some disagreements among established researchers.[52] In part, the divergence stems from use of different animal models.[53] Further complicating factors include the length of exposure to alcohol in the diet and the composition of both the control and the ethanol-containing experimental diets.[53,54]

Epidemiological Studies

Epidemiological studies among countries with high alcohol intake but low rates of alcoholic cirrhosis, and others with high alcohol intake and high rates of alcoholic cirrhosis, have suggested several dietary factors as potential reasons.[54] For example, the U.S. and New Zealand have estimated rates of 14.1 and 12.2 per 100,000 cirrhosis deaths, respectively, based on per capita alcohol consumption. Actual deaths, however, in New Zealand were 2.7, compared with 9.3 in the U.S.. This represents over a threefold difference in the actual rates in the two countries. The potential differences in dietary factors were identified as saturated fat, polyunsaturated fat, cholesterol, and mortality from ischemic heart disease. This study, along with other studies, suggests that those factors contributing to ischemic heart disease might be protective against the development of alcohol liver disease.[54] Some animal studies have suggested that medium-chain triglycerides and vitamin E might reduce the severity of established experimental alcoholic liver disease.[55] Animal studies have also suggested that other dietary factors such as level of carbohydrates, level of fat, type of fat, and carbohydrate:fat ratio can modulate the degree of liver damage in chronic alcohol rat models.[56–60]

Animal Models

Various animal models and experimental diets have been applied to epidemiological studies over the years. The use of animal models was at first quite challenging because most animals refuse to drink sufficient quantities of alcohol to induce liver damage. The first animal model was developed by adding alcohol to the only available drinking water. The second method was developed by Lieber and DeCarli to introduce a liquid form of diet to the rats and was given with or without alcohol.[61,62] Neither method demonstrated the pure effects of alcohol in the development of liver cirrhosis. The third model was developed by direct infusion of liquid diet into the stomach and was termed as the total enteral nutrition (TEN) model. This method allows a large quantity of alcohol to be infused directly into the stomach. This experimental diet technique has allowed testing of many dietary factors in high alcohol intake.[56,57,59,61] This method remains the sole predictable means of producing a high degree of liver necrosis and cirrhosis by producing a high blood alcohol level. Infusion of liquid diet and alcohol directly into the gut allows careful control of both levels of alcohol and nutrients.[53,56,58,59] Using the rat model for alcoholic studies, many investigators have used carbohydrates or fats as substitutes for alcohol kilocalories.[56,59,63] In rat models, overnight fasting must be avoided because alcohol intake on an empty stomach leads to greater damage, as well as to changes in mucosal enzyme activity.[64,65]

Transport rate may also be affected by composition of the diet. Diets including a high saturated fat content, for example, are associated with higher maximal transport rates. Low concentrations of ethanol (<200 mM) do not significantly affect sodium-coupled nutrient uptake.[66] Higher ethanol concentrations, conversely, inhibit such transport. Although mechanisms by which ethanol reduces intestinal glucose transport are not fully understood, they are assumed to involve interference with active transport across the brush-border membrane (BBM). Recent studies have suggested that inhibition of glucose transport stems from an effect of ethanol on passive diffusion, resulting in a more prompt equilibrium of the sodium gradient. This process consequently reduces the uptake velocities of sodium-dependent transport systems.[66]

Acute exposure of the intestinal mucosa to ethanol will adversely affect uptake of those nutrients that use the sodium-dependent gradient for their transport across the BBM (e.g., L-amino acids,[67] glucose,[68,69] and galactose[70]). On the other hand, acute or chronic ethanol has been shown to increase the polarization of the membrane itself, thereby creating a higher electrical driving force for Na$^+$-coupled movement across the BBM.[71,72]

It has been generally accepted that food ingestion causes a decrease in absorption rate and an increase in first-pass metabolism, thereby producing a lower and delayed peak in blood alcohol levels. Two recent clamping studies by Ramchandani et al. suggest that food intake results in increased alcohol elimination rates.[73] Their findings suggest that healthy men have a greater increase in clearance in the fed state than women, perhaps as high as 45% greater clearance. Meal composition, whether high fat, high carbohydrate, or high protein, did not appear to cause these increases to differ significantly. Potential mechanisms for the greater alcohol clearance are food-induced hepatic blood flow and increased activity of alcohol-metabolizing enzymes.[73]

Carbohydrates

Acute doses of ethanol will inhibit the sodium-dependent transport of glucose and other hexoses across the jejunum, both *in vivo* and *in vitro*.[74,75] Acute studies of gut sections from rats that were administered chronic ethanol, followed by a diet rich in polyunsaturated fats, found significantly reduced glucose uptake. Another study that found no discernible change in the active absorption of glucose might reflect the inherent ability of the enterocyte to metabolize glucose.[76] Such inhibitory effects by ethanol upon BBM sugar transport are not yet fully understood. These effects, however, could relate to a variety of factors that include direct conformational effects on the hexose transporter, increased fluidity of the BBM, or perhaps the existence of different carriers for sugars.

Chronic ethanol administration shows enhanced absorption of these nutrients. This enhancement is likely caused by the increased membrane permeability resulting from the increased presence of mature enterocytes by a higher passive membrane permeability to glucose, or to the presence of an increased maturity among the enterocyte population at the villous surface.[77–79] Galactose uptake is also enhanced, possibly due to the enhanced potential difference across the isolated BBM in one study,[74] but not in one other.[78] The composition of diet, however, may again play a vital role in the increased saccharide absorption and jejunal uptake of glucose and galactose. Each of these phenomena is demonstrated in ethanol-fed rats that were given a diet supplemented with saturated fats.

At least one carbohydrate food group, soy milk products—including fermented soy milk—has been shown to inhibit ethanol absorption and enhance ethanol metabolism in rats.[80] Isoflavones may be the active factors. Soy milk products may also suppress ethanol-induced cell injury.[80]

Lipids

There is little evidence to indicate that acute ethanol consumption inhibits the transport of lipids across the intestinal mucosa. Changing the composition of the diet, however, with regard to polyunsaturated and saturated fat content may alter transport of both species. This appears to be the case, especially in rats that were fed ethanol supplemented with highly unsaturated fats (e.g., linoleic acid).

Conflicting reports exist regarding the transport of lipids after chronic ethanol ingestion. Nevertheless, most animal studies indicate that—provided a nutritious diet particularly rich in protein is administered—no malabsorption of lipids occurs.[81] Ethanol does alter lipid metabolism within the enterocyte. Here, it increases triglyceride content in the mucosa. Alterations in the uptake of most medium- and long-chain fatty acids and cholesterol could be detected when chronic ethanol feeding was combined with a diet rich in polyunsaturated fat.

Amino Acids

It is important that experimental conditions for any studies of amino acid uptake and transfer in the presence of ethanol reflect the nutritional status often observed among chronic misusers of alcohol (i.e., reduction in body weight and a high caloric intake). In addition, the experiment must control for the fact that ethanol ingestion enhances nitrogen loss in the urine of both rats[82] and humans.[83] It is also important to recognize the morphological changes in the jejunum as described previously. In the face of a good nutritional state, any inhibition of active transport of amino acids related to ethanol will be compensated by the enhanced diffusion of amino acids across the intestinal mucosa.

Acute ethanol administration can inhibit the active transport of amino acids in animals.[74,84] Indeed, the absorptive capacity of the membrane for amino acids appears to be maintained, despite gross changes to the morphology of the jejunum following chronic ethanol consumption.[84] Because high alcohol concentrations increase membrane permeability, efflux of amino acids from the blood will actually increase in the presence of low luminal amino acid concentrations.[82]

EFFECT OF ETHANOL INGESTION ON PARTICULAR NUTRIENTS

Alcohol ingestion can affect several nutrients by one or more mechanisms. Most noticeably, the effect on thiamin is the most important due to the severity and speed at which a major deficiency can develop. This happens with or without the presence of other drugs. In the presence of drugs, however, other serious but perhaps undetected deficiencies can develop.

Thiamin

Acute ethanol ingestion lowers the maximal rate of intestinal thiamin absorption both in alcoholics and in healthy individuals. In rats, studies using either intact intestinal loops or everted jejunal segments show parallel results. In both systems, the active (low concentration) and the passive (high concentration) absorption of thiamin were susceptible to ethanol inhibition. Because thiamin intake among alcoholics may be extremely low, however, the critical process is active absorption of the vitamin. This absorption process may be independently affected by the combination of ethanol and malnutrition in humans.[85] It has been further suggested that the observed decrease in maximal thiamin absorption may be explained by damage to receptor sites from prolonged receipt of alcohol, by nutritional deficiency, or by a synergistic combination of both factors.[86]

Neurological complications of alcoholism, such as Wernicke–Korsakoff syndrome and polyneuropathy, often develop from direct toxicological effects and from nutrient deficiencies secondary to poor intake or interference with nutrient metabolism. Not all chronic alcohol users carry the same degree of risk for neurotoxicology. A genetic predisposition to thiamin deficiency has been described in Wernicke's encephalopathy.[87] A survey of head-injury patients at risk of Wernicke–Korsakoff syndrome in Scotland revealed that just over half could be classified as alcoholic.[88] These patients were given carbohydrate loads, but less than 30% of the patients were given thiamin, and both the dose and duration of thiamin therapy was judged to be inadequate. Failure to provide adequate thiamin supplements to alcoholics treated for head injuries adds another insult to a damaged brain.

Riboflavin

About 17% of chronic alcoholics demonstrate riboflavin deficiency. Neither animal nor human clinical studies have indicated impairment in riboflavin absorption by either acute or chronic administration of alcohol. Studies so far have indicated that a low dietary intake of this vitamin is the only mechanism suspected to cause the deficiency.[89]

Biotin

Chronic ethanol feeding significantly decreases biotin transport in everted intestinal sac loops, when the vitamin is fed at physiological doses. There was, however, little effect on the absorption of biotin when the nutrient was administered at pharmacologic doses. This contrast indicates selective inhibition by alcohol of the carrier-mediated process for biotin uptake.[90]

Folate

Ethanol will inhibit folate transportation out of the gastrointestinal (GI) lumen in proportion to intestinal ethanol concentration.[91] Studies in human subjects have indicated that when the diet is adequate, ethanol will not adversely affect folate absorption.[92] Chronic ethanol studies using a minipig model (minipigs were administered ethanol for one year) showed decreased hydrolysis of PteGlu but an unchanged uptake of PteGlu.[93] By contrast, a decreased intestinal absorption of folate was identified in well-nourished monkeys after chronic ethanol feeding.[94]

In Americans, it has been postulated that excessive alcohol consumption is the major cause of folate deficiency along with thiamin, B_6, vitamin A, and zinc deficiencies.[95] Because folate status can be negatively impacted with a large number of drugs, the alcoholic patient is particularly at risk of folate deficiency in drug regimens.[95] Herbert has identified six major causes of folate deficiency and states that all may occur concurrently in chronic alcoholism.[96] Anemia in alcoholics is likely caused by a lack of folate.[95]

Vitamin B_6

Anemia in alcoholics may be secondary to B_6 or pyridoxine deficiency. This vitamin is essential for the activity of alanine transaminase (ALT) and may account for the lowered ratio to other liver enzymes in chronic alcoholic liver disease.[95] The pyridoxine deficiency seen in chronic alcoholism is thought to be due to excess acetaldehyde displacing the active form of the vitamin, leading to an increased excretion of the vitamin in the urine.[46,98]

Vitamin C

Absorption of ascorbic acid is reduced when this vitamin is ingested simultaneously with ethanol.[95] The proximal cause of deficiency in alcoholic patients, however, is likely to be inadequate intake. Also, because L-ascorbate is absorbed by the sodium-gradient–dependent transport mechanism, any change in the movement of sodium across the membrane will also alter ascorbic acid status. Chronic alcohol use often occurs in smokers, and the ascorbic acid requirement for smokers has been estimated to be at least twice as much as for nonsmokers.[95]

Vitamin A

Patients suffering from alcohol liver disease exhibit very low levels of hepatic vitamin A. The level of vitamin A in fatty livers is significantly lower than in normal livers and significantly lower than in the livers of patients with chronic, persistent hepatitis. One study indicated that in patients with alcoholic hepatitis, liver vitamin A levels were more than 10 times below normal. Those patients with cirrhosis, who participated in the same study, showed levels 30 times below normal. Thus, chronic alcohol consumption can reduce vitamin A concentrations. Malnutrition also provides another concomitant factor that can contribute to hepatic vitamin A depletion in patients with alcohol liver disease. Although vitamin A supplements may be beneficial to the alcoholic, there is a narrow therapeutic window between meeting the increased needs for vitamin A and avoiding the adverse effects that vitamin A and beta carotene supplements can create.[95,97–99]

Calcium

Acute alcohol ingestion in both nonalcoholic humans and rats does not interfere with calcium transport.[100,101] Chronic alcohol ingestion, however, can inhibit duodenal absorption of calcium.[102] Acute doses of ethanol will adversely affect the carrier at the BBM, inhibiting calcium transport at physiological concentration. There is, however, little effect on the system at pharmacological concentrations. Exactly how this phenomenon occurs remains unknown, but inhibition of energy metabolism and physiochemical alterations in enterocyte membrane have been implicated.

Zinc and Iron

The intestinal absorption of zinc is a homeostasis regulated process located on the apical membrane of the enterocyte. The importance of zinc has long been recognized in chronic alcoholic patients.[103] In chronic alcohol users, zinc deficiency may well be due to several factors (e.g., poor dietary intake, decreased intestinal absorption, and increased urinary excretion).[95]

Chronic users of alcohol exhibit alterations in the acid content of the stomach, as well as in the gastric juices, and the pancreatic, biliary, and other GI secretions. Any or all of these could influence the form of iron present in the GI lumen, as well as its uptake by the BBM. The mechanisms by which ethanol influences uptake and transfer of iron into the enterocyte remain unknown. Physiologically, alcoholic gastritis may produce occult bleeding and lead to iron deficiency anemia in chronic alcoholism. This anemia can be further complicated by low protein and low folate intakes. High intakes of alcohol have been associated with iron overload in some populations.[95] The clinical signs of human iron toxicity with high intakes of alcohol have been confirmed in a rat study, which demonstrated that high intakes of iron and alcohol led to greater hepatocyte damage and iron storage.[104]

Phosphorus and Magnesium

Phosphorus status has been problematic in refeeding of malnourished alcoholics recovering from alcoholic bouts. As in any severe malnourished state, rapid refeeding without adequate phosphorus can lead to hypophosphatemia.[105]

Magnesium was termed "nature's physiological calcium channel blocker" by Iseri and French.[106] Clinical signs of magnesium depletion include muscle cramps, hypertension, and coronary and cerebral vasospasms.[102] Ma et al. have associated serum and dietary magnesium with these signs in alcoholics along with other disease states.[107] Excessive alcohol intake in baboons has been shown to cause renal magnesium wasting which, if a diet is marginal in magnesium content, could impose a risk for magnesium depletion. Nearly all alcoholics have some symptoms of magnesium depletion.[108]

ALCOHOL AND DISEASE INDUCTION

Although alcohol is a toxin that damages many parts of the body, the two organs hit hardest by chronic alcohol abuse are the liver and the brain.[109] This is partly due to toxicological effects, but nutritional deficiencies also contribute to the damage. These deficiencies are due not only to poor intake, but also to the negative impact of alcohol on nutrient absorption and metabolism.[109] At different times in the literature, the primary responsibility has shifted back and forth between toxicology and nutrient deficiencies. Experimental animal data have allowed a bridge to be built between this classic dichotomy of nutritional and toxic effects of alcohol.[49] Although still not fully understood, the interrelationships are complex but appear to be modifiable to a certain degree by dietary and supplement manipulations.

Alcohol Liver Disease (ALD)

ALD represents one major cause of health problems and deaths in Western countries today. The most common form of ALD is fatty liver. More serious ALD includes alcohol hepatitis. This disorder is characterized by persistent liver inflammation and eventually by liver cirrhosis leading to progressive liver injury. Approximately 10–35% of heavy drinkers will develop alcoholic hepatitis, and 10–20% will develop liver cirrhosis.[51,110] In the Unites States, liver cirrhosis stands as the seventh leading cause of death among middle-aged adults.[82] In one prospective study of 280 alcoholics, more than half of those diagnosed with cirrhosis and two-thirds of those with both cirrhosis and alcoholic hepatitis died within 48 months of enrollment.[71]

Alcohol Metabolism

Most (about 70%) of a bolus of alcohol can be absorbed from the stomach, passing directly by the portal vein to the liver. This process represents first-pass metabolism, exactly as described for some drugs in Chapter 2. The rate of alcohol metabolism is then dependent on whether the ethanol was ingested with or without food. The presence of food affects gastric emptying, therefore, food will influence the rate of alcohol metabolism. Gastric emptying is influenced, in turn, by the type of food. An empty stomach will produce the fastest rate of alcohol metabolism. Three pathways exist for ethanol metabolism in the liver: (1) the alcohol dehydrogenase (ADH) pathway in cytosol (the soluble fraction of cell contents), (2) the cytochrome P_{450} ethanol oxidizing system located in the endoplasmic reticulum, and (3) catalase enzymes located in the peroxisomes.[95]

Alcohol Dehydrogenase (ADH) Pathway

ADH represents the major alcohol metabolism pathway. It is an enzyme that catalyzes the conversion of alcohol to acetaldehyde. Five different classes of human ADH have been identified.[35] Class I is composed of isozymes α, β, and γ subunits. These are, in turn, encoded by ADH1, ADH2, ADH3 gene loci. Most class I isozymes showing low K_m for ethanol are localized in the liver, but some are also present in the gastrointestinal tract and the kidney. Class II consists of a single form with π subunits that is encoded by ADH4 gene. It is also located in the liver and has a high K_m for ethanol. Class III is formed by χ subunits encoded by ADH5. It has very low activity with ethanol. Class IV was described first in stomach mucosa, consisting of a homodimer with σ subunits encoded by ADH7. Class IV shows a high affinity for ethanol metabolism. One new class of human ADH may be present in both liver and gastric tissues, and it would be encoded by ADH6.[111]

Gastric ADH

Three different forms of ADH exist in the human stomach, characterized by either high or low K_m for ethanol.[108] Gastric ADH with high K_m for ethanol can become active after alcohol consumption. Significant gastric alcohol metabolism may then ensue.[112,113] The result is metabolism of ethanol in advance of the first-pass (liver and portal circulation) mechanism. It is remarkable that 80% of Japanese people show a deficiency in one of the gastric ADH isozymes.[114] Women also tend to exhibit a lower gastric ADH activity than men after alcohol consumption.[115] As a result, blood alcohol levels can be higher in any person with ADH isozyme deficiency. This increase in blood levels among women is compounded by differences in body composition between men and women. In addition, first-pass metabolism can decrease the bioavailability of alcohol when a low level of alcohol has been consumed. Some commonly used drugs inhibit gastric ADH activity *in vitro*. These include the H_2 histamine-blocker cimetidine[116–117] and the nonsteroidal anti-inflammatory agents.[118] Inhibition of gastric ADH activity in the liver can result in increased blood alcohol levels.

Microsomal Ethanol Oxidizing System (MEOS)

Morphologic changes in alcohol-fed rats that had proliferation of the smooth endoplasmic reticulum first indicated an interaction between alcohol and the microsomal fraction of the hepatocyte.[119] This system could then be induced in liver microsomes *in vitro* and was induced *in vivo* by chronic ethanol feeding. It was named the microsomal ethanol oxidizing system (MEOS). The MEOS shares many properties with other microsomal drug-metabolizing enzymes. These properties include use of cytochrome P_{450}, NADPH, and O_2.[61,62,120,121] This sharing goes far toward explaining many alcohol–drug interactions. After long-term alcohol consumption, MEOS activity can increase, with induction of a specific P_{450} cytochrome pathway (namely CYP2E1). This particular pathway metabolizes ethanol and other hepatotoxic agents such as acetone, pyrazole, and pyridine. Ethanol-induced CYP2E1 isozyme is the most efficient in ethanol oxidation among the various cytochromes P_{450}.[122] Although CYP2E1 has a moderately high K_m for ethanol (8–10 mM), its activity is exquisitely induced by chronic ethanol exposure. Thus, it is the main enzyme involved in microsomal oxidation of ethanol at high blood alcohol levels. Some other cytochromes P_{450}, such as CYP2A12, CYP2B, and CYP3A in rodents, also make contributions to alcohol metabolism. Two studies have investigated the possibility that enterocytes will be able to metabolize ethanol in the presence of the P_{450} enzymes.[122,123] In one study, microsomes isolated from the small intestine of the chronically treated rats demonstrated an enhanced alcohol metabolism. In the second, a decrease in CYP1A and CYP3A was detected immunologically in rats treated with alcohol by intragastric infusion.[123]

Catalase

Catalase is capable of oxidizing alcohol *in vitro* in the presence of a H_2O_2-generating system.[124] Under normal conditions when peroxide is not being produced, however, catalase does not appear to play a major role. It certainly cannot account for an ADH-independent pathway for alcohol metabolism.

SUMMARY

In summary, alcohol can profoundly influence both drug metabolism and nutritional status. Table 9.1 lists those medications that present the greatest risk when consumed with large amounts of alcohol. Table 9.2 lists those nutrients most affected by excessive or prolonged alcohol intake. The field of alcoholism is in the process of investigating the effects of alcohol on nutrients beyond those traditionally associated with chronic alcohol use. Dietary factors can clearly interfere with drug metabolism, and the presence of alcohol in the diet can further complicate the food, drug, and nutrient interactions.

Table 9.1   Drugs That Pose Serious Risks When Combined with Excessive Alcohol Consumption

Drug Class	Generic Name of Example	Common Brand Name
Analgesics	acetaminophen	Tylenol®
	aspirin	Bayer Aspirin®
	ibuprofen	Motrin®
	indomethacin	Indocin®
Anesthetic gases	enflurane	Ethrane®
	halothane	Fluothane®
Anesthetic agents	droperidol	Inapsine®
	ketamine	Ketalar®
	midazolam	Versed®
	propofol	Diprivan®
	thiopental	Sodium Pentothal®
Antibiotics	ciprofloxacin	Cipro®
	griseofulvin	Grisactin®
	metronidazole	Flagyl®
Anticoagulants	warfarin	Coumadin®
Antidepressants		
Tricyclics	amitriptyline	Elavil®
	doxepin	Sinequan®
	imipramine	Tofranil®
Other	trazodone	Desyrel®
	citalopram	Celexa®
	fluoxetine	Prozac®
	paroxetine	Paxil®
	sertraline	Zoloft®
Antidiabetic agents	chlorpropamide	Diabenese®
	glipizide	Glucotrol®
	glyburide	Micronase®
	tolbutamine	Orinase®
Antihistamines	chlorpheniramine	Chlor-Trimeton®
	diphenhydramine	Benadryl®
	hydroxyzine	Vistaril®
	promethazine	Phenergan®
Antipsychotic agents	chlorpromazine	Thorazine®
	prochlorperazine	Compazine®
	trifluoperazine	Stelazine®
	haloperidol	Haldol®
Antiseizure agents	phenytoin	Dilantin®
	phenobarbital	Luminal®
Antiulcer agents	cimetidine	Tagamet®
	ranitidine	Zantac®
Cardiovascular agents	nitroglycerin	NitroStat®
	reserpine	Reserpoid®
	methyldopa	Aldomet®
	hydralazine	Apresoline®
	guanethidine	Ismelin®
	propranolol	Inderal®
Immunosuppressant agents	cyclosporine	Sandimmune®
	glatiramer	Copaxone®
	interferon alpha-2a	Roferon-A®
	hydroxychloroquine	Plaquenil®
Opioids		
Synthetic agents and	fentanyl	Duragesic®
semisynthetic agents	hydromorphone	Dilaudid®
	meperidine	Demerol®
	propoxyphene	Darvon®, Darvocet®

Table 9.1   Drugs That Pose Serious Risks When Combined with Excessive
             Alcohol Consumption *(Continued)*

Drug Class	Generic Name of Example	Common Brand Name
Natural products	codeine	Tylenol #3®, Empirin #3®
	morphine	MS-Contin®
Sedative/hypnotic agents		
Barbituric acid derivatives	pentobarbital	Nembutal®
	phenobarbital	Luminal®
	secobarbital	Seconal®
Benzodiazepines	flurazepam	Dalmane®
	diazepam	Valium®

Note: This table is for illustration only. It is not intended to be complete. Consult
          appropriate drug literature or a drug information center before prescribing
          any drug product in the face of known or suspected, significant acute or
          chronic ethanol intake.

Table 9.2   Nutrients That Are Likely to Be Deficient or
             Submarginal in Heavy Users of Alcohol[a]

Nutrient	Mechanism	Reference
Folate	Inadequate intake	DRI[a]
	Malabsorption	
	Intestinal absorption	
	Hepatobiliary interference	
	Increased requirement	
	Increased renal excretion	
Niacin	Deficiency: poor intake	DRI[a]
	Toxicity: high intake	
Thiamin	Wernicke–Korsakoff syndrome	DRI[a]
	inadequate intake	
Vitamin B$_6$	Low plasma PLP levels	DRI[a]
Magnesium	Low intracellular levels	DRI[b]
Phosphorus	Refeeding syndrome	DRI[b]
Vitamin A	Low hepatocyte level	DRI[c]
Vitamin C	Low absorption	DRI[a]
Calcium	Low duodenal absorption	DRI[b]
Zinc	Low intake and absorption	DRI[c]
	High excretion	
Iron	Low absorption	DRI[c]
	Occult bleeding	

[a] *Source:* Food and Nutrition Board, Institute of Medicine, *Dietary References for Thiamin, Riboflavin, Vitamin B$_6$, Folate, Vitamin B$_{12}$, Pantothenic Acid, Biotin, and Choline,* National Academy Press, Washington, D.C., 1998.
[b] *Source:* Food and Nutrition Board, Institute of Medicine, *Dietary Reference Intakes for Calcium, Phosphorus, Magnesium, Vitamin D, and Fluoride,* National Academy Press, Washington, D.C., 1997.
[c] *Source:* Food and Nutrition Board, Institute of Medicine, *Dietary Reference Intakes for Vitamin A, Vitamin K, Arsenic, Boron, Chromium, Copper Iodine, Iron, Manganese, Molybdenum, Nickel, Silica, Vanadium, Zinc,* National Academy Press, Washington, D.C., 2001.

REFERENCES

1. Caetano, R., Prevalence, incidence and stability of drinking problems among whites, blacks and Hispanics: 1984–1992, *J. Stud. Alcohol,* 58, 565–572, 1997.
2. Caetano, R. and Clark, C.L., Trends in alcohol-related problems among whites, blacks, and Hispanics: 1984–1995, *Alcohol Clin. Exp. Res.,* 22, 534–538, 1998.
3. Ciraulo, D.A. and Barnhill, J., Pharmacokinetic mechanisms of ethanol-psychotropic drug interactions, *National Institute of Drug Abuse Res. Monogr.,* 68, 73–88, 1986.
4. Cooke, A.R. and Clark, E.D., Effect of first part of duodenum on gastric emptying in dogs: response to acid, fat, glucose, and neural blockade, *Gastroenterology,* 70, 550–555, 1976.
5. Edelbroek, M.A. et al., Effects of erythromycin on gastric emptying, alcohol absorption and small intestinal transit in normal subjects, *J. Nucl. Med.,* 34, 582–588, 1993.
6. Gisolfi, C.V. et al., Effect of beverage osmolality on intestinal fluid absorption during exercise, *J. Appl. Physiol.,* 85, 1941–1948, 1998.
7. Guslandi, M., Gastric effects of leukotrienes, *Prostaglandins Leukot. Med.,* 26, 203–208, 1987.
8. Holt, S., Observations on the relation between alcohol absorption and the rate of gastric emptying, *Can. Med. Assoc. J.,* 124, 267–277, 297, 1981.
9. Horowitz, M. et al., Relationships between gastric emptying of solid and caloric liquid meals and alcohol absorption, *Am. J. Physiol.,* 257, G291–298, 1989.
10. Jian, R. et al., Effect of ethanol ingestion on postprandial gastric emptying and secretion, biliopancreatic secretions, and duodenal absorption in man, *Dig. Dis. Sci.,* 31, 604–614, 1986.
11. Johnson, R.D. et al., Cigarette smoking and rate of gastric emptying: effect on alcohol absorption, *Br. Med. J.,* 302, 20–23, 1991.
12. Kalogeris, T.J., Reidelberger, R.D., and Mendel, V.E., Effect of nutrient density and composition of liquid meals on gastric emptying in feeding rats, *Am. J. Physiol.,* 244, R865–R871, 1983.
13. Kaufman, S.E. and Kaye, M.D., Effect of ethanol upon gastric emptying, *Gut,* 20, 688–692, 1979.
14. Kechagias, S., Jonsson, K.A., and Jones, A.W., Impact of gastric emptying on the pharmacokinetics of ethanol as influenced by cisapride, *Br. J. Clin. Pharmacol.,* 48, 728–732, 1999.
15. Mushambi, M.C. et al., Effect of alcohol on gastric emptying in volunteers [published erratum appears in *Br. J. Anaesth.,* 72, 253, 1994], *Br. J. Anaesth.,* 71, 674–676, 1993.
16. Pedrosa, M.C. et al., Gastric emptying and first-pass metabolism of ethanol in elderly subjects with and without atrophic gastritis, *Scand. J. Gastroenterol.,* 31, 671–677, 1996.
17. Romankiewicz, J.A., Effects of antacids on gastrointestinal absorption of drugs, *Primary Care,* 3, 537–550, 1976.
18. Schvarcz, E. et al., Accelerated gastric emptying during hypoglycaemia is not associated with changes in plasma motilin levels, *Acta Diabetol.,* 34, 194–198, 1997.
19. Schwartz, J.G. et al., Gastric emptying of beer in Mexican-Americans compared with non-Hispanic whites, *Metabolism,* 45, 1174–1178, 1996.
20. Sun, W.M. et al., Effects of nitroglycerin on liquid gastric emptying and antropyloroduodenal motility, *Am. J. Physiol.,* 275, G1173–G1178, 1998.
21. Sun, W.M. et al., Effects of glyceryl trinitrate on the pyloric motor response to intraduodenal triglyceride infusion in humans, *Eur. J. Clin. Invest.,* 26, 657–664, 1996.

22. Tachiyashiki, K. and Imaizumi, K., Effects of vegetable oils and C18-unsaturated fatty acids on plasma ethanol levels and gastric emptying in ethanol-administered rats, *J. Nutr. Sci. Vitaminol.* (Tokyo), 39, 163–176, 1993.

23. Tomlin, J. et al., The effect of liquid fiber on gastric emptying in the rat and humans and the distribution of small intestinal contents in the rat, *Gut,* 34, 1177–1181, 1993.

24. Verschuren, P.M. and Nugteren, D.H., Evaluation of jojoba oil as a low-energy fat, 2. Intestinal transit time, stomach emptying and digestibility in short-term feeding studies in rats, *Food. Chem. Toxicol.,* 27, 45–48, 1989.

25. Seitz, H.K., Alcohol effects on drug-nutrient interactions, *Drug Nutr. Interact.,* 4, 143–163, 1985.

26. Thomson, A.D. and Majumdar, S.K., The influence of ethanol on intestinal absorption and utilization of nutrients, *Clin. Gastroenterol.,* 10, 263–293, 1981.

27. Gloria, L. et al., Nutritional deficiencies in chronic alcoholics: relation to dietary intake and alcohol consumption, *Am. J. Gastroenterol.,* 92, 485–489, 1997.

28. Molina, J.A. et al., Alcoholic cognitive deterioration and nutritional deficiencies, *Acta Neurol. Scand.,* 89, 384–390, 1994.

29. Sankaran, H., Larkin, E.C., and Rao, G.A., Induction of malnutrition in chronic alcoholism: role of gastric emptying, *Med. Hypotheses,* 42, 124–128, 1994.

30. Watzl, B. and Watson, R.R., Role of alcohol abuse in nutritional immunosuppression, *J. Nutr.,* 122, 733–737, 1992.

31. Stowell, L.I., Nutritional aspects of alcohol, in *Human Metabolism of Alcohol,* Vol. I, *Pharmacokineteics, Medicolegal Aspects, and General Interest,* Crow, K.E. and Batt, R.D., Eds., CRC Press, Boca Raton, FL, 1989, pp. 187–201.

32. Linnoila, M., Mattila, M.J., and Kitchell, B.S., Drug interactions with alcohol, *Drugs,* 18, 299–311, 1979.

33. Mattila, M.J., Alcohol and drug interactions, *Ann. Med.,* 22, 363–369, 1990.

34. Sellers, E.M. and Holloway, M.R., Drug kinetics and alcohol ingestion, *Clin. Pharmacokinet.,* 3, 440–452, 1978.

35. Utermohlen, V., Diet, nutrition and drug interactions, in *Modern Nutrition in Health and Disease,* 9th ed., Shils, M.E. et al., Eds., Williams & Wilkins, Baltimore, 1999.

36. Stinson, F.S. et al., Main findings from the 1992 national longitudinal alcohol epidemiologic survey (NLAES), in *U.S. Alcohol Epidemiologic Data Release Manual,* Vol. 6, National Institute on Alcohol Abuse and Alcoholism, Division of Biometry, Rockwell, MD, 1998.

37. Frezza, M. et al., High blood alcohol levels in women: the role of decreased gastric alcohol dehydrogenase activity and first-pass metabolism, [published errata appear in *New Engl. J. Med.,* 322, 1540, 1990 and 323, 553, 1990], *New Engl. J. Med.,* 322, 95–99, 1990.

38. Erickson, C.K., A pharmacologist's opinion—alcoholism: the disease debate needs to stop, *Alcohol Alcoholism,* 27, 325–328, 1992.

39. Erickson, C.K., Review of neurotransmitters and their role in alcoholism treatment, *Alcohol Alcoholism,* 1, S5–S11, 1996.

40. Ross, R. et al., Age, ethnicity, and comorbidity in a national sample of hospitalized alcohol-dependent women veterans, *Psychiatr. Serv.,* 49, 663–668, 1998.

41. Suzuki, K., Matsushita, S., and Ishii, T., Relationship between the flushing response and drinking behavior among Japanese high school students, *Alcohol Clin. Exp. Res.,* 21, 1726–1729, 1997.

42. Rosenwaike, I. and Hempstead, K., Differential mortality by ethnicity: foreign-born Irish, Italians and Jews in New York City, 1979–81, *Soc. Sci. Med.,* 29, 885–889, 1989.

43. Kampov-Polevoy, A., Garbutt, J.C., and Janowsky, D., Evidence of preference for a high-concentration sucrose solution in alcoholic men, *Am. J. Psychiatry,* 154, 269–270, 1997.

44. Kampov-Polevoy, A.B. et al., Preference for higher sugar concentrations and tridimensional personality questionnaire scores in alcoholic and nonalcoholic men, *Alcohol Clin. Exp. Res.,* 22, 610–614, 1998.

45. Stewart, R.B. et al., Consumption of sweet, salty, sour, and bitter solutions by selectively bred alcohol-preferring and alcohol-nonpreferring lines of rats, *Alcohol Clin. Exp. Res.,* 18, 375–381, 1994.

46. Dufour, M.C., Archer, L., and Gordis, E., Alcohol and the elderly, *Clin. Geriatr. Med.,* 8, 127–141, 1992.

47. Halsted, C.H., Alcohol: medical and nutritional effects, in *Present Knowledge in Nutrition,* 7th ed., Ziegler, E.E. and Filer, L.J., Jr., Eds., ILSI Press, Washington, D.C., 1996.

48. Lieber, C.S., Herman Award Lecture, 1993: a personal perspective on alcohol, nutrition and the liver, *Am. J. Clin. Nutr.,* 58, 430–442, 1993.

49. Lieber, C.S., Alcohol, liver, and nutrition, *J. Am. Coll. Nutr.,* 10, 602–632, 1991.

50. Lieber, C.S., Alcohol and the liver: 1994 update, *Gastroenterology,* 106, 1085–1105, 1994.

51. Bunout, D., Nutritional and metabolic effects of alcoholism: their relation with alcoholic liver disease, *Nutrition,* 15, 583–589, 1999.

52. Lieber, C.S. and DeCarli, L.M., Recommended amounts of nutrients do not abate the toxic effects of an alcohol dose that sustains significant blood levels of ethanol, *J. Nutr.,* 119, 2038–2040, 1989.

53. French, S.W., Nutrition in the pathogenesis of alcoholic liver disease, *Alcohol Alcoholism,* 28, 97–100, 1993.

54. Nanji, A.A. and French, S.W., Dietary factors and alcoholic cirrhosis, *Alcohol Clin. Exp. Res.,* 10, 271–273, 1986.

55. Nanji, A.A. et al., Medium chain triglycerides and vitamin E reduce the severity of established experimental alcoholic liver disease, *J. Pharmacol. Exp. Ther.,* 277, 1694–1700, 1996.

56. Korourian, S. et al., Diet and risk of ethanol-induced hepatotoxicity: carbohydrate-fat relationships in fat, *Toxicol. Sci.,* 47, 110–117, 1999.

57. Tsukamoto, H. et al., Severe and progressive steatosis and focal necrosis in rat liver induced by continuous intragastric infusion of ethanol and low fat diet, *Hepatology,* 5, 224–232, 1985.

58. Tsukamoto, H. et al., Cyclical pattern of blood alcohol levels during continuous intragastric infusions in rats, *Alcohol Clin. Exp. Res.,* 9, 31–37, 1985.

59. Hakkak, R., Ronis, M.J., and Badger, T.M., Effects of enteral nutrition and ethanol on cytochrome P_{450} distribution in small intestine of male rats, *Gastroenterology,* 104, 1611–1618, 1993.

60. Ronis, M.J. et al., Effects of short-term ethanol and nutrition on the hepatic microsomal monooxygenase system in a model utilizing total enteral nutrition in the rat, *Alcohol Clin. Exp. Res.,* 15, 693–699, 1991.

61. Lieber, C.S. and DeCarli, L.M., Ethanol oxidation by hepatic microsomes: adaptive increase after ethanol feeding, *Science,* 162, 917–918, 1968.

62. Lieber, C.S. and DeCarli, L.M., Hepatic microsomal ethanol oxidizing system: *in vitro* characteristics and adaptive properties *in vivo, J. Biol. Chem.,* 245, 2505–2512, 1970.

63. Tsukamoto, H. et al., Ethanol-induced liver fibrosis in rats fed high-fat diet, *Hepatology,* 6, 814–822, 1986.
64. Murray, D. and Wild, G.E., Effects of fasting on Na-K-ATPase activity in rat small intestinal mucosa, *Can. J. Physiol. Pharmacol.,* 58, 643–649, 1980.
65. Debham, E.S. and Thomson, C.S., Effects of fasting on the potential difference across the brush border membrane of enterocytes in rat small intestine, *J. Physiol.,* 355–449, 1984.
66. O'Neill, B. et al., Ethanol selectively affects Na systems, Na+ gradient dependent intestinal transport system, *F.E.B.S. Lett.,* 194, 183, 1986.
67. Beesley, R.C., Ethanol inhibits Na-gradient dependent uptake of L-amino acids into intestinal brush membrane vesicles, *Dig. Dis. Sci.,* 31, 987–992, 1986.
68. Tillotson, L.G. et al., Inhibition of Na-stimulated glucose transport function and perturbation of intestinal microvillous membrane vesicles by ethanol and acetaldehyde, *Arch. Biochem. Biophys.,* 207, 360–370, 1981.
69. Chang, T., Lewis, J., and Glazko, A.J., Effects of ethanol and other alcohols on the transport of amino acids and glucose by everted sacs of rat small intestine, *Biochem. Biophys. Acta,* 135, 1000–1007, 1967.
70. Thomson, A.B.R., Acute exposure of rabbit jejunum to ethanol. *In vitro* uptake of hexoses, *Dig. Dis. Sci.,* 29, 267–274, 1984.
71. Chendid, A. et al., The VA cooperative group, Prognostic factors in alcoholic liver disease, *Am. J. Gastroenterol.,* 82, 210–216, 1991.
72. Al-Balooi, F., Debham, E.S., and Mazzanti, R., Acute and chronic exposure to ethanol and the electrophysiology of the brush border membrane of rat small intestine, *Gut,* 30, 1698–1703, 1989.
73. Ramchandani, V.A., Effect of food and food composition on alcohol elimination rates in healthy men and women, *J. Clin. Pharmacol.,* 41, 1345–1350, 2001.
74. Bode, J.C., Alcohol and the gastrointestinal tract, *Adv. Intern. Med. Pediatr.,* 45, 1–75, 1980.
75. Lieber, C.S., Medical disorders of alcoholism: pathogenesis and treatment, in *Problems in Internal Medicine,* Smith, L.D., Ed., WB Saunders, Philadelphia, 1982, pp. 22, 363.
76. Debham, E.S., Effect of sodium concentration and plasma sugar concentration on hexose absorption by rat jejunum *in vivo, Pflugers Arch.,* 393, 104–160, 1982.
77. Mazzanti, R. and Jenkins, W.J., Effect of ethanol ingestion on enterocyte turnover in rat small intestine, *Gut,* 28, 52–55, 1987.
78. Mazzanti, R., Debham, E.S., and Jenkins, W.J., Effect of ethanol intake on lactase activity and active galactose absorption in rat small intestine, *Gut,* 28, 56–60, 1987.
79. Thomson, A.B.R., Keelan, M., and Clandinin, M.T., Feeding rats a diet enriched with saturated fatty acids prevents the inhibitory effects of acute and chronic ethanol exposure on the *in vitro* uptake of hexoses and lipids, *Biochim. Biophys. Acta,* 1082, 122–128, 1991.
80. Kano, M. et al., Soymilk products affect ethanol absorption and metabolism in rats during acute and chronic ethanol intake, *J. Nutr.,* 132, 238–244, 2002.
81. Rodrigo, C., Antezana, C., and Baraona, E., Fat and nitrogen balances in rats with alcohol-induced fatty liver, *J. Nutr.,* 101, 1307–1310, 1971.
82. World, M.J., Ryle, P.R., and Thomson, A.D., Alcoholic nutrition and the small intestine, *Alcohol Alcoholism,* 20, 89–124, 1985.
83. McDonald, J.T. and Margen, S., Wine versus ethanol in human nutrition, I. Nitrogen and caloric balance, *Am. J. Clin. Nutr.,* 29, 1093–1103, 1976.

84. Bode, J.C., Alcohol and the gastrointestinal tract, in *Ergebnisse der Inneren Medizin und Klinderheilkunde,* Frick, P.K. et al., Eds., Springer-Verlag, Berlin, 1980.

85. Thomson, A.D., Vitamin deficiency and its role in alcoholic tissue damage, *J. Gastroenterol. Haematol.,* 2, 411, 1990.

86. Thomson, A.D. and Leevy, C.M., Observations on the mechanism of thiamin hydrochloride absorption in humans, *Clin. Sci.,* 43, 153–163, 1972.

87. Martin, P.R., McCool, B.A., and Singleton, C.K., Genetic sensitivity to thiamin deficiency and development of alcoholic organic brain disease, *Alcohol Clin. Exp. Res.,* 170, 31–37, 1993.

88. Ferguson, R.K., Soryal, I.N., and Pentland, B., Thiamin deficiency in head injury: a missed insult? *Alcohol Alcoholism,* 32, 493–500, 1997.

89. Bonjour, J.P., Vitamins and alcoholism, V. Riboflavin, VI. Pantothenic acid, VIII. Biotin, *Int. J. Vit. Res.,* 50, 425–440, 1980.

90. Said, H.M. et al., Chronic ethanol feeding and acute ethanol exposure *in vitro*: effect on intestinal transport of biotin, *Am. J. Clin. Nutr.,* 52, 1083–1086, 1990.

91. Said, H.M. and Strum, B.M., Effect of ethanol and other aliphatic alcohols on the intestinal transport folate, *Digestion,* 35, 129–135, 1986.

92. Halsted, C.H., Robles, E.A., and Mezey, E., Decreased jejunal uptake of labeled folic acid (3H-PGA) in alcoholic patients: roles of alcohol and malnutrition, *New Engl. J. Med.,* 285, 701–706, 1971.

93. Reisenauer, A.M. et al., Folate absorption in alcoholic pigs; in vivo intestinal perfusion studies, *Am. J. Clin. Nutr.,* 50, 1429–1435, 1989.

94. Tamura, T. et al., Hepatic folate metabolism in the alcoholic monkey, *J. Lab. Clin. Med.,* 97, 654–661, 1981.

95. Lieber, C.S., The influence of alcohol on nutritional status, *Nutr. Rev.,* 46, 241–245, 1988.

96. Herbert, V., Folic acid, in *Modern Nutrition in Health and Disease,* 9th ed., Shils, M.E. et al., Eds., Williams & Wilkins, Baltimore, 1999.

97. Lieber, C.S., Mechanisms of ethanol-drug-nutrient interactions, *Clin. Toxicol.,* 32, 631–681, 1994.

98. Leo, M.A. et al., Beta-carotene beadlets potentiate hepatotoxicity of alcohol, *Am. J. Clin. Nutr.,* 66, 1461–1469, 1997.

99. Leo, M.A., Sato, M., and Lieber, C.S., Effect of hepatic vitamin A depletion on the liver in humans and rats, *Gastroenterology,* 84, 562–572, 1983.

100. Verdy, M. and Caron, D., Ethanol et absorption du calcium chez l'humain, *Biol. Gastroenterol.* (Paris), 6, 157–160, 1973.

101. Krawitt, E.L., Effect of acute ethanol administration on duodenal calcium transport, *Proc. Soc. Exp. Med.,* 146, 406–408, 1974.

102. Krawitt, E.L., Sampson, W., and Katagirl, C.A., Effect of 1,25-dihydroxycholecalciferol on ethanol mediated suppression of calcium absorption, *Calcified Tissue Res.,* 18, 119–124, 1975.

103. McClain, C.J. and Su, L.C., Zinc deficiency in the alcoholic: a review, *Alcohol Clin. Exp. Res.,* 7, 5–10, 1983.

104. Stal, P. and Hultcrantz, R., Iron increases ethanol injury in rat liver, *J. Hepatology,* 17, 108–115, 1993.

105. Food and Nutrition Board, Institute of Medicine, Dietary Reference Intakes for calcium, phosphorus, magnesium, and vitamin D, National Academy Press, Washington, D.C., 1997.

106. Iseri, L.T. and French, J.H., Magnesium: nature's physiologic calcium blocker, *Am. Heart J.,* 108, 188–193, 1984.

107. Ma, J. et al., Association of serum and dietary magnesium with cardiovascular disease, hypertension, diabetes, insulin, and carotid arterial wall thickness, The athersclerosis risks in community study, *J. Clin. Epidemiol.,* 48, 927–940, 1995.
108. Abbott, L., Nadler, J., and Rude, R.K., Magnesium deficiency in alcoholism: possible contribution to osteoporosis and cardiovascular disease in alcoholics, *Alcohol Clin. Exp. Res.,* 18, 1076–1082, 1994.
109. Lieber, C.S., Interactions of alcohol and nutrition: introduction to a symposium, *Alcohol. Clin. Exp. Res.,* 7, 2–4, 1983.
110. Sutton, R. and Shields, R., Alcohol and oesophageal varices, *Alcohol Alcoholism,* 30, 581–589, 1995.
111. Hernandez-Munoz, R. et al., Human alcohol dehydrogenase: its inhibition by H_2-receptor antagonists and its effect on the bioavailability of ethanol, *Alcohol Clin. Exp. Res.,* 14, 946–950, 1990.
112. Julkunen, R.J.K., DiPadova, C., and Lieber, C.S., First pass metabolism of ethanol: a gastrointestinal barrier against the systemic toxicity of ethanol, *Life Sci.,* 37, 567–573, 1985.
113. Julkunen, R.J.K. et al., First pass metabolism of ethanol: an important determinant of blood levels after alcohol consumption, *Alcohol,* 2, 437–441, 1985.
114. Baroaona, E. et al., Lack of alcohol dehydrogenase activities isoenzymes activities in stomachs of Japanese subjects, *Life Sci.,* 49, 1929, 1991.
115. Lieber, C.S., Diseases of the Liver, in *Modern Nutrition in Health and Disease,* 9th ed., Shils, M.E. et al., eds., Williams & Wilkins, Baltimore, 1999.
116. Caballeria, J. et al., Effects of cimetidine on gastric alcohol dehydrogenase activity and blood ethanol levels, *Gastroenterology,* 96, 388–392, 1989.
117. Caballeria, J. et al., Effects of H_2 receptor antagonists on gastric alcohol dehydrogenase activity, *Dig. Dis. Sci.,* 36, 1673–1679, 1991.
118. Roine, R. et al., Aspirin increases blood alcohol concentrations in humans after ingestion of ethanol, *J. Am. Med. Assoc.,* 264a, 2406–2408, 1990.
119. Iseri, O.A., Gottieb, L.S., and Lieber, C.S., The ultrastructure of ethanol-induced fatty liver, *Am. J. Pathol.,* 48, 535–555, 1966.
120. DiPadova, C. et al., Effects of ranitidine on blood alcohol levels after ethanol ingestion: comparison with other H_2 receptor antagonists, *J. Am. Med. Assoc.,* 267, 83–86, 1992.
121. Lasker, J.M. et al., Purification and characterization of human liver cytochrome P_{450} ALC, *Biochem. Biophys. Res. Commun.,* 148, 232–238, 1987.
122. Ioannides, C., Cytochrome P_{450}, in *Metabolic and Toxicological Aspects,* CRC Press, Boca Raton, FL, 1996.
123. Seitz, H., Korsten, M., and Lieber, C.S., Ethanol oxidation by intestinal microsomes: increased activity after chronic ethanol administration, *Life Sci.,* 25, 1443–1448, 1979.
124. Keilin, D. and Hartree, E.F., Properties of catalase: catalysis of coupled oxidation of alcohols, *Biochem. J.,* 39, 293–301, 1945.

CHAPTER **10**

Nutrition and Drug Regimens in Older Persons

Albert Barrocas, Charles W. Jastram, and Beverly J. McCabe

CONTENTS

0-8493-1531-X/03/$0.00+$1.50
© 2003 by CRC Press LLC

DRUG USAGE OVERVIEW

Outside the critical care units in American hospitals, individuals most at risk of adverse food and drug interactions are older persons for whom polypharmacy is a way of life. Polypharmacy is a term defining the use of multiple drug regimens and is often set at five or more medications taken daily by an individual.[1] The increased risk has been associated with multiple chronic diseases, multiple specialists, and the aging process. Older adults are the greatest consumers of prescribed medications, estimated to account for over 30% of all prescription drugs, ranging from 7.5 to 17.9 medications per person every year.[1,2] Cornish estimates that a new prescription is given 80% of the time when an older person sees a physician.[2] The picture is quite similar for over-the-counter (OTC) drugs, with the elderly being the largest consumers.[1,3]

Besides multiple chronic diseases and polypharmacy, older adults are also most likely to vary widely in nutritional status. Food intake may be marginal for many reasons including economics, social isolation, limited ability to shop for and prepare food, depression, anorexia, fatigue, and other aspects of chronic diseases. A number of drugs have side effects that interfere with food intake, nutrient absorption, metabolism, and nutrient requirements. Lewis et al.[4] proposed eight classes of drug–nutrient interactions in a study of drug–nutrient interactions in three extended-care facilities as shown in Table 10.1. Clearly food and drug interactions in the elderly are influenced strongly by nutritional status. Thus, nutritional assessment is an integral part of overall care.

NUTRITIONAL ASSESSMENT OVERVIEW

Despite its recognized importance, nutrition evaluation has only recently gained sufficient recognition to be performed as a separate activity or as a central part of a

Table 10.1 Drug–Nutrient Interactions in Long-Term Care Facilities

Class	Adverse events
Tube feeding	Precipitation of acidic liquid formula leading to blockage
	Weight changes due to fluid overload
	Abnormal serum glucose levels
	Diarrhea secondary to broad-spectrum antibiotics
Gastrointestinal	Malabsorption of drug secondary to drug administered with food (interference interaction)
	Absence of food when drug absorption is promoted by intake or when food protects the gut lining (meal-omission interaction)
Appetite altering	Some drugs can lead to increase in appetite
	Some drugs can lead to decrease in appetite
Incompatibility	Toxic interaction of drug with alcohol
	Toxic interaction of drug with pressor amines in food
Loss of therapeutic efficacy	Protein in diet accelerates drug clearance
Loss of metabolic control	Alteration of glycemic control
Drug-induced nutrient	Antinutrient effect by binding/interfering with nutrient
Deficiency	Increased excretion of nutrient
	Decreased absorption of nutrient
Inappropriate supplements/ Inappropriate restrictions	Extra nutrient intake overrides drug effects
	Nutrient restricted diet leads to toxic drug levels

Source: Adapted from Lewis, C.W., Frongillo, E.A., Jr., and Roe, D.A., *J. Am. Diet. Assoc.*, 95, 309–315, 1995. With permission.

comprehensive geriatric assessment.[5] The additional need for a clinical assessment of nutrition and drug interaction remains largely unappreciated by many healthcare professionals.[6] Demographic projections of the large increases in older persons, especially rapid increases in those over the age of 85, mandates that healthcare providers become well versed and experienced in detection of early nutrition derangements in the 21st century.[7] Few can argue with the assertion that the elderly represent the most frail individuals in our society, consuming the largest portion of healthcare services and dollars.[8] Since the 1970s, the federal government has estimated that over 85% of chronic diseases and disabilities experienced by the elderly could be prevented or ameliorated through nutrition interventions.[9] Many older persons can lead productive, happy, and independent lives if these conditions are identified early and appropriate interventions initiated. Use of these programs will assist in shifting the current healthcare paradigm from "rescue and repair" to "disease prevention and health promotion."[9] The results can be a better quality of life for the elderly and a more cost-effective healthcare delivery, which have been recognized as a goal in Healthy People 2010.[10] The required assessment and interventions can be accomplished with minimal effort and with currently available tools in almost any setting by any physician or other healthcare providers.

COST-EFFECTIVE PREVENTION IN THE ELDERLY

In general, prevention can be stratified into three levels: primary, secondary, and tertiary levels.[7,8] Primary prevention usually refers to health promotion in healthy persons through the reduction of risk factor exposure or alteration of susceptibility to these risk factors. Primary prevention are immunization, healthy diets, and exercise programs.[8] Secondary prevention is used to indicate early detection and treatment in those individuals who have a risk factor without overt symptoms of the disease such as weight control in individuals with family history of type 2 diabetes, screenings for cancer, hypertension, and nutrition.[7] Tertiary prevention refers to minimizing the effects of established diseases and improving outcomes. Nutritional assessment, interventions, and drug–nutrient interaction counseling are examples of secondary and tertiary prevention.[9]

The provision of appropriate counseling to prevent drug–nutrient interactions is very cost effective because these interactions can reduce the effectiveness of expensive drugs or lead to additional treatment costs resulting from adverse events.[11] The elderly constitute only about 13% of the population, but they are involved in nearly 40% of adverse drug reactions.[6,12,13] This chapter reviews screening and assessment tools and techniques for nutrition interventions, including likely food and drug interactions for monitoring and counseling of older persons.

BASIC DEFINITIONS IN NUTRITION ASSESSMENT

Three major terms related to nutrition assessment are important to distinguish: nutrition survey, nutrition screening, and nutrition assessment. A nutrition survey looks at large groups or populations based on random samplings. Two major nutrition surveys are commonly done by the U.S. government to monitor nutrition of Americans:

1. National Health and Nutrition Examination Surveys (NHANES) conducted by the U.S. Public Health Service Reference
2. Continuing Survey of Food Intakes by Individuals (CSFII) Reference

Nutrition screening has been defined as "the process of identifying characteristics known to be associated with dietary or nutritional problems."[14,15] Nutrition screening assists in differentiating between individuals at risk for nutritional problems or those who already have poor nutritional status. The screen leads to an in-depth nutrition assessment that may result in a medical diagnosis, treatment, and nutrition counseling as a specific component of a comprehensive healthcare plan. Nutrition assessment consists of the measuring dietary and other nutritional related indicators that identify the presence, nature, and the extent of impaired nutritional status. With these indicators, interventions can be designed to improve nutritional care and other health care.[9,16] Table 10.2 outlines some common factors and some elements by which these risks are assessed.

INCORPORATION OF NUTRITIONAL ASSESSMENT INTO THE TRADITIONAL HISTORY/PHYSICAL/LABORATORY EXAMINATION

Most individuals at nutritional risk do not present with specific complaints about nutrition. The elderly, in particular, present with symptoms of chronic diseases that influence or are influenced by nutritional health.[17–19] Thus, signals or triggers of

Table 10.2 Risk Factors Associated with Poor Nutritional Status in Older Americans Including Elements by Which Risk Is Assessed

Inappropriate Food Intake	Dependency/Disability
Personal Factors	**Personal Factors**
Meal/snack frequency	Functional status
Quantity/quality	activities of daily living
milk/milk products	instrumental activities of daily living
meat/meat substitutes	Disabling conditions
fruit/vegetables	lack of manual dexterity
bread/cereals	use of assistive devices
fats	Inactivity/immobility
sweets	Advanced age
Dietary Modification	**Poverty**
Self-imposed	Low Income
Prescribed	source
Compliance	adequacy
Impact	Food expenditure/resources
	Economic assistance program reliance
Acute/Chronic Disease or Conditions	Food
Alcohol use/abuse	Housing
Abnormalities of body weight	Medical
Oral health problems	Adequacy
Pressure sores/ulcers	Cognitive or emotional impairment
Sensory impairment	Depression
	Dementia
Chronic Medication Usage	Other
Prescribed/self-administered	
	Social Isolation
Polypharmacy	Support systems
Nutritional supplements	Availability
Quackery	Utilization
	Living arrangements
	Cooking/food storage
	Transportation
	Other

Source: Adapted from Nutrition Screening Initiative, *Incorporating nutrition screening and interventions into medical practice: a monograph for physicians,* The Nutrition Screening Initiative, Washington, D.C., 1994, 16, 20, 29–31. With permission.

nutrition problems need to be incorporated into the standard history/physical/laboratory examination, regardless of the chief complaint.[20] Special consideration needs to be given to concerns encountered in the assessment of older individuals. These include accuracy of history, medical conditions, polypharmacy, previous surgery, family and social needs, dietary history, review of systems, physical examination, and nutrition screening critical points.

History

Accuracy of the historical information obtained from the older person may be questionable due to declining memory or reluctance to provide information. The older person may fear that giving certain information may change the home situation or result in recommendation for a transfer to other facilities or restriction on activities. If possible, a caregiver or family member who knows the patient's history can assist in the interview. Previous records from other institutions, physicians, and other health professionals may help.[21]

Medical

Certain diseases and conditions, acute or chronic, are more likely to trigger nutritional problems and can serve as signals for further nutrition assessment.[21-24] These include cardiovascular and cerebrovascular diseases, dementia, depression, diabetes, obesity, osteoporosis, cancer, and chronic obstructive pulmonary disease. Digestive disorders that interfere with absorption or digestion of nutrients may lead to decreased intake, anorexia, or evacuation problems. Acute diseases may suggest increased nutrient needs and impaired food intake in the older person whose usual intake was already marginal due to many factors. Questions regarding other mental and cognitive conditions such as anxiety, memory deficits, and educational level may identify additional factors that impact on the individual's ability to shop, prepare, or eat food. Identification of chronic disabilities may determine functional capacity and the length of time that the individual has been unable to perform certain activities. Activities of daily living (ADL) and instrumental activities of daily living (IADL) are two commonly used parameters in the assessment of the elderly.[23] Assessment of oral health can also identify factors that reduce the enjoyment of food and discourage adequate intake of protective foods such as many vegetables, fruits, and whole grain products.

If medical conditions warrant, assessment for the need for aggressive nutrition support should be performed. Protein–calorie malnutrition and folate and vitamin B_{12} deficiencies are commonly associated with underlying medical disorders (e.g., heart disease, cancer, chronic obstructive pulmonary disease, pancreatic inflammation, and bowel disease) that should be diagnosed and treated. Nutrition support should usually be provided while attempting to treat the underlying condition associated with or causing malnutrition. Medical indications for tube feeding and/or parenteral nutrition support usually include: (1) weight loss greater than 10% that is continuing, (2) inadequate dietary intake, or (3) mid-arm muscle circumference below the 10th percentile, despite use of early interventions to improve oral intake. Other indicators of poor nutritional status, such as body mass index (BMI) less than 22, triceps skinfold less than the 10th percentile, or serum albumin less than 3.5 g/dL, should be evaluated, explained, and monitored if estimated dietary intakes are adequate. If nutrient intakes are judged to be inadequate, such changes constitute evidence of the need for nutrition support.

Polypharmacy

No medical history can be complete without a detailed list of past and current medications. Polypharmacy is common, and adverse drug–drug or food–drug interactions may go unnoticed. Specific questions need to include the use of mail-ordered or Internet-ordered medications in addition to prescribed or nonprescription medications and supplements. Individuals may purposely minimize the amount of medications they are consuming or not reveal that they continue to obtain prescriptions from former physicians. Taking medications prescribed for friends or relatives is not uncommon in this age group. Ideally, a medication review will include an inventory of the bathroom medicine cabinet, night table, kitchen cabinet, and other drug storage areas. Pharmacists frequently conduct "brown bag" reviews in which the patients bring all medications to them.

Specific questions about use of herbal products or other dietary supplements are needed because individuals are unlikely to tell health professionals about their use without direct questioning.[25,26] In a study of older Wisconsin adults, approximately half of females and 42% of males aged 65 to 84 years reported current and regular use of herbals.[25] This represented a doubling of usage in a 10-year period. Between 1990 and 1997, the use of at least one alternative medicine therapy among the general public increased from 33.8 to 42.1%.[26] Less than 40% of these patients informed their physicians about the use of these therapies. In general, older adults are even more likely to use alternative therapies than younger adults.[27] Clinicians may well find that dietary and herbal supplement use by the elderly is the rule rather than the exception in the 21st century.

Assessment of Medication Knowledge and Practices of Older Adults

All members of the healthcare team should and can be involved in a thorough assessment of the nutritional and medication knowledge and practices of older adults. Table 10.3 is one example of a model instrument for medication assessment proposed by DeBrew et al. with five sections: administration and storage, purchasing habits, attitudes, lifestyle habits, home/environment, and medication profile.[1] In an evaluation of this instrument, the greatest knowledge deficits about drug action, administration, and side effects were observed for medications that had been prescribed shortly before or during a recent hospitalization.

Surgical

Questions about previous surgeries, especially those involving the gastrointestinal tract, are important in identifying specific nutritional risks for maldigestion and malabsorption. Asking whether the patient was able to eat, whether parenteral or enteral nutrition support was provided, and how much weight was lost prior to or after the surgery can provide additional clues of nutrition problems.[21,22,28]

Additional questions about oral surgeries, procedures, and problems are especially important since these may contribute to avoidance of foods, less enjoyment of food, or simply smaller intake. Specific goals in *Healthy People 2010* include preventing the loss of permanent teeth and the erosion of gingival tissue.[10]

Family

Family history can also identify diseases that can directly influence nutrition or be influenced by nutrition.[9] Familial diseases such as anemias, cardiovascular dis-

Table 10.3 Medication Assessment Tool of Knowledge and Habits in Older Adults, and Medication Profile Tool

Medication Assessment

Please check the appropriate response:

Administrator: "I need to see all of your medications. Please show me those you take every day, and those you take occasionally. Don't forget to show me eye drops, insulin, laxatives, vitamins, herbal products, antacids, ointments, or any other over-the-counter drugs you some-times use. Are there any other medications that you regularly take that are not here today?" (Attach copy/copies of each medication profile).

I. Medication administration and storage

    ☐ Yes   ☐ No   Can patient open a pill bottle? (Have patient demonstrate.)

    ☐ Yes   ☐ No   Can patient break a pill in half? (Either have patient demonstrate or omit.)

    ☐ Yes   ☐ No   Does someone help you take your medicine?

    ☐ Yes   ☐ No   Do you use any type of system to help you take your pills, such as a pillbox or a calendar? If yes, list: _____

    ☐ Yes   ☐ No   Do you have problems swallowing your pills?

                              Where do you store your medicine? _____

II. Medication purchasing habits

    Where do you purchase your medicines? _____

    ☐ Yes   ☐ No   Does the drug store you use deliver the medicines to your home? If no, how do you get your medicines? _____

    ☐ Yes   ☐ No   Do you always use the same drug store? If no, explain: _____

    ☐ Yes   ☐ No   Do financial difficulties ever prevent you from buying your medicine?

III. Attitudes

    ☐ Excellent   How would you describe your health? _____

    ☐ Good   What do you see as your health needs? _____

    ☐ Fair   _____

    ☐ Poor   _____

    ☐ Yes   ☐ No   Does taking your medicines upset your daily routine? If yes, explain: _____

    ☐ Yes   ☐ No   Do side effects from your medications upset your daily routine?

    ☐ Yes   ☐ No   Do your medicine(s) help you?

    ☐ Don't Know

    ☐ Yes   ☐ No   Do you ever share your medicines with anyone else?

IV. Lifestyle habits

    Times per week

    _____ How often do you drink coffee, tea, colas, or eat chocolate?

    _____ How often do you use cigarettes, snuff, or other tobacco products?

    _____ How often do you consume beer, wine, or liquor?

    _____ How often do you use recreational drugs such as marijuana?

V. Home environment

    Who else stays at your residence? (List relationship and age.) _____

    ☐ Yes   ☐ No   If someone else lives in home, does that person participate in your health care? If yes, explain: _____

VI. Medication profile

    Record each medication separately on the form below. (Attach additional sheets as necessary.)

Table 10.3 **Medication Assessment Tool of Knowledge and Habits in Older Adults, and Medication Profile Tool (*Continued*)**

		Medicine name: _____
		Dosage: _____
		Route: _____
		Expiration Date exactly as printed on label: _____
☐ Yes	☐ No	Can you read the name, dosage, and expiration date of this medicine?
		Why do you take this medicine? _____
		How long have you taken the dosage? _____
		When do you take the medicine? _____
		How many do you take? _____
		Do you know what the side effects are? List: _____
☐ Yes	☐ No	Does the medicine cause you any problems or side effects?
		What do you do if you experience side effects (stop the pills, call the doctor, etc.)? _____

Source: DeBrew, J.K., Barba, B.E., and Tesh, A.S., *Home Healthcare Nurse,*16, 688–689, 1998. With permission.

eases, dementias, depression, endocrine diseases, and inherited metabolic diseases particularly impact nutrition status. Drug–nutrient history of family members may provide additional information in assessing nutritional risks, such as iron overload in families with hemachromatosis or development of B vitamin deficiencies in family members on long-term regimens of diuretics or antidepressants.

Social

Factors that disrupt a person's eating patterns, create undue stress, provide exposure to environmental risks, or interfere with normal activities or exercise patterns need to be identified.[20,23] Assessment of living arrangements, social support network, daily activities, adequacy of resources, and high-risk lifestyles such as smoking and alcohol use may also provide clues as to nutrition needs and dietary adequacy.

Dietary History

Perhaps the most important nutrition assessment component is a report of weight change per unit of time. It is important to determine whether weight gains or losses were intentional, when onset occurred, and what attempts have been made to modify the changes.[23] A dietary assessment can be conducted by several methods. In clinical settings a usual dietary intake for one day with a crosscheck of food group frequency provides a clue as to usual diet patterns. A 3-day food record that the patient or caregiver keeps can also provide good insight into both food quality and quantity. Questions about finances may reveal an inability to purchase an adequate diet or use of food assistance programs. Questions about food purchasing, food preparation, food handling, food storage, and eating habits may reveal food safety and health risks centering around food choices. An often-overlooked important aspect of the dietary history is fluid intake. Thirst mechanisms of the older person may be impaired, and dehydration is a risk factor. Often older patients will report limited intake of food and water due to the multiple medications that they have to ingest on a daily basis. This may be especially problematic when unexpected expenses, such as high energy bills, force the elderly to choose between purchasing food or purchasing medication. Either choice is likely to produce a reduced beneficial effect.

Review of Systems

The review of systems often reveals many subtle symptoms of nutrition derangements, which are reported by the patient but ascribed to a nonnutritional etiology, inasmuch as malnutrition often mimics the aging process. Further questioning of the individuals may yield more specific correlation of the findings with eating patterns or habits.

Physical Exam

As is the case with the history, the performance of a routine physical exam can reveal clues concerning the individual's nutritional status. Specific physical findings that relate to nutritional status and are critical points in evaluating nutritional status can be found in Appendix E.1.

Nutrition Screening Initiative

For more than 10 years, the Nutrition Screening Initiative (NSI), a national multiprofessional/multiorganizational group, has provided a plethora of background literature containing tools for nutrition screening, assessment, and interventions. This information, in part abstracted in this chapter, is available through numerous sources including the Internet (http://www.aafp.org/NSI) or by writing directly to Nutrition Screening Initiative, 1010 Wisconsin Avenue, NW, Suite 800, Washington, D.C. 20007.

IDENTIFYING THOSE WHO NEED NUTRITION SUPPORT

Several evaluation instruments developed by the Nutrition Screening Initiative can be used to identify individuals needing nutrition support. These include two types of tools that differ in administration and complexity. The first tool termed the *determine* checklist is self-administered or caregiver-administered as an awareness tool. The second set of tools is the levels I and II screens, which are administered by a social or healthcare professional.

Statements from the DETERMINE checklist or level I screen include the following:[20]

1. I have an illness or condition that made me change the kind and/or amount of food I eat.

Table 10.4 Nutrition Support Screening Alerts

If an older individual indicates that the following questions listed on the checklist, level I and level II screens are descriptive of his or her condition or life situations, nutrition counseling and support interventions may help solve any nutritional problems and improve nutritional status.

Determine Your Nutritional Health Checklist Alerts

I have an illness or condition that made me change the kind and/or amount of food I eat.
Without wanting to, I have lost or gained 10 pounds in the last 6 months.
I am not always physically able to shop, cook, and/or feed myself.

Level I Screen Alerts

Has lost or gained 10 pounds or more in the past 6 months
Body mass index <22 or >27
Is on a special diet
Has difficulty chewing or swallowing
Has pain in mouth, teeth, or gums
Usually or always needs assistance with preparing food, shopping for foods

Level II Screen Alerts

Has lost or gained 10 pounds or more in the past 6 months
Body mass index <22 or >27
Is on a special diet
Has difficulty chewing or swallowing
Usually or always needs assistance with preparing or shopping for food
Has pain in mouth, teeth, or gums
Midarm muscle circumference <10th percentile
Triceps skinfold < 10th percentile or > 95th percentile
Serum albumin below 3.5 g/dl
Serum cholesterol below 160 mg/dl
Clinical evidence of mental/cognitive impairment
Clinical evidence of depressive illness
Clinical evidence of type 1 or type 2 diabetes, heart disease, high blood pressure, stroke, gastrointestinal disease, kidney disease, chronic lung disease, liver disease, osteoporosis, osteomalacia

Source: Adapted from Nutrition Screening Initiative, *Incorporating nutrition screening and interventions into medical practice: a monograph for physicians,* The Nutrition Screening Initiative, Washington, D.C., 1994, 16, 20, 29–31. With permission.

2. I eat fewer than two meals per day.
3. I eat few fruits or vegetables or milk products.
4. I have three or more drinks of beer, liquor, or wine almost every day.
5. I have tooth or mouth problems that make it hard for me to eat.
6. I don't always have enough money to buy the food I need.
7. I eat alone most of the time.
8. I take three or more different prescribed or over-the-counter drugs a day.
9. Without wanting to, I have lost or gained 10 pounds in the last 6 months.
10. I am not always physically able to shop, cook, and/or feed myself.

Affirmative responses to these questions are summed and tabulated. Table 10.4 presents the screening alerts that suggest nutrition counseling and support interventions.

Some of the level II screen parameters include the following:[20]

1. Has lost or gained 10 pounds or more in the past 6 months
2. Body mass index <22
3. Body mass index >27
4. Is on a special diet
5. Has difficulty chewing or swallowing
6. Usually or always needs assistance with preparing food, shopping for food
7. Has pain in mouth, teeth, or gums
8. Midarm muscle circumference <10th percentile
9. Triceps skinfold <10th percentile
10. Triceps skinfold >95th percentile
11. Serum albumin below 3.5 g/dL
12. Serum cholesterol below 160 mg/dL
13. Clinical evidence of mental/cognitive impairment
14. Clinical evidence of depressive illness
15. Clinical evidence of insulin-dependent diabetes, adult onset diabetes, heart disease, high blood pressure, stroke, gastrointestinal disease, kidney disease, chronic lung disease, liver disease, osteoporosis, osteomalacia

In addition to these parameters, screening alerts pertaining to medications used that are associated with increased risks for food–drug interactions are included. See Table 10.5 for medications screening alerts and Table 10.6 for drug–nutrient interaction screen.

NUTRITION SUPPORT, SUPPLEMENTATION, AND REPLACEMENT

The provision of nutrition to the older American spans a continuum of modalities from usual food intake to the most sophisticated intravenous nutrition. It also spans a continuum of environments from the home setting of the free-living, independent individual to the totally dependent, bedridden, institutionalized older American. Also, those who come in contact with the older American represent a wide spectrum of caregivers from family members to subspecialists in the fields of medicine and rehabilitation. This means no simple set of instructions or procedures will suffice to prevent nutrient–drug interactions or malnutrition in all older adults.

OVERVIEW OF NUTRITION SUPPORT

The goals of nutrition support interventions for the elderly are (1) to maintain or improve nutritional status, (2) to determine and institute nutrient modifications in order to prevent or treat nutrient deficiencies and to manage disease, and (3) to use the most physiologic, efficient, and cost-effective methods.[9] Nutrition support interventions are indicated for older individuals who cannot eat normally or otherwise are at risk for malnutrition or are malnourished. The interventions are needed in a variety of settings, including the home. Sometimes, major medical problems must take priority over nutritional deficits and must be managed simultaneously or

Table 10.5 Medication Use Screening Alerts for Older Adults

If an older individual indicates that the following questions listed on the checklist, level I and level II screens are descriptive of his or her condition or life situation, medication use interventions may help solve nutritional problems and improve nutritional status.

Determine Your Nutritional Health Checklist Alerts

I take three or more different prescribed or over-the-counter drugs a day.
I have three or more drinks of beer, liquor, or wine almost every day.
Without wanting to, I have lost or gained 10 pounds in the past 6 months.

Level I Screen Alerts

Three or more prescription drugs, OTC medications, and/or vitamin/mineral supplements daily
Has lost or gained 10 pounds or more in the past six months
Has poor appetite
Has difficulty chewing or swallowing
Usually or always needs assistance with walking or moving about, traveling outside the home, preparing food, or shopping for food or other necessities

Level II Screen Alerts

Has lost or gained 10 pounds or more in the past 6 months
Has poor appetite
Has difficulty chewing or swallowing
Usually or always needs assistance with walking or moving about, traveling outside the home, preparing food, or shopping for food and other necessities
Three or more prescription drugs, OTC medications, or vitamin/mineral supplements daily
Clinical evidence of mental/cognitive impairment
Clinical evidence of depression

Source: Adapted from Nutrition Screening Initiative, *Incorporating nutrition screening and interventions into medical practice: a monograph for physicians,* The Nutrition Screening Initiative, Washington, D.C., 1994, 16, 20, 29–31. With permission.

even before nutritional intervention can be optimized; such priorities include management of infection, control of blood pressure, metabolic derangements, and correction of fluid and electrolyte imbalance.

In stable, long-term care patients, chronic undernutrition is a frequent problem, despite the lack of acute disease processes. Patients who require long-term care may have inadequate dietary and fluid intakes because of dementia or the need for help with feeding.[23,28,29] That need for help may be a significant factor even in less dependent nursing home patients, not only for adequate energy and fluid intake but also for nutrient density. Inadequate energy and fluid intake may negatively impact on drug metabolism. Suboptimal body cell mass and body composition or changing body composition may affect drug binding and distribution creating problems with food and drug interactions.

INDICATIONS FOR NUTRITION SUPPORT

A nutrition support intervention is indicated for older individuals who because of anatomic, physiologic, or mental health problems cannot meet their nutritional

Table 10.6 Drug–Nutrient Interaction Screen

1. Does the patient take any of the drugs included on the following list, that can adversely affect nutritional status?
   a. Digoxin
   b. Diuretics
   c. Nonsteroidal antiinflammatory drugs
   d. Sulfasalazine
   e. Phenytoin
   f. Cancer chemotherapeutic agents
   g. Bile acid sequestrants (e.g., cholestyramine or colestipol)
   h. Other
   If the patient is taking a drug that may adversely affect their nutritional status, biochemical assessment of nutritional status and blood counts are required on a regular basis.
2. Is the patient currently receiving food, formula, or nutrient supplements that impair drug absorption (e.g., Sustacal or Ensure) at the time when that drug is given? To answer this question, you may want to check with a pharmacist or the American Dietetic Association Handbook on Drug–Nutrient Interactions.
   If yes, then the time to give the food, formula, or nutrient should be changed.
3. Is the patient eating foods that are likely to cause reactions when consumed with the patient's present medications?
   If yes, then advise the patient to avoid such foods.
4. Does the patient consume more than two alcoholic beverages a day?
   Since alcohol can adversely affect drug and nutrient interactions, advise patient not to drink.
5. Has the effectiveness of this patient's drug therapy declined following a diet change?
   If yes, then obtain the drug levels; if below the therapeutic level, then the physician should modify the dose if the present diet is necessary, otherwise, return patient to the previous diet.
6. Has this patient's nutritional status declined since the current drugs were prescribed?
   If yes, then perhaps the drug caused the change; to improve the patient's nutritional status, either (1) discontinue the drug; (2) give a nutrient supplement in order to meet higher drug-related nutritional requirements; or (3) make referral to dietitian for in-depth assessment of nutrient intake.
7. Has the patient received instruction on when to take his/her medications in relation to food?
   If no, give instructions orally and in writing.
8. Do both the patient and the caregiver understand these instructions?
   If no, counsel the patient and the caregiver.
9. Is the patient receiving a drug that could increase the risk of chronic disease including diabetes and chronic heart disease?
   If yes, then monitor blood glucose and lipid levels.
10. Does the patient have impaired liver or kidney function?
    If yes, reduction in drug dosage is indicated and the patient will need careful monitoring because slow elimination of drugs increases the risk of toxicity and drug-induced nutritional deficiency.

See *Handbook on Drug and Nutrient Interactions* by Daphne Roe, American Dietetic Association, Chicago, IL 1992

Source: The Nutrition Screening Initiative, *Nutrition Interventions Manual for Professionals Caring for Older Americans, Executive Summary,* Nutrition Screening Initiative, Washington, D.C., 1992, 31. With permission.

needs by eating a nutritionally balanced diet normally; that is, individuals who cannot, should not, or will not eat sufficiently. Nutrition counseling interventions provide individualized guidance on appropriate food and nutrition intakes for those with special needs and are an integral component of nutrition support interventions. Such counseling may include advice about increasing or decreasing nutrients in the diet; changing the timing, size, or composition of meals; modifying the texture of foods; and, in certain instances, changing the route of the administration from oral to tube to intravenous.[30]

Nutrition support interventions include modification of nutrient content, nutrient density, consistency, or form. Nutrition support regimens may include use of medical nutritional products such as oral supplements or total enteral feedings. Nutrition support can also be provided by an enterally placed tube or intravenous catheter. Even in the absence of overt protein–energy malnutrition, there may be indications for nutritional support whether in independent living or in acute or chronic institutional settings. A wide variety of older individuals can benefit from nutrition support interventions. Some are severely ill, but most suffer from chronic conditions or diseases often associated with the aging process. Modified foods will be more costly than normal foods, but may avoid even more expensive medical care and hospitalizations. Parenteral or enteral feeding when used appropriately can be financially advantageous. Indications for nutrition support are discussed in the following sections.

Cannot Eat Enough

Older individuals who are chronically ill or functionally dependent have difficulty accessing a complete diet and may be classified as individuals who cannot eat enough—those who have experienced a stroke, are being treated for cancer, have dementia, have had bone fractures, are chronically depressed, or are residing in an institutional environment, for example. Chronically ill individuals who are taking an array of medications often have appetite changes, taste changes, and altered nutrient needs that limit consumption of a complete diet. Other individuals who cannot eat enough include those who have dysphagia, malabsorption, or maldigestion; are recovering from surgery; or have chewing or other swallowing disorders.

Cannot Eat

Individuals who are acutely ill or injured, have had recent surgery, or have gastrointestinal obstruction fall into the category of those who cannot eat at all. Otherwise healthy patients who remain heavily sedated or in a coma for more than seven days need special consideration of nutrition support beyond simple dextrose and electrolyte administration.

Should Not Eat

Individuals who should not eat because of severe diarrhea, malabsorption, obstruction, surgery of the gastrointestinal tract, radiation enteritis, or metabolic disease require more specialized nutrition support intervention. Often, parenteral nutrition is the best option, although early enteral feeding is often a viable option for postsurgical patients.

Will Not Eat

Individuals who will not eat adequate amounts of nutrients by the normal oral routes may suffer from conditions such as anorexia, dementia, depression, the side effects of drugs, or perceived intolerance.

ENERGY AND PROTEIN REQUIREMENTS

Physiologic, socioeconomic, and psychologic factors affect dietary intake and therefore nutritional status. This section briefly summarizes what is known or hypothesized regarding how energy and protein requirements of older individuals may differ from those of younger adults.

Energy Requirements

One of the outcomes of nutritional screening and assessment is to arrive at a nutritional diagnosis and a determination of the nutritional needs of the patient. Energy needs may be determined through cumbersome complex direct measurements of metabolic rates or through indirect measurements or estimations of energy expenditure. Because the most sophisticated direct measures of metabolic rates may not be practical outside of research or academic settings, estimations of energy needs must often suffice.

Resting energy expenditure (REE), the largest component of total energy expenditure for most individuals, is the energy expended by a person at rest. It varies with the amount and composition of metabolically active tissue, which in turn varies with age. Lean body (fat-free) mass, the most metabolically active body compartment, declines with age. A proportional decrease occurs in REE. The energy (caloric) requirements of older persons are less than those of younger persons. Energy requirements, however, are not based on chronologic age alone. Rates of decline in energy expenditure vary widely among individuals and differ according to factors such as body size, body composition, and activity level.

Table 10.7 provides two common methods of estimating energy and protein requirements. These may be adjusted for various medical conditions, body alterations (e.g., obesity or amputation), and for various physical and exercise lifestyles.

Protein Requirements

Protein metabolism changes with age. A loss of total body protein occurs largely because of decreased skeletal muscle mass. Whether protein requirements in older persons are higher or lower is controversial. Arguments for decreasing protein intake are based on whether the aging kidney can handle higher filtration loads associated

Table 10.7 Formulas for Estimating Energy and Protein Needs
of Older Persons

A. Empiric Formula for Daily Energy and Protein Needs in Older Persons

Activity/Stress	Resting	Moderate
Energy	20–25 kcal/kg	25–30 kcal/kg
Protein	1 g/kg	1.5 g/kg

B. Harris–Benedict Equation to Estimate Calorie Requirements

Harris–Benedict Equation (HBE) for basal energy expenditure
Men: $66.47 + 13.75W + 5.0H - 6.76A$
Women: $665.10 + 9.56W + 1.85H - 4.68A$

Note: W = weight in kg; H = height in cm; A = age in years.

with higher protein intakes. Little evidence, however, supports this concern in individuals who are free of renal disease.

Although most studies suggest that healthy older adults have a recommended dietary allowance (RDA) of 0.8 g protein per kilogram of body weight, a study of older men and women with minor chronic diseases suggested that this level was insufficient to maintain adequate nitrogen balance in about 50% of subjects.[27] Other studies of protein intake and exercise suggest that maintenance or building of lean tissue in the elderly requires a higher level of protein.[31,32] From a practical perspective, 1 g/kg body weight is easier to remember and use and may be more appropriate for the chronically ill older person. Protein requirements may increase with surgery, infection, trauma, and other metabolically stressful situations, as in younger persons. The presence of pressure sores or the immobilization of an individual in restraints, a wheelchair, or a bed may increase the protein requirements of an older adult for maintenance of nitrogen equilibrium. Protein requirements may be estimated using the energy requirements yielded by the Harris–Benedict equation. Healthy individuals usually require about 10–12% of kilocalories to come from protein sources.

NUTRITION SUPPORT — WALKING THE TALK

Individuals at risk for malnutrition should receive a nutritionally dense, well-balanced diet and should be encouraged to eat as much as possible within the limits of their disabilities, oral health status, and medical conditions.[16, 20–22] Food is an important part of life, and elderly individuals should be encouraged to maintain their normal diets as long as possible. Supplementation may be necessary. See Table 10.8 for screening alerts for nutrition support.[20]

Even in the critically ill elderly patient, the optimal route of nutrition delivery is the gastrointestinal tract; intraluminal nutrients maximize intestinal mass and function. Figure 10.1 provides a nutrition support route decision tree. When selecting alternate feeding regimens, the route and formula selected should be the most cost effective and best physiologic choice. The oral route should be maximized by the use of frequent feedings as appropriate, desirable flavors, avoidance of malodorous

Table 10.8 Nutrition Support Interventions for Four Stages of Nutrition Support

Stage	Characteristics	Recommendations[a]
Stage one	Inadequate/inappropriate diet	More frequent meals/snacks
	Change in nutrient content/density	Encourage nutrient-dense foods
Stage two	Eating/chewing difficulties	Modify food consistency—chop, blend, puree
	Unable to feed self	Use oral medical nutritional supplements, fortified puddings, beverages
Stage three	Unable to meet nutritionally needs orally	Select enteral formula to meet needs
	Unable to swallow sufficient supplements	May use "recreational" feeding (a small amount given for psychological satisfaction or first step toward oral feeding)
Stage four	Unable to use gastrointestinal tract or meet needs through enteral nutrition	Establish parenteral nutrition plan; may use "recreational" feeding

[a] For more detailed screening alerts and recommendations for various caregivers, see Nutrition Support Interventions in *Nutrition Interventions Manual for Professionals Caring for Older Americans, Executive Summary*, Nutrition Screening Initiative, Washington, D.C. 1994, page 31; and *Incorporating nutrition screening and interventions into medical practice: A monograph for physicians,* The Nutrition Screening Initiative, Washington, D.C., 1994, 16, 20, 29–31. With permission.

products, as well as palatable, calorically dense oral formulas when needed, such as puddings and medical nutritional supplements.

The timing of feeding is important, and a schedule of eating should be established. This schedule should also incorporate the appropriate timing of medications. While the older individual is awake, every opportunity should be taken to offer the patient additional nutrients. In individuals with dementia or with short-term memory loss from other causes, multiple frequent feedings are often better accepted and tolerated than traditional meals. Consideration of potential drug–nutrient interactions are, however, extremely important to recognize in frequent feeding schedules. For the patients with dementia, certain days are more difficult than others. Preferred foods or favorite meals may be substituted for the regular menu to encourage food intake on these days.

FOUR STAGES OF NUTRITION SUPPORT

It is convenient to consider nutrition support in four stages as shown in Table 10.8. The first stage is the alteration of usual food intake by modification of nutrient content and density. Recommended actions may include increasing the number of times a day the person eats or incorporating high-nutrient foods into the diet. The second stage is the modification of food consistency and the use of medical nutritional supplements. The third stage is enteral tube feeding, and the fourth stage is parenteral nutrition.[9]

Evaluation of dysphagia is receiving appropriately increased attention. Modification of textures and consistencies of food may enhance swallowing. Different

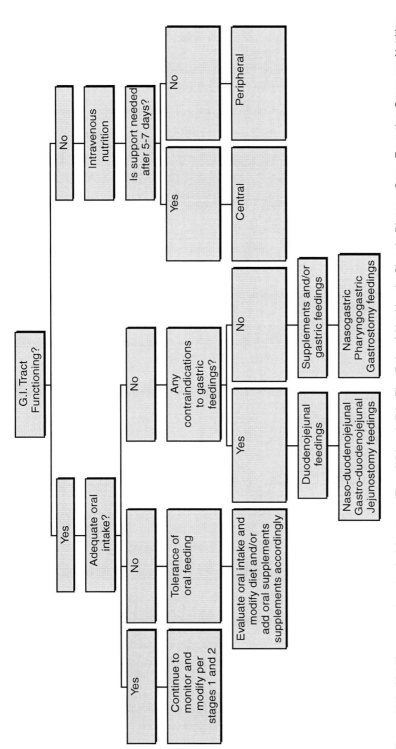

Figure 10.1 Nutrition support route decision tree. (From White, J. Ed., *The Role of Nutrition in Chronic Disease Care, Executive Summary*, Nutrition Screening Initiative, 5, 18, 24, 33, 43, 50, 62, 71, 1997. With permission.)

swallowing problems are best treated with various food consistencies. As a general rule, foods of similar consistency should be presented at any given time. Some individuals can swallow only food that is softened or moistened with thick liquids; others may only tolerate thin liquids. In some instances, commercially available thickening agents can be added to liquid supplements to facilitate their safe ingestion. These thickening agents, which are basically carbohydrates and, hence, digestible, do provide some kilocalories and have not been shown to interfere with nutrient bioavailability. Little or no study of the potential effect of these substances on drugs has been reported.

It is important in evaluation of dysphagia/aspiration to incorporate the status of the esophagus and stomach. Often modified barium swallows are performed that reveal penetration (aspiration) and the study is terminated with a recommendation that the patient be placed nothing by mouth (NPO) and a percutaneous endoscopic gastrostomy (PEG) tube inserted without a complete evaluation of gastric functioning. In many elderly individuals gastroesophageal reflux disease (GERD), gastroparesis, or gastric outlet obstruction may be present from a variety of etiologic factors (i.e., diabetes, neurological deficits, GERD, peptic ulcer disease) or medications (e.g., anticholinergics, smooth muscle relaxants).

In these individuals, gastric feedings would be fraught with the potential of aspiration, similar to that associated with eating. Thus, in situations where dysphagia/aspiration leading to the documentation of aspiration by modified barium swallow, these individuals should have a small bore nasogastric tube inserted, through which Gastrograffin® or barium is introduced into the stomach to assess gastrointestinal motility, esophageal reflux, and "retro" aspiration potential.

Nutritional Supplements

Many nutritional supplements are available. Carbohydrate and protein powders can be added to the patient's usual diet to increase the caloric and nutrient density without changing the flavor, texture, or color. Medical nutritional supplements available in grocery stores and pharmacies can provide protein, carbohydrates, and fats, as well as vitamins and minerals. The supplement chosen should be effective for the purpose intended; a nutritional supplement from the shelf of a health food store or a mail-order catalog may not qualify. Consultation with a registered dietitian or other qualified healthcare professional is obviously indicated in selecting such supplements. This recommendation is particularly important for long-term care patients with chronic cardiac, renal, pulmonary, and hepatic disease. Supplements must, therefore, fit the therapeutic needs of such individuals.

Many older individuals, especially African-Americans, Asian-Americans, and Latinos are lactose intolerant or have conditions that temporarily render them lactose deficient (e.g., severe malnutrition, sprue, bacterial overgrowth, chemotoxicity). These individuals may need lactose-free or low-lactose nutritional supplements in place of milkshakes, custards, or cream soups.

Oral supplementation of patient's diets with commercial medical nutritional supplements has been shown to be useful in cancer patients, long-term care patients, and homebound individuals. The addition of nutritional supplements significantly improved overall nutrient intake and helped correct nutritional deficiencies. Fiber-supplemented formulas for individuals who will be on a full liquid diet for a prolonged period of time or who have constipation, diverticulosis, or anorectal disease may be indicated.[33]

When considering alternatives to oral feedings such as enteral and parenteral nutrition, ethical and legal issues are often encountered. These are often reduced through appropriate open and honest communication among all parties involved. The patient, when possible, should be the principal decision maker.[19]

Enteral Tube Feeding

Aggressive nutritional support via enteral tube feeding can restore nutritional status in individuals who are unable to ingest adequate nutrients by mouth.[34] Enteral feeding by tube provides a reasonably safe, cost-effective method of providing protein, calories, vitamins, minerals, trace elements, and fluid while preserving or restoring a functional bowel.[8,14,31]

Long-term enteral support can be safe and effective for extended periods of time. It is most successful if administered at volumes and rates tailored to meet the patient's tolerance and caloric and nutritional needs.

Feeding Routes

The simplest normal approach to the gastrointestinal tract is through nasally inserted tubes. Technologic advances over the past 25 years have resulted in the development of soft biocompatible tubes that are well tolerated for prolonged periods. The flexibility of these tubes, however, means easy malpositioning or dislodgement. Most incorporate a tungsten or other nonmercury metal tip. Nasogastric, nasoduodenal, and nasojejunal tubes for feeding are generally used for short-term (less than 3 months) access. For individuals unable to be fed through the nasoenteric route and for patients on long-term tube feeding, various invasive and minimally invasive procedures or ostoenteric routes have been developed. These include cervical pharyngostomies, gastrointestinal tract endoscopic tubes (percutaneous endoscopic gastrostomies [PEG], percutaneous endoscopic gastrojejunostomy [PEGJ], or surgically placed entry, including laparoscopy or laparoscopically placed, gastrostomy, and jejunostomy).

In some instances, long double-lumen nasogastroduodenal tubes provide access to the GI tract for postpyloric feeding while simultaneously suctioning the stomach in patients with gastric atony or aspiration risk. Similarly, dual lumen gastrostomy tubes with provision for both gastric decompression and transpyloric feeding are available.

Enteral Formulas

A number of commercially prepared formulas are available for enteral feeding. These formulas have varying concentrations of protein, carbohydrates, and fat and may differ in caloric density, calorie-to-nitrogen ratio, electrolyte content, vitamin and mineral content, and osmolarity. They also may differ in degree of hydrolysis of the protein source as well as in the source of other macronutrients. These formulas (containing whole protein, fat, and carbohydrates) and the specialty formulas, with rare exceptions, meet the dietary reference intakes (DRIs) for essential nutrients when provided in amounts that meet energy needs. The choice of formula should be based on clinical efficacy and cost effectiveness; that is, the least expensive product that best meets the patient's needs. Formula selection should optimally coincide with the GIT functional status in the individual. As a general rule, the more complete the formula, the more physiologic, palatable, isotonic, and less expensive.

Some general guidelines can help in selection of formulas for enteral as well as parenteral nutrition support. First, the selected product should meet the older patient's nutritional need at the appropriate rate, volume, and osmolality through the route selected. Second, product literature should be read for information regarding the nutrient concentrations and other product attributes. Third, product information should be based on sound scientific research. Fourth, dietitians, physicians, pharmacists, and nurses, particularly those who are members of nutrition support teams, can provide timely and expert advice regarding formula selection.

Selecting a formula for use with long-term tube-fed patients requires consideration of energy, protein, vitamin, mineral, and fluid needs. Although energy needs may be low owing to a decrease in energy output and a slower basal metabolic rate, requirements for other nutrients remain the same, with only small variations. The challenge this represents is that small volumes of formula sometimes do not provide the levels of protein, vitamins, minerals, trace elements, and fluid needed to maintain nutritional status. Commercially available formulas have been designed for use in the older American to provide appropriate levels of macronutrients and micronutrients within restricted volumes. Inadequate volumes of enteral formulas may be a factor in the inadequate hydration of tube-fed older individuals; many are susceptible to disorientation and confusion as a result of dehydration.[29]

As a general rule, fluid requirements for individuals older than 50 years of age are approximately 1500 ml/d. The fluid requirements can be met by providing at least 1 ml/kcal ingested, 30 ml/kg of body weight, or 125% of the volume of the formula.

The most important criterion for effectiveness of nutrition support is clinical tolerance and meeting nutritional goals (energy). The required energy intakes, generally estimated at 30 kcal/kg, are adjusted according to clinical response and nutritional parameters such as weight gain, anthropometry, and serum albumin level.

Complications

Complications of enteral nutritional support include mechanical clogging of the tube, aspiration of stomach contents, vomiting, and bloating. Proper product selection, administration, and patient monitoring can often prevent or alleviate these symptoms. The most common complications that occur are diarrhea and cramping abdominal pain. These are sometimes due to rapid infusion and can be ameliorated by reducing the flow rate, but other more frequent causes should be suspected. One frequent and overlooked cause of diarrhea is the hyperosmolarity of medications such as potassium chloride, antibiotics, and additives such as sorbitol delivered through the feeding tube. Other causes include bacterial overgrowth and hypooncotic acid factitious diarrhea from a fecal impaction. Metabolic, fluid, and electrolyte abnormalities may occur and include hyperglycemia and glycosuria, hyperosmolar coma, edema, congestive heart failure, hyponatremia, hyperkalemia, hypercalcemia, and essential fatty acid deficiency. These complications are rare when appropriate formulations are administered and tolerated. Older patients usually exhibit increasing glucose intolerance with advancing age. The hyperglycemia and glycosuria can be treated by reducing flow rate, providing formulas designed for patients with hyperglycemia, and administering insulin, if necessary.[5]

Parenteral Nutrition Support

Some elderly patients require parenteral (intravenous) nutrition for some or all of their needs for at least a time. Individuals who are candidates for parenteral nutrition are those who cannot meet their nutritional goal by the oral or tube feeding enteral route.

Peripheral Venous Route

The peripheral venous route may be used for periods of 5 to 7 days in a small subset of patients who are neither severely catabolic nor depleted and in whom the return of gastrointestinal function is expected within days. The peripheral route is limited by the availability of veins and the need to change sites, usually every 48 h. Atrophic skin changes and easy bruising, often seen in the older adult, limit the route's usefulness. In addition, osmolalities should not exceed 900 mOsm/L. Dextrose concentrations greater than 10% may be associated with the development of phlebitis and thrombosis. Although intravenous lipid emulsions have been able to provide additional kilocalories to spare proteins, these solutions seldom provide the optimal daily requirements of kilocalories. Nevertheless, the peripheral route is a useful short-term modality when the rate of the patient's GI recovery is uncertain.[5]

Central Venous Route

The mainstay of parenteral nutrition remains the central intravenous route, which is necessary to access veins of large diameter and high flow such as the superior vena cava and to provide the hypertonic solutions of total parenteral nutrition (TPN). Many different parenteral solutions and enteral products are now available. General guidelines for formulas are detailed in Chapter 8.

Complications

Complications may arise from formula feeding, and these are outlined in Table 10.9. Special consideration to long-term use of these feedings is needed in older patients, especially in home health care. Thus, the development of an interdisciplinary care plan (ICP) is particularly critical in successful outcomes of such therapies. This care plan can be incorporated into a therapy agreement when the various

Table 10.9 Potential Complications of Total Parenteral Nutrition

Medical/Catheter Related

Air embolism
Catheter tip dislodgment
Contaminated TPN solution
Hemothorax
Incorrect catheter positioning
Pneumothorax (early or late)
Sepsis—catheter exit site or catheter tip
Venous tear
Venous thrombosis

Metabolic

Biliary sludge/stones
Essential fatty acid deficiency
Hepatic dysfunction
Hyperammonemia
Hyperglycemia or hypoglycemia
Hypocalcemia
Hypophosphatemia
Metabolic bone disease
Prerenal azotemia
Trace mineral deficiencies: zinc, copper, chromium
Vitamin deficiency: B vitamins and vitamin C
Vitamin toxicity: vitamin A and vitamin D

procedures, the individual responsible for each task, the potential complications, the monitoring, and the approximate costs included along with the goals of the therapy are outlined. The agreement should then be signed by the patient, a family member or other caregiver, the physician, the home infusion company, and, where applicable, the home health agency or others involved in the home nutrition support. The interdisciplinary care plan is essential for the reimbursement of home therapy and can be very important to the well-being of the patient and the caregivers. Included in ICP are the precautions necessary for the safe and effective use of medications with the nutrition therapy.

ADVERSE DRUG EFFECTS ON NUTRITIONAL HEALTH

Potential for food-drug interactions in nutrition support have been discussed in Chapter 8. In the elderly, the risks for adverse events increase significantly.[6] Multifactorial risks in elderly rise with the existence of multiple disease conditions and polypharmacy.[32] Ten of the most common disease states in older persons are presented in Table 10.10. The drugs commonly used to treat these disease states and the nutrition-related adverse effects are summarized. Bolding of selected events indicate those most likely to occur in older patients. The number of adverse events and the potential impact on nutritional status make monitoring of older patients' drug regimens and nutritional status critical in promoting a better quality of life and better health care for our senior citizens.

CONCLUSIONS

The elderly population is at high-risk for malnutrition, drug-nutrient interactions and adverse effects on nutritional status. In many instances these negative outcomes can be ameliorated through early, cost-effective nutritional assessment and interventions.

Nutrition support in the acute or long-term institutional and home care settings can be successful in older patients. Careful attention must be given to lifestyle factors, gastrointestinal function, unique nutrient needs, tube site location, feeding regimen, disease-specific requirements, and polypharmacy. Likewise, ethical and legal issues should be considered when dealing with non-volitional nutrition support in the elderly. Oral, enteral, and parenteral nutritional support may be used singly or together, as needed in a rational sequence, through the four stages of nutrition support; these stages represent a gradual increase in complexity and cost paralleling progressive inability to use regular foods and the GI tract. Regardless of the stages of nutrition support, scrutiny of the drugs (prescribed and over the counter) that the older person is receiving will minimize polypharmacy, drug-nutrient interactions and adverse drug effects on nutritional health.

Potential for food–drug interactions in nutrition support have been discussed in Chapter 8. In the elderly, the risks for adverse events increase significantly.[6] Multi-factorial risks in elderly rise with the existence of multiple disease conditions and polypharmacy.[32] Ten of the most common disease states in older persons are presented in Table 10.10. The drugs commonly used to treat these disease states and the nutrition-related adverse effects are summarized. Bolding of selected events indicate those most likely to occur in older patients. The number of adverse events and the potential impact on nutritional status make monitoring of older patients' drug regimens and nutritional status critical in promoting a better quality of life and better health care for our senior citizens.

Table 10.10 Drugs Used in the Treatment of Specific Diseases or Conditions with the Potential to Negatively Impact Nutritional Status in Older Patients

Disease States or Conditions	Drug Categories	Nutrition-Related Adverse Effects (Items Appearing in Bolded Type Occur with Greater Frequency)
Cancer (CA)	Corticosteroids, e.g., cortisone (Cortone®), hydrocortisone (Cortef®, Solu-Cortef®), methylprednisolone (Medrol®, Solu-Medrol®), prednisone (Deltasone®), prednisolone (Prelone™), triamcinolone (Aristocort®), or dexamethasone (Decadron®)	Abdominal distention, anorexia, increased appetite, diarrhea, ulcerative esophagitis, GI bleeding, **hypocalcemia, hyperglycemia or hypoglycemia, hypokalemia,** hypertension, muscle mass loss, nausea, **osteoporosis,** pancreatitis, **sodium and fluid retention,** vomiting, weight gain
	Hormonal oncologics, e.g., methyltestosterone (Android®), diethylstilbesterol (DES®), anastrozole (Arimidex®), bicalutamide (Casodex®), estramustine (Emcyt®), flutamide (Eulexin®), toremifene (Fareston®), letrozole (Femara®), fluoxymesterone (Halotestin®), leuprolide (Lupron®), megestrol (Megace®), nilutamide (Nilandron®), tamoxifen (Nolvadex®), goserelin (Zoladex®)	Anorexia, anemia, increased appetite, diarrhea, edema, **fluid retention,** glossitis, **nausea, vomiting,** weight gain
	Immunotherapeutics, e.g., interferon alpha 2a (Roferon A®), interferon alpha 2b (Intron A®), rituximab (Rituxan®), trastuzumab (Herceptin®), denileukin diftitox (Ontak®), gemtuzumab, ozogamien (Mylotarg®)	**Anorexia, diarrhea,** edema, **nausea, vomiting, stomatitis,** taste perversion, weight loss
	Chemotherapeutic agents: alkylating agents, e.g., inelphalan (Alkeran®), cyclophosphamide (Cytoxan®), ifosfamide/mesna (Ifex/Mesnex®), busulfan (Myleran®) antibiotic agents, e.g., daunorubicin (Cerubidine®), daunorubicin liposomal (Daunoxome®), doxorubicin (Adriamycin®), doxorubicin liposomal (Doxil®), idarubicin (Idamycin®), plicamycin (Mithracin®), mitomycin (Mutamycin®), pentostatin (Nipent®), mitoxantrone (Novantrone®), bleomycin (Blenoxane®) antimetabolites, e.g., fluorouracil (5-FU), fludarabine (Fludara®), mercaptopurine (Purinethol®) mitotic inhibitors, e.g., irinotecan (Camptosar®), etoposide (VePesid®), topotecan (Hycamtin®), radiopharmaceuticals, other cytotoxic agents	Abdominal discomfort, anorexia, diarrhea, oral and GI ulceration, **nausea,** stomatitis, **vomiting** (premedication with antiemtics will sometimes relieve/reduce severity of nausea and vomiting)

Condition	Drug	Side effects
Chronic obstructive pulmonary disease (COPD)	Antibiotics (a more extensive list of antibiotics is available in the pneumonia section of this chart), e.g., cephalosporins, fluoroquinolones, macrolides, penicillins, tetracyclines, sulfonamides	**Abdominal pain/cramping,** anemia, **anorexia,** black hairy tongue, constipation, **diarrhea,** dry mouth **dysguesia, dyspepsia, flatulence, gastritis, glossitis,** heartburn, nausea, oral candidiasis, stomatitis, **vomiting**
	Anticholinergics, e.g., ipratropium bromide (Atrovent®), atropine sulfate	**Constipation,** dizziness, drowsiness, **dry mouth, dyspepsia,** headache, **nausea,** nervousness, confusion
	Bronchodilators, sympathomimetics, e.g., albuterol (Proventil®), bitolterol (Tornalate®), levalbuterol (Xopenex®), metaproterenol (Alupent®), pirbuterol (Maxair®), salmeterol (Serevent®), terbutaline (Bricanyl®), isoproterenol (Isuprel®), ethylnorepinephrine, ephedrine, epinephrine	Anorexia, **anxiety,** arrhythmias, diarrhea, **dyspepsia,** headache, heartburn, hyperglycemia, hypokalemia, irritability, **nausea, vomiting,** tachycardia, vomiting
	Bronchodilators, xanthine derivatives, e.g., aminophylline, oxytriphylline (Choledyl®), theophylline (Theo-Dur®)	**Aspiration, diarrhea,** dysrhythmias, headache, hyperglycemia, insomnia, irritability, **multiple drug/food interactions, nausea, peptic ulcer disease, reflux,** tachycardia, **vomiting**
	Cromolyn Sodium (Intal®), Nedocromil Sodium (Tilade®)	**Abdominal pain,** anemia, **diarrhea,** dizziness, **dry or irritated throat, dyspepsia, nausea,** swollen parotid gland, **unpleasant taste**
	Corticosteriods, inhaled, e.g., beclomethasone (Beclovent®), dexamethasone (Decadron®), flunisolide (Aerobid®), triamcinolone (Azmacort®), budesonide (Pulmocort®)	Dysphonia, dry mouth, facial edema, **fungal infections (oral cavity), sore mouth/throat,** wheezing
	Corticosteroids, e.g., cortisone (Cortone®), hydrocortisone (Cortef®, Solu-Cortef®), methylprednisolone (Medrol®, Solu-Medrol®), prednisone (Deltasone®), prednisolone (Prelone™), triamcinolone (Aristocort®), or dexamethasone (Decadron®)	Abdominal distention, anorexia, increased appetite, diarrhea, ulcerative esophagitis, GI bleeding, **hypocalcemia, hyperglycemia or hypoglycemia, hypokalemia,** hypertension, muscle mass loss, nausea, **osteoporosis,** pancreatitis, **sodium and fluid retention,** vomiting, weight gain
	Lipoxygenase inhibitors, e.g., zafirlukast (Accolate®), zileoton (Zyflo®), montelukast (Singulair®)	**Diarrhea,** dizziness, **dyspepsia, headache,** lower abdominal pain, **nausea,** systemic infections
	Mucolytics, e.g., acetylcysteine (Mucomyst®)	Drowsiness, **nausea, stomatitis, vomiting**
Congestive heart failure (CHF)	Angiotensin converting enzyme (ACE) inhibitors, e.g., benazepril (Lotensin®), captopril (Capoten®), enalapril (Vasotec®), enalaprilat (Vasotec I.V.®), fosinopril (Monopril®), lisinopril (Zestril®, Prinivil®), moexipril (Univasc®), perindopril (Aceon®), quinapril (Accupril®), ramipril (Altace®), trandolapril (Mavik®)	**Abdominal pain,** anemia, anorexia, **chronic cough,** constipation, diarrhea, dry mouth, dysguesia, dyspepsia, **fatigue,** glossitis, headache, **nausea,** oliguria, **vomiting**
	Cardiac glycosides, e.g., digitoxin (Crystodigin®), digoxin (Lanoxin®)	Abdominal pain, **anorexia, diarrhea,** headache, **nausea, vomiting**

Table 10.10 Drugs Used in the Treatment of Specific Diseases or Conditions with the Potential to Negatively Impact Nutritional Status in Older Patients (Continued)

Disease States or Conditions	Drug Categories	Nutrition-Related Adverse Effects (Items Appearing in Bolded Type Occur with Greater Frequency)
CHF (continued)	Diuretics: loop, e.g., bumetanide (Bumex®), ethacrynic acid (Edecrin®), furosemide (Lasix®), torsemide (Demadex®)	Anemia, **anorexia**, cramping, constipation, **diarrhea**, dysphagia, **fluid/electrolyte imbalance**, glycosuria, hyperglycemia, hyperuricemia, **nausea**, oral and gastric irritation (take with food or milk), **vomiting**
	Diuretics: potassium sparing, e.g., amiloride (Midamor®), spironolactone (Aldactone®), triamterene (Dyrenium®)	Abdominal pain, **anorexia**, appetite changes, constipation, **diarrhea**, dry mouth, dyspepsia, **fluid/electrolyte imbalance**, flatulence, gas pain, headache, heartburn, **nausea** (take with food or immediately after meals), thirst, **vomiting**
	Diuretics: thiazide and related compounds, e.g., chlorthalidone (Hygroton®), indapamide (Lozol®) hydrochlorothiazide (Hydrodiuril®), metolazone (Diulo®, Mykrox®)	**Abdominal pain, anorexia, bloating, cramping**, dry mouth, **epigastric distress**, fluid/electrolyte imbalance, **headache, glucosuria, hyperglycemia, hyperurecemia, nausea** (take with food or milk), **vomiting**
	Hydralazine (Apresoline®)	**Anorexia**, constipation, **diarrhea, headache, nausea**, paralytic ileus, **vomiting**
	Nitrates, e.g., isosorbide dinitrate (Isordil®), isosorbide mononitrate (Ismo®, Imdur®), nitroglycerin (Nitro-Bid®)	Abdominal pain, **diarrhea, dyspepsia, headache**, incontinence, **nausea**, tooth disorder, **vomiting**
Coronary heart disease (CHD)	Angiotensin converting enzyme (ACE) inhibitors, e.g., benazepril (Lotensin®), captopril (Capoten®), enalapril (Vasotec®), enalaprilat (Vasotec I.V.®), fosinopril (Monopril®), lisinopril (Zestril®, Prinivil®), moexipril (Univasc®), perindopril (Aceon®), quinapril (Accupril®), ramipril (Altace®), trandolapril (Mavik®)	**Abdominal pain**, anemia, anorexia, **chronic cough**, constipation, diarrhea, dry mouth, dysguesia, dyspepsia, **fatigue**, glossitis, headache, **nausea**, oliguria, **vomiting**
	Antiplatelet agents/anticoagulants, e.g., aspirin (lower doses recommended for the elderly)	**Anemia, anorexia, dyspepsia, gastric irritation and bleeding, heartburn, nausea**, thirst, dim vision
	Oral anticoagulant, e.g., warfarin (Coumadin®)	Abdominal cramping, anorexia, **diarrhea**, nausea, mouth ulcers, sore mouth, vomiting, vitamin K deficiency (lower doses recommended for the elderly) (multiple food/drug interactions)

Drug	Side effects
Beta adrenergic blockers, e.g., acebutolol (Sectral®), atenolol (Tenormin®), betaxolol (Kerlone®), bisoprolol (Zebeta®), carteolol (Cartrol®), metoprolol (Lopressor® Toprol XL®), nadolol (Corgard®), penbutolol (Levatrol®), pindolol (Visken®), propranolol (Inderal®), timolol (Blocadren®), labetalol (Normodyne® Trandate®), carvedilol (Coreg®)	Anorexia, appetite disorder, bloating, constipation, **depression,** diarrhea, dry mouth, **dyspepsia, fatigue,** flatulence, gastritis, heartburn, hyper/hypoglycemia (diabetics): nausea, serum lipid elevations, **sleep disturbances,** taste distortion, vomiting, weight gain/loss
Bile acid sequestrants, e.g., cholestyramine (Questran®), colestipol (Colestid®), colesevelam (Welchol®)	Abdominal pain/distention/cramping, anorexia, belching, bloating, **constipation,** diarrhea, flatulence, gastric bleeding, **heartburn,** indigestion, **nausea,** steatorrhea, vomiting
Estrogens (postmenopausal), e.g., conjugated estrogens (Premarin®), esterified estrogens (Estrace®, Menest®), estropipate (Ogen®), estradiol (Estraderm®, Vivelle®),	**Abdominal cramps, bloating,** depression, dizziness, edema, headache, **nausea,** reduced carbohydrate tolerance, **vomiting, weight change**
Fibrate derivatives, e.g., Gemfibrozil (Lopid®), fenofibrate (Tricor®)	**Abdominal pain,** anemia, constipation, **diarrhea, dyspepsia,** fatigue, headache, nausea, **vertigo,** vomiting
HMG-CoA reductase inhibitors, e.g., lovastatin (Mevacor®), simvastatin (Zocor®), pravastatin (Pravachol®), fluvastatin (Lescol®), atorvastatin (Lipitor®)	**Abdominal pain/cramping, constipation, diarrhea,** dizziness, dry mouth, dysguesia, **dyspepsia, flatulence,** headache, **nausea, vomiting**
Nicotinic acid (niacin) (take with meals)	**Flushing, gastric upset,** hyperglycemia, peptic ulcer, pruritis, blurred vision, xerostomia
Dementia	
Antianxiety agents (benzodiazepines), e.g., alprazolam (Xanax®), triazolam (Halcion®), oxazepam (Serax®), midazolam (Versed®), lorazepam (Ativan®), estazolam (Prosom®), temazepam (Restoril®), diazepam (Valium®), chlordiazepoxide (Librium®), clorazepate (Tranxene®), flurazepam (Dalmane®)	**Anorexia,** increased appetite, constipation, **diarrhea, dry mouth,** flatulence, sore gums, **nausea,** salivation, burning tongue, **vomiting** (take with meals, avoid alcohol)
Hypnotics/Antianxiety agents (nonbenzodiazepines), e.g., buspirone (BuSpar®), hydroxyzine (Vistaril®), butabarbital (Butisol®), pentobarbital (Nembutal®), phenobarbital (Luminal®), secobarbital (Seconal®), amobarbital/secobarbital (Tuinal®), zaleplon (Sonata®), zolpidem (Ambien®)	

Table 10.10 Drugs Used in the Treatment of Specific Diseases or Conditions with the Potential to Negatively Impact Nutritional Status in Older Patients (*Continued*)

Disease States or Conditions	Drug Categories	Nutrition-Related Adverse Effects (Items Appearing in Bolded Type Occur with Greater Frequency)
Dementia (continued)	Anticonvulsants (barbiturates), e.g., Phenobarbital (Luminal®)	**Anorexia, constipation,** cramps, **diarrhea,** dry mouth, gastric upset, hyperglycemia, sore gums, hiccups, **nausea,** salivation, **vomiting,** weight loss (take with meals, avoid alcohol)
	Anticonvulsants (benzodiazepines), e.g., lorazepam (Ativan®), diazepam (Valium®) chlordiazepoxide (Librium®), clonazepam (Klonopin®)	
	Anticonvulsants (miscellaneous), e.g., carbamazepine (Tegretol), fosphenytoin (Cerebyx®, valproic acid (Depakene®), divalproex sodium (Depakote®, phenytoin (Dilantin®), felbamate (Felbatol®), tiagabine (Gabitril®), Levetiracetam (Keppra®), lamotrigine (Lamictal®), primidone (Mysoline®), gabapentin (Neurontin®), topiramate (Topamax®), ethosuximide (Zarontin®), zonisamide (Zonegran®)	
	Antidepressants (SSRIs), e.g., fluoxetine (Prozac®), fluvoxamine (Luvox®, paroxetine (Paxil®), sertraline (Zoloft®), citalopram (Celexa®), citalopram oxalate (Lexapro®	Abdominal pain, **altered weight and appetite,** constipation, **confusion,** dental caries, **diarrhea, dry mouth,** dyspepsia, flatulence, **nausea,** thirst, vomiting (avoid alcohol)
	Antidepressants (tricyclic), e.g., amitriptyline, clomipramine (Anafranil®), desipramine (Norpramin®), doxepin (Sinequan®), imipramine (Tofranil®), nortriptyline (Pamelor®), protriptyline (Vivactil®), trimipramine (Surmontil®	Abdominal cramps, anorexia, **constipation, confusion, dry mouth,** dysphagia, **epigastric distress,** flatulence, gastric motility disorders, glossitis, **nausea,** salivation, stomatitis, peculiar taste, **vomiting** (avoid alcohol)
	Antidepressants (MAO-I), e.g., phenelzine (Nardil®), tranylcypromine (Parmate®)	
	Antidepressants (miscellaneous), e.g., amoxapine (Asendin®), bupropion (Wellbutrin®, Zyban®), trazodone (Desyrel®), venlafaxine (Effexor®), maprotiline (Ludiomil®), mirtazapine (Remeron®), nefazodone (Serzone®)	

Condition	Drug	Effects
	Antipsychotics, e.g., chlorpromazine (Thorazine®), thioridazine (Mellaril®), mesoridazine (Serentil®), loxapine (Loxitane®), molindone (Moban®), perphenazine (Trilafon®), fluphenazine (Prolixin®), haloperidol (Haldol®), thiothixene (Navane®), pimozide (Orap®), trifluoperazine (Stelazine®), clozapine (Clozaril®), risperidone (Risperdol®), quetiapine (Seroquel®), olanzapine (Zyprexa®)	**Anorexia**, constipation, diarrhea, **dry mouth**, gastric motility disorders, fecal impaction, **nausea**, obstipation, salivation, **vomiting** (avoid alcohol)
	Cholinesterase inhibitors, e.g., donepezil (Aricept®), tacrine (Cognex®), rivastigmine (Exelon®), galantamine (Reminyl®)	Abdominal pain, **anorexia, constipation, diarrhea**, dizziness, dyspepsia, flatulence, headache, **nausea, vomiting** (take with food or meals)
Diabetes mellitus (DM)	Insulin, e.g., human insulin (Humulin®, Novolin®), beef or pork insulin (Iletin®), insulin lispro (Humalog®)	**Hypoglycemia** (can usually be prevented or ameliorated with careful monitoring along with diet and exercise), hypersensitivity, **insulin resistance (obesity)**, lipodystrophy, lipohypertrophy
	Sulfonylureas, e.g., first generation—acetohexamide (Dymelor®), chlorpropamide (Diabinese®), tolazamide (Tolinase®), tolbutamide (Orinase®) (not recommended for the elderly); second generation—glyburide (DiaBeta®), glipizide (Glucotrol®), glimepiride (Amaryl®)	Diarrhea, dizziness, **epigastric fullness**, headache, **heartburn, hypoglycemia, nausea**, taste alterations, vomiting (avoid alcohol and salicylates) glipizide absorption is delayed by food, take 30 minutes prior to meals
	Biguanides, e.g., metformin (Glucophage®)	**Anorexia, bloating, diarrhea, flatulence**, lactic acidosis (in patients with renal dysfunction), metallic taste, nausea, subnormal vitamin B_{12} levels, **vomiting** (take with meals)
	Meglitinides, e.g., nateglinide (Starlik®), repaglinide (Prandin®)	Headache, chest pain, rhinitis, sinusitis, **nausea, vomiting, diarrhea**, constipation, dyspepsia
	Sugar/starch blocker, e.g., acarbose (Precose®), miglitol (Glyset®)	Abdominal discomfort, bloating, flatulence (take with meals)
	Thiazolidinediones, e.g., pioglitazone (Actos®), rosiglitazone (Avandia®)	Diarrhea, increased risk of infection
	Glucagon	Hypokalemia, nausea, vomiting
Failure to thrive (FTT)	Alcohol	Consistent with excessive alcohol intake
	Dronabinol (Marinol®)	Abnormal thinking, anorexia, diarrhea, depression, dizziness, euphoria, fecal incontinence, **nausea, somnolence, vomiting**
	Megesterol acetate (Megace®)	Increased appetite, edema, hyperglycemia, nausea, vomiting, weight gain (adipose)

Table 10.10 Drugs Used in the Treatment of Specific Diseases or Conditions with the Potential to Negatively Impact Nutritional Status in Older Patients (Continued)

Disease States or Conditions	Drug Categories	Nutrition-Related Adverse Effects (Items Appearing in Bold Type Occur with Greater Frequency)
FTT (continued)	Cyproheptadine (Periactin®)	Anorexia, increased appetite, constipation, diarrhea, **epigastric distress**, nausea, vomiting, weight gain
Hypertension (HTN)	Antiadrenergic agents—centrally acting, e.g., methyldopa (Aldomet®), clonidine (Catapres®), guanfacine (Tenex®), guanabenz (Wytensin®)	Anorexia, **constipation**, diarrhea, distention, **dry mouth**, dyspepsia, dysphagia, epigastric pain, flatus, fluid retention, malaise, **nausea**, **sedation**, **sore or "black" tongue**, **taste distortion**, vomiting, **weight gain**
	Antiadrenergic agents—peripherally acting, e.g., reserpine (Serpasil®), doxazosin (Cardura®), prazosin (Minipress®), terazosin (Hytrin®)	**Abdominal pain**, **constipation**, **depression**, diarrhea, drowsiness, **dry mouth**, dyspepsia, **edema**, epigastric pain, fatigue, flatulence, hypoglycemia, **nausea**, taste distortion, **vomiting**, weight gain
	Angiotensin II receptor antagonists, e.g., candesartan (Atacand®), eprosartan (Teveten®), irbesartan (Avapro®), losartan (Cozaar®), telmisartan (Micardis®), valsartan (Diovan®)	**Aguesia**, **anemia**, anorexia, constipation, dental pain, depression, **diarrhea**, **dizziness**, dry mouth, dysguesia, **dyspepsia**, flatulence, gastritis, hyperkalemia, sleep disturbance, vomiting
	Angiotensin converting enzyme (ACE) inhibitors, e.g., benazepril (Lotensin®), captopril (Capoten®), enalapril (Vasotec®), enalaprat (Vasotec I.V.®), fosinopril (Monopril®), lisinopril (Zestril® Prinivil®), moexipril (Univasc®), perindopril (Aceon®), quinapril (Accupril®), ramipril (Altace®), trandolapril (Mavik®)	**Abdominal pain**, anemia, anorexia, **chronic cough**, constipation, diarrhea, dry mouth, dusguesia, dyspepsia, **fatigue**, glossitis, headache, **nausea**, oliguria, **vomiting**
	Beta adrenergic blockers, e.g., acebutolol (Sectral®), atenolol (Tenormin®), betaxolol (Kerlone®), bisoprolol (Zebeta®), carteolol (Cartrol®), metoprolol (Lopressor®, Toprol XL®), nadolol (Corgard®), penbutolol (Levatrol®), pindolol (Visken®), propanolol (Inderal®), timolol (Blocadren®), labetolol (Normodyne®, Trandate®), carvedilol (Coreg®)	Anorexia, appetite disorder, bloating, constipation, **depression**, diarrhea, dry mouth, **dyspepsia**, **fatigue**, flatulence, gastritis, heartburn, hyper/hypoglycemia (diabetics), nausea, serum lipid elevations, **sleep disturbances**, taste distortion, vomiting, weight gain/loss

Drug	Effects
Calcium channel blocking agents (dihydropyridines), e.g., amlodipine (Norvasc®), felodipine (Plendil®), isradipine (Dynacirc®), nicardipine (Cardene®), nifedipine (Procardia®, Adalet®), nisoldipine (Sular®)	**Abdominal discomfort,** anemia, **constipation, cramps, diarrhea, dizziness,** drowsiness, **dry mouth,** dysguesia, **dyspepsia,** flatulence, **headache, nausea,** vomiting
Calcium channel blocking agents (others), e.g., bepridil (Vascor®), diltiazem (Cardizem®, Dilacor®, Tiazac®), verapramil (Calan®, Isoptin®)	Anemia, **anorexia,** cramping, constipation, **diarrhea,** dysphagia, **fluid/electrolyte imbalance,** glycosuria, hyperglycemia, hyperuricemia, **nausea,** oral and gastric irritation (take with food or milk), **vomiting**
Diuretics: loop, e.g., bumetanide (Bumex®), ethacrynic acid (Edecrin®), furosemide (Lasix®), torsemide (Demadex®)	Abdominal pain, **anorexia,** appetite changes, constipation, **diarrhea,** dry mouth, dyspepsia, **fluid/electrolyte imbalance,** flatulence, gas pain, headache, heartburn, **nausea** (take with food or immediately after meals), thirst, **vomiting**
Diuretics: potassium sparing, e.g., amiloride (Midamor®), spironolactone (Aldactone®), triampterene (Dyrenium®)	**Abdominal pain, anorexia, bloating, cramping,** dry mouth, **epigastric distress,** fluid/electrolyte imbalance, **headache, glucosuria, hyperglycemia, hyperurecemia, nausea** (take with food or milk), **vomiting**
Diuretics: thiazide and related compounds, e.g., chlorthalidone (Hygroton®), indapamide Lozol®), hydrochlorothiazide (hydrodiuril®), metolazone (Diulo®, Mykrox®, Zaroxolyn®)	**Anorexia,** constipation, **diarrhea, headache, nausea,** paralytic ileus, **vomiting**
Vasodilators, e.g., minoxidil Loniten®), hydralazine (Apresoline®)	Abdominal distention, **acid regurgitation, anorexia, constipation, diarrhea,** dysphagia, **esophageal ulceration, flatulence,** gastritis, headache, **nausea,** stomatitis (take with water, sit upright, for at least 30 minutes)
Osteoporosis — Biphosphonates, e.g., risedronate (Actonel®), pamidronate (Aredia®), etidronate (Didronel®), alendronate (Fosamax®), tiludronate (Skelid®), zoledronic acid (Zometa®)	Abdominal pain, **anorexia,** increased appetite, constipation, diarrhea, dry mouth, dyspepsia, epigastric discomfort, flatulence, gastritis, **nausea,** salty taste, vomiting
Calcitonin-salmon (Calcimar®, Miacalcin®)	Abdominal pain, decreased absorption or minerals (iron, phosphorus), **anorexia, constipation,** dry mouth, flatulence, **nausea,** polyuria, thirst, **vomiting** (take with meals or immediately following meals to increase absorption of calcium)
Calcium salts, e.g., calcium citrate (Citracal®), calcium carbonate (Tums®), calcium gluconate, calcium lactate	**Abdominal cramps, bloating,** depression, dizziness, edema, headache, **nausea,** reduced carbohydrate tolerance, **vomiting, weight change**
Estrogens (postmenopausal), e.g., conjugated estrogens (Premarin®), esterified estrogens (Estrace®, Menest®), estropipate (Ogen®), estradiol (Estraderm®, Vivelle®)	

Table 10.10 Drugs Used in the Treatment of Specific Diseases or Conditions with the Potential to Negatively Impact Nutritional Status in Older Patients (Continued)

Disease States or Conditions	Drug Categories	Nutrition-Related Adverse Effects (Items Appearing in Bolded Type Occur with Greater Frequency)
Osteoporosis (continued)	Fluoride (sodium salt)	**Abdominal pain, diarrhea,** fractures, gastric distress, headache, **nausea, salivation,** mottled teeth, **vomiting** (milk/milk products decrease the absorption of sodium fluoride)
	Vitamin D, e.g., calcitriol (Rocaltrol®), doxercalciferol (Hectoral®), dihydrotachysterol (DHT), ergocalciferol, paricalcitol (Zemplar®)	Abdominal cramps, **anorexia,** bone pain, constipation, diarrhea, dry mouth, **headache, lethargy,** muscle pain, **nausea, somnolence,** metallic taste, excessive thirst, vertigo, vomiting, **weakness, weight loss**
Pneumonia	Aminoglycoside antibiotics, e.g., amikacin (Amikin®), gentamicin (Garamycin®), tobramycin (Nebcin®)	Anemia, diarrhea, headache, hypocalcemia, hypokalemia, hypomagnesemia, hyponatremia, **nausea, nephrotoxicity, ototoxicity, vomiting**
	Cephalosporin antibiotics, e.g., cefaclor (Ceclor®), cefamandole (Mandol®), cefadroxil (Duricef®), cefazolin (Ancef®), cefepime (Maxipime®), cefixime (Suprax®), cefmetazole (Zefazone®), cefonicid (Monocid®), cefoperazone (Cefobid®), cefotaxime (Claforan®), cefotetan (Cefotan®), cefoxitin (Mefoxin®), cefpodoxime proxetil (Vantin®), cefprozil (Cefzil®), ceftazidime (Fortaz®), ceftizoxime (Cefizox®), ceftriaxone (Rocephin®), cefuroxime (Zinacef®), cfuroxime axetil (Ceftin®), cephalexin (Keflex®), loracarbef (Lorabid®)	Abdominal pain, **anorexia,** cholestasis, colitis, **diarrhea,** dizziness, **dysguesia,** dyspepsia, flatulence, glossitis, headache, heartburn, **nausea,** stomach cramps, **vomiting**
	Fluoroquinolone antibiotics, e.g., ciprofloxacin (Cipro®), enoxacin (Penetrex®), gatafloxacin (Tequin®), lomefloxacin (maxaquin®), levofloxacin (Levaquin®), moxifloxacin (Avelox®), norfloxacin (Noroxin®, sparfloxacin (Zagam®), trovafloxacin (Trovan®)	**Abdominal pain,** anorexia, constipation, colitis, **diarrhea,** dizziness, **dysguesia,** dyspepsia, dysphagia, flatulence, **GI bleeding,** headache, **nausea, vomiting**
	Lincosamide antibiotics, e.g., clindamycin (Cleocin®)	Abdominal pain, anorexia, **colitis, diarrhea,** dizziness, dysguesia, dyspepsia, flatulence, esophagitis, glossitis, metallic taste, **nausea,** stomatitis, vomiting (food delays absorption)
	Macrolide antibiotics, e.g., clarithromycin (Biaxin®), erythromycin, azithromycin (Zithromax®)	**Abdominal pain, abnormal taste,** anorexia, colitis, **diarrhea,** dyspepsia, headache, **nausea, vomiting** (food delays absorption)

Penicillin antibiotics, e.g., penicillin G (Pentids®), penicillin V (V-Cillin-K®), ampicillin (Polycillin®), amoxicillin (Amoxil®), amoxicillin/clavulanate (Aumentin®), cloxacillin (Cloxapen®), dicloxacillin (Dynapen®), nafcillin (Unipen®), oxacillin (Prostaphlin®), ticarcillin (Ticar®), ticarcillin/clavulanate (Timentin®), piperacillin (Pipracil®), piperacillin/tazobactam (Zosyn®)	Abdominal pain, abnormal taste, anorexia, colitis, cramps, **diarrhea**, dry mouth, flatulence, **glossitis**, rectal bleeding, nausea, **sore mouth/tongue, stomatitis**, vomiting (food delays absorption)
Tetracycline antibiotics, e.g., doxycycline (Vibramycin®), minocyclin (Minocin®), tetracycline (Sumycin®)	**Anorexia**, black hairy tongue, colitis, **diarrhea**, dysphagia, epigastric distress, **esophageal ulcers**, glossitis, monial overgrowth, **nausea**, sore throat, stomatitis, **vomiting** (food delays absorption)
Miscellaneous antibiotics: cotrimoxazole (Bactrim®)	Abdominal pain, **anorexia**, diarrhea, colitis, **headache**, glossitis, **nausea**, stomatitis, **vomiting**
metronidazole (Flagyl®)	**Anorexia**, diarrhea, constipation, cramping, colitis, epigastric distress, glossitis, **headache**, metallic taste, **nausea** (avoid alcohol, take with food)
vancomycin (Vancocin®)	Dizziness, nausea, ototoxicity, vertigo, **vomiting**
Antivirals, e.g., amantadine (Symmetrel®), rimantadine (Flumadine®), oseltavivir (Tamiflu®), zanamivir (Relenza®)	Anorexia, constipation, **dizziness**, dysguesia, **dyspepsia**, dysphagia, dry mouth, headache, nausea, stomatitis

Source: Adapted from *The Role of Nutrition in Chronic Disease Care, Executive Summary*, White, J., Ed., Nutrition Screening Initiative, Washington, D.C., 1997, 5, 18, 24, 33, 43, 50, 62, 71. With permission.

REFERENCES

1. DeBrew, J.K., Barba, B.E., and Tesh, A.S., Assessing medication knowledge and practices of older adults, *Home Healthcare Nurse,* 16, 686–691, 1998.
2. Cornish, J., Color coding patient medications, *Caring,* 11, 46–51, 1992.
3. Conn, V., Self management of over-the-counter medications by older adults, *Public Health Nursing,* 96, 29–35, 1992.
4. Lewis, C.W., Frongillo, E.A., and Roe, D.A., Drug–nutrient interactions in three long-term care facilities, *J. Am. Diet. Assoc.,* 95, 309–315, 1995.
5. Barrocas, A. et al., Enteral and parenteral nutrition, *Probl. Crit. Care,* 5, 411–471, 1991.
6. Blumberg, J. and Couris, R., Pharmacology, nutrition, and the elderly: interactions and implications, in *Geriatric Nutrition. A Handbook for Health Professionals,* 2nd ed., Chernoff, R., Ed., Aspen Publishers, Gaithersburg, MD, 1999, p. 359.
7. McCabe, B.J. and Dorsey, J.N., Health promotion and disease prevention in the elderly, in *Geriatric Nutrition. A Handbook for Health Professionals,* Chernoff, R., Ed., Aspen Publishers, Gaithersburg, MD, 1999.
8. Kramer, A.M., Fox, P.D., and Morgenstern, N., Geriatric care approaches in health maintenance organizations, *J. Am. Geriatr.,* 40, 1055–1067, 1992.
9. Barrocas, A. et al., Nutritional assessment: practical approaches, *Clin. Geriatr. Med.,* 11, 695–713, 1995.
10. USDHHS, *Healthy People 2010: Tracking Healthy People 2010,* Washington, D.C., U.S. Government Printing Office, November, 2000. Also available with updates at http://www.cdc.gov/nchs.
11. Roe, D.A., Medications and nutrition in the elderly, *Primary Care Clin. Office Pract.,* 21, 135–147, 1994.
12. Young, F.E., Clinical evaluation of medicine used by the elderly, *Clin. Pharmacol. Ther.,* 42, 666–669, 1987.
13. Diehl, M. et al., Examination of priorities for therapeutic drug utilization review, *J. Geriatr. Drug Ther.,* 6, 65–85, 1991.
14. Joint Commission on Accreditation of Healthcare Organizations, *1995 Accreditation Manual for Hospitals,* JCAHO, Oakbrook Terrace, IL.
15. Joint Commission on Accreditation of Healthcare Organization, 1994 Accreditation Manual for Health Care Organization, JCAHO, Oakbrook Terrace, IL, 1994, p. 171.
16. Barrocas, A., The nutrition needs of the geriatric patient, *The Connector,* Wisconsin Society of Parenteral and Enteral Nutrition, 1994.
17. *A Physician's Guide to Nutrition in Chronic Disease Management,* Nutrition Screening Initiative, Washington, D.C., 2002.
18. *A Physician's Guide to Nutrition in Chronic Disease Management for Older Adults,* Expanded Version, Nutrition Screening Initiative, Washington, D.C., 2003, http://www.aafp/x16705.xml, last accessed January 14, 2003.
19. Barrocus, A. et al., Ethical and legal issues in nutrition support of the geriatric patient: the can, should, and must of nutrition support, *Nutr. Clin. Pract.,* 18, 2003, in press.
20. *Nutrition Interventions Manual for Professionals Caring for Older Americans, Executive Summary,* Nutrition Screening Initiative, Washington, D.C., 1992, p. 31.
21. Ham, R.J., The signs and symptoms of poor nutritional status, *Primary Care,* 21, 33–67, 1994.
22. Barrocas, A., *Nutritional assessment, a handbook of hospital nutrition,* Cutter Medical, 1984.

23. *Incorporating nutrition screening and interventions into medical practice: a monograph for physicians,* Nutrition Screening Initiative, Washington, D.C., 1994, pp. 16, 20, 29–31.

24. *The Role of Nutrition in Chronic Disease Care, Executive Summary,* White, J., Ed., Nutrition Screening Initiative, Washington, D.C., 1997, pp. 5, 18, 24, 33, 43, 50, 62, 71.

25. Mares-Perlman, J.A. et al., Nutrient supplements contribute to the dietary intake of middle- and older-aged adult residents of Beaver Dam, Wisconsin, *J. Nutr.,* 123, 176–188, 1993.

26. Eisenberg, D.M. et al., Trends in alternative medicine use in the United States, 1990–1997, *J. Am. Med. Assoc.,* 280, 1569–1575, 1998.

27. Lyle, B.J. et al., Supplement users differ from nonusers in demographic, lifestyle, dietary, and health characteristics, *J. Nutr.,* 128, 2355–2362, 1998.

28. Szauter, K.M., Mullen, K.D., and McCollough, A.J., Nutrition in critically ill patients with gastrointestinal and hepatic diseases, *Probl. Crit. Care,* 3, 469, 1989.

29. Weinsier, R.L. and Morgan, S.L., *Fundamentals of Clinical Nutrition,* Mosby, St. Louis, MO, 1993, pp. 134–135.

30. *Report of the 14th Ross Roundtable on Medical Issues,* Laboratory utilization for nutrition support: current practices, requirements, expectations, Columbus, OH, Ross Laboratories, 1994.

31. Morse, M.H. et al., Protein requirements of elderly women: nitrogen balance responses to three levels of protein intake, *J. Gerontol.,* 56, M724–M730, 2001.

32. Campbell, W.W. et al., Increased protein requirements in elderly people: new data and retrospective reassessments, *Am. J. Clin. Nutr.,* 60, 501–509, 1994.

33. The Nutrition Institute of Louisiana™, *Healthy Hand-y Hints for Sensible Eating,* 1994.

34. *Intervention manual for professionals caring for older Americans,* The Nutrition Screening Initiative, Washington, D.C., 1991.

35. Johnson, L.E., Challenges to practical nutritional assessment of older adults in non-hospital settings, *Nutr. Clin. Pract.,* 15, S24–S31, 2000.

CHAPTER 11

Obesity and Appetite Drugs

Tiffany R. Bolton

CONTENTS

As the second leading cause of preventable death in the U.S. today, excess weight and obesity have become a major public health issue.[1] Approximately 97 million adults are overweight or obese in the U.S.[2] Over the past several decades, the prevalence of this health problem has steadily been on the rise as described by the National Health and Nutrition Examination Surveys (NHANES).[3,4,5] The most recent NHANES data for the period of 1988–1994 show that approximately 55% of Americans older than 20 years are either overweight or obese.[4,6] In addition, substantial proportions of children (14%) and adolescents (12.9%) are also overweight.[5] Individuals who are overweight or obese are at increased risk for comorbid diseases, which are often chronic and may cause significant functional disability. These diseases include hypertension, hyperlipidemia, type 2 diabetes, stroke, osteoarthritis, gallbladder disease, sleep apnea, and respiratory problems, as well as cancers of the endometrium, breast, prostate, and colon.[6,7] The link between obesity and increased health risks translates into increased medical care and disability costs. Each year in the U.S., the total economic cost attributable to obesity is close to $100 billion.[6] This figure can be expected to rise as the prevalence of obesity and comorbid disorders increases.

DEFINING OBESITY

Obesity is defined as an excess of total body fat.[2] Several expensive methods can be used for assessing total body fat (i.e., underwater weighing, MRI, DEXA); however, the most clinically useful and practical approach is calculation of body mass index (BMI).[6] This parameter is useful in assessing accurate body weight status, degree of adiposity, and risk for obesity-related conditions. BMI is a weight–height ratio that is easily calculated by dividing the body weight by the square of the height; therefore, BMI = kg/m^2. Table 11.1 presents the most recent BMI classification system developed by the 1998 National Heart, Lung, and Blood Institute Expert Panel on Obesity.[6] BMI values ≥ 25 kg/m^2 in obese and overweight adults are associated with rapid increases in morbidity and mortality. Increases in BMI have been directly correlated with increased risks of hypertension, type 2 diabetes, coronary heart disease, and detrimental changes in serum lipids.[6]

Waist circumference and waist–hip ratio are other measurements used to determine health risk. A waist circumference >40 inches in men and >35 inches in women has been correlated with increased risk for obesity-related conditions such as diabetes and cardiovascular disease.[6] Elevated waist–hip ratios in men (>1.0) or women (>0.8) resulting from a high proportion of abdominal and visceral fat, are also associated with an increased risk for ischemic heart disease, stroke, and death. In contrast,

Table 11.1 BMI Classification

Classification	BMI kg/m^2	Obesity Class
Underweight	<18.5	
Normal	18.5–24.9	
Overweight	25.0–29.9	
Obesity	30.0–34.9	I
	35.0–39.9	II
Extreme Obesity	≥ 40	III

Source: NHLBI Expert Panel, *Clinical Guidelines on the Identification, Evaluation, and Treatment of Overweight and Obesity in Adults. The Evidence Report,* National Heart, Lung, and Blood Institute, Bethesda, MD, 1998.

typical female, or gynoid (gluteofemoral), distribution of fat with a low waist–hip ratio is not generally associated with these problems.[6,8]

ETIOLOGY OF OBESITY

In the vast majority of individuals, the etiology of obesity is unknown. It is likely a combination of several factors that contribute in various degrees in different individuals. Obesity may result from physiologic, genetic, or psychologic causes; endocrine and metabolic abnormalities; or a combination of several of these issues. Regardless of the etiology, obesity, generally stated, results from an imbalance between food (energy) intake and energy expenditure. Only when the cycle of energy intake is equal to energy expenditure can weight be maintained.[9]

MANAGEMENT OF OBESITY

Weight-reduction therapies are aimed at affecting one or more steps in the energy intake, storage, and expenditure cycle. Typical treatment strategies include diet restriction, exercise, behavior modification, pharmacologic procedures, and even invasive procedures.[10] There is no single standard weight-loss strategy that is effective for all individuals suffering from obesity. Weight-reduction programs must be designed to fulfill the needs and fit the lifestyle of each individual. The critical element or goal for any program is to have energy expenditures exceed caloric demands. These changes must be maintained to achieve the desired weight. According to the most recent recommendations by National Heart, Lung, and Blood Institute Expert Panel on Obesity, lifestyle therapy should be tried for at least 6 months before considering pharmacotherapy. For patients who are mildly overweight, behavior modification and dietary intervention should be adequate. Patients with a BMI of ≥ 27 kg/m^2 with concomitant obesity-related risk factors or diseases, or those with a BMI ≥ 30 kg/m^2 without diagnosed complications, may be candidates for drug therapy in conjunction with exercise and behavior modification. The risk factors or diseases considered important enough to warrant pharmacotherapy at a BMI of 27–29.9 kg/m^2 are hypertension, dyslipidemia, coronary heart disease, type 2 diabetes, and sleep apnea. Adults with a BMI ≥ 40 kg/m^2 or BMI ≥ 35 kg/m^2 with comorbid conditions are candidates for surgical interventions.[6]

Current guidelines recommend that the initial goal of weight-loss therapy should be to reduce body weight by approximately 10% from baseline. A reasonable rate of weight loss is typically 1–2 lb/week for a period of 6 months, at which time efforts to maintain the new weight should be put into place.[6] Studies have shown that with the loss of only 5–10% of initial body weight, health risks such as insulin resistance, hypertension, and hyperlipidemia can be reduced.[9,11] If a patient is initially successful in reducing his or her body weight by 10%, further weight loss can be attempted if indicated through repeated assessment.[6] Unfortunately, numerous individuals seek therapy for obesity primarily for cosmetic purposes and have unreasonable goals and expectations for weight loss. The benefits associated with weight loss are not sustained if the weight is regained. Over 80% of individuals who lose weight will gradually regain it; therefore, a weight maintenance program consisting of dietary therapy, physical activity, and behavior therapy should be continued indefinitely.[6] Drugs may also be used to maintain weight loss; however, safety and efficacy beyond 1 to 2 years of total treatment have not been established.

This chapter focuses on over-the-counter (OTC) preparations and prescription medications approved for the short- and long-term management of obesity. Many of these agents are designed to suppress appetite. It is currently believed specific areas of the hypothalamus act as the regulatory center for obesity where the balance of hunger and satiety is regulated through food intake. Appetite suppressants are centrally acting agents that reduce appetite by augmenting either catecholamine or serotonin action in the brain. Alternatively, weight-reduction programs can also include orlistat/Xenical®, a digestive inhibitor that decreases energy intake by interfering with the breakdown and digestion of dietary fat.

OVER THE COUNTER MEDICATIONS

Although many ingredients and herbal products are included in OTC weight-loss formulations, most are not generally recognized to be safe and effective by the Food and Drug Administration (FDA). In 1991, the FDA issued a final rule establishing that 111 active ingredients in OTC weight control products are not generally recognized as safe and effective.[12] These products are listed in Table 11.2. Until recently, consumers were able to purchase two OTC medications that were FDA approved for weight loss: phenylpropanolamine (PPA) and benzocaine. Unfortunately, PPA was removed from the market in 2000 after its use was linked to hemorrhagic stroke.[13]

Phenylpropanolamine

PPA is a sympathomimetic agent structurally similar to amphetamine and ephedrine. It is an adrenergic agonist that mimics norepinephrine to enhance catecholamine neurotransmission, leading to increased sympathetic activity and reduced appetite.[14] PPA was one of the most commonly used nonprescription drugs in the U.S. It was used in formulations as a decongestant and as an appetite suppressant. As an appetite suppressant (e.g., Acutrim® and Dexatrim®), it was FDA-approved for short-term weight control (8–12 weeks) in combination with reduced caloric intake. The usual adult oral dosage of PPA as conventional capsules or tablets was 25 mg three times daily or 37.5 mg twice daily, administered 30 min before meals with one or two full glasses of water. The recommended dosage of the extended release capsules or tablets was 75 mg once daily, administered in midmorning with a full glass of water.[14]

During the 1970s, a total of 30 reports were published in the literature that described the occurrence of intracranial hemorrhage after PPA ingestion. This literature was in addition to 22 spontaneous reports that were submitted to the FDA

Table 11.2 Ingredients Recognized by the FDA as Not Generally Safe and Effective in the Treatment of Obesity

Alcohol	Corn syrup	Liver concentrate	Rice polishings
Alfalfa	Corn silk, potassium	Lysine	Saccharin
Alginic acid	extract	Lysine hydrochloride	Sea minerals
Anise oil	Cupric sulfate	Magnesium	Sesame seed
Arginine	Cyanocobalamin	Magnesium oxide	Sodium
Ascorbic acid	(vitamin B$_{12}$)	Malt	Sodium bicarbonate
Bearberry	Cystine	Maltodextrin	Sodium caseinate
Biotin	Dextrose	Manganese citrate	Sodium chloride
Bone marrow, red	Docusate sodium	Mannitol	(salt)
Buchu	Ergocalciferol	Methionine	Soybean protein
Buchu, potassium	Ferric ammonium	Methycellulose	Soy meal
extract	citrate	Monoglycerides and	Sucrose
Caffeine	Ferric pyrophopshate	diglycerides	Thiamin
Caffeine citrate	Ferrous fumarate	Niacinamide	hydrochloride
Calcium	Ferrous gluconate	Organic vegetables	(vitamin B$_1$)
Calcium carbonate	Ferrous sulfate (iron)	Pancreatin	Thiamine
Calcium caseinate	Flax seed	Pantothenic acid	mononitrate
Calcium lactate	Folic acid	Papain	(vitamin B$_1$
Calcium	Fructose	Papaya enzymes	mononitrate)
pantothenate	Guar gum	Pepsin	Threonine
Carboxymethylcellu-	Histidine	Phenacetin	Tricalcium phosphate
lose sodium	Hydrastis	Phenylanine	Tryptophan
Carrageenan	canadensis	Phosphorus	Tyrosine
Cholecalciferol	Inositol	Phytolacca	Uva ursi, potassium
Choline	Iodine	Pineapple enzymes	extract
Chondrus	Isoleucine	Plantago seed	Valine
Citric acid	Juniper, Potassium	Potassium citrate	Vegetable
Cnicus benedictus	extract	Pyridoxine	Vitamin A
Copper	Karaya gum	hydrochloride	Vitamin A acetate
Copper gluconate	Kelp	(vitamin B$_4$)	Vitamin A palmitate
Corn oil	Lactose	Riboflavin	Vitamin E
	Lecithin		Wheat germ
	Leucine		Xanthan gum
			Yeast

Source: Federal Register, Washington, D.C., 56, 37792–37799, Aug. 8, 1991.

between 1969 and 1991, which also suggested an association. Typically, the hemorrhagic strokes occurred in patients who were young women between 17 and 45 years of age who were using appetite suppressant or cough/cold products that contained PPA. Many were first-time users of the medication.[15]

Because of the rising concern over the years about PPA and risk for hemorrhagic stroke, the FDA conducted a research study with PPA manufacturers to clarify whether any increase in risk existed. This collaborative effort, known as the Hemorrhagic Stroke Project, did find an association between PPA use and stroke in women. Women who took appetite suppressants or nasal decongestants containing PPA were at an increased risk of hemorrhagic stroke, particularly during the 3 days after initiation of therapy. Men were also considered to be at risk.[15] Although the FDA believed the overall incidence of hemorrhagic stroke to be low, they felt that the benefits of PPA did not warrant the risk for such a serious adverse effect. Therefore, in November 2000, the FDA requested that all drug companies discontinue marketing products containing PPA.[13,16]

Benzocaine

Benzocaine (Diet Ayds,® Slim-Mint,® or Trocaine®) is a local anesthetic that is used for topical treatment of skin irritations and for oral use in various throat lozenges, sprays, and cough syrups. The role of benzocaine in obesity is to discourage snacking and promote weight loss by producing numbing of the oral cavity and gastrointestinal mucosa. Its anesthetic action dulls the taste of food thereby helping the individual eat less.[17] Although several studies have documented the efficacy of benzocaine in weight loss,[18–22] only two have been double-blinded and placebo controlled.[21,22] These trials, one using benzocaine lozenges and the other using benzocaine gum, present opposite conclusions regarding benzocaine's effectiveness.

In a 6-week study, 52 subjects were randomized to diet and placebo, or diet and benzocaine lozenges. One or two lozenges, each containing 5 mg of benzocaine, were to be taken prior to mealtime, between meals, and after meals with fluids. No difference in cumulative weight loss was observed between the two groups during the first 2 weeks. However, during weeks four and six, the benzocaine group had a statistically significant mean cumulative weight loss as compared with those receiving placebo (6.71 vs. 2.5 lbs).[21]

Another study involving 37 patients compared benzocaine gum (6 mg benzocaine per piece), PPA 75 mg, the combination of benzocaine gum and PPA, and placebo. At the end of the 12-week trial, benzocaine alone produced less weight loss than the placebo and the PPA groups, although this was not statistically significant. In addition, weight loss was not enhanced when benzocaine was combined with PPA. Thus, the authors concluded that benzocaine gum was ineffective for weight loss.[22] Regardless of the lack of conclusive data, benzocaine is FDA approved as an adjunct to a weight-reduction regimen based on caloric restriction. A dose of 6–15 mg as gum, lozenges, or candy should be administered just prior to food consumption. Patients should not exceed 45 mg/d.[23]

Although rare, cyanotic reactions such as methemoglobinemia have been reported following benzocaine administration. Although these reactions occur primarily among infants, they have also been reported in adults. In addition, anaphylactic reactions have occurred a few minutes after ingesting throat lozenges containing benzocaine. Obese individuals who routinely take preparations containing benzocaine over a long period of time may be predisposed to drug-induced hypersensitivity.[24]

OTC Product Selection Guidelines

The nonprescription weight-loss market in the U.S. is flooded with many hundreds of products that promise to shed pounds quickly and easily. Few data, however, support their efficacy or safety as agents for weight reduction and long-term maintenance of weight loss. Healthcare professionals should stress that weight cannot be reduced without a concerted effort to change one's eating and exercise lifestyle and to maintain the new behavior long term. Nonprescription obesity control products should be considered only as short-term adjuncts to a planned weight-reduction program. These agents can initially play a role to aid in the curtailment of calories until the individual's dietary and exercise habits have changed.

Ingredients such as ephedrine, caffeine, benzocaine, chromium, psyllium, chitosan, and herbal preparations are frequently included in weight-control products as single components or in combination. Popular herbal ingredients include ma huang, St. John's wort, guarana, and kola nut. The methods by which these agents reportedly induce weight loss include stimulatory effects (ephedrine, ma huang, caffeine, guarana, and kola nut), serotonergic regulation of satiety (St. John's wort), induction of thermogenesis (ephedrine, ma huang), and bulk formation to decrease hunger and fat absorption (psyllium and chitosan).[25]

Herbal products are not without adverse effects and drug interactions. Cardiovascular status can become compromised when patients with preexisting cardiac disease (e.g., hypertension and angina) take agents such as ephedrine, ma huang, guarana, and kola nut.[26] Heart attacks, stroke, and death have been associated with ephedrine.[27] Thus, benzocaine may be a more appropriate choice for patients with cardiovascular disease, thyroid disease, and diabetes. Patients who are taking monoamine oxidase inhibitors (MAOIs) should not use ephedrine-like products or St. John's wort due to the risk of hypertensive crisis. In addition, serotonin syndrome may occur when St. John's wort is administered with other serotonergic agents.[28]

When recommending a nonprescription product for weight control, the healthcare professional should inquire about previous diet control regimens the patient has attempted so that other nonprescription diet management adjuncts may be considered. In addition, the patient should be interviewed for concomitant disease states or drug interactions that may prevent them from taking an OTC preparation. Users of nonprescription or herbal weight-loss products should be cautioned about adverse effects, drug interactions, and the potential impurities of herbal products.[28,29] Patients should be encouraged to consult their physicians when initiating an OTC weight-loss product, so appropriate monitoring for safety and efficacy can be performed.

PRESCRIPTION APPETITE SUPPRESSANT DRUGS

Appetite suppressants are centrally active agents that exert their effects directly on the hypothalamic feeding center through either noradrenergic or serotonergic activity. Noradrenergic agents (e.g., amphetamine, benzphetamine, phendimetrazine, diethylpropion, mazindol, and phentermine) mimic norepinephrine to enhance catecholamine release, leading to increased sympathomimetic activity and reduced appetite. Serotonergic compounds (e.g., fenfluramine and dexfenfluramine) release serotonin into the synaptic clefts of nerve endings and inhibit its reuptake. This may affect food intake by reducing an individual's food-seeking behavior, thus reducing snacking episodes, or it may reduce the amount of food consumed at each meal. Until September 1997, the combination of fenfluramine and phentermine (fen-phen) was a widely used treatment for obesity. Fenfluramine and dexfenfluramine were voluntarily withdrawn from the market and are currently unavailable. Sibutramine is another centrally acting agent that recently received FDA approval for the management of obesity. It possesses noradrenergic and serotonergic activity by inhibiting the reuptake of both norepinephrine and serotonin.

Noradrenergic Agents

Amphetamine was the first noradrenergic agent to be introduced for the treatment of obesity. Amphetamines, and closely related compounds such as methamphetamine and phenmetrazine, have a high potential for abuse; thus, their use is no longer recommended in the treatment of obesity.[30] In a search for safer agents, other derivatives of amphetamine were produced that reduced the risk for central nervous system (CNS) stimulation and abuse but retained appetite suppressing effects. These drugs are included in Table 11.3. In a review of the safety and efficacy of this group of drugs, the FDA examined clinical data from 10,000 patients reported in 200 double-blind studies. At the end of 20 weeks, patients taking either drug or placebo had equal dropout rates. Patients taking drugs averaged about 0.5 lb (0.25 kg) per week greater weight loss.[31] Several sources have reviewed the use of benzphetamine, phendimetrazine diethylproprion, mazindol, and phentermine in the treatment of obesity.[30,32] Except for phentermine, many of these medications are used infrequently in clinical practice.

Phentermine is structurally similar to amphetamine, but it has less severe central nervous system stimulation and lower abuse potential.[33] It is available in both immediate-release and sustained-release formulations in dosage strengths ranging from 8 mg to 37.5 mg. Effective appetite suppression is attained after a single morning dose of 15–37.5 mg before breakfast or 10–14 h before retiring. It may also be given in a dose of 8 mg three times daily one-half hour before meals.[33] Patients may not tolerate the stimulatory effects of phentermine; therefore, its use as a single agent may be limited. Phentermine was extensively used in combination with fenfluramine before fenfluramine was removed from the market. By combining these medications, the stimulatory effects of phentermine are counteracted by the lethargic effects caused by fenfluramine. This combination has been demonstrated to be more effective in causing weight loss than either agent alone.[34–42]

No one agent of the amphetamine-like anorectics has been shown to be superior over the others[31]; therefore, drug selection is usually made by trial and error. Patients will often tolerate agents from one chemical class better than another. Duration of action can be helpful in choosing a medication for a given patient. Patients who overeat in the evening will not benefit from medications that are typically administered in the morning. Long-acting preparations are inappropriate when patients indulge in eating during particular times of the day. In both situations, short-acting medications are preferred.

The conventional belief among practitioners is that patients develop a tolerance to this class of drugs, as demonstrated by decreasing weight loss with continued use. Current FDA recommendations suggest that the use of amphetamine-like appetite suppressants should be limited to short-term use (2–3 months). It appears, however, that these agents sustain weight loss for as long as they are used, in most patients. After discontinuation, a rapid rebound of weight and increased appetite occurs.[43,44]

Table 11.3 Agents Used for the Treatment of Obesity

Drug (Trade Name)	Schedule[a]	Dosage
Noradrenergic Agents		
Amphetamine (Biphetamine®)	Rx, II[b]	5–10 mg TID before meals 10–15 mg QD (morning)
Dextroamphetamine (Dexedrine®)	Rx, II[b]	5–10 mg TID before meals
Methamphetamine (Desoxyn®)	Rx, II[b]	5 mg TID before meals 10–15 mg QD (midmorning)
Phenmetrazine (Preludin®)	Rx, II[b]	75 mg QD (midmorning)
Benzphetamine (Didrex®)	Rx, III	25–50 mg QD (midmorning)
Phendimetrazine (Bontril®, Plegine®, Prelu-2®)	Rx, III	35 mg BID or TID before meals 105 mg QD before breakfast
Phentermine (Ionamin®, Fastin®, Adipex-P®)	Rx, IV	8 mg TID before meals 15–37.5 mg QD before breakfast or 10–14 h before retiring
Diethylpropion (Tenuate®, Tenuate Dospan®)	Rx, IV	25 mg TID before meals 75 mg QD (midmorning)
Mazindol (Sanorex®, Mazinor®)	Rx, IV	1 mg TID before meals 2 mg QD (one hour before lunch)
Phenylpropanolamine (Dexatrim®, Acutrim®)	OTC[c]	25 mg TID before meals 75 mg QD in the morning
Serotonergic Agents		
Dexfenfluramine (Redux®)	Rx, IV[c]	15 mg BID
Fenfluramine (Pondimin®)	Rx, IV[c]	20–40 mg TID before meals
Noradrenergic/Serotonergic Agents		
Sibutramine (Meridia®)	Rx, IV	10 mg QD
Digestive inhibitor		
Orlistat (Xenical®)	Rx	120 mg TID with each meal containing fat

[a] Food and Drug Administration (FDA) assigns drugs to legend (Rx, prescription only) or to over-the-counter (OTC) status. Drug Enforcement Administration (DEA) assigns drugs to federal control schedules (I, II, III, IV, V) on the basis of accepted medical use and demonstrated potential for abuse.

[b] Amphetamines are not recommended for the treatment of obesity because of their high potential for abuse or dependence.

[c] Withdrawn from the market.

These newer findings suggest that tolerance may not be significant at doses usually employed, and long-term treatment may be appropriate for selected patients.

Commonly reported side effects of the amphetamine-like anorectics include restlessness, insomnia, tremors, tachycardia, nausea, diarrhea, constipation, dry mouth, and mydriasis.[33,44] Dry mouth can be minimized by sucking on sugarless hard candy. Patients who have problems with insomnia from long-acting preparations can minimize this effect by taking the medication early in the day. Elevated blood pressure and cardiac arrhythmias may also occur.[33,44] These agents have many drug interactions. Pharmacists should be alert to concomitant use with OTC preparations containing other adrenergic agents (i.e., pseudoephedrine, and phenylephrine), MAOIs (i.e., phenelzine, tranylcypromine, and isocarboxazid), and caffeine. The combination of these agents increases the pressor effect of the amphetamine-like anorectics and may result in severe hypertensive episodes. Tricyclic antidepressants may decrease the effects of the anorexiants; therefore, an increased dose may be necessary.[44]

Serotonergic Agents

Many human physiologic systems involve the important neurotransmitter serotonin. Serotonin activity is linked to sleep–wake cycles, sensitivity to pain, blood pressure, mood, and eating behaviors. Serotonergic agents, such as fenfluramine (Pondimin®) and dexfenfluramine (Redux®), increase central serotonin levels via reuptake inhibition and possibly by increasing serotonin release. Elevated levels of serotonin results in decreased food consumption and prolonged time between food intake. A major difference between serotonergic and noradrenergic appetite suppressants is the serotonergic agents' lack of stimulatory effects on the central nervous system and abuse potential compared to the noradrenergic compounds.[33] Fenfluramine and dexfenfluramine were FDA-approved for the management of obesity.

Fenfluramine

Fenfluramine is an orally active, racemic mixture (D,L-fenfluramine) that is similar chemically, but not pharmacologically, to amphetamine. It is the most widely studied serotonergic drug for obesity management. Short-term therapy with fenfluramine produces weight loss significantly greater than diet, exercise, and behavioral modification alone; therefore, it was used extensively as monotherapy for many years.[45–50]

Low doses of phentermine (15–30 mg/d) combined with fenfluramine (30–60 mg/d) were a frequently prescribed combination known as Fen-Phen. The combination capitalized on their pharmacodynamic differences, resulting in weight loss equivalent to that achieved with full doses of either agent alone and better appetite control. This combination in conjunction with dietary management, exercise, and behavioral modification has been shown to induce and maintain weight loss on a long-term basis (>1 yr).[34–42]

Fenfluramine and phentermine in combination, however, have been associated with abnormal echocardiograms, valvular heart disease, and primary pulmonary hypertension. As a result, fenfluramine was withdrawn from the worldwide market in 1997.[51] The FDA did not request the withdrawal of phentermine because valvular abnormalities were not documented when phentermine was used alone.

Dexfenfluramine

Dexfenfluramine is the d-isomer of fenfluramine. There have been both short- and long-term studies investigating the efficacy of dexfenfluramine in obesity in conjunction with diet and exercise. In most studies, it has produced weight loss for up to 6 months and prevented weight regain when given for an additional 6-month period. Effective doses in these studies were 15–30 mg twice daily.[52–60] Additional effectiveness was also noted when dexfenfluramine was given in combination with phentermine.[61] As a derivative of fenfluramine, it was also withdrawn from the worldwide market because of potential cardiovalvular morphology alterations.[51]

Sibutramine

Sibutramine is the first centrally acting antiobesity agent to inhibit reuptake of norepinephrine, serotonin, and dopamine. By working on multiple pathways of reuptake inhibition, sibutramine causes weight loss by decreasing food intake through the enhancement of postingestion satiety. This mechanism of action is unlike the amphetamines, which directly stimulate the release of noradrenergic neurotransmitters. Sibutramine is indicated for the management of obesity, including weight loss and the maintenance of weight loss in patients with a BMI of ≥ 30 kg/m^2, or ≥ 27 kg/m^2 with concomitant risk factors such as hypertension, diabetes mellitus, and dyslipidemia. Sibutramine should be used as adjunctive therapy in combination with a low-calorie diet, exercise, and behavior modification.[62]

Sibutramine is rapidly absorbed from the gastrointestinal tract after oral administration and undergoes extensive first-pass metabolism in the liver resulting in the formation of two active amine metabolites (M1 and M2). Through these metabolites, sibutramine exerts its pharmacological actions. Metabolites M1 and M2 inhibit neurotransmitter reuptake to varying degrees. Reuptake inhibition appears to be greatest for norepinephrine and, to a lesser extent, serotonin and dopamine.[62,63]

The pharmacokinetic profile of sibutramine and its active metabolites support once-daily dosing. Sibutramine may be administered with or without food. No major pharmacokinetic changes have been observed, and no dosage adjustments are necessary in obese patients based on age, gender, race, or mild or moderate renal or hepatic impairment.[62]

Sibutramine, administered once daily, has established its superiority to placebo in producing weight loss in combination with other nonpharmacologic therapies. In placebo-controlled clinical trials, a clear dose–response relationship has been demonstrated in doses from 1 to 30 mg daily.[64–75] Sibutramine dosages of ≥ 10 mg/d produced significantly better results than the placebo ($p < 0.05$) in obese patients with or without concomitant disease.[64,66–75] In some studies, a dosage of 5 mg/d also demonstrated significant efficacy when compared with placebo.[64–66,72,73,75] Most trials involved similar inclusion criteria: overweight or obese adults from 18 to 65 years of age with a BMI between 27 and 40 kg/m^2.

Based upon long-term clinical trials (6–12 months), dose-related weight loss with sibutramine becomes apparent within the first month of treatment and is maximal by 6 months.[69–73,75] Weight loss is maintained with continued treatment up to one year; thus, the drug is indicated for long-term treatment of obesity. In these clinical trials, patients experienced modest weight loss (2–7 kg) with sibutramine in the recommended dosage range of 10–15 mg daily. A 5% reduction in total body weight was achieved by 45–67% of sibutramine-treated patients on 10–15 mg/d, with 12–39% experiencing a 10% reduction in total body weight. Weight loss in these trials was accompanied by dose-related reductions in BMI and waist circumference, which are also useful predictors of risk for comorbidities. As with other centrally active appetite suppressants, weight regain of up to 10–25% of previously lost weight occurs within 1 to 6 weeks of medication discontinuance. This suggests that long-term maintenance therapy with sibutramine may be required.

The recommended starting dose of sibutramine is 10 mg daily, with a recommended dosage range of 5–15 mg daily. The 5-mg dose should be reserved for patients who do not tolerate the recommended initial starting dose. Analyses of numerous variables from clinical trials have indicated that 60% of patients who lose greater than 1% of initial body weight (or at least 1.8 kg) within the first 4 weeks of starting sibutramine at a given dose along with a reduced-calorie diet lose at least 5% of their initial body weight by the end of 6 months to 1 year of treatment on that dose. Eighty percent of patients who do not achieve at least a 1.8 kg weight loss within the first 4 weeks of starting sibutramine at a given dose are less likely to achieve successful outcomes. If this extent of weight loss is not apparent after 1 month of treatment, the physician should consider increasing the dose or discontinuing sibutramine. Doses larger than 15 mg/d are not recommended.[62]

Sibutramine has been studied in patients with obesity-related diseases, such as hypertension,[76] type 2 diabetes,[77,78] and hyperlipidemia.[79–81] In these trials, patients treated with sibutramine reportedly demonstrated weight loss without compromising, and usually with improvement of, the concomitant disease state. These observations were based on measurements such as blood pressure, serum glucose, and lipid profiles. In obese patients with type 2 diabetes, once-daily doses of sibutramine produced significant weight loss, particularly in the android (upper body) regions, and reductions in BMI. The changes in lean body mass, fasting blood sugars, and HbA were not statistically significant compared with placebo.[77] In obese patients with controlled mild to moderate hypertension, treatment with sibutramine significantly decreased weight, BMI, and waist circumference with no worsening of hypertensive status.[76]

Sibutramine has been compared with only one other antiobesity agent: dexfenfluramine. Two clinical trials assessing these agents involved 278 obese patients with a BMI of at least 27 kg/m^2.[82,83] The overall efficacy and tolerability of both agents was considered equivalent,[83] or not significantly different,[82] after 12 weeks of therapy with sibutramine 10 mg/d or with dexfenfluramine 15 mg twice daily.

The most common adverse effects associated with sibutramine are headache (30.3%), dry mouth (17.2%), loss of appetite (13%), constipation (11.5%), and insomnia (10.7%).[62] Adverse effects that have raised the most concern are increases in blood pressure and heart rate. According to the manufacturer, significant increases in blood pressure and pulse rate of approximately 1–3 mm Hg and 4–5 beats/min, respectively, have been noted with sibutramine at doses of 5–20 mg/d.[62] Baseline blood pressure should be established prior to beginning therapy and close monitoring at regular intervals is required when using this agent. Product labeling indicates that sibutramine should not be used in patients with a history of uncontrolled hypertension, stroke, coronary artery disease, congestive heart failure, or arrhythmias. At this time, primary pulmonary hypertension and cardiac valve problems have not been reported with sibutramine use.

Product labeling recommends that sibutramine not be used in patients receiving a selective serotonin reuptake inhibitor (SSRI) (i.e., fluoxetine, fluvoxamine, paroxetine, sertraline, or venlafaxine) or monoamine oxidase inhibitor (i.e., phenelzine, tranylcypromine, or isocarboxazid).[62] Because sibutramine inhibits serotonin reuptake, combination therapy with these agents may cause serotonin syndrome or hypertensive crisis. Caution should be exercised when sibutramine is administered concomitantly with other agents that may increase blood pressure. These include decongestants; cough, cold, and allergy medications that contain agents such as ephedrine; or pseudoephedrine. The coadministration of sibutramine with other prescription or nonprescription weight-loss agents cannot be recommended at this time due to a lack of safety and efficacy data.

Digestive Inhibitor

Orlistat

Excessive dietary fat intake has been identified as a contributor to the development of obesity.[84] Fat is an extremely dense energy source providing 9 kcal/g compared to 4 kcal/g with carbohydrates and protein. In addition, the metabolic costs of synthesizing fat from dietary carbohydrates are much greater than from dietary fat. The excessive storage of body fat comes most extensively from the excessive and calorically dense dietary fat. Thus, diets emphasizing reduced fat content are frequently used in weight-loss programs. Orlistat/Xenical® is a new drug that enhances weight loss by interfering with the breakdown and digestion of dietary fat, leading to malabsorption. It is unlike any other antiobesity agent currently on the market.

Orlistat is a hydrogenated derivative of lipstatin, a natural lipase inhibitor produced by *Streptomyces toxytricini*. Orlistat selectively binds to and inhibits gastrointestinal (gastric, pancreatic, and carboxylester) lipases, which are key enzymes in the hydrolysis of long-chain triglycerides. As a result of lipase inhibition, free fatty acids and cholesterol are prevented from being absorbed through the intestinal mucosal wall. Intact triglycerides and other nonabsorbed lipids pass through the gastrointestinal (GI) tract and are excreted in the feces.[85,86] This persistent lowering of dietary fat absorption has been shown to reduce body weight in patients with obesity.

Several dose-ranging studies have evaluated the impact of orlistat on fecal fat excretion.[87,88] Orlistat demonstrates dose-dependent reductions in fat absorption in conjunction with daily diets providing from 20–48% of daily calories from fat. Administration of orlistat at doses between 10 and 400 mg three times daily results in 5–35.8% fecal loss of ingested fat beyond that which occurs with a placebo.[87] The dose–response relationship is steep at doses less than 120 mg TID and begins to plateau at higher doses. No additional increases in fecal fat excretion occur with doses above 400 mg/d. Clinically, as much as a 30% reduction in fat absorption occurs with the recommended dose of 120 mg three times daily.[87,88]

Several large, long-term trials (1–2-yr duration) involving overweight and obese patients have established that orlistat, in conjunction with a hypocaloric diet, is effective in promoting weight loss.[89–93] After 1 year of treatment, a dose of 120 mg TID induced a mean weight loss ranging from 7.9 to 10% (7–10 kg) vs. 4.2 to 6.6% (4.1–6.4 kg) with placebo in obese nondiabetic individuals.[90–93] In a study involving obese patients with type 2 diabetes, the mean weight reduction was 6.2% (6.19 kg).[94] At the conclusion of 1 year of treatment, 51–69% of those treated with orlistat and diet and 31–49% of the placebo-treated patients lost at least 5% of their baseline body weight. More orlistat than placebo patients (29–39% vs. 11–25%, respectively) also lost at least 10% of their initial body weight.[90–93] Orlistat was also significantly more effective than placebo in 2-year studies that were designed to evaluate its effects on weight regain.[90–93] During the second year of treatment when patients were switched from a hypocaloric diet to a eucaloric diet, placebo recipients regained significantly more weight than orlistat recipients. The end result after 2 years of treatment was significantly greater weight loss in the patients taking orlistat as compared with those receiving placebo.

The effects of orlistat on risk factors for cardiovascular disease have also been investigated.[89–93,95,96] The drug has been associated with significant improvements in lipid profiles (total cholesterol and LDL cholesterol) relative to placebo in nondiabetic obese patients. In a study of obese patients with type 2 diabetes, weight loss and improved lipid profiles were greater in patients treated with orlistat compared with placebo recipients. The magnitude of this change was reported to be greater than that expected from weight loss alone, indicative of a pharmacological action of orlistat on fat absorption.[94] Certain aspects of blood pressure and glycemic control in type 2 diabetics and nondiabetic patients were also improved in recipients of orlistat vs. placebo.[97]

Orlistat causes few systemic effects because of its minimal absorption, and it is generally well tolerated. Gastrointestinal symptoms are the most commonly observed adverse events associated with the use of orlistat (incidence ≥5%) and are primarily a manifestation of inhibited fat absorption. Oily fecal spotting, flatus with discharge, fecal urgency, and oily stool can occur during early orlistat therapy. The majority of gastrointestinal events occur within the first week of therapy, tend to be mild and transient, and improve with continued use. These complaints may increase if orlistat is taken with a high-fat diet containing >30% of daily kilocalories from fat, or with any single meal with a very high fat content. Patients taking orlistat should be counseled to maintain a low-fat diet in an attempt to minimize the occurrence of gastrointestinal adverse effects.[98,99] Although orlistat has not been shown to cause gallstone formation, it is contraindicated in patients with cholestasis. Its use is also contraindicated in patients with malabsorption syndrome. Urinary oxalate levels may become elevated in patients taking orlistat; therefore, the medication should be used cautiously in patients with a history of hyperoxaluria or calcium oxalate nephrolithiasis. Orlistat inhibits pancreatic carboxylester lipase and may, therefore, affect the absorption of fat-soluble vitamins (A, D, E, and K). Vitamin supplementation should be considered during therapy with this agent. A multivitamin should be taken once daily at least 2 h before or after the administration of orlistat.[98,100]

Despite its mechanism of action, orlistat does not appear to affect the pharma-cokinetics and/or pharmacodynamics of numerous other agents. Medications docu-mented to have minimal interactions when administered concurrently with orlistat include oral contraceptives,[101] digoxin,[102] glyburide,[103] phenytoin,[104] pravastatin,[105] warfarin,[106] extended-release nifedipine,[107,108] captopril,[108] atenolol,[108] furosemide,[108] and ethanol.[109] Although no clinical studies have evaluated the impact of simulta-neously using orlistat- and Olestra®-containing products, this combination may increase the risk of gastrointestinal side effects in some patients. The safety and efficacy of using orlistat in combination with other weight-loss agents has not been established. Combination therapy cannot be recommended at this time.

Like other weight-loss medications currently on the market, orlistat does not provide a miracle cure for obesity and is not intended for use in individuals who wish to lose only 5–10 pounds. Orlistat should be used only in patients who are obese (BMI ≥ 30 or ≥ 27 with other risk factors) and in combination with dietary changes, exercise, and behavioral modification. Orlistat in 120-mg doses should be administered three times daily with each main meal containing fat (during or up to 1 h after the meal). The drug must be taken with foods that contain fat in order to exert its effect. If a meal is occasionally missed or contains no fat, the dose of orlistat can be omitted.[98] The effectiveness of orlistat is dependent upon continuous use of the product and a change in the patient's eating habits. Some patients may require long-term therapy to maintain their weight loss. The acceptable tolerability profile of orlistat and its lack of systemic adverse effects make it an attractive option in the treatment of obese patients with preexisting cardiovascular disease who may not be candidates for centrally acting appetite suppressants.

SUMMARY

Obesity has emerged as a critical health issue over the last several decades, and its prevalence is expected to increase. Obesity significantly increases the risk for comorbid disorders and premature mortality. A weight loss of at least 5–10% of initial body weight is sufficient to achieve clinically meaningful improvements in obesity-related comorbidities. Weight loss and weight maintenance plans should include a combination of dietary therapy, increased physical activity, and behavior therapy.

Drug therapy can also be used as an adjunct to these strategies. Prescription weight-loss drugs are appropriate for patients with a BMI of ≥ 30 with no concomitant obesity-related risk factors or diseases, and for patients with a BMI of ≥ 27 with concomitant obesity-related risk factors or diseases. Nonpharmacological therapy is the treatment of choice in patients who are less obese without obesity-related risk factors or diseases.[6]

Drug therapy has undergone multiple changes in the last several years. Phenyl-propanolamine, a popular OTC product used for the short-term treatment of obesity, was recently withdrawn from the market after it was determined that users were at increased risk for hemorrhagic stroke. With the recognition that obesity is a chronic disorder, the focus on drug therapy has shifted from short- to long-term administration. Dexfenfluramine and fenfluramine alone, as well as the combination of phentermine/fenfluramine, were the first agents to be used extensively on a long-term basis. Dexfenfluramine and fenfluramine were removed from the market in 1997 after the discovery of life-threatening side effects. At that time, the only other prescription agents were the amphetamine-like derivatives (e.g., phentermine), which are approved only for short-term use. Newer agents, sibutramine and orlistat, have demonstrated effectiveness that lasts at least 1 year and should be considered as first-line therapy options for the long-term treatment of obesity.

All classes of antiobesity medications are effective, but they produce only modest weight loss. The net weight loss attributable to drug therapy has been reported to range from 2 to 10 kg (4.4 to 22 lb), with a majority of the weight loss occurring within the first 6 months of therapy. As treatment extends beyond 6 months, weight loss tends to plateau.[6] Current recommendations suggest that weight-loss medications be used for a trial period of several weeks to determine their efficacy in a given patient. Long-term response is less likely if patients do not achieve at least a 2 kg (4.4 lb) weight loss during the first month of therapy. If a patient does not respond to a medication, the physician should reassess the patient's compliance with the entire weight-loss program and consider increasing the medication dose. If the patient experiences serious adverse effects or continues to be unresponsive to the medication, the medication should be discontinued and an alternative medication should be considered. In patients who respond adequately to weight-loss medications, continued assessment to evaluate the drug's safety should occur. If the patient is not experiencing any serious adverse effects, the medication can be continued indefinitely, keeping in mind that drug safety and efficacy beyond 1 to 2 years of treatment have not been established.

Although combination drug therapy may be efficacious in certain patients, the risk of adverse effects is increased. Until additional trials are conducted evaluating the safety of this practice, antiobesity medications should be used as single agents. During the first year of treatment with a medication, patients should be closely monitored for side effects, particularly during the first 3 months.[6]

The physician, pharmacist, dietician, or other healthcare professional can be vital in helping patients avoid drug interactions with their weight-loss medication. Many consumers have a great interest in herbal, natural, or food supplement products and may use these agents as an adjunct to a weight-loss program. Products such as chromium, ma huang, St. John's wort, white willow bark, and guarana and tea extracts have potential weight-loss properties. The manufacturing and labeling of these products are not strictly regulated by the FDA; therefore, the preparations may have inconsistent amounts of active ingredients and unpredictable and potentially harmful effects when used singly or combined with other medications. Herbal medications should not be recommended as part of a weight-loss program. OTC cough, cold, and allergy products should be selected with care in patients receiving nonprescription or prescription appetite suppressants. Many of the ingredients in OTC preparations can exert effects on blood pressure when combined with herbal products, amphetamine derivatives, and sibutramine. Concomitant use with certain antidepressant medications should also be avoided.

All health professionals involved in monitoring a patient's progress on a weight-loss program can play an important role in the management of obesity. Patients must realize that no magic cures exist for obesity, and partial success is better than total failure. Physicians, dieticians, and pharmacists are in the position to put the many components of a weight-loss program into perspective. Using educational and reinforcing techniques, healthcare professionals can assist the obese patient to achieve lasting results.

REFERENCES

1. McGinnis JM, Foege WH. Actual causes of death in the United States. *JAMA*. 1993; 270:2207–2212.
2. Kuczmarski RJ, Carroll MD, Flegal KM, Troiano RP. Varying body mass index cutoff points to describe overweight prevalence among U.S. adults: NHANES III (1988–1994). *Obes Res*. 1997;5:542–548.
3. Flegal KM, Carroll MD, Kuczmarski RJ, Johnson CL. Overweight and obesity in the United States: prevalence and trends, 1960–1994. *Int J Obes*. 1998;22:39–47.
4. Kuczmarski RJ, Flegal KM, Campbell SM, Johnson CL. Increasing prevalence of overweight among US adults. *JAMA*. 1994;272(3):205–210.
5. Division of Health Examination Statistics, National Center for Health Statistics, Division of Nutrition and Physical Activity, National Center for Chronic Disease Prevention and Health Promotion, CDC. Update: prevalence of overweight among children, adolescents, and adults — United States, 1988–1994. *MMWR*. 1997; 46(9):199–201.
6. NHLBI Obesity Education Initiative Expert Panel on the Identification, Evaluation, and Treatment of Overweight and Obesity in Adults. *Clincial Guidelines on the Identification, Evaluation, and Treatment of Overweight and Obesity in Adults. The Evidence Report*. Bethesda, MD: National Heart, Lung, and Blood Institute. 1998.
7. Pi-Sunyer FX. Medical hazards of obesity. *Ann Intern Med*. 1993;119:655–660.
8. Bray GA. Pathophysiology of obesity. *Am J Clin Nut*. 1992;55:488S–94S.
9. Stunkard AJ. Current views on obesity. *Am J Med*. 1996;100:230–236.
10. Caterson ID. Management strategies for weight control: eating, exercise and behaviour. *Drugs*. 1990;39 (Suppl 3):20–32.
11. Goldstein DJ. Beneficial health effects of modest weight loss. *Int J Obes*. 1992;16:397–415.
12. Department of Health and Human Services, Food and Drug Administration. Weight control drug products for over-the-counter human use; certain active ingredients. *Federal Register*. 1991;56(Aug 8th):37792–37799.
13. Food and Drug Administration. Washington, DC: U.S. Department of Health and Human Services 2000 Nov 6. (Talk Paper T00-58).
14. The American Society of Health-System Pharmacists. Phenylpropanolamine hydrochloride. In: McEvoy GK, editor. *American Hospital Formulary Service*. Bethesda: The American Society of Health-System Pharmacists. 1998;1062–4.
15. Kernan WN, Viscoli CM, Brass LM, Broderick JP, Brott T, Feldmann E et al. Phenylpropanolamine and the risk of hemorrhagic stroke. *NEJM*. 2000;343:1826–32.
16. Food and Drug Administration science background safety of phenylpropanolamine. Nov 6, 2000. Retrieved July 7, 20002, from http://www.fda.gov/cder/drug/infopage/ppa/science.htm.

17. A Nasal Decongestant and a Local Anesthetic for Weight Control? *Medical Letter on Drugs and Therapeutics.* 1979;21(16):65–66.
18. Plotz M. Obesity. *Med Times.* 1958;86:860–863.
19. Gould WL. Obesity and hypertension: the importance of a safe compound to control appetite. *North Carolina Med J.* 1950;11:327–334.
20. McClure CW, Brusch CA. Treatment of oral syndrome obesity with non-traditional appetite control plan. *JAMWA.* 1973;28:239–248.
21. Collipp PJ. The treatment of exogenous obesity by medicated benzocaine candy: a double blind placebo study. *Obesity/Bariatric Med.* 1981;10(5):123–125.
22. Greenway F, Heber D, Raum W, Morales S. Double-blind, randomized, placebo-controlled clinical trials with non-prescription medications for the treatment of obesity. *Obes Res.* 1999;7(4):370–378.
23. Drug Facts and Comparisons. St. Louis, MO: Facts and Comparisons, 2000.
24. Hutchison TA, Shahan DR and Anderson ML (Eds): DRUGDEX® System. MICROMEDEX, Inc., Englewood, Colorado (Edition expires May 2000).
25. American Society of Health System Pharmacists. ASHP therapeutic position statement on the safe use of pharmacotherapy for obesity management in adults. *Am J Health-Syst Pharm.* 2001;58:1645–55.
26. The review of natural products. St. Louis, MO: *Facts and Comparisons, 2002.*
27. Centers for Disease Control and Prevention. Adverse events associated with ephedrine-containing products — Texas, December 1993–September 1995. *MMWR Morb Mortal Wkly Rep.* 1996;45:689–92.
28. Miller LG. Herbal medicinals. *Arch Intern Med.* 1998;158:2200–11.
29. Winslow LC, Kroll DJ. Herbs as medicines. *Arch Intern Med.* 1998;158:2192–99.
30. National Task Force on the Prevention of Obesity. Long-term pharmacotherapy in the management of obesity. *JAMA.* 1996;276:1907–1915.
31. Obesity in perspective: a conference/sponsored by the John E. Fogarty International Center for Advanced Study in the Health Sciences, National Institutes of Health, Bethesda, MD, Oct. 1–3, 1973; George A Bray, editor. Washington DC: US Government Printing Office, DHEW publication number (NIH75-708).
32. Bray GA. Use and abuse of appetite-suppressant drugs in the treatment of obesity. *Ann Intern Med.* 1993;119;707–713.
33. Silverstone T. Appetite suppressants. *Drugs.* 1992;43(6):820–836.
34. Weintraub M. Long-term weight control: the National Heart, Lung, and Blood Institute funded multimodal intervention study. *Clin Pharmacol Ther.* 1992;51:581–585.
35. Weintraub M, Sundaresan PR, Madan M, Schuster B, Balder A, Lasagna L et al. Long-term weight control study I (weeks 0 to 34). *Clin Pharmacol Ther.* 1992;51:586–594.
36. Weintraub M, Sundaresan PR, Schuster B, Ginsberg G, Madan M, Balder A et al. Long-term weight control study II (weeks 34 to 104). *Clin Pharmacol Ther.* 1992;51:595–601.
37. Weintraub M, Sundaresan PR, Schuster B, Moscucci M, Stein C. Long-term weight control study III (weeks 104 to 156). *Clin Pharmacol Ther.* 1992;51:602–607.
38. Weintraub M, Sundaresan PR, Schuster B, Averbuch M, Stein C, Cox C et al. Long-term weight control study IV (weeks 156 to 190). *Clin Pharmacol Ther.* 1992;51:608–614.
39. Weintraub M, Sundaresan PR, Schuster B, Averbuch M, Stein C, Byrne L. Long-term weight control study V (weeks 190 to 210). *Clin Pharmacol Ther.* 1992;51:615–618.

40. Weintraub M, Sundersan PR, Cox C. Long-term weight control study VI. *Clin Pharmacol Ther.* 1992;51:619–633.
41. Weintraub M. Long-term weight control study: conclusions. *Clin Pharmacol Ther.* 1992;51:642–646.
42. Weintraub M, Hasday JD, Mushlin AI, Lockwood DH. A double-blind clinical trial in weight control: use of fenfluramine and phentermine alone and in combination. *Arch Intern Med.* 1984;144:1143–1148.
43. Stunkard AJ. Anorectic agents: a theory of action and lack of tolerance in a clinical trial. In Garattini S, editor. *Anorectic agents: mechanisms of action and tolerance.* New York: Raven Press, 1981.
44. The American Society of Health-System Pharmacists. Amphetamines general statement. In: McEvoy GK, editor. *American Hospital Formulary Service.* Bethesda: The American Society of Health-System Pharmacists. 1998;1902–1905.
45. Elliott BW. A collaborative investigation of fenfluramine: anorexigenic with sedative properties. *Current Ther Res.* 1970;12(8):502–515.
46. Sainani GS, Fulambarkar AM, Khurana BK. A double-blind clinical trial of fenfluramine in the treatment of obesity. *Br J Clin Prac.* 1973;27(4):136–138.
47. Tisdale SA, Ervin DK. Anorectic effectiveness of differing dosage forms of fenfluramine. *Current Ther Res.* 1976;19(6):589–594.
48. Wurtman J, Wurtman R, Mark S, Tsay R, Gilbert W, Growdon J. d-Fenfluramine selectively suppresses carbohydrate snacking by obese subjects. *Int J Eat Disorders.* 1985;4(1):89–99.
49. Weintraub M, Sriwatanakul K, Sundaresan PR, Weis OF, Dorn M. Extended-release fenfluramine: patient acceptance and efficacy of evening dosing. *Clin Pharmacol Ther.* 1983;33(5):621–627.
50. Lele RD, Joshi VR, Nathwani AN. A double-blind clinical trial of fenfluramine. *Br J Clin Pract.* 1972;26:79–82.
51. U.S. Department of Health and Human Services. Cardiac valvulopathy associated with exposure to fenfluramine or dexfenfluramine: interim public health recommendations. *MMWR.* 1997;46(45):1061–1066.
52. Turner P. Dexfenfluramine its place in weight control. *Drugs.* 1990;39(suppl 3):53–62.
53. McTavish D, Heel RC. Dexfenfluramine a review of its pharmacological properties and therapeutic potential in obesity. *Drugs.* 1992;43(5):713–733.
54. Swinburn BA, Carmichael HE, Wilson MR. Dexfenfluramine as an adjunct to a reduced-fat, ad libitum diet: effects on body composition, nutrient intake and cardiovascular risk factors. *Int J Obes.* 1996;20:1033–1040.
55. Enzi G, Crepaldi G, Inelman EM, Bruni R, Baggio B. Efficacy and safety of dexfenfluramine in obese patients: a multicenter study. *Clin Neuropharm.* 1988;11(1):S173–S175.
56. Noble RE. A six-month study of the effects of dexfenfluramine on partially successful dieters. *Curr Ther Res.* 1990;47(4):612–619.
57. Marbury TC, Angelo JE, Gulley RM, Krosnick A, Sugimoto DH, Zellner SR. A placebo-controlled, dose response study of dexfenfluramine in the treatment of obese patients. *Curr Ther Res.* 1996;57(9):663–674.
58. Holdaway IM, Wallace E, Westbrooke L, Gamble G. Effect of dexfenfluramine on body weight, blood pressure, insulin resistance and serum cholesterol in obese individuals. *Int J Obes.* 1995;19:749–751.
59. Finer N. Body weight evolution during dexfenfluramine treatment after initial weight control. *Int J Obes.* 1992;16(suppl 3):S25–S29.

60. Guy-Grand B, Apfelbaum M, Crepaldi G, Cries A, Lefebvre P, Turner P. International trial of long-term dexfenfluramine in obesity. *Lancet.* 1989;2:1142–1144.

61. Khan MA. The effect of adding phentermine to weight management therapy in patients with declining response to dexfenfluramine alone. *Obes Res.* 1997;5:22S.

62. Knoll Pharmaceutical. Meridia (sibutramine) Product information. Mt. Olive, NJ, 1998.

63. McNeely W, Goa KL. Sibutramine a review of its contribution to the management of obesity. *Drugs.* 1998;56(6):1093–1124.

64. Kaiser PE. Hinson JL. Sibutramine: dose response and plasma metabolite concentrations in weight loss (abstract). *J Clin Pharmacol.* 1994;34:1019.

65. Weintraub M, Rubio A, Golik A, Byrne L, Scheinbaum ML. Sibutramine in weight control: a dose-ranging, efficacy study. *Clin Pharmacol Ther.* 1991;50:330–337.

66. Bray GA, Ryan DH, Gordon D, Heidingsfelder S, Cerise F, Wilson K. A double-blind randomized placebo controlled trial of sibutramine. *Obes Res.* 1996;4:263–270.

67. Drouin P, Hanotin C, Courcier S, Leutenegger E. A dose ranging study: efficacy and tolerability of sibutramine in weight loss (abstract). *Int J Obes Relat Metab Disord.*1994;18(suppl 2):60.

68. Jones SP, Newman BM, Romanec FM. Sibutramine hydrochloride: weight loss in overweight subjects (abstract). *Int J Obes Relat Metab Disord.* 1994;18(suppl 2):61.

69. Jones SP, Smith IG, Kelly F, Gray JA. Long-term weight loss with sibutramine (abstract). *Int J Obes Relat Metab Disord.* 1995;19(suppl 2):S41.

70. Jones AP, Heath MJ. Long-term weight loss with sibutramine: 5% responders (abstract). *Int J Obes Relat Metab Disord.* 1996;20(suppl 4):157.

71. Apfelbaum M, Vague P, Ziegler O, Hanotin C, Thomas F, Leutenegger E. Long-term maintenance of weight loss after a very-low-calorie diet: a randomized blinded trial of the efficacy and tolerability of sibutramine. *Am J Med.* 1999;106:179–184.

72. Bray GA, Blackburn GL, Ferguson JM, Greenway FL, Jain A, Kaiser PE et al. Sibutramine-dose response and long-term efficacy in weight loss, a double-blind study (abstract). *Int J Obes Relat Metab Disord.* 1994;18(suppl 2):60.

73. Mendels J, Blackburn GL, Bray GA, Ferguson JM, Greenway FL, Jain A et al. Sibutramine and long-term weight loss: percent of patients losing 5 and 10% of baseline weight (abstract). *Int J Obes Relat Metab Disord.* 1994;18(suppl 2):61.

74. Hanotin C, Thomas F, Jones SP, Leutenegger E, Drouin P. Efficacy and tolerability of sibutramine in obese patients: a dose-ranging study. *Int J Obes Relat Metab Disord.* 1998;22:32–38.

75. Bray GA, Blackburn GL, Ferguson JM, Greenway FL, Jain AK, Mendel CM et al. Sibutramine produces dose-related weight loss. *Obes Res.* 1999;7:189–198.

76. Hazenberg BP, Johnson SG, Kelly F. Sibutramine in the treatment of obese subjects with hypertension (abstract). *Int J Obes Relat Metab Disord.* 1996;20(suppl 4):S156.

77. Griffiths J, Brynes AE, Frost G, Bloom SR, Finer N, Jones SP et al. Sibutramine in the treatment of overweight non-insulin dependent diabetics (abstract). *Int J Obes Relat Metab Disord.* 1995;19(suppl 2):41.

78. Shepherd G, Fitchet M, Kelly F. Sibutramine: a meta-analysis of the change in fasting plasma glucose in patients with a high baseline fasting value (abstract). *Int J Obes Relat Metab Disord.* 1997;21(suppl 2):S54.

79. Fitchet M, Shepherd G, Kelly F. Sibutramine: a meta-analysis of chages in fasting serum lipids in placebo controlled studies (abstract). *Int J Obes Relat Metab Disord.* 1997;21(suppl 2):S53.

80. Oya M, Dominguez R, Heath M. The effect of sibutramine induced weight loss in obese subjects with hyperlipidemia (abstract). *Int J Obes Relat Metab Disord.* 1997;21(suppl 2):S54.
81. Hansen DL, Toubro S, Astrup A. Effects of sibutramine on blood lipids (abstract). *Int J Obes Relat Metab Disord.* 1997;21(suppl 2)S55.
82. Kelly F, Wade AF, Jones SP, Johnson SG. Sibutramine hydrochloride vs dexfenfluramine: weight loss in obese subjects (abstract). *Int J Obes Relat Metab Disord.* 1994;18(suppl 2):S61.
83. Hanotin C, Thomas F, Jones SP, Leutenegger E, Drouin P. A comparison of sibutramine and dexfenfluramine in the treatment of obesity. *Obes Res.* 1998;6(4):285–291.
84. Golay A, Bobbioni E. The role of dietary fat in obesity. *Int J Obes.* 1997;21(suppl 3):S2–S11.
85. Guerciolini R. Mode of action of orlistat. *Int J Obes.* 1997;21(suppl 3):S12–S23.
86. Drent ML, van der Veen EA. Lipase inhibition: a novel concept in the treatment of obesity. *Int J Obes.* 1993;17:241–244.
87. Hauptman JB, Jeunet FS, Hartman D. Initial studies in humans with the novel gastrointestinal lipase inhibitor Ro 18-0647 (tetrahydrolipstatin). *Am J Clin Nutr.* 1992;55:309S–313S.
88. Zhi J, Melia AT, Guerciolini R, Chung J, Kinberg J, Hauptman JB et al. Retrospective population-based analysis of the dose-response (fecal fat excretion) relationship of orlistat in normal and obese volunteers. *Clin Pharmacol Ther.* 1994;56:82–85.
89. Hill JO, Hauptman J, Anderson JW, Fujioka K, O'Neil PM, Smith DK et al. Orlistat, a lipase inhibitor, for weight maintenance after conventional dieting: a 1-y study. *Am J Clin Nutr.* 1999;69:1108–1116.
90. Davidson MH, Hauptman J, DiGirolamo M, Foreyt JP, Halsted CH, Heber D et al. Weight control and risk factor reduction in obese subjects treated for 2 years with orlistat. *JAMA.* 1999;281(3):235–242.
91. Sjostrom L, Rissanen A, Anderson T, Boldrin M, Golay A, Koppeschaar HPF et al. Randomised placebo-controlled trial of orlistat for weight loss and prevention of weight regain in obese patients. *Lancet.* 1998;35(2):167–172.
92. Hauptman J, Lucas C, Boldrin MN, Collins H, Segal KR. Orlistat in the long-term treatment of obesity in primary care settings. *Arch Fam Med.* 2000;9:160–7.
93. Rossner S, Sjostrom L, Noack R, Meinders AE, Noseda G. Weight loss, weight maintenance, and improved cardiovascular risk factors after 2 years treatment with orlistat for obesity. *Obesity Res.* 2000;8(1):49–61.
94. Hollander PA, Elbein SC, Hirsch IB, Kelley D, McGill, Taylor T et al. Role of orlistat in the treatment of obese patients with type 2 diabetes. *Diabetes Care.* 1998;21:1288–1294.
95. Tonstad S, Pometta D, Erkelens DW, Ose L, Moccetti T, Schouten JA et al. The effect of the gastrointestinal lipase inhibitor, orlistat, on serum lipids and lipoproteins in patients with primary hyperlipidaemia. *Eur J Clin Pharmacol.* 1994;46(5):405–410.
96. Reitsma JB, Cabezas MC, Bruin TWA, Erkelens DW. Relationship between improved postprandial lipemia and low-density lipoprotein metabolism during treatment with tetrahydrolipstatin, a pancreatic lipasc inhibitor. *Metabolism.* 1994;43:293–298.
97. Pataky Z, Golay A. Effect of treatment with orlistat for one-year on blood pressure in obese patients (abstract). *Int J Obes.* 1999;23(suppl 5):S175.
98. Roche Laboratories. Xenical (orlistat) Product Information. Nutley, NJ, 1999.
99. Canovatchel W. Long-term tolerability profile of orlistat, an intestinal lipase inhibitor (abstract). *Diabetologia.* 1997;40(suppl 1):A196.

100. Melia AT, Doss-Twardy SG, Zhi J. The effect of orlistat, an inhibitor of dietary fat absorption, on the absorption of vitamins A and E in healthy volunteers. *J Clin Pharmacol.* 1996;36:647–653.

101. Hartmann D, Guzelhan C, Zuiderwijk PBM, Odink J. Lack of interaction between orlistat and oral contraceptives. *Eur J Clin Pharmacol.* 1996;50:421–424.

102. Melia AT, Zhi J, Koss-Twardy SG, Min BH, Smith BL, Freundlich NL et al. The influence of reduced dietary fat absorption induced by orlistat on the pharmacokinetics of digoxin in healthy volunteers. *J Clin Pharmacol.* 1995;35:840–843.

103. Zhi J, Melia AT, Koss-Twardy SG, Min B, Guerciolini R, Freundlich NL et al. The influence of orlistat on the pharmacokinetics and pharmacodynamics of glyburide in healthy volunteers. *J Clin Pharmacol.* 1995;35:521–525.

104. Melia AT, Mulligan TE, Zhi J. The effect of orlistat on the pharmacokinetics of phenytoin in healthy volunteers. *J Clin Pharmacol.* 1996;36:654–658.

105. Oo CY, Akbari B, Lee S, Nichols S, Hellmann CP. Effect of orlistat, a novel anti-obesity agent, on the pharmacokinetics and pharmacodynamics of pravastatin in patients with mild hypercholesterolaemia. *Clin Drug Invest.* 1999;17:217–223.

106. Zhi J, Melia AT, Guercioline R, Koss-Twardy SG, Passe SM, Rakhit A et al. The effect of orlistat on the pharmacokinetics and pharmacodynamics of warfarin in healthy volunteers. *J Clin Pharmacol.* 1996;36:659–666.

107. Melia AT. Lack of effect of orlistat on the bioavailability of a single dose of nifedipine extended release tablets (Procardia XL) in healthy volunteers. *J Clin Pharmacol.* 1996;36:352–355.

108. Weber C, Tam YK, Schmidtke-Schrezenmeier G, Jonkmann JHG, ban Brummelen P. Effect of the lipase inhibitor orlistat on the pharmacokinetics of four different antihypertensive drugs in healthy volunteers. *Eur J Clin Pharmacol.* 1996;51:87–90.

109. Melia AT, Zhi J, Zelasko R, Hartmann D, Guzelhan C, Guerciolini R. The interaction of the lipase inhibitor orlistat with ethanol in healthy volunteers. *Eur J Clin Pharmacol.* 1998;54:773–777.

CHAPTER 12

Nonprescription Drug and Nutrient Interactions

Beth Miller and Nancy Carthan

CONTENTS

Self-care is becoming increasingly popular among consumers. More and more consumers are using over-the-counter (OTC) products to treat common complaints and minor illnesses. Retail sales of OTC products have grown from $1.9 billion in 1964 to more than $16.6 billion in 1997. Because of this growth, clinicians should assume that OTC medication use is a common patient self-care behavior. In addition, because consumers are more willing to self-medicate without the advice or knowledge of their healthcare provider, drug–drug and drug–nutrient interactions are increasing concerns. This is especially true because the market share for OTC medications has been shifting from pharmacies to convenience stores, discount stores, and small grocery stores.[1,2]

So why are consumers more willing to self-care? One reason may be the cost savings. In 1997, OTC medication availability saved Americans more than $20 billion in healthcare costs. This sum encompassed office visits, prescription costs, time lost from work, and insurance costs. Self-care has been defined as "the practice of activities that individuals initiate and perform on their own behalf in maintaining life, health, and well-being." A 1992 survey lists the ten most common conditions treated with OTC products, which are headache, athlete's foot, the common cold, chronic dandruff, upset stomach, lip problems, premenstrual symptoms, menstrual symptoms, dry skin, and sinus problems. Six of these conditions rely primarily on orally ingested drugs for self-treatment.[1,3,4,5]

Prescription medications are being switched to OTC status with increasing frequency. More than 600 OTC products have ingredients or dosages previously available by prescription only. The U.S. Food and Drug Administration (FDA) has a division that reviews proposed OTC drugs. Drug approval for OTC use requires that the drug be on the market long enough to establish it to have "an acceptable safety margin, a low potential for misuse and abuse, the ability for the average consumer to self-diagnose, self-recognize, and self-treat the condition, and a label adequate to be understood by the lay consumer." Benefits of having OTC availability include decreased costs and enhanced patient autonomy; however, the potential risks of self-diagnosis may include inappropriate use, unnecessary use, or delay in treatment that could lead to increased costs and morbidity.[6]

Healthcare professionals need to be cognizant of drug–nutrient interactions in order to educate patients who self-medicate with OTC products. A nutrient is defined as a chemical substance needed for growth and maintenance of normal cells in both plants and animals. It should be understood that diet and nutrition can affect therapeutic response and these interactions have varying degrees of clinical significance. The interaction in some cases may be advantageous when it lessens side effects or increases therapeutic efficacy. On the other hand, drug–nutrient interactions can result in therapeutic failure. Testing for drug–nutrient interactions is still relatively new and has been reviewed in only a small percentage of drugs—the majority being prescription medications. As a result, health professionals often must make educated guesses about the effects of food on drug therapy.[7–11]

EFFECT OF FOOD/NUTRIENTS ON MEDICATION ABSORPTION

Food intake in relation to drug administration can have a significant impact on drug dissolution and absorption. The presence of food changes gastric motility, changes the gastrointestinal pH, and provides substances for drug and nutrient chelation and adsorption. Typically, when food is present in the stomach, drugs are absorbed more slowly; however, a clear distinction must be made between decreased rate of absorption and decreased amount of drug absorbed. A decreased absorption rate allows for increased nutrient interactions and possible delays in therapeutic efficacy without changing the overall bioavailability of the drug.[12–15]

The interaction of aspirin with food is an example of a nutrient delaying onset of activity without altering bioavailability. A study in 25 subjects found that food roughly halved the serum salicylate level 10 and 20 min after a 650-mg dose when compared with placebo. Additional studies have confirmed this finding. It is likely that the aspirin is adsorbed onto the food and the food itself delays gastric emptying. Food intake markedly slows the absorption of aspirin and thus the time to onset of therapeutic effect. On the other hand, a delay in absorption may be beneficial.

Cimetidine is given with food to assist in maintaining a therapeutic blood concentration. A fraction of cimetidine is absorbed while food is present, allowing the remaining drug to be dissolved once the gut is cleared. Thus, therapeutic levels are maintained throughout the dosing interval.[13,16–18]

Although it is frequently assumed that food reduces drug absorption, lipophilic drugs are, in many cases, more readily used when taken with a high-fat meal. The increased residency in the gut improves drug dissolution. Water-insoluble drugs (such as the prescription drugs spironolactone and griseofulvin) are better absorbed when taken directly after a meal. Owing to their lipophilic nature, supplements for vitamins A, E, D, and K have enhanced absorption when taken with a high-fat meal.[19,20]

Chelation is an additional factor that influences drug absorption. Chelation involves the formation of a complex between certain dietary components, especially divalent or trivalent cations (e.g., Ca, Mg, Al, Fe, and Zn) and certain drugs. The complex is a less soluble substance; therefore, absorption of the nutrient and drug is decreased. Antacids containing aluminum, magnesium, and calcium or foods rich in copper, calcium, magnesium, zinc, and iron are most often responsible for chelation. To prevent chelation, antacids should be dosed 2–3 h apart from foods containing these nutrients. Tannins, a component of strong tea, coffee, and some wines, form complexes with iron and other heavy metals, which are then not absorbed. It may be prudent to avoid taking iron supplements at the same time as these liquids.

Specific nutrients and food components also influence the rate of drug absorption. A high-carbohydrate meal slows the absorption of many drugs. Fiber and calcium can bind with a drug to prevent absorption. The absorption of acetaminophen is slowed by the presence of pectin, a fiber. Acidic juices and cola may cause rapid dissolution of some drugs. A drug with its primary activity in the intestines may be broken down too early if administered with an acidic beverage. Thus, the drug's efficacy is greatly reduced. In contrast, juice with a high vitamin C content enhances the absorption of iron supplements.[21,22]

EFFECT OF FOOD/NUTRIENTS ON MEDICATION METABOLISM

The metabolism of many substances including drugs occurs primarily through the mixed-function oxidase system and the conjugating system of the cell cytosol. The mixed-function oxidase system catalyzes oxidative reactions (phase I) of a number of drug classes as well as endogenous substance, fatty acids, and prostaglandins. More than 30 isoenzymes of the system have been identified as belonging to the cytochrome P_{450} series (CYP_{450}). The major enzymes responsible for drug metabolism are CYP3A4, CYP2D6, CYP1A2, and the CYP2C. In the conjugating system, drugs are primarily converted to glucoronides, ester sulfates, or glutathione conjugates (phase II). Phase I and II reactions occur in the liver as well as in the intestinal mucosa.[23,24]

Dietary components of food may alter this hepatic metabolism by induction or inhibition of the mixed-function oxidase system. Induction of the enzyme system results in an increased metabolism of a parent drug to metabolites and thus a decrease in the availability of the parent drug. As a result, enzyme induction commonly produces lower blood levels of the parent drug. Lower blood levels may result in decreased efficacy of the drug. If the parent drug, however, must be converted by the enzyme system to an active metabolite, induction may be associated with increased toxicity due to higher concentrations of the metabolite. High-protein, low-carbohydrate diets induce the mixed-function oxidase system and promote metabolism of drugs that are substrates of this system. Indoles found in cruciferous vegetables, such as cabbage and Brussels sprouts, and chemicals in charcoal-broiled meats significantly induce chemical oxidations of medications as well. Smoked and preserved meats likely also contain chemicals oxidized by CYP_{450} isoenzymes.[22,23]

On the other hand, bioflavanoids and other substances found naturally in fruits and vegetables may inhibit drug hepatic metabolism. Inhibition of the mixed-function oxidase system typically results in elevated serum levels of the parent drug, prolonged therapeutic efficacy, and increased incidence of adverse effects. Several components of grapefruit juice and whole grapefruit are assumed to be responsible for inhibition of the CYP_{450} isoenzymes 1A2 and 3A4. An appreciable increase of systemic availability of certain medications can occur when administered with grapefruit juice. Acetaminophen and naproxen are substrates of these isoenzymes; therefore, grapefruit juice may theoretically increase drug levels. In contrast, charbroiled food is an inducer of 1A2 and 3A4 and may decrease the efficacy of acetaminophen and naproxen. Minimal clinical significance, however, has been found with interactions between OTC products and grapefruit juice.[23,24]

Nutrients have also been shown to influence hepatic blood flow. Any drug absorbed in the intestine is taken directly to the liver. The enterohepatic circulation is a fundamental process in all pharmacokinetic processes involving orally ingested drugs. A number of drugs undergo biotransformation during this first pass through the gut wall and liver, with its complex enzyme systems. These biotransformations occur prior to drug transportation into circulation. Protein may increase the rate of blood flow to the liver and, therefore, increase the metabolism of a drug. Increased metabolism, as with induction of the mixed-function oxidase system, leads to changes in the amount of parent drug available. Blood levels, efficacy, and side effects of a drug may be increased or decreased as a result.[3,5,14,22] (See Table 12.1.)

EFFECT OF FOOD/NUTRIENTS ON MEDICATION EXCRETION

Food and nutrients may alter the renal excretion of some drugs. At high urinary pH values, weakly acidic drugs largely exist as ionized lipid-soluble molecules that cannot diffuse back across the renal tubule into blood and are lost in the urine. The converse is true for weak bases. Salicylic acid offers a useful example applicable to drugs likely to be affected by diet-related increases in urinary pH. Alkaline urine causes the salicylic acid to be reabsorbed from the urine. Drugs excreted from acidic urine but reabsorbed from alkaline urine include antihistamines, ascorbic acid, and nicotine. The clinical significance of this is usually small. Most drugs are transformed by the liver to inactive metabolites, and few are excreted unchanged in the urine.[3,7,25]

Table 12.1 Nutrient Effects on Drugs

Nutrients Involved	Drug Affected	Effect on Drug	Recommendation
Starches, clay, egg yolks	Iron	Decreased absorption	
Coadministration of food	Riboflavin	Increased absorption	
Coadministration of food	Thiamine	Delayed absorption	
Coadministration with pectin (fiber)	Acetaminophen	Delayed absorption and onset	
Coadministration of food	Cimetidine	Delayed absorption and onset	
Coadministration of food	Aspirin	Delayed absorption and onset	
Coadministration of food	Pseudoephedrine	Delayed absorption and onset	
Coadministration of food	Ibuprofen, ketoprofen, naproxen	Food delays absorption and onset but not significant; may cause GI upset, bleeding, ulceration or perforation	Administer with food to decrease GI upset
Coadministration of food	Famotidine	Slightly increased absorption	
Coadministration of food	Potassium	Delayed absorption and onset	

EFFECT OF MEDICATION ON FOOD/NUTRIENT ABSORPTION

Alterations in gastric pH due to drugs, such as antacids and H_2 antagonists, may influence the absorption of other drugs and nutrients. Prolonged use of antiulcer drugs, such as omeprazole, lansoprazole, pantoprazole, famotidine, ranitidine, nizatidine, or cimetidine, may decrease the absorption of vitamin B_{12}, thiamin, and iron. Drugs that change the pH in the different regions of the intestines may also influence nutrient absorption. Potassium chloride found in salt substitutes lowers the pH in the ileum, impairing vitamin B_{12} absorption. Antacids can produce an increase in gastric pH to alkaline levels (i.e., >7.2). The absorption of calcium, iron, magnesium, zinc, and folacin decreases in such an environment. Calcium carbonate given in 500-mg or greater doses increases the rate of absorption of folic acid due to an increased dissolution rate. Aluminum in aluminum hydroxide antacids can combine with phosphorus to form an insoluble complex that is excreted in the feces, with decreased phosphate absorption and blood levels. This interaction may be valuable in the treatment of hyperphosphatemia but harmful in the face of symptomatic hypophosphatemia. Aluminum antacids can also precipitate bile acids, leading to decreased absorption of vitamin A. Bisacodyl, a stimulant laxative, should not be taken with milk. The dissolution of this enteric-coated tablet is pH dependent. The milk may cause the drug to dissolve in the stomach, rather than in the small intestine, resulting in severe abdominal cramping and gastrointestinal irritation.[14,22]

Many OTC products interfere with gastric motility and thus the absorption of nutrients. Antacids and anticholinergic drugs affect bowel motility and thus the rate at which the nutrient moves through the gastrointestinal tract. Aluminum antacids may relax the gastric smooth muscle and cause a delay in gastric emptying. Anticholinergic drugs, such as antihistamines, slow peristalsis, thus slowing gastric emptying. The decreased transit time may result in more nutrient–drug interactions and a slow therapeutic response. On the other hand, laxatives may stimulate peristalsis, causing nutrients to be moved through the gut more quickly. Prolonged use of stimulant laxatives (e.g., bisacodyl) or saline laxatives (e.g., milk of magnesia) may decrease absorption of electrolytes such as calcium and potassium.[1,2,26]

Mineral oil acts as a physical barrier to the absorption of fat-soluble vitamins A, D, E, and K, as well as beta carotene and phosphorus. Mineral oil used as a laxative coats the lining of the small intestines. The body does not absorb it. Many nutrients, particularly fat-soluble vitamins, are dissolved in the mineral oil and are never absorbed. A variety of metabolic abnormalities such as low serum calcium and phosphate may result due to decreased vitamin D absorption. Mineral oil is rarely used, particularly in elderly patients, due to the risk of lipid pneumonitis from aspiration of oil droplets.[1,7]

Drugs may also directly affect nutrient absorption by damaging the mucosal wall of the small intestines, thus preventing a drug from being absorbed. Aspirin is a typical example of a drug that induces mucosal damage in the gut. Aspirin and other nonsteroidal products cause direct gastric irritation by breaking the gastric mucosal barrier. They also block the prostaglandins that produce gastric mucosal secretions to protect the stomach. As a result, blood is lost through the gastrointestinal tract. This gastrointestinal mucosal damage alters the absorption of iron and calcium. Chronic salicylate ingestion is a common cause of iron deficiency anemia.[4,13,15,18,19]

EFFECT OF MEDICATION ON FOOD/NUTRIENT METABOLISM

Cimetidine, an H_2 antagonist, inhibits the activity of cytochrome P_{450}, thereby slowing the metabolism of many substances that are substrates of the mixed-function oxidase system. Ranitidine has a lesser affinity to CYP_{450} than cimetidine. Therefore, clinically significant drug interactions are less likely to occur when ranitidine is chosen in place of cimetidine. Nizatidine and famotidine represent other H_2 antagonists that do not appear to produce interactions via this mechanism. Thus, it is reasonable to anticipate that the action of agents metabolized via this pathway would remain at normal levels or increase. The potential exists for nutrients metabolized via the liver to reach increased levels due to cimetidine-induced inhibition. No interactions between them have been documented at this time. Cimetidine may have an additional role in drug–nutrient interactions. Cimetidine (but not the other H_2 antagonists) decreases hepatic blood flow and thereby increases the bioavailability of nutrients or other drugs.[22,23,24]

Although not currently documented with OTC products, drugs may increase the metabolism of certain nutrients, resulting in higher dietary requirements. Anticonvulsants, phenobarbital, and phenytoin increase the metabolism of folic acid and

Table 12.2 Drug Effects on Nutrients

Drug Involved	Nutrient Involved	Effect on Nutrient	Recommendation for Drug
Alcohol	Magnesium, potassium, zinc, folate, thiamine	Increased renal excretion	Consume more foods rich in these nutrients
Aluminum hydroxide	Phosphate	Less absorption	Dose on empty stomach
Aspirin	Iron, potassium	Fecal iron loss, potassium depletion	Take with low-mineral carbohydrate snack
Bisacodyl	Potassium, sodium	Less absorption	Dose on empty stomach
Cimetidine	Calcium, magnesium, aluminum (antacids)	Decreased absorption	Take 2 hr before or after antacid
Mineral oil	Calcium, phosphate, potassium, vitamins A, E, D, K, beta carotene	Less absorption—drug is a physical barrier to absorption	Dose on empty stomach
Vitamin A	Aluminum (antacid)	Decreased absorption	Take 2 hr before or after antacid
Anticholinergics	All nutrients	Impaired GI motility	
Laxatives (phenolphthalein)	Potassium, calcium		

vitamins D and K. Drugs may also antagonize vitamin conversion to active forms. The antituberculosis drug, isoniazid, inhibits the conversion of B_6 to its active form. Vitamin B_6 deficiency could result in peripheral neuropathy if not supplemented appropriately. It is likely that interactions involving OTC medications and metabolism of certain nutrients will become more prevalent as the number of OTC products increases.[1,13,22] (See Table 12.2.)

EFFECT OF MEDICATION ON FOOD/NUTRIENT EXCRETION

Laxatives are the primary drug class that causes increased excretion of nutrients. Malabsorption of nutrients by the increased gastric motility from laxatives can sometimes lead to significant metabolic imbalances. This is discussed in more detail in Chapter 7. Another mechanism of increased nutrient excretion is through increased urinary loss of electrolytes. Loop diuretics increase the excretion of Na, K, Cl, Mg, and Ca. Persons using diuretics are frequently instructed to take the medication with a banana or orange juice. The fruit aids in replacing electrolyte nutrients lost to the increased urinary excretion secondary to appropriate diuresis.[8,16,20,22,26]

REFERENCES

1. Lamy, P.P., Over-the-counter medication: the drug interactions we overlook, *J. Am. Geriatr. Soc.*, 30, S69–S75, 1982.

2. Lowe, N.K. and Ryan-Wenger, N.M., Over-the-counter medications and self-care, *The Nurse Pract.,* 24, 34–44, 1999.

3. Anderson, K.E., Influences of diet and nutrition on clinical pharmacokinetics, *Clin. Pharmacokinet.,* 14, 325–346, 1988.

4. Berchtold, P., Weihrauch, T.R., and Berger, M., Food and drug interactions on digestive absorption, *World Rev. Nutr. Diet.,* 43, 10–33, 1984.

5. Griffin, J.P., Drug interactions occurring during absorption from the gastrointestinal tract, *Pharm. Ther.,* 15, 79–88, 1981.

6. Lipsky, M.S. and Waters, T., The "prescription to OTC switch" movement: its effects on antifungal vaginitis preparation, *Arch. Fam. Med.,* 8, 297–300, 1999.

7. Hathcock, J.N., Metabolic mechanisms of drug-nutrient interactions, *Fed. Proc.,* 44, 124–129, 1985.

8. Hathcock, J.N., Nutrient–drug interactions, *Clin. Geriatr. Med.,* 3, 297–307, 1987.

9. Kirk, J.K., Significant drug–nutrient interactions, *Am. Fam. Phys.,* 51, 1175–1182, 1995.

10. Knapp, H.R., Nutrient–drug interactions, in *Present Knowledge in Nutrition,* 7th ed., Ziegler, E.K. and Filer, J.R., Eds., ILSI Press, Washington, D.C., 1996, pp. 540–545.

11. Lamy, P.P., Effects of diet and nutrition on drug therapy, *J. Am. Geriatr. Soc.,* 30, S99–S112, 1982.

12. Roe, D.A., Food, formula, and drug effects on the disposition of nutrients, *World Rev. Nutr. Diet.,* 43, 80–94, 1984.

13. Roe, D.A., Interactions of drugs with food and nutrients, in *Nutritional Biochemistry and Metabolism with Clinical Applications,* 2nd ed., Linder, M.C., Ed., Elsevier, New York, 1991, pp. 559–571.

14. Walter-Sack, I. and Klotz, U., Influence of diet and nutritional status on drug metabolism, *Clin. Pharmacokinet.,* 31, 47–64, 1996.

15. Wood, J.H., Effect of food on aspirin absorption, *Lancet,* 2, 212, 1967.

16. Roe, D.R., Nutrients and drug interactions, *Nutr. Rev.,* 42, 141–154, 1994.

17. Royer, R.J. et al., Food and drug interactions, *World Rev. Nutr. Diet.,* 43, 117–128, 1984.

18. Volans, G.N., Effects of food and exercise on the absorption of effervescent aspirin, *Br. J. Clin. Pharmacol.,* 1, 137–141, 1974.

19. Melander, A., Influence of food and different nutrients on drug bioavailability, *World Rev. Nutr. Diet.,* 43, 34–44, 1984.

20. Pronsky, Z.M., *Food Medication Interactions,* 10th ed., Powers & Moore's Food–Medication Interactions, Pottstown, PA, 1997.

21. Trovato, A., Nuhlicek, D.N., and Midtling, J.E., Drug–nutrient interactions, *Am. Fam. Phys.,* 44, 1651–1658, 1991.

22. Yamreudeewong, W., et al., Drug–food interactions in clinical practice, *J. Fam. Pract.,* 40, 376–384, 1995.

23. Levein, T.L. and Baker, D.E., Cytochrome P_{450} drug interactions, *Pharm. Lett.,* 150–400, 1999.

24. Michalets, E.L., Clinically significant cytochrome P_{450} drug interactions, *Pharmacotherapy,* 18, 84–112, 1998.

25. Holman, S.H., *Essentials of Nutrition for the Health Professions,* J.B. Lippincott Co., Philadelphia, 1987, pp. 327–335.

26. Murray, J.J. and Healy, M., Drug-mineral interactions: a new responsibility for the hospital dietitian, *Perspec. Pract.,* 91, 66–73, 1991.

CHAPTER 13

Herbal and Dietary Supplement Interactions with Drugs

Bill J. Gurley and Dorothy W. Hagan

CONTENTS

As early as 1652, American colonists recognized the potential for fraud, safety risks, and adulteration of the food supply and passed laws to protect the public.[1] Prior to the establishment of the Food and Drug Administration (FDA) by the U.S. Congress in 1938, the U.S. Pharmacopeia (USP) played a strong role in regulating herbals. Standards were published as a result of The U.S. Pharmacopeial Convention, and, thus, the USP became the only quasigovernmental regulation of the purity of medicinal herbs. Compliance was seen by the designation of USP on the label of a product. The National Formulary (NF) was a second and similar publication. Products complying with the rules could be designated NF. As medical practice moved from herbal to chemical products, items were deleted from these compendiums.

In 1938, when congress passed the Food, Drug and Cosmetic Act (FDCA) and created the Food and Drug Administration (FDA), authority was mandated to reg-

ulate food and drugs. The FDCA defined both drugs and foods but left plant medicinals undefined. The ambiguity of herbal products led the FDA to generally categorize herbals as (1) generally recognized as safe (GRAS), (2) unsafe or ineffective,
or (3) lack of adequate information to determine safety and efficacy. The nutrition
labeling and education act of 1990 mandated labeling of dietary supplements and
defined health claims. Additional amendments and legislation modified the FDCA
and led to the Dietary Supplement Health and Education Act (DSHEA) of 1994. A
provision in DSHEA is now being acted on by the USP with the goal of generating
informational monographs and standards for manufacture. DSHEA legislation, however, ultimately created an environment for selling unregulated herbal and botanical
products in the U.S.

One problem consistently observed in evaluating plant medicines is the definition
of herbs and botanicals. The Herb Trade Association in 1976 defined herbs as "a
plant, plant part, or extract thereof used for flavor, fragrance, or medicinal purposes."[1]
In 1991, the World Health Organization (WHO) defined herbal medicines as follows:

> Finished, labeled medicinal products that contain as active ingredients aerial or
> underground parts of plants, or other plant material, or combinations thereof; whether
> in the crude state or as plant preparations. Plant material also includes juices, gums,
> fatty oils, essential oils, and any other substances of this nature. Herbal medicines
> may contain excipients in addition to the active ingredients. Medicines containing
> plant materials combined with chemically-defined active substances, including iso-
> lated constituents of plants, are not considered to be herbal medicines.[2]

The DSHEA provides a legal definition for dietary supplements as "dietary
substances for use by man to supplement the diet by increasing total dietary intake"
including "a concentrate, metabolite, constituent, extract, or combination" of these
ingredients. Dietary supplements include vitamins, minerals, herbs, or other botanicals and thus include the nutrition-science-based use of vitamins, minerals, protein,
carbohydrate, and fat products and the historical-based herbals and botanicals.

Herbals, botanicals, and dietary supplements fall somewhere between a food and
a drug. Dietary supplements are more expansive in definition and include vitamins,
minerals, amino acids or proteins, fats, and carbohydrate preparations. Herbals and
botanicals include concentrated forms such as extracts, powder forms, or combinations of herbs in formulated products. Separate and distinct from dietary supplements
are functional foods, which are also referred to in the literature as pharmafoods,
nutraceuticals, designer foods, phytochemicals, and chemopreventative agents.[3] Dietitians view carbohydrates, protein, fat, vitamins, and minerals as a part of food and,
thus, a source of essential nutrients. Pharmacists view derivatives of plants and often
even essential nutrients as drugs.

Following the implementation of DSHEA in 1994, the scientific/medical community has undertaken identification of those supplements that constitute an interaction risk. Prospective investigations into the pharmacological mechanism(s) underlying herb–drug interactions have been delayed and confounded by a variety of
factors. Among these are the rapid influx of products into the marketplace that exhibit
unique and complex phytochemical compositions; consumer willingness to self-

medicate with dietary supplements; lack of premarket safety and efficacy testing; and problems associated with product quality. In general, the types of interactions that have been identified appear to be pharmacokinetic and/or pharmacodynamic in character.

Pharmacokinetic herb–drug interactions can stem from phytochemical-mediated alterations in the activity of xenobiotic metabolizing enzymes (human cytochrome P_{450} alleles [CYPs], transferases) or transport proteins (e.g., P-glycoproteins [P-gp], human organic cation transport proteins [OCTP], human organic anion transporting polypeptides [OATP]). Together, these proteins are principal determinants in the absorption, distribution, and elimination of many chemicals including drugs. CYPs present in the liver and small intestine are involved in the oxidative metabolism of drugs and other xenobiotics. In the gut and liver P-gp functions as an efflux pump, actively transporting substances back into the intestinal lumen or into the bile canaliculi. Other transport proteins/polypeptides facilitate the uptake of organic anions or cations across cell membranes of various organs. Thus, botanical dietary supplements that modulate drug metabolizing enzyme activity and/or transporter function can adversely affect the bioavailability or clearance for drugs that are substrates for the affected proteins. The end result may be either diminished drug efficacy or enhanced toxicity.

Pharmacodynamic interactions, on the other hand, appear to result from phytochemicals whose pharmacological action either diminishes or exacerbates the effects of conventional medications by mechanisms unrelated to altered metabolism or transport.

The concept that botanical supplements could interact with conventional medications is understandable given that food–drug interactions have been recognized for a variety of fruits and vegetables that constitute part of the normal human diet.[4,5] Many food–drug interactions have phytochemical-mediated pharmacokinetic components. For example, furanocoumarins present in grapefruit juice inhibit intestinal CYP3A4 and have been shown to increase the oral bioavailability of medications that are CYP3A4 substrates (e.g., felodipine, midazolam, cyclosporine).[4,5] Furanocoumarins and bioflavonoids present in fruit juices are also inhibitors of intestinal OATP and, when ingested concomitantly, can reduce the oral bioavailability of the OATP substrate, fexofenadine.[6] Similarly, cruciferous vegetables (e.g., broccoli, cabbage, watercress) contain appreciable amounts of glucosinolates that appear capable of inhibiting CYP1A2 and CYP2E1[7,8] while inducing various phase II enzymes.[7]

The previous examples are merely a sampling of the wide variety of plant-derived chemicals that have been identified as potential modulators of mammalian enzyme and transport systems. One major class in particular, polyphenols (e.g., anthocyanins, coumarins, flavonoids, lignans, tannins), are not only ubiquitous in herbs, vegetables, fruits, flowers, and leaves of many plants, but, when consumed in large amounts, can be potent inhibitors[8–11] or inducers[10,12–13] of CYP enzymes and transport proteins.[14,15] Several excellent reviews detailing the effects of one major subclass of polyphenols, the bioflavonoids, on CYP and P-gp activity further support this premise.[4,10,16] Thus, botanical dietary supplements are not only likely candidates for phytochemical-mediated drug interactions, but, when formulated as concentrated plant extracts and intended for prolonged use, they pose an even greater risk for interacting with conventional medications.

The following discussion focuses on several dietary supplements known or suspected of interacting with conventional medications and their purported mechanism(s). Each example illustrates some aspect of the complex nature of botanical supplement/drug interactions and the variables, known and unknown, that must be considered when evaluating the likelihood of such interactions.

ST. JOHN'S WORT (*HYPERICUM PERFORATUM*)

Extracts of *H. perforatum* have been touted for their antidepressant activity, although the efficacy of many St. John's Wort products remains questionable.[17] Nevertheless, some small clinical trials have demonstrated efficacy comparable to tricyclic antidepressants and the selective serotonin reuptake inhibitors (SSRIs), but with a more favorable short-term safety profile than conventional antidepressive agents.[18–20] When used as a single agent, a favorable risk/benefit ratio has made St. John's Wort one of the most readily consumed dietary supplements in the world.[18] In turn, the popularity of St. John's Wort has also contributed to its distinction as being one of the most problematic dietary supplements with regard to herb–drug interactions.

The preponderance of evidence from case reports and prospective studies clearly indicates that St. John's Wort reduces the efficacy of conventional medications that are CYP3A4 and/or P-gp substrates (e.g., cyclosporine, digoxin, indinavir, simvastatin, oral contraceptives).[21–24] Phenotype assessment studies employing the CYP3A4 probe, midazolam, and the 14C-erythromycin breath test confirm that St. John's Wort extracts induce both intestinal and hepatic CYP3A4 activity.[25–28] Further verification comes from Western blot analysis of human duodenal biopsy samples that reveal increased CYP3A4 expression following sustained supplementation with St. John's Wort.[26] Phenotypic trait assessments using digoxin and fexofenadine also indicate that prolonged *Hypericum* administration induces P-gp and possibly OATP function.[26–29] Western blot analysis of human intestinal biopsies[26] and flow cytometry/reverse transcriptase polymerase chain reaction studies on human peripheral blood lymphocytes[30] verify that P-gp expression increases severalfold in subjects treated with St. John's Wort.

St. John's Wort contains numerous phytochemicals including naphthodianthrones (e.g., hypericin, pseudohypericin), flavonoids (e.g., hyperoside, quercetin, I3,II8-biapigenin, rutin), and tannins, but CYP3A4 induction appears to be mediated by a prenylated phloroglucinol, hyperforin. Hyperforin is a high-affinity ligand for the human steroid X receptor (SXR), an orphan nuclear receptor selectively expressed in the liver and intestine that mediates the induction of CYP3A4 gene transcription.[12,31] (SXR and receptor-mediated transcriptional activation of the CYP3A4 gene have been the subject of recent reviews.[32–34]) According to one estimate, hyperforin is the most potent SXR activator discovered to date,[12] with a half-maximal effective concentration (EC50) of 23 nM—a value well below plasma concentrations often achieved in humans (~100–300 nM). Moreover, SXR acts as a xenobiotic-responsive transcription factor not only for CYP3A genes but also for multiple drug resistance

1 gene (MDR1), the gene encoding P-glycoprotein.[35,36] Thus, hyperforin, is the likely causative agent for *Hypericum*-mediated P-gp induction.

Some evidence suggests that gender may be a contributing factor to CYP3A4 induction by St. John's Wort. Gurley et al. observed that 28 d of St. John's Wort supplementation produced a significantly greater increase in CYP3A4 activity among female participants that was unrelated to body mass index, weight-adjusted hyperforin dose, or plasma hyperforin concentrations.[28] The precise reason for this apparent sexual dimorphism is unclear; however, previous studies hint at an elevated basal expression of CYP3A4 in female subjects.[37,38] This finding raises the question as to whether women are more susceptible to interactions involving St. John's Wort. The significance of this observation is heightened by studies showing that St. John's Wort increases the clearance of the oral contraceptive, norethindrone, and produces breakthrough bleeding after prolonged use.[24,39] Moreover, women represent the largest demographic with regard to dietary supplement use, including St. John's Wort.[40,41]

Duration of use and hyperforin content appear to dictate the degree of CYP3A/P-gp induction. Administration of St. John's Wort for less than 7 days appears to have little effect on the pharmacokinetics of CYP3A4 or P-gp substrates,[42–44] while supplementation periods of longer duration significantly reduce oral bioavailability, area under the curve (AUC), maximum plasma concentration (C_{max}), and average steady state concentration (C_{ss}) values.[23–29] This probably reflects the time dependency of receptor-mediated CYP3A/P-gp induction. Owing to hyperforin's oral bioavailability and moderate elimination half-life (~9 h), the typical recommended dose of St. John's Wort (300 mg, three times daily) is adequate for achieving steady-state hyperforin concentrations in human plasma.[45] Exposure to the substance, however, is often product dependent. Considerable variability in hyperforin content exists between brands and among individual lots of St. John's Wort supplements.[46–48] This is due, in part, to the chemical instability of hyperforin,[49] but more so because products are often standardized to contain a consistent quantity of hypericin (0.3%), a compound not capable of inducing CYP3A or P-gp.[12] As a result, product label claims for hypericin content are not indicative of hyperforin—a condition that may render some brands more prone to interactions than others. Most studies evaluating St. John's Wort's effect on CYP enzymes provide no data regarding hyperforin content or plasma hyperforin concentrations. A lack of effect stemming from an absence of hyperforin could partially explain the noninteraction noted for St. John's Wort and the CYP3A4 substrate, carbamazepine.[50]

Induction of other CYP isoforms by St. John's Wort appears to be selective. Studies using probe drug cocktails to assess multiple CYP phenotypes suggest that St. John's Wort is capable of inducing both human and murine CYP2E1[28,44] but has little effect on CYP1A2, CYP2D6, and CYP2C9 activity.[25,28,43,51] Currently, it is unclear whether CYP2E1 induction by St. John's Wort occurs at the transcriptional or posttranscriptional level or even whether the effect is attributable to hyperforin. CYP2E1 plays an important role in the metabolic activation of a variety of drugs, chemical carcinogens, and other toxicants.[52] Thus, it is conceivable that long-term usage of St. John's Wort may predispose some consumers to drug toxicity or certain cancers. To date, few interactions involving St. John's Wort and CYP2E1 substrates have been reported. This lack of interaction probably stems from the paucity of orally administered drugs that are CYP2E1 substrates; nevertheless, several inhaled anesthetics (e.g., enflurane, isoflurane, methoxyflurane) are metabolized by CYP2E1, and a potential interaction may exist for these agents.

Given that more than 70% of all conventional medications are substrates for CYP3A4, CYP2E1, and P-gp, the potential for pharmacokinetic drug interactions is enormous. The end result is a reduced therapeutic effect, the severity of which is exemplified by acute organ rejection in transplant recipients maintained on cyclosporine who self-medicate with St. John's Wort.[53–54] Cancer patients may be another special population vulnerable to interactions with St. John's Wort. Botanical supplement use is prevalent among cancer patients,[55–56] and recently an interaction with St. John's Wort and the camptothecin analog, irinotecan, was reported.[57] In a randomized, crossover study involving cancer patients, administration of a St. John's Wort product for 21 days reduced irinotecan active metabolite concentrations by 50% following intravenous infusion of the parent drug. Because irinotecan and its active metabolite are P-gp substrates that undergo biliary secretion,[58] the interaction probably stems from induced P-gp expression within the hepatobiliary tree. Consideration must also be given to stimulated P-gp expression in tumors. Development of drug resistance in many cancers is attributable to P-gp and other multidrug resistance proteins that act as efflux pumps for chemotherapeutic agents.[59] Thus, it is conceivable that prolonged supplementation with St. John's Wort may not only reduce the effectiveness of cancer chemotherapy but also promote active drug resistance in tumors.

Unlike hyperforin, other *H. perforatum* constitutents are not potent ligands of SXR[12,31] and probably do not figure heavily into interactions linked to CYP3A or P-gp induction. *In vitro* binding assays do suggest that hypericin and I3,II8-biapigenin are inhibitors of human CYP3A4, CYP1A2, CYP2C9, and CYP2D6.[60,61] Hypericin is orally bioavailable and exhibits an elimination half-life of approximately 40 h following multiple dosing of *Hypericum* extracts.[62] Hypericin steadystate plasma concentrations (~17 nM), however, are approximately two orders of magnitude below the IC50 values determined for human CYPs, making it an unlikely participant in CYP-mediated drug interactions. Although I3,II8-biapigenin is a potent inhibitor of human CYP3A4 *in vitro* (~80 nM),[60] too little is known about its absorption, distribution, metabolism, and excretion to render any conclusions about an interaction potential. This paucity of knowledge regarding phytochemical disposition in humans also holds true for many of the other components in *H. perforatum* extracts. An inhibitory effect on human CYP liver microsomes was also demonstrated for methanolic fractions of St. John's Wort extracts, but no specific ligands were identified.[63]

Interactions between St. John's Wort and selective neurotransmitter reuptake inhibitors (e.g., paroxetine, sertraline, nefazodone) that cause symptoms of central serotonin excess may be characterized as pharmacodynamic.[39] Again, hyperforin and another phlorglucinol derivative, adhyperforin, appear to mediate this effect through a novel monoamine reuptake inhibition mechanism.[64–67] Additive effects from other components (e.g., hypericin, biapigenin) exhibiting high binding affinities for various enzymes (e.g., dopamine-β-hydroxylase) and receptors (benzodiazepine, GABA, sigma) in the brain may also figure into these interactions.[67,68]

GARLIC (*ALLIUM SATIVUM*)

The putative antihypercholesterolemic effect of garlic supplements makes them one of the most widely used botanical supplements in the U.S. Their efficacy, however, remains equivocal due to conflicting results from numerous published clinical trials.[69] This is probably a function of the type of product used, its quality, and poor characterization of the phytochemical agent(s) responsible for garlic's serum lipid lowering effect.

Three general categories of garlic supplements are available commercially (garlic oil, dehydrated garlic powder, and aged garlic extract), each with their own unique composition of purported bioactive components.[70,71] Within these products, a plethora of organosulfur compounds, steroid saponins, and other phytochemicals have been identified.[70–72] Of these, the oil-soluble organosulfur compounds, including allyl thiosulfinates (allicin), alkyl sulfides (diallyl sulfide), vinyldithiins, and ajoene, have received the most attention. Allicin has long been touted as the agent responsible for garlic's hypocholesterolemic effects, yet the compound is unstable in the gastrointestinal tract, is not bioavailable, and is rarely found in commercial products.[70,71] Its degradation products, diallyl sulfide, diallyl disulfide, diallyl trisulfide, dithiin, and ajoene, may contribute to the lowering of serum cholesterol levels; however, many products, particularly those containing garlic oil, have relatively poor efficacy.[73,74] In addition, many *in vivo* studies indicate that garlic oil and individual alkyl sulfides, most notably diallyl sulfide, inhibit murine and human CYP2E1.[7,28,75–78] This is likely a result of the CYP2E1-catalyzed biotransformation of diallyl sulfide to diallyl sulfoxide and diallyl sulfone, in which the latter is a mechanism-based inhibitor of the enzyme.[77] Despite inhibition of human CYP2E1, few interactions involving garlic products and CYP2E1 substrates have been reported, a consequence that probably reflects the paucity of drugs metabolized by this enzyme. Conversely, prolonged administration of diallyl sulfide and diallyl disulfide induced other hepatic and intestinal murine CYP subfamilies (CYP2B, CYP1A, CYP3A), in addition to various transferases (glutathione transferase, uridine 5′-diphosphate (UDP)-glucuronyl transferase).[7,75,76]

Aged garlic extracts, on the other hand, do not appear to inhibit human CYP2E1 as evidenced by lack of an effect on acetaminophen metabolism in healthy volunteers.[79] This may stem from a dearth of oil-soluble organosulfur compounds in aged garlic extracts and a preponderance of water-soluble components (e.g., S-allyl cysteine, saponins).[71] The shift from oil- to water-soluble ingredients arises from the aging process, which makes aged garlic extracts distinct from the other types of garlic products. To date, however, little data are available on the effect aged garlic extracts may have on other CYP enzymes or drug transporters. Only one *in vitro* assessment of an aged garlic extract on human CYP and P-gp activity has been reported.[80] Modest inhibitory effects on CYP2C9, 2C19, 3A4, and P-gp were observed, while CYP2D6 was unaffected.[80] In this study, similar effects were also noted for odorless garlic powder products, garlic oil products, and a freeze-dried garlic supplement indicating that both oil- and water-soluble components have the potential to inhibit drug metabolism and transport.

Only a few prospective human *in vivo* studies have investigated the interaction potential of garlic supplements, and, owing to the variety of products evaluated, the results have been mixed.[28,78,81–82] Prolonged garlic oil supplementation (500 mg, three times daily for 28 d) inhibited human CYP2E1 activity by almost 40%; however, no modulatory effects were noted for CYP1A2, CYP2D6, or CYP3A4.[28] Four weeks of supplementation with aged garlic extract (10 mL daily) had little impact on acetaminophen pharmacokinetics.[79] In contrast, 21 d of twice daily supplementation with garlic powder reduced by 50% the mean area under the curve (AUC), 8-h trough concentrations, and mean maximum concentrations (C_{max}) of the protease inhibitor, saquinavir.[81] The authors concluded that the garlic powder supplement might have induced intestinal CYP3A4 and/or P-gp because saquinavir is a substrate for both proteins. A similar, although less dramatic, effect on ritonavir AUC was observed after a 4-d course of garlic extract (5 mg, twice daily).[82] These four examples appear to corroborate earlier studies in murine systems where specific alkyl sulfides were capable of selectively inducing certain CYPs while inhibiting, or possibly down-regulating, CYP2E1.[75,76] Although much emphasis has been placed on the organosulfur constituents of garlic, identification of the specific component(s) responsible for CYP induction in humans remains to be determined.

Taken together, these disparate findings imply that garlic–drug interactions are product specific and may reflect differences in the type, quantity, and bioavailability of garlic phytochemicals, as well as duration of use. Because garlic supplement dosage forms can exhibit significant differences in phytochemical content and dissolution rate,[67,68,80,83] the occurrence and severity of CYP/P-gp-mediated garlic–drug interactions is difficult to predict.

Purported interactions involving garlic and warfarin probably do not involve a pharmacokinetic mechanism because warfarin is not a CYP2E1 substrate and, to date, this enzyme appears to be the only human isoform inhibited by garlic *in vivo.*[28] Such interactions may be characterized as pharmacodynamic because *in vitro* evidence suggests that garlic products can also affect blood coagulability.[84,85] The organosulfur compounds ajoene,[86,87] alkyl sulfides,[85] and thiosulfinates[88] have been shown to inhibit platelet aggregation, while certain steroid saponins in garlic promote fribrinolysis.[72] Not unexpectedly, variability in phytochemical content, dose, and duration of use will also factor into the potential for garlic supplements to elicit pharmacodynamic drug interactions.

GINKGO BILOBA

Case reports documenting possible interactions between Ginkgo biloba and anticoagulants appear to be attributable to inhibition of platelet activating factor by various ginkgolides.[89,90] Based on recent studies using probe drug cocktails to assess CYP phenotype, a pharmacokinetic basis for these interactions appears to be less plausible. Clinically insignificant changes in CYP1A2, CYP2C19, CYP2D6, CYP2E1, and CYP3A4 phenotypes were noted after prolonged oral administration (12 or 28 d) of Ginkgo biloba supplements to healthy human volunteers.[28,91] These findings corroborate earlier studies using antipyrine, a nonspecific probe of hepatic microsomal drug oxidation.[92] Comparisons of *in vitro*[61,93] vs. *in vivo*[94–96] data also indicate that oral administration of Ginkgo biloba yields plasma concentrations of ginkgolides, bilobalides, and other phytohemicals that are several orders of magnitude below that necessary for marked inhibition of human CYP isoforms.

Conversely, a 12-day course of Ginkgo biloba in healthy volunteers inhibited N-acetyltransferase by 43%,[91] while prolonged administration of a different brand increased mean plasma nifedipine (CYP3A4 substrate) concentrations 53%, suggestive of CYP3A4 inhibition.[97] Disparity among Ginkgo biloba products with regard to phytochemical composition, dissolution rate, and bioavailability could explain some of the inconsistencies among studies.[98–99]

PANAX GINSENG

Like Ginkgo biloba, Panax ginseng appears to have little effect on CYP-mediated drug metabolism and is probably less prone to cause pharmacokinetic interactions. Ginsenosides and other saponins found in various ginseng species are absorbed following oral administration,[100] yet the attainment of serum concentrations capable of modulating CYP activity *in vivo* appears unlikely. This was evident for several ginsenosides where the IC50 concentrations for recombinant human CYP isoforms were several orders of magnitude higher than that for ketoconazole, a potent inhibitor of CYP3A.[101] Further support comes from studies examining Panax ginseng supplementation on human CYP probe drug phenotypes that found the herb to have little or no modulatory effect on CYP1A2, CYP2C9, CYP2D6, CYP2E1, or CYP3A4 *in vivo*.[28,93,102] Additional evidence can be found in animal studies that cite no effect of ginseng on warfarin pharmacokinetics.[103]

In contrast, long-term ginseng supplementation was shown to produce modest increases in nifedipine plasma concentrations, implying an inhibitory effect on CYP3A4.[97] Panax ginseng has also been shown to enhance blood alcohol clearance in healthy volunteers,[104] an effect possibly attributed to induction of alcohol dehydrogenase.[105] Again, substantial variability in ginsenoside content has been reported among commercial ginseng preparations, indicating that clinically significant effects on CYP and other drug metabolizing enzymes could be brand specific.[106] Still other factors that may impinge on the variability of ginseng supplements and their drug interaction potential include differences in processing methods[107] and metabolism by human intestinal bacteria.[108]

MILK THISTLE (*SILYBUM MARIANUM*)

The popularity of milk thistle is due to the purported hepatoprotectant properties of silymarin, a mixture of flavanolignans (e.g., silibinin A, silibinin B, silichristin, silidianin, taxifolin) extracted from the seeds of *Silybum marianum*. Indicated for the treatment and prevention of various liver diseases, silymarin has a good safety profile, but its mechanism of action is unclear.[109] Another uncertainty is the drug interaction potential of silymarin. Two groups using *in vitro* models have recently documented inhibitory effects of either milk thistle extract or silibinin on human drug metabolizing enzymes.[110,111] Of the enzymes investigated, only CYP3A4, CYP2C9, and uridine diphosphoglucuronsyl transferase were inhibited at concentrations similar to those observed *in vivo*. Reports detailing the pharmacokinetics of silibinin in humans have yielded varied results.[109,112] Oral administration of silymarin extract in doses from 120 to 360 mg produced serum concentrations of silibinin and its glucuronide and sulfate conjugates in the range of 100 to 1400 ng/mL, while bile concentrations reached 100 times those of serum, indicating extensive biliary secretion.[109] Thus, when administered orally, concentrations of silymarin components may be sufficiently high to compete for CYP binding sites in the liver and gut wall.

In vivo evidence for CYP-mediated milk thistle interactions, however, is less compelling. Administration of silymarin (Legalon, 70 mg, three times daily) for 28 days to healthy volunteers had no effect on the pharmacokinetics of aminopyrine or phenylbutazone.[113] Following 21 days of milk thistle extract administration (153 mg silymarin, three times daily) no clinically significant changes in the pharmacokinetics of indinavir (partial CYP3A4 substrate) were noted in human subjects.[114] Similarly, 28 days of milk thistle extract supplementation to human volunteers (110 mg silymarin, twice daily) reduced midazolam clearance (CYP3A4 substrate) an average of only 13%.[115] This seeming lack of *in vitro/in vivo* correlation may stem from poor bioavailability, large interindividual variations in silibinin absorption, lower CYP binding affinities of silibinin conjugates, poor dissolution characteristics of milk thistle dosage forms, or interproduct variability in silymarin content.[109,116]

Interestingly, enhanced activity of phase II enzymes (e.g., glutathione S-transferase, quinone reductase) has been noted in mice following prolonged administration of large silibinin doses.[117] Whether similar effects occur in humans, however, remains to be determined.

LICORICE (*GLYCYRRHIZA GLABRA*)

Licorice extract is a common ingredient in many multicomponent dietary supplements. When ingested, the sweet tasting glycoside found in licorice, glycyrrhizin, is hydrolyzed by bacterial β-glucuronidases in the intestine to yield the aglycone, glycyrrhetic acid.[118] As a potent inhibitor of 11 β hydroxysteroid dehydrogenase, glycyrrhetic acid increases access of cortisol to the mineralocorticoid receptor causing sodium retention and potassium depletion.[118,119] Accordingly, chronic ingestion of licorice extract may interfere with various medications, including antihypertensives and antiarrhythmic agents. Unlike many other phytochemicals, the pharmacokinetics of glycyrrhetic acid is well characterized.[120] Its absorption is slow and formulation dependent. Circulating plasma concentrations of glycyrrhetic acid can range from 100 to 2000 nM—levels capable of inhibiting 11-β-hydroxysteroid dehydrogenase.[118] In the liver, glycyrrhetic acid is conjugated and eliminated via biliary secretion, and subject to enterohepatic cycling[120]; therefore, liver dysfunction may exacerbate the onset and severity of mineralocorticoid side effects. Few prospective studies have examined licorice's effect on drug pharmacokinetics. In one such study, inhibition of 11-β-hydroxysteroid dehydrogenase was the suspected cause of decreased prednisolone clearance among healthy volunteers.[121] As with many dietary supplements, there is large intersubject variability with regard to glycyrrhetic acid absorption, elimination, toxicity, and interaction potential, much of which is likely related to product quality and pattern of usage.[118,122,123]

EPHEDRA (MA HUANG)

Ephedra, also known by its Chinese name, ma hung, is a natural source of ephedrine alkaloids (e.g., ephedrine, pseudophedrine, and methylphedrine) and is a common component of dietary supplements marketed as weight loss aids, energy boosters, and exercise performance enchancers. Ephedra-containing dietary supplements are rarely formulated as single ingredient products. Along with ephedrine alkaloids most ephedra-containing products also contain natural sources of caffeine (e.g., guarana, kola nut, green tea), additional stimulants (synephrine), and a host of other botanicals and amino acids.[124] The pharmacokinetics of ephedrine following ingestion of supplements formulated as concentrated ephedra extracts is indistinguishable from that of synthetic ephedrine found in conventional dosage forms.[125,126] Thus, ephedrine and other sympathomimetic amines create a risk of interaction with conventional stimulants, hypoglycemic agents, antihypertensives, and monamine oxidase inhibitors, yet ephedra-containing supplements also pose a serious health hazard in their own right, due in part to interactions among the individual phytochemical components.

From a pharmacodynamic standpoint, ephedrine and caffeine potentiate each other's cardiovascular and central nervous system stimulant effects, thereby increasing the risk of adverse events in susceptible individuals.[124] Because of this enhanced health risk, the FDA has not allowed ephedrine/caffeine combinations in conventional OTC products since 1983.[124] Other phytochemical components in ephedra-containing dietary supplements appear to exacerbate ephedrine/caffeine pharmacodynamics. Catechins, a class of polyphenolic compounds found in high concentrations in guarana and green tea, enhance the sympathetic activity of ephedrine and caffeine by inhibiting catechol-O-methyltransferase.[127] Catechins are also readily absorbed into the systemic circulation and elicit their own inotropic effect on the heart.[128,129] Another common ingredient, *Citrus aurantium* (bitter orange) extract, provides an additional source of sympathomimetics (synephrine, octopamine) and has been shown to be arrythmogenic in laboratory animals.[124,130] Recently, it was shown that multicomponent ephedra-containing dietary supplements containing caffeine, catechins, and *Citrus aurantium* are more toxic in animal models than ephedra alone.[131] Taken together, these findings lend credence to adverse events reported in the medical literature and those submitted to the FDA's MEDWATCH program.[131–133]

DISCONNECT BETWEEN *IN VITRO* AND *IN VIVO* FINDINGS

From the preceding discussion, it is apparent that the ability to predict herb–drug interactions in humans is often impaired by discrepancies between *in vitro* and *in vivo* findings. This disconnect is best exemplified by St. John's Wort and milk thistle. *In vitro* results indicated that St. John's Wort inhibited various human CYP enzymes, but *in vivo* studies showed it to be a potent inducer of CYP3A4 and CYP2E1. Only after nuclear receptor binding studies were performed was it recognized that hyperforin was a potent ligand for SXR. Similarly, it was demonstrated that milk thistle inhibited CYP3A4 activity *in vitro*, yet *in vivo* studies have failed to corroborate this finding. On the other hand, *in vitro/in vivo* data appear to correlate well for supplements like garlic, ginseng, and *Ginkgo biloba,* at least with regard to CYP inhibition. In short, herb–drug interactions are often difficult to predict.

Reasons for this disconnect are varied, but much of the blame lies with DSHEA. The act exempts manufacturers of botanical dietary supplements from premarket safety and efficacy testing required of the conventional pharmaceutical industry. Accordingly, *a priori* investigations into potential herb–drug interactions are not compulsory for dietary supplement manufacturers. This is troublesome because, unlike conventional drug products, botanical supplements are complex mixtures of diverse phytochemicals where the individual, let alone collective, pharmacological activity is often unknown. Little is also known about the pharmacokinetics of individual phytochemicals—an inadequacy that can affect the utility of *in vitro* data as a predictor of outcomes *in vivo.*

Often formulated as concentrated extracts, botanical supplements can exhibit significant interproduct and intraproduct variability with regard to content, dissolution, and bioavailability, each of which can affect the extrapolative value of *in vivo* studies to separate brands. In other words, different brands may have different prospectives for interaction. Variability in manufacturer recommended dose and duration of use are also factors for consideration, not to mention the ingestion of multiple supplements. One final issue is contamination of botanical supplements with conventional medications.[134] Although not widespread, adulteration of botanical supplements with undeclared pharmaceutical agents does occur and should be taken into account when evaluating herb–drug interactions. In summary, the potential for clinically significant interactions between herbs and drugs varies for a multitude of reasons.

CULINARY HERBS AND MINERAL SUPPLEMENTS

In general, culinary herbs used to flavor foods are not likely to induce a clinically significant reaction because of the small quantity used in a dish or in a serving. Table 13.1 presents a list of culinary herbs for which a potential exists for interactions.[135] On the other hand, when herbs are dried, ground, or otherwise concentrated and then made into a beverage, the potential for interactions with drugs increases. For example, the yeast extract, Marmite®, has been reported to cause a tyramine-induced hypertensive reaction when made into a beverage but has not been reported when used as a toast spread. The source of a dietary supplement can also make a difference. For example, Marmite® is derived from residual brewer's yeast following fermentation of beer or ale. Brewer's yeast grown specifically for a dry dietary supplement has not been found to contain any tyramine. See Appendix D for the differences in tyramine content of the two different types of brewer's yeast.

Table 13.1 Culinary Herbs That May Interact with Drugs[135]

Culinary Herb	Active Substance(s)	Potential Drug Interaction
Anise[137] (*Pimpinella anisum*)	Volatile oil Caffeic acid derivatives Flavonoids Fatty oil Proteins	Potential estrogen-like effect
Balm, Lemon[136–137] (*Melissa officinalis*)	Volatile oils Glycosides Caffeic acid derivatives Flavonoids Triterpene acids	Inhibits certain thyroid hormones
Brewer's yeast[136] (*Saccharomyces cerevisiae*)	B vitamins Polysaccharides Proteins Amines Sterols	Monoamine oxidase inhibitors may interact and result in an increase in blood pressure
Cocoa[136–138] (*Theobroma cacao*)	Purine alkaloids—theobromine and caffeine Fat Proteins Catechin tannins—tyramines Proanthocyanidins oxaluric acid	Monoamine oxidase inhibitors may interact and result in an increase in blood pressure May interact with oral contraceptives and quinolone antibiotics, thus increasing stimulating effect of herb
Coffee[136,138] (*Coffea Arabica*)	Purine alkaloids—caffeine, theobromine, and theophyllin Trigonelliline Carbonization products of hemicelluloses Caffeic and ferulic acid ester of quinic acid Norditerpene glycoside ester	May decrease resorption of some drugs May interact with oral contraceptives and quinolone antibiotics thus increasing stimulating effect of herb
Cola[136–140] (*Cola acuminata*)	Purine alkaloids—caffeine Catechin tannins Oligomeric proanthocyanidins Starch	May increase the effect of psychoanaleptic drugs Enhances effect of aspirin

Table 13.1 Culinary Herbs That May Interact with Drugs[135] (Continued)

Culinary Herb	Active Substance(s)	Potential Drug Interaction
Cranberry[137] (*Vaccinium macrocarpon*)	Anthocyanin Catechin Triterpenoids Carbohydrates	May interact with medications that affect the kidney or urinary tract
Fennel[136–137] (*Foeniculum vulgare*)	Volatile oil—transanethole, fenchon, and estragole Hydroxycoumrins Pyranocoumarins Flavonoids Fatty oil	May potentiate the effect of hormone replacement therapy
Fenugreek[136–138] (*Trigonella foenum-graecum*)	Mucilages Proteins Protease inhibitors Steroid saponins Steroid saponin-peptide ester Flavonoids Volatile oil	May interact with monoamine oxidase inhibitors, diabetes, heart, hormone, and blood thinning medications
Flaxseed[136–137] (*Linum Usitatissimum*)	Mucilages Cyanogenic glycosides Essential fatty acids Proteins Ballast Lignans Phenylpropane derivatives	Effects absorption of other drugs
Garlic[136–138] (*Allium sativum*)	Alliins Fructosans (polysaccharides) Saponins	May interfere with blood sugar lowering medications May interfere with anticoagulants—warfarin and aspirin
Ginger[136–138] (*Zingiber officinale*)	Volatile oil Arylalkane Gingerols Shogaols Gingerdiols Diarylheptanoids	May interfere with anticoagulant, diabetes, and heart medications

Herb	Constituents	Interactions
Guarana [137–138] (*Paullinia cupana*)	Purine alkaloids—caffeine Tannins Cyanolipides Saponins Starch Proteins	May potentiate the effect of other caffeine herbs and beverages May interact with clozapine, benzodiazepines, beta blockers, lithium, monoamine oxidase inhibitors, phenylpropanolamine, some quinolone antibiotics, oral contraceptives, cimetidine, furafylline, verapamil, disulfiram, fluconazole, mexiletine, and phenytoin
Guar Gum [139] (*Cyamopsis tetragonolobus*)	Fiber	Decreases absorption of penicillin V and digoxin
Hops [136–138] (*Humulus lupulus*)	Acylphloroglucinols Beta-bitter acids Volatile oil Resins Phenolic acid Tannins Flavonoids	May enhance effects of sedatives and estrogenic hormones
Horehound [136–137] (*Ballota nigra*)	Diterpenes, marrubiin Volatile oil Caffeic and ferulic acid derivatives Tannin	May interfere with heart rhythms and heart medications
Horseradish [136–137] (*Armoracia rusticana*)	Allylisothiocyanate Butylthiocyanate Mustard oil Mustard oil glycosides	May interfere with hypothyroid medications, such as thyroxine
Kombucha1 [137] Manchurian Mushroom	Sugar Alcohol Gluconic acid Lactic acid Yeasts	May interfere with immunosuppressants
Licorice [136–139] (*Glycyrrhiza glabra*)	Triterpene saponins Flavonoids Isoflavonoids Cumestan derivatives Sterols Volatile oil	Interacts with thiazide diuretics Potentiates the use of digitalis glycosides Alters metabolism of cortisol May interfere with hormone medications

Table 13.1 Culinary Herbs That May Interact with Drugs[135] (*Continued*)

Culinary Herb	Active Substance(s)	Potential Drug Interaction
Lovage[136–137] (*Levisticum officinale*)	Volatile oil Hydroxycoumarins Coumarin Furocoumarins Polyynes	May interact with diuretic therapy and sedatives
Marshmallow[136–137] (*Althaea officinalis*)	Mucilage Pectins Starch	May interfere with blood sugar lowering medications May delay absorption of other drugs
Mate[136,138,2,3] (Ilex paraguariensis)	Purine alkaloids—caffeine and theobromine Caffeic acid derivatives Flavonoids Triterpene saponins Nitrile glycosides	May potentiate the effect of other caffeine herbs and beverages May interfere with clozapine, benzodiazepines, beta blockers, lithium, and monoamine oxidase inhibitors
Nutmeg[136–138] (*Myristica fragrans*)	Volatile oil—myristicin Fatty oil Saponins Sterols	May potentiate psychiatric drugs
Olive oil[1,136] (*Olea europaea*)	Iridoide monoterpenes Triterpenes Flavonoids Essential fatty acids	May influence blood sugar lowering medications and interact with anticoagulant therapy
Oregano[136–137] (*Origanum vulgare*)	Volatile oil Flavonoids Caffeic acid derivatives	May interfere with fertility drugs
Papaya[136–137] (*Carica papaya*)	Proteolytic enzymes (papain) and other enzymes Lipases Polyketide alkaloids Glucosinolates Cyanogenic glycosides Saponins Proteolytic ferments (ficin)	Increases effect of anticoagulants—warfarin

Herb	Constituents	Interaction
Psyllium[136-139] (Plantago afra, plantago isphagula)	Mucilages Iridoide monoterpenes Fatty oil	Delays absorption of drugs
Red pepper[137] (Capsicum annum, Capsicum frutescens)	Capsaicinoids—capacin Vitamin C	May increase liver metabolism of other medications May interfere with high blood pressure medications and monoamine oxidase inhibitors
Rhubarb[137] (Rheum Palmatum)	Anthracene derivatives Tannins Flavonoids Naphthohydroquinone glycosides	Increased effect of cardiac glycosides due to potassium loss
Sage[137] (Salvia officinalis)	Volatile oil—thujone caffeic acid derivatives Diterpenes Flavonoids Triterpenes Tannins	May interact with estrogenic medications
Shitake[137] mushrooms (Lentinula edodes)	Vitamins Carbohydrates Proteins Lentinan	May enhance action of AZT (zidovudine)
Tea[136-137] (Camellia sinensis)	Purine alkaloids—caffeine, theobromine, and theophylline Triterpene saponins Catechins Caffeic acid derivatives Anorganic ions Volatile oil Tannins	May inhibit thiamin use May potentiate the effect of other caffeine herbs and beverages May interact with clozapine, benzodiazepines, beta blockers, lithium, monoamine oxidase inhibitors, phenylpropanolamine, some quinolone antibiotics, oral contraceptives, cimetidine, furafylline, verapamil, disulfiram, fluconazole, mexiletine, and phenytoin
Thyme[136-137] (Thymus vulgaris)	Volatile oils—thymol and carvacrol Caffeic acid derivatives Flavonoids Triterpenes	May interfere with thyroid medications

Table 13.1 Culinary Herbs That May Interact with Drugs[135] (*Continued*)

Culinary Herb	Active Substance(s)	Potential Drug Interaction
Tonka Beans[136–137] (*Dipteryx odorata*)	Coumarin Fatty oil	Acts synergistically with coumarin and other anticoagulants
Turmeric[137] (*Curcuma domestica*)	Volatile oil Curcuminoids—curcumin Starch	May enhance anticoagulant therapy
Wintergreen[136–137] (*Gaultheria procumbens, Pyrola rotundifolia*)	Volatile oil—methyl salicylate Hydroquinone derivatives Naphthacene derivatives Tannins Mucilage	May enhance anticoagulant therapy

Source: From Hagan, D., *The World According to Herbs: Culinary and Medicinal Uses: A CD-ROM*, 1999. With permission.

Mineral salts are another type of dietary supplements with a high nonprescription use that may interact with prescription drugs. Single nutrient supplements that are frequently taken on top of a multivitamin and mineral supplement and an adequate diet are also potential reactors with drugs. Table 13.2 lists the documented interactions between drugs and dietary supplements such as mineral salts and nutrients.[136]

Table 13.3 provides a list of documented interactions between herbs and drugs with identification of the active substance(s), specific drugs, mechanism of action, and contraindications for use. This is not intended as an exclusive list but rather a brief summary of examples.[137–141] As more supplements are used by more people taking multiple drugs, documentation of interactions will continue to expand. Health professionals need to work together to solicit information on herbal and dietary supplement usage and to be prepared to counsel patients on the potential for these interactions.

Table 13.2 Documented Interactions between Dietary Supplements and Drugs[135-136,142]

Dietary Supplement	Specific Drug	Drug Category	Mechanism for Interaction on Drug
		Mineral Salts	
Aluminum chloride	Flecanide	Antiarrhythmic	Decreases excretion
Aluminum hydroxide	Amphetamine	Miscellaneous	Increase excretion
	Aspirin	Analgesic	Increases excretion
	Indomethacin	Analgesic	Decreases absorption
	Ticlopidine	Anticoagulant	Decreases absorption
	Captopril	Antihypertensive	Alters metabolism (decreases bioavailability)
	Ciprofloxacin	Antiinfective	Alters metabolism
	Ethambutol	Antiinfective	Decreases absorption
	Isoniazid	Antiinfective	Decreases absorption; alters metabolism
	Ketoconazole	Antiinfective	Decreases absorption
	Clorazepate	Antipsychotic/antianxiety	Decreases absorption
	Chlorpromazine	Antipsychotic/antianxiety	Decreases absorption
	Tetracyclines	Antiinfective	Decreases absorption
	Propranolol	Beta-adrenergic blocking agent	Decreases absorption
	Cholecalciferol	Vitamin	Increase absorption of aluminum
	Ferrous Sulfate	Mineral	Decrease absorption
	Digoxin	Cardiac glycoside	Decrease absorption
	Theophyllin	Xanthine drug	Alters metabolism
	Cimetidine	Miscellaneous	Alters metabolism
	Citric acid	Miscellaneous	Increase absorption
	Levodopa	Miscellaneous	Increase absorption
	Misoprostol	Miscellaneous	Unknown
	Penicillamine	Miscellaneous	Decreases absorption
	Prednisolone	Miscellaneous	Decreases absorption
Calcium carbonate	Atenolol	Beta-adrenergic blocking agent	Decreases absorption
	Chlorothiazide	Diuretic	Alters metabolism and decreases excretion
	Levothyroxine	Miscellaneous	Decreases absorption

Supplement	Drug	Drug Class	Effect
Calcium chloride	Digitalis	Cardiac glycoside	Alters metabolism
Calcium gluconate	Verapamil	Antiarrhythmic	Alters metabolism
Ferrous sulfate	Tetracyclines	Antiinfective	Decreases absorption
	Levodopa	Miscellaneous	Decreases absorption
	Levothyroxine	Miscellaneous	Decreases absorption
Magnesium carbonate	Captopril	Antihypertensive	Alters metabolism (decreases bioavailability)
	Ferrous sulfate	Mineral	Decrease absorption
Magnesium hydroxide	Aspirin	Analgesic	Increases excretion
	Ticlopidine	Anticoagulant	Decreases absorption
	Captopril	Antihypertensive	Alters metabolism (decreases bioavailability)
	Ciprofloxacin	Antiinfective	Alters metabolism
	Ketoconazole	Antiinfective	Decreases absorption
	Chlorpromazine	Antipsychotic/antianxiety drug	Decreases absorption
	Clorazepate	Antipsychotic/antianxiety drug	Decreases absorption
	Digoxin	Cardiac glycoside	Decrease absorption
	Ferrous sulfate	Mineral	Decrease absorption
	Theophyllin	Xanthine drug	Increase absorption
	Cimetidine	Miscellaneous	Alters metabolism
	Levodopa	Miscellaneous	Increases absorption
	Levodopa	Miscellaneous	Increases absorption
	Misoprostol	Miscellaneous	Unknown
	Penicillamine	Miscellaneous	Decreases absorption
Magnesium sulfate	Nifedipine	Antiarrhythmic	Lowers blood pressure
Magnesium trisilate	Digoxin	Cardiac glycoside	Decrease absorption
Potassium chloride	Captopril	Antiarrhythmic	Alters metabolism
	Spironolactone	Diuretic	Decrease excretion
Sodium bicarbonate	Flecainide	Antiarrhythmic	Decreases excretion
	Methotrexate	Antineoplastic	Increases excretion
	Amphetamine	Miscellaneous	Decrease excretion
Charcoal	Aspirin	Analgesic	Decrease absorption
	Disopyramide	Antiarrhythmic	Decrease bioavailability
	Flecainide	Antiarrhythmic	Decrease absorption

Table 13.2 Documented Interactions between Dietary Supplements and Drugs[135–136,142] (Continued)

Dietary Supplement	Specific Drug	Drug Category	Mechanism for Interaction on Drug
Charcoal (continued)	Carbamazepine	Anticonvulsant	Decrease absorption
	Phenytoin	Anticonvulsant	Decrease absorption
	Nortriptyline	Antidepressant	Decrease absorption
	Promazine	Antipsychotic/antianxiety	Decrease absorption
	Digoxin	Cardiac glycoside	Decrease absorption
	Furosemide	Diuretic	Decrease absorption
	Glipizide	Hypoglycemic	Decrease absorption
	Phenobarbital	Sedative/hypnotic	Decrease absorption
	Theophylline	Xanthine drug	Decrease absorption
	Nizatidine	Miscellaneous	Decrease absorption
		Nutrients	
Ascorbic acid	Warfarin	Anticoagulant	Alters metabolism
	Aspirin	Analgesic	Decrease excretion
	Ethinyl estradiol	Miscellaneous	Alters absorption
	Ferrous Sulfate	Nutrient	Increases absorption of iron
DHEA[1,142] dehydroepiandosterone	Hormones	Miscellaneous	Alters metabolism
Fish oil[142]	Heparin	Anticoagulant	Alters metabolism
	Warfarin	Anticoagulant	Alters metabolism
	Dipyridamole	Anticoagulant	Alters metabolism
	Sulfinpyrazone	Anticoagulant	Alters metabolism
	Aspirin	Analgesic	Alters metabolism
	Ticlopidine		Alters metabolism
Folic Acid	Phenytoin	Anticonvulsant	Alters metabolism of folate
	Sulfasalzine		Decrease absorption of folate
L-phenylalanine	Monoamine oxidase inhibitors		
L-tyrosine	Monoamine oxidase inhibitor		

Melatonin

Supplement	Drug	Category	Effect
Tryptophan	Fluoxetine	Antidepressant	Alters metabolism
	Tranylcypromine	Antidepressant	Alters metabolism
Pyridoxine	Isoniazid	Antiinfective	Alters metabolism of B_6
	Phenobarbital	Sedative/hypnotic	Alters metabolism
	Levodopa	Miscellaneous	Alters metabolism
Cyanocobalamine	Omeprazole	Miscellaneous	Decrease absorption
Niacin	Aspirin	Analgesic	Alter metabolism
Nicotinic acid	Lovastatin		Unknown
Vitamin D	Phenytoin	Anticonvulsant	Alters metabolism of vitamin
Vitamin E	Warfarin	Anticoagulant	Alters metabolism
Zinc	Tetracycline		

Source: Zucchero, F.J., Hogan, J.J., and Sommer, C.D., *Evaluations of Drug Interactions*, First DataBank, Inc., San Bruno, CA, 1999. With permission.

Adapted from http://www.firstdatabank.com. Hagan, D.W. et al., *The World According to Herbs: Culinary and Medicinal Uses*, CD-ROM, 1999.

Table 13.3 Documented Interactions between Herbs and Drugs[1,3,137,138,140]

Herb	Active Substance	Specific Drug	Mechanism	Contraindications
Adonis[1] (*Adonis vernalis*)	Cardioactive steroid glycosides	Quinidine Calcium Saluretics Laxatives Long-term use of Glucocorticoids	Enhances effect of drugs	Avoid with digitalis glycoside Avoid in potassium deficiency
Aloe[1] (*Aloe barbadensis*)	Anthraquinones	Cardiac glycosides Antiarrhythmic drugs Thiazide diuretic Corticosteroids Licorice	Increases effect through loss of potassium	Avoid with gastrointestinal inflammation Avoid using with children, pregnant and lactating women, and elderly
Belladonna[1] (*Atropa belladonna*)	Tropan alkaloids — atropine and hyoscyamine Hydroxycoumarins Tannins	Amantadine hydrochloride Quinidine Tricyclic antidepressants Atropine Scopolamine	Drugs enhance effect of herb	Avoid large doses[3] Avoid use in tachycardic arrhythmias, prostate adenomas, glaucoma, acute edema of lungs, megacolon, and mechanical stenosis of gastrointestinal tract[4]
Broom[1,138] (*Cytisus scoparius*)	Quinolizidine alkaloids — sparteine Biogenic amines Flavonoids Isoflavonoids	Monoamine oxidase inhibitors	Amines interact leading to a sudden change in blood pressure or hypertensive crisis	Avoid using on patients with high blood pressure
Buckthorn[1] (*Rhamnus cathartica*)	Anthracene derivatives Tannins Flavonoids	Cardiac glycosides Thiazide diuretics Corticosteroids Licorice	Enhanced effect of drug due to loss of potassium	
Buckthorn bark[1] (*Rhamnus frangula*)	Anthracene derivatives Naphthaquinone derivatives Peptide alkaloids	Cardiac glycosides Thiazide diuretics Corticosteroids Licorice	Enhanced effect of drug due to loss of potassium	

Herb	Constituents	Drug	Effect	Comments
Bugleweed[1] (*Lycopus virginicus*)	Caffeic acid derivatives, Flavonoids	Thyroid hormone preparations	Inhibits peripheral deiodination of T4; Lowers prolactin levels	Do not use for an enlarged thyroid; Interferes with diagnostic procedures using radioactive iodine[4]
Cascara sagrada[1] (*Rhamnus purshianus*)	Anthracene derivatives, Aglycones	Cardiac glycosides, Thiazide diuretics, Corticosteroids, Licorice, Antiarrhythmics	Enhanced effect of drug due to loss of potassium	Avoid use with intestinal obstruction, gastrointestinal inflammations, and abdominal pain; Avoid during pregnancy and lactation
Castor oil[1] (*Ricinus communis*)	Fatty oil, Proteins, Lectins, Pyridine alkaloids, Triglycerides, Tocopherols	Cardioactive steroids	Enhanced effect of drug due to loss of potassium	Avoid use during pregnancy, lactation, and in children under 12; Avoid use for intestinal obstruction, gastrointestinal inflammation, and abdominal pain
Chaste tree[1] (*Vitex agnus-castus*)	Iridoid glycosides, Flavonoids, Volatile oil, Fatty oils	Dopamine antagonists	Decreases dopaminergic effect of herb	Avoid use in pregnancy and during lactation
Cinchona[1] (*Cinchona pubescens*)	Quinoline alkaloids, Catechin tannins	Anticoagulants	Increases effect resulting in thrombocytopenia	Avoid use in pregnancy and during lactation
Feverfew[1,138] (*Tanacetum parthenium*)	Volatile oil, Sesquiterpene lactones, Flavonoids, Polynes	Antithrombotic medications — aspirin, heparin, and warfarin	Interferes with prostaglandin metabolism	
Foxglove[1] (*Digitalis purpurea*)	Cardioactive steroid glycosides, Steroid saponin, Anthraquinones	Arrhythmogenic medications — sympathomimetics, methylxanthines, phosphodiesterase inhibitors, quinidine, Digitoxin, Digoxin	Available primarily as standardized drug; if used in herb form, could cause an additive effect or overdose	

Table 13.3 Documented Interactions between Herbs and Drugs[1,3,137,138,140] (*Continued*)

Herb	Active Substance	Specific Drug	Mechanism	Contraindications
Ginkgo[1] (*Ginkgo biloba*)	Flavonoids Biflavonoids Proanthocyanidins Trilactonic diterpenes Trilactonic sesquiterpene	Antithrombotic medications	Inhibits platelet activating factor	
Henbane[1,137] (*Hyoscyamus niger*)	Tropane alkaloids Flavonoids Fatty oil	Tricyclic antidepressants Amantadine Anithistamines Phenothiazines Procainamide Quinidine	Enhanced anticholinergic effect	
Hibiscus[137] (*Hibiscus sabdariffa*)	Fruit acids Anthocyans Flavonoids Muscilages	Chloroquine	Herb reduces effectiveness of drug	
Kava[1,138] (*Piper methysticum*)	Kava lactones Chalcones	Alprazolam Central nervous system depressants Alcohol Levodopa	Herb enhances effect of drug	Avoid during pregnancy and lactation
Khat[140]	Alkaloids Tannins	Ampicillin	Decreases bioavailability of drug	
Kyushin[140]	Cardiotonic steroids — bufalin	Digoxin	Alters metabolism of drug	
Lily-of-the-Valley[1] (*Convllaria majalis*)	Cardioactive steroid glycosides	Quinidine Calcium salts Saluretics Laxatives Glucocorticoids	Herb enhances effects of drug	

Herb	Constituents	Drugs	Interaction	Precautions
Ma huang[1,137,138] (*Ephedra sinica*)	Alkaloids of the 2-aminophenylpropane type	Cardiac glycosides Halothane Guanethidine Monoamine oxidase inhibitors Secale alkaloid derivative — oxytocin	Affects heart rhythm Enhances sympathomimetic effect Potentiates the sympathomimetic effect of ephedrine Leads to development of high blood pressure	Avoid in children and individuals with heart conditions, high blood pressure, thyroid disorders, diabetes, prostate enlargement, anorexia and bulimia, and insomnia
Niauli[1] (*Melaleucea viridiflora*)	Cineol	Coadministered drugs metabolized by the liver	Decreases effect of drugs due to induction of liver enzymes	
Oak Bark[1,137–138] (*Quercus robur*)	Tannins Catechins and leucocyanidins	Alkaloid and alkaline drugs	Interaction inhibits absorption of drug	
Oleander Leaf[1,3] (*Nerium odoratum*)	Cardiac steroids	Quinidine Calcium salts Saluretics Laxatives Glucocorticoids	Increases effects of drugs	
Rauwolfia[1] (*Rauwolfia serpentina*)	Indole alkaloids Starch	Alcohol Neuroleptics Barbiturates Digitalis glycosides Levodopa Sympathomimetics	Synergistic effect Decreases effect of drug Increases blood pressure	Avoid use in depression, ulceration, pheochromocytoma, pregnancy, and lactation
Rhubarb Root[1,137,138] (*Rheum palmatum*)	Anthracene derivatives Tannins Flavonoids Naphthohydroquinone glucosides	Cardiac glycosides	Increased effect due to potassium loss	Avoid use with intestinal obstruction, gastrointestinal inflammations, and abdominal pain Avoid during pregnancy, lactation, and with children
Scopolia[1,137] (*Scopolia carniolica*)	Tropane alkaloids Hydroxycoumarins Caffeic acid derivatives[140]	Tricyclic antidepressants Amantadine Quinidine	Enhances effect of drug	Avoid in angle-closure glaucoma, prostate cancer, tachycardias, narrowing of gastrointestinal tract, and megacolon

Table 13.3 Documented Interactions between Herbs and Drugs[1,3,137,138,140] (Continued)

Herb	Active Substance	Specific Drug	Mechanism	Contraindications
Senna[1,137–138] (Cassia species)	Anthracene derivatives Naphthacene derivatives	Cardiac glycosides Thiazide diuretics Corticosteroids Licorice Antiarrhythmics	Enhanced effect of drug due to loss of potassium	Avoid during pregnancy and lactation Avoid with bowl obstructions and abdominal pain
Squill[1,137,138] (Drimia maritima)	Cardioactive steroid glycosides Mucilage	Quinidine Calcium Saluretics Laxatives Glucocorticoids Methylxanthines Phosphodiesterase inhibitors Sympathomimetic agents	Enhances effect of drug Increases risk of arrhythmias	Avoid use in heart block, arrhythmias, and electrolyte imbalance
Uva-Ursi,[1,137,138] (Arctostaphylos uva-ursi)	Hydroquinone glycosides Tannins Iridoide monoterpenes Flavonoids Triterpenes	Urine acidifiers	Reduces effect of drugs which cause acidic urine	Avoid use during pregnancy, lactation, and with children
Yohimbe[1,3,138] (Pausinystalia yohimbe)	Indole alkaloids Tannins	Yohimbine Blood pressure medications Monoamine oxidase inhibitors Antidepressants Antihistamines	Enhanced or synergistic effect	Avoid nonprescription use of this drug herb

REFERENCES

1. Blumenthal, M. et al., *The Complete German Commission E Monographs, Therapeutic Guide to Herbal Medicines,* American Botanical Council, Austin, TX, Boston, MA, 1998, p. 684.

2. Akerele, O., Summary of WHO guidelines for the assessment of herbal medicine, *HerbalGram,* 28, 13–16, 1993.

3. Block, A. and Thompson, C.A., Position of the American Dietetic Association: phytochemicals and functional foods, *J. Am. Diet. Assoc.,* 95, 493–496, 1995.

4. Wilkinson, G.R., The effects of diet, aging and disease-states on presystemic elimination and oral drug bioavailability in humans, *Adv. Drug. Deliv. Rev.,* 27, 129–159, 1997.

5. Ioannides, C., Effect of diet and nutrition on the expression of cytochromes P450, *Xenobiotica,* 29, 109–154, 1999.

6. Dresser, G.K. et al., Fruit juices inhibit organic anion transporting polypeptide-mediated drug uptake to decrease the oral availability of fexofenadine, *Clin. Pharmacol. Ther.,* 71, 11–20, 2002.

7. Smith, T.J. and Yang, C.S., Effect of organosulfur compounds from garlic and cruciferous vegetables on drug metabolism enzymes, *Drug Metab. Drug Int.,* 17, 23–49, 2000.

8. Leclercq, I., Desager, J., and Horsmans, Y., Inhibition of chlorzoxazone metabolism, a clinical probe for CYP2E1, by a single ingestion of watercress, *Clin. Pharmacol. Ther.,* 64, 144–149, 1998.

9. Zhai, S. et al., Comparative inhibition of human cytochromes P450 1A1 and 1A2 by flavonoids, *Drug Metab. Dispos.,* 26, 989–992, 1998.

10. Obermeier, M.T., White, R.E., and Yang, C.S., Effects of bioflavanoids on hepatic P450 activities, *Xenobiotica,* 25, 575–584, 1995.

11. Eaton, E.A. et al., Flavonoids, potent inhibitors of the human p-form phenolsulfotransferase: potential role in drug metabolism and chemoprevention, *Drug Metab. Dispos.,* 24, 232–237, 1996.

12. Moore, L.B. et al., St. John's wort induces hepatic drug metabolism through activation of the pregnane X receptor, *Proc. Natl. Acad. Sci.,* 97, 7500–7502, 2000.

13. Canivenc-Lavier, M. et al., Comparative effects of flavonoids and model inducers on drug metabolizing enzymes in the rat liver, *Toxicology,* 114, 19–27, 1996.

14. Conseil, G. et al., Flavonoids: a class of modulators with bifunctional interactions at vicinal ATP- and steroid-binding sites on mouse P-glycoprotein, *Proc. Natl. Acad. Sci.,* 95, 9831–9836, 1998.

15. Ohnishi, A. et al., Effect of furanocoumarin derivatives in grapefruit juice on the uptake of vinblastine by Caco-2 cells and on the activity of cytochrome P450 3A4, *Br. J. Pharmacol.,* 130, 1369–1377, 2000.

16. Hodek, P., Trefil, P., and Stiborova, M., Flavonoids-potent and versatile biologically active compounds interacting with cytochromes P450, *Chem.-Biol. Interact.,* 139, 1–21, 2002.

17. Hypericum Depression Trial Study Group, Effect of *Hypericum perforatum* (St. John's wort) in major depressive disorder: a randomized controlled trial, *J. Am. Med. Assoc.,* 141, 807–141, 814, 2002.

18. Schulz, V., Incidence and clinical relevance of the interactions and side effects of *Hypericum* preparations, *Phytomed.,* 8, 152–160, 2001.

19. Brenner, R., et al., Comparison of an extract of *Hypericum* (LI160) and sertraline in the treatment of depression: a double-blind, randomized pilot study, *Clin. Ther.,* 22, 411–419, 2000.

20. Linde, K. et al., St. John's wort for depression—an overview and meta-analysis of randomized clinical trials, *Br. Med. J.,* 313, 253–258, 1996.

21. Fugh-Berman, A. and Ernst, E., Herb–drug interactions: review and assessment of report reliability, *Br. J. Clin. Pharmacol.,* 52, 587–595, 2001.

22. Izzo, A.A. and Ernst, E., Interactions between herbal medicines and prescribed drugs: a systematic review, *Drugs,* 61, 2163–2175, 2001.

23. Sugimoto, K. et al., Different effects of St. John's wort on the pharmacokinetics of simvastatin and pravastatin, *Clin. Pharmacol. Ther.,* 70, 518–524, 2001.

24. Gorski, J.C. et al., The effect of St. John's wort on the efficacy of oral contraception, *Clin. Pharmacol. Ther.,* 71, P25, 2002

25. Wang, Z. et al., The effects of St. John's wort (*Hypericum perforatum*) on human cytochrome P450 activities, *Clin. Pharmacol. Ther.,* 70, 317–326, 2001.

26. Dürr, D. et al., St. John's wort induces intestinal P-glycoprotein/MDR1 and intestinal and hepatic CYP3A4, *Clin. Pharmacol. Ther.,* 68, 598–604, 2000.

27. Dresser, G.K. et al., St. John's wort induces intestinal and hepatic CYP3A4 and P-glycoprotein in healthy volunteers, *Clin. Pharmacol. Ther.,* 69, P23, 2000.

28. Gurley, B.J. et al., Cytochrome P450 phenotypic ratios for predicting herb–drug interactions in humans, *Clin. Pharmacol. Ther.,* 72, 276–282, 2002.

29. Johne, A. et al., Pharmacokinetic interaction of digoxin with an herbal extract from St. John's wort (*Hypericum perforatum*), *Clin. Pharmacol Ther.,* 66, 338–345, 1999.

30. Hennessy, M. et al., St. John's wort increases expression of P-glycoprotein: implications for drug interactions, *Br. J. Clin. Pharmacol. J. Biol.,* 53, 75–82, 2002.

31. Wentworth, J.M. et al., St. John's wort, a herbal antidepressant, activates the steroid X receptor, *J. Endocrinol.,* 166, R11–R16, 2000.

32. Moore, J.T. and Kliewer, S.A., Use of the nuclear receptor PXR to predict drug interactions, *Toxicology,* 153, 1–10, 2000.

33. Xie, W. and Evans, R.M., Orphan nuclear receptors: the exotics of xenobiotics, *J. Biol. Chem.,* 276, 37739–37742, 2001.

34. Gibson, G.G. et al., Receptor-dependent transcriptional activation of cytochrome P4503A genes: induction mechanisms, species differences and interindividual variations in man, *Xenobiotica,* 32, 165–206, 2002.

35. Geick, A., Eichelbaum, M., and Burk, O., Nuclear receptor response elements mediate induction of intestinal MDR1 by rifampin, *J. Biol. Chem.,* 276, 14581–14587, 2001.

36. Synold, T.W., Dussault, I., and Forman, B.M., The orphan nuclear receptor SXR coordinately regulates drug metabolism and efflux, *Nature Med.,* 7, 584–590, 2001.

37. Watkins, P.B. et al., Erythromycin breath test as an assay of glucocorticoid-inducible liver cytochromes P-450, *J. Clin. Invest.,* 83, 688–697, 1989.

38. Tanaka, E., Gender-related differences in pharmacokinetics and their clinical significance, *J. Clin. Pharm. Ther.,* 24, 339–346, 1999.

39. Barnes, J., Anderson, L.A., and Phillipson, J.D., St John's wort (*Hypericum perforatum* L.): a review of its chemistry, pharmacology and clinical properties, *J. Pharm. Pharmacol.,* 53, 583–600, 2001.

40. Beckman, S.E., Sommi, R.W., and Switzer, J., Consumer use of St. John's wort: a survey on effectiveness, safety, and tolerability, *Pharmacotherapy,* 20, 568–574, 2000.

41. Redvers, A. et al., How many patients self-medicate with St. John's wort? *Psychiat. Bull.,* 25, 254–256, 2001.

42. Markowitz, J.S. et al., Effect of St. John's wort (*Hypericum perforatum*) on cytochrome P-450 2D6 and 3A4 activity in healthy volunteers, *Life Sci.,* 66, 133–139, 2000.

43. Ereshefsky, B. et al., Determination of SJW differential metabolism at CYP2D6 and CYP3A4, using dextromethorphan probe methodology [poster 130], paper presented at the NCDEU 39 Annual Meeting, Boca Raton, FL, 1999.
44. Bray, B.J. et al., Short term treatment with St. John's wort, hypericin or hyperforin fails to induce CYP450 isoforms in the Swiss Webster mouse, *Life Sci.*, 70, 1325–1335, 2002.
45. Biber, A. et al., Oral bioavailability of hyperforin from *Hypericum* extracts in rats and human volunteers, *Pharmacopsychiatry*, 31, 36–43, 1998.
46. Liu, F.F. et al., Evaluation of major active components in St. John's wort dietary supplements by high-performance liquid chromatography with photodiode array detection and electrospray mass spectrometric confirmation, *J. Chromatogr. (A)*, 888, 85–92, 2000.
47. De Los Reyes, G.C. and Koda, R.T., Determining hyperforin and hypericin content in eight brands of St. John's wort, *Am. J. Health Syst. Pharm.*, 59, 545–547, 2002.
48. Ganzera, M., Zhao, J., and Khan, I.A., Hypericum perforatum—Chemical profiling and quantitative results of St. John's wort products by an improved high-performance liquid chromatography method, *J. Pharm. Sci.*, 91, 623–630, 2002.
49. Verotta, L. et al., Hyperforin analogues from St. John's wort (*Hypericum perforatum*), *J. Natl. Prod.*, 63, 412–415, 2000.
50. Burstein, A.H. et al., Lack of effect of St. John's wort on carbamazepine pharmacokinetics in healthy volunteers, *Clin. Pharmacol. Ther.*, 68, 605–612, 2000.
51. Roby, C.A., Dryer, D.A., and Burstein, A.H., St. John's wort: effect on CYP2D6 activity using dextromethorphan–dextrorphan ratios, *J. Clin. Psychopharmacol.*, 21, 530–532, 2001.
52. Raucy, J.L., Risk assessment: toxicity from chemical exposure resulting from enhanced expression of CYP2E1, *Toxicology*, 105, 217–223, 1995.
53. Barone, G.W. et al., Herbal supplements: a potential for drug interactions in transplant recipients, *Transplantation*, 71, 239–241, 2001.
54. Ernst, E., St. John's wort supplements endanger the success of organ transplantation, *Arch. Surg.*, 137, 316–319, 2002.
55. Ernst, E. and Cassileth, B.R., The prevalence of complementary/alternative medicine in cancer, *Cancer*, 83, 777–782, 1998.
56. Ernst, E., The role of complementary and alternative medicine in cancer, *Lancet Oncol.*, 1, 176–180, 2000.
57. Mathijssen, R.H. et al., Modulation of irinotecan (CPT-11) metabolism by St. John's wort in cancer patients, paper presented at the American Association for Cancer Research Annual Meeting, 2002, San Francisco, abstract 2443.
58. Chu, X.Y. et al., Active efflux of CPT-11 and its metabolites in human KB-derived cell lines, *J. Pharmacol. Exp. Ther.*, 288, 735–741, 1999.
59. Kim, R.B., Drugs as P-glycoprotein substrates, inhibitors, and inducers, *Drug Metab. Rev.*, 34, 47–54, 2002.
60. Obach, R.S., Inhibition of human cytochrome P450 enzymes by constituents of St. John's wort, an herbal preparation used in the treatment of depression, *J. Pharmacol. Exp. Ther.*, 294, 88–95, 2000.
61. Budzinski, J.W. et al., An *in vitro* evaluation of human cytochrome P450 3A4 inhibition by selected commercial herbal extracts and tinctures, *Phytomedicine*, 7, 273–282, 2000.
62. Kerb, R. et al., Single-dose and steady-state pharmacokinetics of hypericin and pseudohypericin, *Antimicrob. Agent Chemother.*, 40, 2087–2093, 1996.

63. Carson, S.W. et al., Inhibitory effect of methanolic solution of St. John's wort (*Hypericum perforatum*) on cytochrome P450 3A4 activity in human liver microsomes, *Clin. Pharmacol. Ther.,* 67, 99, 1999.

64. Muller, W.E. et al., Hyperforin represents the neuotransmitter reuptake inhibiting constituent of *Hypericum* extract, *Pharmacopsychiatry,* 31, 16–21, 1998.

65. Singer, A., Wonnemann, M., and Muller, W.E., Hyperforin, a major antidepressant constituent of St. John's wort, inhibits serotonin uptake by elevating free intracellular Na+1, *J. Pharmacol. Exp. Ther.,* 290, 1363–1368, 1999.

66. Jensen, A.G., Hansen, S.H., and Nielsen, E.O., Adhyperforin as a contributor to the effect of *Hypericum perforatum* L. in biochemical models of antidepressant activity, *Life Sci.,* 68, 1593–1605, 2001.

67. Denke, A. et al., Biochemical activities of extracts from *Hypericum perforatum* L. 5th communication: dopamine-beta-hydroxylase-product quantification by HPLC and inhibition by hypericins and flavonoids, *Arzneim Forsch.,* 50, 415–419, 2000.

68. Gobbi, M. et al., *In vitro* binding studies with two *Hypericum perforatum* extracts—hyperforin, hypericin, and biapigenin—on 5-HT6, 5-HT7, GABA(A)/benzodiazepine, sigma, NPY-Y1/Y2 receptors and dopamine transporters, *Pharmacopsychiatry,* 34, S45–S48, 2001.

69. Stevinson, C., Pittler, M.H., and Ernst, E., Garlic for treating hypercholesterolemia: a meta analysis of randomized clinical trials, *Ann. Intern. Med.,* 133, 420–429, 2000.

70. Lawson, L.D., Wang, Z.J., and Hughes, B.G., Identification and HPLC quantitation of the sulfides and dialk(en)yl thiosulfinates in commercial garlic products, *Planta Med.,* 57, 363–370, 1991.

71. Amagase, H. et al., Intake of garlic and its bioactive components. *J. Nutr.,* 131, 955S–962S, 2001.

72. Matsuura, H., Saponins in garlic as modifiers of the risk of cardiovascular disease, *J. Nutr.,* 131, 1000S–1005S, 2001.

73. Simons, L.A. et al., On the effect of garlic oil on plasma lipids and lipoproteins in mild hypercholesterolaemia, *Atherosclerosis,* 113, 219–225, 1995.

74. Berthold, H.K., Sudhop, T., and von Bergman, K., Effect of a garlic oil preparation on serum lipoproteins and cholesterol metabolism: a randomized controlled trial, *J. Am. Med, Assoc.,* 279, 1900–1902, 1998.

75. Haber, D. et al., Differential effects of dietary diallyl sulfide and diallyl disulfide on rat intestinal and hepatic drug-metabolizing enzymes, *J. Toxicol. Environ. Health,* 44, 423–434, 1995.

76. Siess, M., Modification of hepatic drug-metabolizing enzymes in rats treated with alkyl sulfides, *Cancer Lett.,* 120, 195–201, 1997.

77. Yang, C.S. et al., Mechanisms of inhibition of chemical toxicity and carcinogenesis by diallyl sulfide (DAS) and related compounds from garlic, *J. Nutr.,* 131, 1041S–1045S, 2001.

78. Loizou, G.D. and Crocker, J., The effects of alcohol and diallyl sulphide on CYP2E1 activity in humans: a phenotyping study using chlorzoxazone, *Hum. Exp. Toxicol.,* 20, 321–327, 2001.

79. Gwilt, P.R. et al., The effect of garlic extract on human metabolism of acetaminophen, *Cancer Epidemiol. Biol. Prev.,* 3, 155–160, 1994.

80. Foster, B.C. et al., An *in vitro* evaluation of human cytochrome P450 3A4 and p-glycoprotein inhibition by garlic, *J. Pharm. Pharmaceut. Sci.,* 4, 176–184, 2001.

81. Piscitelli, S.C., et al., The effect of garlic supplements on the pharmacokinetics of saquinavir, *Clin. Infect. Dis.,* 34, 234–238, 2002.

82. Choudri, S.H., Gallicano, K., and Foster, B., A study of pharmacokinetic interactions between garlic supplements and ritonavir in healthy volunteers [abstract 1637], in program and abstracts of the 40th Interscience Conference on Antimicrobial Agents and Chemotherapy (Toronto), Washington, D.C., American Society for Microbiology, 2000.

83. Lawson, L.D., Wang, Z.J., and Papadimitriou, D., Allicin release under simulated gastrointestinal conditions from garlic powder tablets employed in clinical trials on serum cholesterol, *Planta Med.,* 67, 13–18, 2001.

84. Bordia, A., Verma, S.K., and Srivastava, K.C., Effect of garlic (*Allium sativum*) on blood lipids, blood sugar, fibrinogen and fibrinolytic activity in patients with coronary artery disease, *Prost. Leuk. Essent. Fat. Acids,* 58, 257–263, 1998.

85. Rahman, K. and Billington, D., Dietary supplementation with aged garlic extract inhibits ADP-induced platelet aggregation in humans, *J. Nutr.,* 130, 2662–2665, 2000.

86. Block, E. and Ahmad, S., (E,Z)-Ajoene: a potent antithrombotic agent from garlic, *J. Am. Chem. Soc.,* 106, 8295–8296, 1984.

87. Srivastava, K.C. and Tyagi, O.D., Effects of a garlic-derived principle (ajoene) on aggregation and arachidonic metabolism in human platelets, *Prost. Leuk. Essent. Fat. Acids,* 49, 587–595, 1993.

88. Briggs, W.H. et al., Differential inhibition of human platelet aggregation by selected Allium thiosulfinates, *J. Agr. Food Chem.,* 48, 5731–5735, 2000.

89. Chung, K.F. et al., Effect of ginkgolide mixture (BN 52063) in antagonizing skin and platelet responses to platelet activating factor in man, *Lancet,* 1, 248–251, 1987.

90. Kim, Y.S. et al., Antiplatelet and antithrombotic effects of a combination of ticlopidine and ginkgo biloba extract, (Egb 761), *Thrombosis Res.,* 91, 33–38, 1998.

91. Sun, H. et al., A "high-throughput" cocktail method for screening the effect of herbal on liver isozyme activities: experience with ginkgo biloba, *Clin. Pharmacol. Ther.,* 71, P100, 2002.

92. Duche, J.C. et al., Effect of ginkgo biloba extract on microsomal enzyme induction, *Int. J. Clin. Pharm. Res.,* 9, 165–168, 1989.

93. He, N. and Edeki, T., Effects of ginseng and ginkgo biloba components on CYP2C9 mediated tolbutamide 4-methyl-hydroxylation in human liver microsomes, *Clin. Pharmacol. Ther.,* 71, P67, 2002.

94. Drago, F. et al., Pharmacokinetics and bioavailability of a ginkgo biloba extract, *J. Ocular Pharmacol. Ther.,* 18, 197–202, 2002.

95. Wojcicki, J. et al., Comparative pharmacokinetics and bioavailability of flavonoid glycosides of ginkgo biloba after a single oral administration of three formulations to healthy volunteers, *Materia Med. Pol.,* 27, 141–146, 1995.

96. Fourtillan, J.B. et al., Pharmacokinetics of bilobalide, ginkgolide A and ginkgolide B in healthy volunteers following oral and intravenous administrations of ginkgo biloba extract (Egb 761), *Therapie,* 50, 137–144, 1995.

97. Smith, M., Lin, K.M., and Zheng, Y.P., An open trial of nifedipine–herb interactions: nifedipine with St. John's wort, ginseng or ginkgo biloba, *Clin. Pharmacol. Ther.,* 69, P86, 2001.

98. Li, C.H. and Wong, Y.Y., The bioavailability of ginkgolides in ginkgo biloba extracts, *Planta Med.,* 63, 563–565, 1997.

99. Kressmann, S., Muller, W.E., and Blume, H.H., Pharmaceutical quality of different ginkgo biloba brands, *J. Pharm. Pharmacol.,* 54, 661–669, 2002.

100. Cui, J.F., Garle, M., and Bjorkhem, I., Determination of aglycones of ginsenosides in ginseng preparations sold in Sweden and in urine preparations from Swedish athletes consuming ginseng, *Scand. J. Clin. Lab. Invest.,* 56, 151–160, 1996.

101. Henderson, G.L. et al., Effects of ginseng components on c-DNA-expressed cyto-chrome P450 enzyme catalytic activity, *Life Sci.*, 65, 209–214, 1999.

102. Anderson, G.D. et al., Lack of effect of soy extract and panax ginseng on the urinary excretion of 6-beta-OH-cortisol/cortisol, *Clin. Pharmacol. Ther.*, 71, P34, 2002.

103. Zhu, M. et al., Possible influences of ginseng on the pharmacokinetics and pharma-cokinetics of warfarin in rats, *J. Pharm. Pharmacol.*, 51, 175–180, 1999.

104. Lee, F.C. et al., Effects of panax ginseng on blood alcohol clearance in man, *Clin. Exp. Pharmacol. Physiol.*, 14, 543–546, 1987.

105. Choi, C.W., Lee, S.I., and Huh, K., Effects of ginseng on the hepatic alcohol metab-olizing enzyme system activity in chronic alcohol-treated mice, *Korean J. Pharma-col.*, 20, 13–21, 1984.

106. Harkey, M.R. et al., Variability in commercial ginseng products: an analysis of 25 preparations, *Am. J. Clin. Nutr.*, 73, 1101–1106, 2001.

107. Park, I.H. et al., Cytotoxic dammarane glycosides from processed ginseng, *Chem. Pharm. Bull.*, 50, 538–540, 2002.

108. Bae, E. et al., Metabolism of 20(S)- and 20(R)-ginsenoside Rg3 by human intestinal bacteria and its relation to in vitro biological activities, *Biol. Pharm. Bull.*, 25, 58–63, 2002.

109. Saller, R., Meier, R., and Brignoli, R., The use of silymarin in the treatment of liver diseases, *Drugs*, 61, 2035–2063, 2001.

110. Venkataramanan, R. et al., Milk thistle, an herbal supplement, decreases the activity of CYP3A4 and uridine diphosphoglucuronsyl transferase in human hepatocyte cul-tures, *Drug Metab. Dispos.*, 28, 1270–1273, 2000.

111. Beckmann-Knopp, S. et al., Inhibitory effects of silibinin on cytochromes P-450 enzymes in human liver microsomes, *Pharmacol. Toxicol.*, 86, 250–256, 2000.

112. Weyhenmeyer, R., Mascher, H., and Birkmayer, J., Study on dose-linearity of the pharmacokinetics of silibin diastereomers using a new stereospecific assay, *Int. J. Clin. Pharmacol. Ther. Toxicol.*, 30, 134–138, 1992.

113. Leber, H.W. and Knauff, S., Influence of silymarin on drug metabolizing enzymes in rat and man, *Arzneim Forsch.*, 26, 1603–1605, 1976.

114. Piscitelli, S.C. et al., Effect of milk thistle on the pharmacokinetics of indinavir in healthy volunteers, *Pharmacotherapy*, 22, 551–556, 2002.

115. Gurley, B.J., Personal communication.

116. Schulz, H.U. et al., Investigation of dissolution and bioequivalence of silymarin products, *Arzneim Forsch.*, 45, 61–64, 1995.

117. Zhao, J. and Agarwal, R., Tissue distribution of silibinin, the major active constituent of silymarin, in mice and its association with enhancement of phase II enzymes. implications in cancer chemoprevention, *Carcinogenesis*, 20, 2101–2108, 1999.

118. Størmer, F.C., Reistad, R., and Alexander, J., Glycyrrhizic acid in licorice—evaluation of health hazard, *Food Chem. Toxicol.*, 31, 303–312, 1993.

119. Serra, A. et al., Glycyrrhetinic acid decreases plasma potassium concentrations in patients with anuria, *J. Am. Soc. Nephrol.*, 13, 191–196, 2002.

120. Ploeger, B. et al., The pharmacokinetics of glycyrrhizic acid evaluated by physiolog-ically based pharmacokinetic modeling, *Drug Metab. Rev.*, 33, 125–147, 2001.

121. Chen, M. et al., Effect of oral glycyrrhizin on the pharmacokinetics of prednisolone, *Endocrinol. Jpn.*, 37, 331–341.118, 1991.

122. Cantelli-Forti, G. et al., Interaction of licorice on glycyrrhizin pharmacokinetics, *Environ. Health Perspect.*, 102, 65–68, 1994.

123. Bernardi, M. et al., Effects of prolonged ingestion of graded doses of licorice by healthy volunteers, *Life Sci.*, 55, 863–872, 1994.

124. Gurley, B.J., Gardner, S.F., and Hubbard, M.A., Content versus label claims in ephedra-containing dietary supplements, *Am. J. Health Syst. Pharm.,* 57, 963–969, 2000.

125. Gurley, B.J. et al., Ephedrine pharmacokinetics after the ingestion of nutritional supplements containing *Ephedra sinica* (ma huang), *Ther. Drug Monit.,* 20, 439–445, 1998.

126. Gurley, B., Extract versus herb: effect of formulation on the absorption rate of botanical ephedrine from dietary supplements containing *Ephedra* (ma huang), *Ther. Drug Monit.,* 22, 497, 2000.

127. Dulloo, A.G. et al., Green tea and thermogenesis: interactions between catechin-polyphenols, caffeine and sympathetic activity, *Int. J. Obesity,* 24, 52–258, 2000.

128. Van Amelsvoort, J.M.M., Plasma concentrations of individual tea catechins after a single oral dose in humans, *Xenobiotica,* 31, 891–901, 2001.

129. Kubota, Y. et al., Safety of dietary supplements: chronotropic and inotropic effects on rat atria, *Biol. Pharm. Bull.,* 25, 197–200, 2002.

130. Calapai, G., Firenzouli, F., and Saitta, A., Antiobesity and cardiovascular toxic effects of Citrus aurantium extracts in the rat: a preliminary report, *Fitoterapia,* 70, 586–592, 1999.

131. Gurley, B.J. and Ali, S., Toxicity of multi-component ephedra-containing dietary supplements, [poster #W4075] paper presented at the American Association of Pharmaceutical Scientists annual meeting, Denver, CO, October 24, 2001.

132. Haller, C.A. and Benowitz, N.L., Adverse cardiovascular and central nervous system events associated with ephedra dietary supplements containing ephedra alkaloids, *N. Engl. J. Med.,* 343, 1833–1838, 2000.

133. Samenuk, D. et al., Adverse cardiovascular events temporally associated with ma huang, an herbal source of ephedrine, *Mayo Clin. Proc.,* 77, 12–16, 2002.

134. Ernst, E., Toxic heavy metals and undeclared drugs in Asian herbal medicines, *Trends Pharmacol. Sci.,* 23, 136–139, 2002.

135. Hagan, D.W. et al., *The world according to herbs: culinary and medicinal uses,* A CD-ROM, 1999.

136. Zucchero, F.J., Hogan, M.J., and Sommer, C.D., *Evaluation of Drug Interactions,* EDI First DataBank, Inc., St. Louis, MO, 2002.

137. Peirce, A., *A Practical Guide to Natural Medicines,* The American Pharmaceutical Associates, A Stonesong Press Book, William Morrow and Co., Inc., New York, 1999.

138. *PDR for Herbal Medicines,* Medical Economics Co., Montvale, NJ, 1998,

139. Brinker, F., *Herb Contraindications and Drug Interactions,* Eclectic Medical Publications, Sandy, OR, 1998.

140. *Monographs on the Medicinal Uses of Plant Drugs,* European Scientific Cooperative on Phytotherapy, Fasicule, 1–2, 1996; Fasicule, 3–5, 1997.

141. Hagan, D.W. et al., *To Herb or Not to Herb? A Guide to Over-the-Counter Herbals and Medicinals,* A CD-ROM, 1998.

142. Miller, L.G. and Murry, W.J., Specific toxicologic considerations of selected herbal products, in *Herbal Medicinals: A Clinician's Guide,* Pharmaceutical Products Press, an imprint of the Haworth Press, Inc., New York, 1998.

CHAPTER **14**

Dietary Counseling to Prevent Food–Drug Interactions

Beverly J. McCabe

CONTENTS

0-8493-1531-X/03/$0.00+$1.50
© 2003 by CRC Press LLC

Effective counseling for food and drug interaction prevention is based on the same premises as all good teaching and tutoring, whether by dietitian, physician, health educator, nurse, or pharmacist. Just as teaching is far more than just telling the student to learn this, counseling is far more than just handling out a list of foods or drugs to avoid and briefly telling the patient what to do. The basis of good teaching starts with solid knowledge on the teacher's part and with willingness to learn on the pupil's part. The teacher first prepares by knowing the subject well enough to guide the pupil in learning. The second step is assessing where the pupil stands in knowledge, willingness to learn, and learning style. The next step is to prepare a learning plan that will lead to the achievement of desired outcomes. The fourth step is to evaluate current learning by having the pupil demonstrate knowledge and skills. The fifth step is to develop a follow-up plan by which knowledge or motivation gaps can be addressed over time. While counseling and teaching may be perceived as differing greatly, effective learning by either approach is enhanced by assessing student readiness, environment, skills, and habits. Table 14.1 compares the traditional

Table 14.1 A Comparison of Traditional Education and Counseling Models

Education	Counseling
Knowledge	Knowledge
Assessment	Assessment
Plan	Establish mutual goals
Evaluate	Evaluate
	Reinforce

S is for SOURCE.

A is for ASSESSMENT.

F is for FOOD LISTS.

E is for EVALUATE.

R is for REVIEW AND REINFORCE.

Figure 14.1 SAFER: A mnemonic model for prevention of food–drug interactions.

viewpoints of education and counseling. Active involvement of the student in development and implementation of a specific plan is essential in effective counseling. Any change in diet behavior is complex and requires time and effort to incorporate into daily life. This chapter provides a model by which diet counseling for some important food–drug interactions can be readily planned, implemented, and evaluated without undue time demands on busy practitioners. The model is briefly outlined in Figure 14.1. The latter part of the chapter presents a critical review of the world literature on biogenic amines, especially tyramine and histamine, associated with clinically significant risks that demand careful attention in dietary counseling. Appendix D.1 and Appendix D.2 present the tyramine and histamine values derived from this review.

SAFER: MNEMONIC MODEL FOR FOOD–DRUG INTERACTIONS

Source: Identify and Evaluate Reliable Sources of Information on Which to Base Counseling

Knowledge of the sources of food components or nutrients involved in potential reactions as well as other drugs that may interact or potentiate a reaction is essential. Thorough knowledge of foods allows the dietitian to avoid undue restrictions imposed in the past. For example, the unnecessary elimination of all foods containing baker's yeast, such as bread and rolls in the tyramine-restricted diet in the past, was an extrapolation of case reports of consumption of a British yeast extract called Marmite® prepared from actual yeast remnants from the brewing process.[1–5] Whereas Marmite had clearly been shown to contain clinically significant amounts of tyramine and more than one case report documented reactions from its consumption, the same is not true of baker's yeast or of brewer's yeast manufactured in the U.S. as a dietary supplement.[4] Knowledge of the reactions involved will assist the dietitian, pharmacist, and physician to reasonably identify potential interactions before a problem is demonstrated in a case report. Calculations based on food analysis done by McCabe and Tsuang provide an example of a process that predicted avocado could cause a cheese reaction in patients on monoamine oxidase inhibitors (MAOIs) but only if consumed in an unusually large amount.[1,2] A pharmacist published a case report of a patient presenting in hypertensive crisis after consuming a quart of guacamole sauce in one setting.[6] Knowledge of the literature develops a scientifically sound approach to diet planning through critical evaluation of case reports and analysis of food.

A computerized search of medical literature will identify case reports, reviews by health practitioners, and experiments that pinpoint the metabolism involved in a food–drug reaction. Lacking, however, may be critical articles from food science literature that describe differences in food processing, food analysis techniques, and analysis of various foods and beverages around the world that provide rational diet planning. Unfortunately, a computerized search of food science literature is not readily available from most personal computers or from most medical libraries. Although excellent food science databases are available at universities with food science departments, most require that the researcher either be at the library itself or have faculty or student status for remote access. Two examples of food science print and computerized databases are *Nutrition Abstracts and Reviews* by CABI and *Food Science and Technology Abstracts* (FSTA) by Silver Platter.[7,8]

Reviewing the Literature to Determine Food Risks

With the possible exception of aged cheeses, few clear answers are available regarding whether a given food contains sufficient amounts of tyramine, a biogenic amine, to risk a hypertensive crisis in individuals on monoamine oxidase inhibitors. Determining the specific foods to absolutely avoid requires knowledge of the literature, professional judgment, and a touch of common sense. The literature contains three sources of information: (1) case reports, (2) laboratory analysis, and (3) review articles with summation and application advice.

Case Reports

Case reports vary from a simple report of a patient presenting to an emergency room in hypertensive crisis with only a verbal diet recall, to case reports in which the suspected food was analyzed and similar samples were subsequently analyzed. A single case report needs to be carefully considered but may well represent only a rare contamination. An adventitious decarboxylating organism in any protein-rich food stored improperly for too long or at inadequate temperatures may produce biogenic amines. Examples of the single case report that suggests food contamination and spoilage are beef liver, chicken liver, and chicken nuggets.[9–11] Subsequent analysis of fresh samples of such foods did not detect any or only insignificant levels of tyramine.[11,12] This type of case report and the subsequent analysis are very helpful in recognizing the importance of buying high-quality foods and maintaining storage within adequate temperature and time guidelines.

Other case studies have led to laboratory analysis of subsequent samples that reveal significant levels of tyramine in fresh samples of the food. Examples of this type of case study include fermented Asian dishes and tap beer.[13,14]

Laboratory Analysis

Articles containing laboratory analysis are generally found in two different categories: medical literature and food science literature. Computerized nutrient software programs most generally contain only 30 common nutrients; a few expensive software programs report 90 nutrients or food constituents.

Medical Literature

The medical literature generally contains analyses conducted in a university laboratory for clinical purposes. These articles usually contain one or more lists of foods and the amount of tyramine found in one or two samples purchased locally. Examples of this type of analysis are those of Shulman et al. and Mosnaim et al.[4,12] Analysis found in the medical literature may be conducted in pharmaceutical research laboratories. The design for such reports is often the purchase of several restaurant meals locally representing one or more ethnic menus. A representative sample of this type of reference is by DaPrada et al.[15] Usually, one sample is reported, and the purpose of the analysis is to determine relative safety of food items for a particular drug regimen. One difficulty with these laboratory analysis articles, particularly the latter type, is that publication is frequently in highly specialized journals that may not be readily available to most practitioners. For example, the most frequent source of tyramine analysis over the past 20 years has been the *Journal of Clinical Psychopharmacology.*

Since interlibrary loans from a medical library or online through the National Library of Medicine of the National Institutes of Health, such as Pubmeds and Loansome Doc, make these more accessible, this is less of a problem.[16] Several search tools enable the practitioner to readily identify articles in the medical literature.

Food Science Literature

The literature in the food science and technology field is not, however, readily available online, nor do most medical or college libraries have food journals. Literature search tools for food science such as Food Science and Technology Abstracts® (FSTA) are available on CD-ROM.[8] Unfortunately, such tools tend to be accessible only on campuses with food science and technology degree programs. Another excellent database, available in print or online, is the Nutrition Abstracts and Reviews, which provides abstracts of many topics in food science and in medical diet therapy taken from the world's food and nutrition journals.[7] Agricola is the search tool of the National Agricultural Library and can be accessed at www.nalusda.gov.[17] This readily available tool is not as user-friendly or efficient as others. A comparison search for "tyramine" yielded 130 references, while FSTA yielded 300 references. A search of one or the other of these food science databases is essential for a thorough review for food analysis articles.

Food science articles with specific analysis fall into four broad categories. The main focus of one category is food analysis methodology. Small numbers of samples, often one only, provide food data as a secondary component of the article. An example of this type is by Moret and Conte, who reported on the use of reversed-phase high-performance liquid chromatography for evaluation of biogenic amines.[18]

The second category of food analysis comprises those focused primarily on the use of analysis techniques in quality control. These articles may report much larger number of samples (often 3–20 samples). These are usually limited to one or two kinds of foods such as fresh beef and pork products or various forms of fish products. Ordonez et al. reported on the formation of biogenic amines in Idiazabal ewe's milk cheese.[19] Another example is the investigation of the relationship between histamine and tyramine in Spanish wine with other characteristics of the fermentation process.[20] Others test the effect of storage temperatures and length of storage on formation of biogenic amines.[21,22]

Technology is the basis for the third category involving the effects of new processing and packaging on microbial growth, organoleptic changes, and safety. An example is modified atmosphere packaging (MAP) used in fish and seafood—foods that are highly perishable. Sivertsvik et al. recently reviewed the benefits of MAP but also the essentiality of continuous proper storage temperature.[23] As exports and imports of fresh meat increase, as they have with the aid of CO_2-MAP for beef and pork, monitoring for biogenic amine formation will be increasingly important.[24–26]

A fourth category of food science articles is the large database studies such as those conducted by the U.S. government and reported in several journal articles in both medical and food science literature. An example of this category is the Food and Drug Administration's total diet studies on aluminum content of the American diet published in food science for adult intakes and in the pediatric medical literature for children and adolescent intakes.[27,28] This type of nutrient assessment considers not only absolute amounts of a food constituent but also frequency of inclusion in the diet.[29] The latter type of data can be helpful in deciding what to emphasize in food–drug interaction counseling or in designing specific food frequency question-naires as a prelude to counseling a specific patient or groups of patients.

The National Agriculture Library does provide online access to food composi-tion data for those nutrients and food dishes found in the continuing survey of intake by individuals (CSFII). The online program is known as the reference intake data and is named according to its release number, the latest one being 17.[30] This database provides data on most nutrients but very limited data on other food constituents such as *trans*-fatty acids and phytoestrogens. This computerized data-base basically replaces older food composition volumes of *Handbook No. 8,* some of which are now out of print. The site allows the search for data on a single food at a time, a slow but reliable online search for nutrients of interest for a number of foods. Use of the CSFII CD-ROM from 1994–1996 allows the researcher to pull the top sources of individual nutrients from a database of over 15,000 diet records.[31] This database has been used to determine the mineral tables in Appendix D.3–Appendix D.9.

Review Articles

Review articles are usually the starting point of students and professionals in beginning a literature search on a new topic and may represent the only article actually read by many busy practitioners on a complex subject. Some review articles represent a compilation of one set of researcher's data with comparison to the findings of others. Examples of this type of review article include reviews by Shalaby, Gardner et al., and Stratton et al.[32–34]

Other reviews have been carefully compiled from the world literature with carefully considered and well-drawn conclusions strengthened by either previous research or extensive practice experience. Review articles may focus on preparing summary tables of food content of a given food constituent or preparing lists of foods to use or not use in specific clinical regimens as the tyramine recommendations in Appendix D.1.

In review articles, it is important to consider the dates of the summarized data and recommendations. A good review article goes beyond merely summarizing past data; it also adds to the general knowledge base by making critical evaluations upon which to establish recommendations. All recommendations are based on current knowledge and may change as more data become available. Recommendations may change when more precise analytic techniques are developed that provide more accurate data.

A Matter of Units

In preparing a review of food analysis data, the reader is immediately faced with the use of multiple units in which the tyramine content are expressed in different articles. The analyses of histamine and tyramine may be reported as milligrams per kilogram, milligrams per 100 g, milligrams per deciliter, micrograms per gram, or parts per million. In order to compare various sources, the amounts need to be converted to common units. Since the numbers remain the same for mg/kg as for μg/g, the conversion between these units is simple. The units mg/100 g and mg/dl are also considered the same for calculation purposes, but they need a conversion factor to be taken to a more common unit such as mg/kg or μg/g. Regulatory limits in foods are often expressed in parts per million, a unit not commonly used by nutrition professionals. This unit represents 1 μg/g or 1 mg/kg.

For practical purposes of combining many analyses into a single table, the unit of μg has several advantages. It represents the smallest common unit for assessing food content. Smaller amounts can be summed more readily without relying on scientific notation. Because the minimum amount of tyramine likely to cause a "cheese" reaction has been designated as 6 mg per day, the summing of micrograms allows easy assessment by converting the minimum level to 6000 μg of tyramine/day.[3–5] Appendix D.1 contains a compiled list of food analyses reported in μg/g or μg/serving of a given food or beverage.

PRIORITIES FOR DIETARY ASSESSMENT AND COUNSELING

Assessment

Assess the patient's current usage of and knowledge about food and nutrient guidelines to determine how to proceed with counseling. A specially designed brief diet history or food frequency form may enable a rapid assessment of dietary practices on which to focus counseling. An example of such a form is given in Appendix E.3 and Appendix E.4 and in various articles in the literature.[35] Assessment, especially in the elderly, may also include functional assessment of ability to hear and understand spoken language, ability to understand and retain complex information, and ability to carry out activities of daily living (ADL).[36] Not only the actual foods used but also food purchasing, food preparation, and food storage habits may need to be assessed. For example, instructions for the tyramine-restricted diet encourage the patient to "Buy Fresh, Cook Fresh, Eat Fresh."[5,37] Although this is very valid advice, this has rarely been translated into practical terms. For patients taking MAOIs, food guidelines designed for the general public may not protect them sufficiently from modest rises in biogenic amines that may occur before expiration dates and cause no problems for the general public. See Appendix C.1 for general guidelines for storage of foods for the general population and for high-risk populations. Certain subgroups of a population may also have decreased tolerance of early spoilage changes, such as the elderly, the immune-suppressed patients, and very young children.[38]

As in any educational endeavor, learning readiness, learning skills, preferred learning modes, previous knowledge, and learners' perceptions can be critical for an effective outcome. Assessment of literacy skills is critical in selecting or preparing written materials to serve as a reinforcement of verbal advice. This assessment also includes the learner's abilities or willingness to prepare logs, charts, or other methods of monitoring compliance or progress in the therapeutic plan. Another essential step is asking about the learning style preferences as to oral, visual, written, observation, practice exercises, or question and answer modes. Some individuals prefer to read materials prior to counseling; others prefer a verbal overview followed by written or other visual modes. Still others wish to be taken carefully through all the required steps.

Knowledge of the learning theories, especially those related to the adult learner, helps to assess, plan for, and counsel on avoiding food–drug interactions. While an in-depth discussion of learning and cognitive theories is beyond the scope of this book, certain theories are more commonly employed as working theories in nutrition counseling. Snetsalaar identifies five specific theories that influence nutrition counselors: person- or client-centered therapy, rational emotive therapy, behavioral therapy, Gestalt therapy, and family therapy.[39] Large clinical trials of nutrition intervention have used stages of change, decisional balance, and self-efficacy constructs.[40–42] The original five stages of change, however, may need to be extended for the complexity of dietary changes.[43] Another construct, termed the theory of planned behavior (TPB), is also being used in clinical trials.[44]

Food List or Diet Plan Development

Once food values have been specifically determined for important food items and for dishes likely to be used by the patient population, a dietary screening tool can be developed for the food constituent of interest (e.g., tyramine). Although a diet history can be taken, a specialized food frequency questionnaire is simpler and faster. In the case of biogenic amines, additional questions such as food purchasing and food storage practices need to be asked. If counseling for specific nutrients, such as vitamin K, divalent ions such as iron or zinc, or monovalent ions such as sodium and potassium, is needed, additional questions must address dietary supplement usage and food-preparation methods. The great majority of most nutrients are consumed in less than 50 foods.[29,45,46] Not only is the amount of the nutrient in a given food important in counseling, but also the frequency of consumption of that given food is important. Appendix D.3–Appendix D.9 contain the foods most likely to contribute the minerals commonly involved in drug interactions.

After identifying the foods of most importance in the specific food–drug interactions of interest, a food frequency questionnaire can be drafted with the food names, frequency of consumption, and serving size. Whereas a particular food may be eaten only once or twice a year, if it is consumed in large quantities such as reported for guacamole, the patient should be encouraged to either eliminate the food or keep the serving size to a modest amount (e.g., half a cup). Timing of intake may also be quite important in determining the effect of a food constituent upon a drug. Some assessment tools should evaluate whether the food is eaten with a meal or alone or how a current drug is taken in relationship to meals or snacks.

In developing any food frequency questionnaire, consideration needs to be given to the usual food habits of the population in which it is to be used.[47] Familiarity with common dishes of the region, restaurants, and grocery store chains as well as food products generally raised in the area all help refine diet history instruments to more effectively assess likely intakes.[48,49] Seasonal variations also need to be considered. For example, fresh garden vegetables in summer create a need for close monitoring for those on anticoagulants. Another consideration is the nutrient analysis and common serving sizes offered at fast food and family restaurant chains. These nutrient values can usually be obtained from food composition books, Internet Web pages of restaurant chains, or by writing the consumer affairs office for a given company. Some chains may actually post food composition information in the restaurants themselves or have an abbreviated nutrition label on the menu. Some publications are dedicated to providing fast food composition data.[46,47] In rural areas or communities with small grocery stores, food marts at gasoline stations, or other locally owned independent establishments, a visit may be required to actually see what is being sold. For example, Although home use of soft drink products may routinely be considered to be a 12-ounce can, in some stores 16- or 20-ounce serving containers may be the smallest offered. Choices available to customers in rural communities may be limited.

Individualized Diet Plan Development

Once personal preferences and habits have been considered in developing an individualized plan for diet counseling, several other factors need to be addressed.

Food economics, availability, transportation, and ability to prepare and store food must come into play. In making recommendations about food intake, local markets must be considered. Choice among fresh fruits and vegetables may be limited, especially in the winter months, if small neighborhood or independent grocers are the only sources. For counseling on sodium restrictions, this limitation may be particularly important. Limited delivery dates for fresh meat, seafood, dairy products, and other highly perishable items may make purchase of very fresh foods more difficult for those on MAOIs regimens.

Another consideration is the availability of adequately functioning refrigerators, freezers, stoves, and microwaves in those homes with limited resources. Even the simplest of food-preparation equipment, such as measuring cups and spoons, may not be available. Food insecurity may mean that some limited resource and fixed income homes may have limited or no food left during the final week of the month. Thus, consistent food intakes for diet counseling for lithium carbonate or for warfarin, in which consistent intakes of sodium and vitamin K, respectively, are recommended, may prove difficult to some individuals. The use of food banks during periods of food insecurity may not provide adequate amounts of the right types of food to meet the diet plan. Food banks are seldom staffed with dietitians to assist individuals with special needs.

The counselor cannot assume that patients can even recognize fresh produce in the grocery store, much less know how to prepare dishes from scratch. Young adults may well have been raised entirely with convenience dishes, fast foods, and ready-to-eat items. This is one reason that simply handing a universal diet sheet to a patient does not represent effective counseling. Individualization and development of a diet plan jointly with the patient are necessary to achieve effective counseling.

Every therapeutic plan, whether for diet, medication, or other forms of therapy, needs to begin with specific goals or objectives to be achieved. The implementation and evaluation of the plan then becomes continuous.

Evaluate and Encourage

After the literature review is completed, a screening tool such as a food frequency questionnaire can be devised to evaluate the usual intake of the nutrient or food component of interest. For example, a tyramine food frequency would need to include those foods most likely to contain tyramine and to be consumed by the patient population. Foods most likely to be restricted on a tyramine-restricted diet would be aged cheeses, fermented sausages, yeast extracts, wine, sauerkraut, and soy sauce.[1–5] A food frequency needs to be evaluated for its applicability to a given population by testing in the population.[47] An example of a patient survey by a tyramine frequency questionnaire was reported by Sweet et al.[35] The monoamine oxidase inhibitor interaction prevention survey (MIPS) lists 42 food items that patients identified as being consumed daily, weekly, monthly, or never. Seven of the items were not tyramine-containing items as a test of inappropriate generalization.[35] A patient's responses identify those foods most likely to create adherence problems.

An instructional plan focusing on the individual's usual habits can then be constructed to effectively avoid food–drug interactions. General concepts such as the importance of freshness in food purchasing, preparation, and consumption can be incorporated. The patient can be asked to practice implementation of the plan by selecting foods from a menu list or identify appropriate foods to substitute, such as American cheese for cheddar cheese in a cheese dish.[50] The patient can also be asked what concerns he or she perceives in following the dietary plan. Another strategy is to ask the patient if he or she has any questions. When answering questions, it is important for the counselor to understand why the question is being asked before answering.[51] A common mistake by some counselors is the rush to provide information without first listening to the patient. For example, a patient may ask if one can have too many sleeping medications, not because of suicide contemplation but because he or she has seen two doctors who have both prescribed a sleeping medication.[51] When patients see multiple doctors, they may receive medications and diet information that are not compatible, incomplete, or counter-productive.[52,53] Evaluation is not complete without the patient providing an evaluation of the plan from his or her perspective. The single greatest prediction of compliance with a therapeutic regimen is how difficult the patient perceives the regimen to be from his or her own framework. Compliance difficulty may be assessed by direct questioning such as, "How difficult do you think it will be for you to carry out this plan?" or "Will this be hard or easy for you to work into your usual day?" If the patient sees the plan as being very hard, then ways to make it less burdensome can be discussed. The patient can be asked to make just one change for now and come back to report how well that change has worked. Making changes slowly and one at a time may produce better compliance.

Encouragement of questions communicates to the patient that it is all right not to know or understand everything right now. Encouragement to return for follow-up is especially crucial in those diet instructions ordered late in the hospital stay or at the end of a long clinic visit for tests and examinations. Termed "suitcase instructions," these are seldom as effective as those that allow adequate time and consider the patient's ability to concentrate. Rather than negatively dismissing a request to return for follow-up, a patient may make special efforts to return when he or she perceives that the counselor is interested in his personal welfare. Trying to retain a patient past his or her caregiver's tolerance is not likely to achieve positive long-term learning or behavior change. Although delay of a weight-loss regimen instruction until a better time may be optional, food–drug interaction instruction may not be optional. Brief instruction with written materials with telephone follow-up or a return visit must be done for some medications.

Review and Reinforce

Confucius is credited with saying, "I hear and I forget. I see and I remember. I do and I understand." Another common axiom is that "teaching begins when telling stops." These bits of folk wisdom suggest that (1) counselors need to provide opportunity to review important points more than once and in more than one mode, (2) use of more than one sense aids memory, and (3) practice is essential for truly grasping the whole concept. Teachers are encouraged to provide some form of visual reinforcement such as handouts, transparencies, or slides along with the verbal lecture or discussion. Three repetitions have been traditionally taught as the requisite amount of teaching for the patient to move the information from short-term to long-term memory. Review of major points by summation is one approach to review and to reinforce initial instruction. Telling, however, is not as effective with adult learners as allowing them to become actively involved in teaching themselves with the counselor there to praise and reinforce successful efforts.

Practice Suggestions

Several methods can be used to evaluate, review, and reinforce appropriate behavior changes. The preferred learning style of the individual comes into play here. Patients might be presented with one or more menus and asked to identify foods that are a good fit with the therapeutic plan or foods that would be best omitted. Photographs of foods, food models, or simple food cards may be used as a mock meal or a day's menus. Sorting or selection from these visual devices might be practiced electronically as well as by paper and pencils or physical sorting. Adult learners with a preferred concrete learning style will likely prefer actively handling the models or photographs. The use of live demonstrations or videotapes provides demonstrations of people actually performing the tasks. This allows those who are often termed *Gestalt* learners to get the big picture first before addressing the details. Adult learners with a preferred abstract learning style, however, may prefer simply to read and to practice with pencil and paper or with the computer. These individuals prefer to take the details and assemble the big picture on their own with the counselor simply acting as facilitator rather than instructor.

Observation of the learner who actively practices essential skills allows the counselor to reinforce positive behaviors and to reteach missed skills. Ideally, practicing the skills allows the learner to self-identify gaps in knowledge or understanding that need more study or review. Success in implementing small steps is important in incorporating the therapeutic plan into daily activities.

Another popular bit of folk wisdom is taken from Lewis Carroll's famous tale, *Alice in Wonderland.* The Mad Hatter states that if you do not know where you are going, you are likely to wind up somewhere else. This seemingly nonsensical statement actually points out that if you do not have a specific goal and if you do not check your progress, you may achieve a different goal than you intended. Whereas you as a counselor may have established a goal for the patient, the patient may have had another goal, or taken an action contrary to your goal. As a counselor, you need to undergo continuous self-review of your patients' outcomes and reassessment of your approach with the patients. A checklist by which the counselor can evaluate his or her own performance and skill development is provided in Appendix E.6.

FOOD AND DRUG INTERACTION EDUCATION

The nutrition practitioner may stop and ask how the time can be found to counsel patients effectively on food and drug interactions if this much time and effort is required. The answer lies in two important planning components: (1) assigning a priority to food–drug counseling and (2) preparing a library of materials and approaches to be readily available.

High Priority for Food–Drug Counseling

Certain food–drug counseling must be done before the patient is placed on the drug regimen outside the hospital setting. These are interactions that may cause potentially serious illness or problems over a short period of time. The hypertensive crisis that biogenic amines may induce in those on MAOI regimens is clearly one such interaction. Sudden large drops in the dietary intake of sodium may result in lithium toxicity. Another is the loss of potential drug action due to diet. Examples of this include warfarin and vitamin K, taking mineral-rich foods or medications at the same time as tetracycline or other antibiotics. Simultaneous intake of alcohol and medication may reduce or drastically enhance the effectiveness of different drugs. Even consumption of food with a medication may reduce the effective serum concentration of drugs, such as an antituberlin, which incompletely eradicates the organism and encourages the development of a drug-resistant strain. A sample of a vitamin K food frequency questionnaire is found in Appendix D.4. Consistency in food intake is important in assisting with correct and effective dosage of many drugs.

Moderate Priority for Food–Drug Counseling

Less critical in the short-term but very serious in the long-term is the chronic use of certain drugs interfering with nutrient status. Drugs that interfere with folate status can lead to serious and often unrecognized nutrient deficiencies. Examples of these are phenytoin, nonsteroidal antiinflammatory drugs (NSAIDs), and methotrexate.[54] A history of use of such drugs should be part of the routine medical and nutritional assessment of all hospital and clinic patients.

Lower Priority for Special Food–Drug Counseling

A third group of food–drug interactions are those that specialized nutrition practitioners need to monitor during daily care of patients in specialty areas such as diabetes, cardiovascular disease, hypertension, and kidney diseases. Thiamin status may be negatively affected in the elderly taking loop diuretics, for example, furosemide. These reactions are less likely to lead to a life-threatening crisis, but may increase nutrient or drug requirements over the long term. For example, a high-sodium diet may increase the level of antihypertensive drug required for blood pressure control (with greater side effects and costs) than would be the case using a mild sodium restriction and a lower drug dose. Critical pathways or protocols can be used to monitor for and to identify the need for additional food–drug counseling.

Development of a Food–Drug Counseling Center, Library, or Committee

Table 14.2 provides a potential model for a food–drug counseling library and center. The model proposes an interdisciplinary resource that could be used by all healthcare professionals. If a hospital already has a poison control center or patient health education center, this might be adapted to serve as the central clearinghouse. An interdisciplinary committee could serve to conduct needs assessment, identify existing educational resources, develop or purchase needed resources, evaluate food–drug counseling techniques and procedures, and review adverse events for future directions.

Table 14.2 Components of a Model Food–Drug Counseling Library or Center

1. Books and journal articles pertaining to food–drug interaction including reading lists of materials available in the medical library or online for reputable Web sites
2. Written patient materials with appropriate reading levels
3. Appropriate dietary and medication screening tools
4. Diet plans illustrating appropriate menus
5. Food models, photographs, or food cards
   a. Types of foods
   b. Serving sizes
   c. Others
6. Videotapes and audiotapes
7. Follow-up technology: mailers, telephone, computer-assisted, interactive television
8. Evaluation program for food–drug counseling
9. Interdisciplinary committee on food–drug interactions and counseling

Sample Literature Review of Biogenic Amines, Food Content, and Drug Interactions

The first biogenic amine of interest to healthcare professionals was tyramine. The discovery of the relationship between the hypertensive crisis termed the cheese reaction involving severe headaches and even deaths of some English patients taking antidepressants, known as MAOIs, initiated this interest.

Current drugs on the U.S. market known to interact with biogenic amines are listed in Table 14.3. Table 14.4 provides a classification of the various biogenic amines found in food. MAOI drugs fall into two broad categories.[55] The first group used are irreversible and nonselective in that both MAO-A and MAO-B isoforms are inhibited.[55–57] These are now used primarily as antidepressants for treatment-resistant depression complicated by anxiety. Being irreversible means that avoidance of tyramine must occur for at least 2 weeks after cessation of the drug regimen. The second group is reversible and selective for MAO-B inhibition only, and is termed reversible inhibition monoamine A or RIMA.[55–57] This new generation has not worked as well as antidepressants of the older type. Only one drug in this group, selegiline, is currently approved in this country, and it is used in the treatment of Parkinson's disease.[54] The RIMA drugs, however, may create some risks when consumed at high dosage levels for an extended period. The antitubercular drug, isoniazid, has been

Table 14.3 Monoamine Oxidase Inhibitor Drugs Currently on the U.S. Market

Therapeutic Classification	Generic Name	Brand Name	Manufacturer	Form	Contents
Antidepressants					
	Isocarboxazid	Marplan®	Oxford	Tablet, 10 mg	Lactose
	Phenelzine sulfate	Nardil®	Parke-Davis	Tablets, 15 mg (as sulfate)	Sucrose
	Tranylcypromine sulfate	Parnate®	SmithKline & Beecham	Tablet, 10 mg (as sulfate)	Mannitol
Anti-Parkinson's	Selegiline	Eldepryl®		Tablet, 5 mg	Lactose

Table 14.4 Classification of Biogenic Amines by Chemical Characteristics, Physiological Consequences, and Manufacturing Interest

Group 1: Aromatic and Heterocyclic Amines

Histamine
Tyramine
β-phenylethylamine
Tryptamine

Group 2: Aliphatic Diamines, Triamines, and Polyamines

Putrescine
Cadaverine
Agmatine
Spermidine
Spermine

Group 3: Aliphatic Volatile Amines

Ethylamine
Methylamine
Isoamylamine
Ethanolamine

Source: Adapted from Mafra, I. et al., *Am. J. Enol. Vitic.,* 50, 128–132. 1999. With permission.

associated with tyramine and with histamine interactions.[1,2,32,33] Ingestion of foods containing unusually high levels of biogenic amines, especially histamine, may produce a foodborne poisoning or intoxication. One type of poisoning thought to be due to very high levels of histamine is termed scombroid fish poisoning.[32] Other biogenic amines may be synergetic with tyramine and histamine.[32–34]

Roles of Biogenic Amines

In small amounts, endogenous amines in this group play a physiologically significant role in man and higher animal species.[28,32,58–60] In larger amounts in foods, these amines may cause mild to severe illnesses, especially in individuals taking medications that inhibit the oxidases that normally render exogenous amines harmless.[58] Biogenic amines are organic bases usually produced by decarboxylation of amino acids or by amination and transamination of aldehydes and ketones.[33] Those amines with biological activity are classified according to their physiological effects in humans as either pyschoactive or vasoactive.[60]

Vasoactive amines such as tyramine, tryptamine, and β-phenylanine act on the vascular system, while psychoactive amines such as histamine, putrescine, and cadaverine act on the nervous system.[32,33] Tyramine and β-phenylethylamine have been implicated as causes of migraine and cluster headaches. Two additional amines found in food are spermine and spermidine.[33] Table 14.4 summarizes the biogenic amines found in food that are of interest to manufacturers due to their effects on food quality.

Another classification of biogenic amines is based on chemical characteristics as well as physiological consequences. Mafra et al. divide the amines into three groups of interest, particularly to the wine industry, as outlined in Table 14.4.[61] They consider Group 1 as only rarely occurring with pronounced toxicological effects or perhaps responsible for only slight alteration of human well-being (e.g., nausea, headache). Group 2 is described as related by the same metabolic pathway and traditionally associated with sanitary conditions of musts or vinification that enhance microbial activity. Group 3 has not been described as having adverse effects on humans but needs to be known and controlled in wines to prevent alteration of organoleptic properties.[61]

Low levels of biogenic amines may be found in virtually all protein-containing foods such as fish, cheese, meat, fruits, vegetables, nuts, and chocolate, as well as in wines and beers.[32,33,58–80] Biogenic amines have been considered endogenous to plant matter but are formed in other foods as a result of microbial action during aging and storage.[32]

The level of biogenic amines present in foods depends on conditions that allow microbiological and biochemical reactions to occur. As food ages and spoilage begins, the levels may rise in the presence of certain organisms.[73–77] Tests that detect the presence of biogenic amines, such as tyramine, histamine, putrescine, and cadaverine, have been proposed as indicators of spoilage of fish and meats.[20,21,73–77] Several researchers have concluded that the presence of tyramine in fresh meat and fish is indicative of poor hygiene and poor quality.[61,71–76]

The detection of low levels is possible in part because methods of analysis now allow highly specific, sensitive, accurate, and reproducible assessments of biogenic amines.[32,33,73–77] This suggests that earlier analysis of some foods and beverages may not be accurate because of matrix interference caused by free amino acids and the low levels at which the amines are found such as a few parts per million (ppm).[76] Various chromatographic methods used to quantitatively determine amines are thin-layer chromatography, ion-exchange chromatography, gas chromatography with a packed column, and others.[18] At least one report suggests that reversed-phase high-performance liquid chromatography (HPLC) is usually considered the most suitable technique for analysis of biogenic amines, but other studies have not really found significant differences by various methods for histamine and tyramine.[18,75,76]

Although wine is not high in protein, free amino acids that serve as precursors for biogenic amines are present.[20,61,78–80] By means of decarboxylation reactions, biogenic amines form from the free amino acids described in Table 14.5.[60,64,65]

The advent of vacuum packaging of various types of fresh and cured meat has led to extended shelf life of food by preserving taste, smell, and appearance.[24–26,72,77] For example, current vacuum packaging technology enables beef products to remain acceptable for consumption for about 45 days. This form of packaging, however, produces an anaerobic environment that allows growth of some proteolytic and decarboxylating bacteria.[77]

Biogenic amines such as tyramine can, however, accumulate to detectable levels even though organoleptic acceptance is prolonged under normal refrigeration temperature.[72] Krizek et al. found significant levels of tyramine (15 µg/g) when fresh vacuum packaged beef was stored for 20 d at 2°C and for 40 d at –2°C.[77] The

Table 14.5 Decarboxylation Reactions Convert Free Amino Acids to Biogenic Amines

Free Amino Acid	Converts to Amine
Arginine	Putrescine, diaminobutane
Histidine	Histamine
Lysine	Cadaverine, diaminopentane
Ornithine	Diaminobutane
Phenylalanine	1-phenylethylamine, tyramine
Tyrosine	Tyramine
Tryptophan	Tryptamine

Source: Adapted from Moret, S. and Conte, L.S., *J. Chromatography A.,* 729, 363–369, 1996 and Soufleros, E., Barrios, M.-L., and Bertrand, A., *Am. J. Enol. Vitic.,* 49, 266–278, 1998. With permission.

tyramine could not be detected more than 6 mm from the surface, and one-third of the amine was removed by washing the meat with tap water.[63] From these studies, it is important to consider that tyramine may not be reduced by cooking, but that rinsing well in tap water has some beneficial effect.

Another recent food marketing approach is the generation of refrigerated ready-to-eat vegetables that present potential spoilage and microbial action to produce biogenic amines.[81] Simon-Sarkadi et al. examined the typical microbial population and amount of biogenic amines in prepackaged salad mixtures containing endive, frisee, and radicchio, as well as Chinese cabbage and iceberg lettuce purchased chilled from German grocery stores.[69] Histamine was detected only in Chinese cabbage, but tyramine was found in small amounts and total biogenic amines increased in all salads stored for 6 days.[69]

Histamine

A heat-stable toxin develops in the flesh of red meat fish, such as tuna, mackerel, and mahi-mahi (dolphin), stored at insufficiently cold temperatures in which degradation of histidine to histamine occurs.[21–23,82,83] This results in a pseudoallergic syndrome with flushing, diarrhea, and vomiting, and even bronchospasm and hypotension in severe cases.[83]

Other types of fish, cheese, and fermented foods, such as wine and beer, fermented vegetables (e.g., sauerkraut, kim chee), dry sausages, soy sauce, and related foods have also been found to contain histamine.[32–34,66–88] Responses to histamine include stimulation of heart muscle, sensory, and motor neurons. The stimulation can manifest itself in cardiac irregularities, extravascular smooth muscle contractions and relaxation, and gastric acid secretion.[32–34,85] Thus, histamine poisoning can produce diverse symptoms. The presence of other biogenic amines may exaggerate the effects by inhibiting histamine metabolizing enzymes.[32,82,83]

Certain drugs appear to be contributing factors in histamine poisoning. Among these drugs are isoniazid, an antituberculosis drug that is most commonly implicated, as well as antihistamine and antimalarials.[32,89–94] A case report of histamine poisoning has been described in a patient on isoniazid who consumed aged cheddar cheese that was later found to contain 40 mg histamine/100 g cheese.[90] For healthy individuals not using a drug that inhibits histamase, the level of histamine in the food has to reach a level of 80–100 mg histamine/100 g of food in order to cause recognized clinical symptoms.[73] Crapo and Himelbloom observed that noticeable signs of spoilage occur in fresh fish before histamine can be detected in such fresh fish as Pacific herring.[82] They found no detectable histamine in fresh pink salmon even after 14 days of spoilage and concluded that the level of histidine was too low to produce detectable amounts of histamine.[22]

The U.S. has set a limit of 50 mg histamine/100 g of tuna as a human health hazard. This hazard action level is set only for tuna and not for other fish with the potential to form high levels of histamine.[34] If signs of decomposition are present, a defect level of 10 mg/100 g tuna has been set. Tuna is considered to be decomposed at a level of 20 mg histamine/100 g tuna, even without any visual or olfactory signs of deterioration.[83] Another report of 42 mg of histamine/100 g of cheese was found in a sample of Swiss cheese implicated in an outbreak.[84] Twenty cases, 14 involving fish and 6 involving cheese, have been reported in the Netherlands.[91] Three incidents of histamine poisoning from Swiss cheese have been reported in the U.S., and one incident from Gruyère cheese in France has been reported.[32]

After fish, reports indicate that cheese most frequently causes histamine poisoning or intoxication. Most microorganisms used in cheese production do not produce histamine, so these cases may represent adventitious organisms.[33] Histamine content of wines ranged from nondetectable (ND) to 30 mg/L in several varieties of European (Austrian) and American (California and New York State) wines, as summarized by Stratton et al.[34] Soufleros et al. also found a similar maximum histamine and tyramine content of 31.6 and 22 mg/L in French wine and a minimum of 0.03 and 0.13 mg/L, respectively.[71] Gloria et al. found a maximum of 23.98 and 8.31 mg/L, respectively, and a minimum value of nondetectable in Oregon red wines.[78] Spanish wines have also been analyzed for histamine and tyramine.[20,71,80] Headaches may be induced at a histamine level of 8 mg/L when these are consumed in large quantities.[92] White wines tended to be lower in histamine than red or rosé California wines.[79] More recent studies suggest that although white wines are not necessarily free of biogenic amines, they are likely to be lower than red or rosé wines.[71,78–80]

The histamine content of Gouda cheese made from pasteurized ewe's milk is lower than cheese made from raw milk.[19] Histamine content increased to a high of 25.6 ppm for 15 d, then declined to 11.5 ppm at 30 d, and declined to nondetectable levels after 30 d. Tyramine levels, on the other hand, continued to increase to a high of 238 ppm by day 180.[19]

Tyramine

Tyramine, tryptamine, and β-phenylethylamine are vasoactive pressor amines that are mildly toxic. Physiological effects of tyramine include peripheral vasoconstriction, increased cardiac output, increased respiration, elevated blood sugar, and the release of norepinephrine.[30] Migraine and cluster headaches may result from tyramine.[92] Others have failed to confirm the relationship between tyramine and headaches.[12] The healthy gut normally detoxifies tyramine in food by the enzyme monoamine oxidase. Two isoforms of this enzyme share about 70% of their amino acids in common but are coded by different genes.[93] Additional differences such as substrate preferences, inhibition specificity, and tissue distribution suggest differing physiological functions.[92–95]

The MAO-A isoform is found predominantly in sympathetic nerve terminals where it preferentially deaminates serotonin, norepinephrine, and epinephrine as well as in intestinal cells where it deaminates dietary monoamines.[94–95] The MAO-B isoform is found predominantly in the liver, platelets, pineal gland, skeletal muscles, and brain where it preferentially deaminates dopamine, phenylethylamine, and benzylamine.[93] Both isoforms deaminate tyramine. Inhibition of one of the isoforms thus produces different effects. The original MAOI drugs were nonspecific and inhibited all monoamines and increased the level of biogenic amine neurotransmitters in the brain.[94] Another common effect is an increase of endogenous and exogenous trace amines (e.g., tyramine, tryptamine) by allowing accumulation to occur. This effect led specifically to the cheese effect during the early use of MAOIs as antidepressants.[94]

Cheese

The formation of biogenic amines in cheeses depends on several factors: starter culture, pasteurization of milk, and ripening times.[19] Storage time and temperature after purchase also contribute to variation in content. Biogenic amines occur naturally in milk in concentrations below 1 ppm (L μg/g). These same compounds can be found in cheese products in much higher amounts. Joosten has proposed that the relatively high tyramine formation in cheese is likely due to decarboxylation activity of indigenous flora of raw milk.[95] Starter cultures produce the characteristic texture and aroma of cheese. If the starter culture exhibits decarboxylase activity, the potential for amine formation is increased. Other microorganisms used in cheese making exhibit amine-degrading activities. Such bacteria are important for surface ripening of cheeses (e.g., Muenster), and the conditions for red smear cheese are favorable for amine breakdown because the pH increases and oxygen is present.[85] Leuschner and Hammes demonstrated reduction in both histamine and tyramine content of Muenster cheeses by manipulation of amine-degrading starter cultures.[85] Thus, the potential exists to revise preparation practices and, thereby, lower the amine content of some cheeses to safer levels.

As shown in Appendix D.1, cheeses vary widely in tyramine content. Fresh cheese types, such as cottage cheese, do not contain detectable amounts of tyramine unless contaminated and stored at inappropriate temperatures too long.[4,12,32–34] For patients taking MAOI drugs, recommend that only appropriate cheeses made from pasteurized milk be used. Most processed and American-style cheeses made in Canada and America have been shown to contain no or low levels of tyramine and histamine, if used in moderation.[4,12] Aged cheeses, however, must be avoided completely.

Raw milk cheeses such as Semicotto Caprino are often manufactured with different protocols and under less than desirable hygienic conditions.[98] A recent analysis by Galgano et al. suggests that Semicotto Caprino cheese has a mean content of histamine and other biogenic amines to be considered a potential hazard for food–drug interactions.[96] An intake of greater than 40 mg of biogenic amines per meal has been considered potentially toxic in certain conditions, including high alcohol intake, gastrointestinal disease, and the use of amine–oxidase inhibiting drugs.[96]

Another traditional sheep and goat cheese is feta cheese, a particular group of cheeses that are matured and stored in brine.[97] Tyramine constituted about 40% of total biogenic amines in feta cheese aged for 120 days—a total of 617 mg/kg of tyramine and 84.6 mg/kg of histamine.[97] The low pH and high salt content of feta cheese does not appear to be favorable to biogenic amine formation if good hygiene and low temperature control are practiced.[97]

One of Americans' favorite ways to consume cheese is in the form of pizza. A recent study by Shulman and Walker analyzed pizzas made with double cheese and double pepperoni from several sources.[98] They conclude that large American pizza store chains provide products that contain insignificant amounts of tyramine when consumed in moderation (about half of a medium pizza).[98] This does not mean, however, that all pizza can be safely consumed. Gourmet pizza made with aged cheese or pizza from a small store with low turnover of cheese, inadequate refrigeration, or poor sanitation may contain significant amounts of tyramine. A further safety caution is to sharply limit or avoid consuming beer with the pizza.

Fish

The canning industry is increasingly using freeze-stored fish, especially those fish harvested seasonally such as albacore (white tuna) off the coast of northern Spain.[21] Freezing is a nonsterilization technique that retards microbial growth. If immediate storage in ice or refrigerated seawater is not done, temperature abuse occurs and histamine formation may occur. Histamine may not only persist but also increase during frozen storage, as may other biogenic amines. Canning does little to reduce amines that have already formed. Ben-Guirey et al. found that the use of high-quality albacore frozen for 9 months resulted in histamine levels below 5 ppm—well below the new U.S. guidelines of 50 ppm.[21]

Other types of fish may not form histamine in detectable amounts even with severe spoilage beyond the level fit for human consumption.[22] During inadequate storage and spoilage, other biogenic amines will form.[22] Fish stored appropriately, however, carries a low risk for tyramine formation.[3,4,12]

Meat and Meat Products

Fresh, good quality meat contains little or no detectable levels of histamine, tyramine or phenylethylamine, although it does contain trace amounts of less important amines.[3,4,12,73,86–89] Indeed, freshness of meat can be judged by a significant increase in tyramine and histamine. Fresh beef stored at 10°C (50°F) begins to have a dramatic rise in tyramine content after the second day and a less dramatic rise after the seventh day when stored at 5°C (41°F).[86] If stored at 0°C (32°F), tyramine levels do not rise until day 20. The authors conclude that a tyramine sensor was useful for estimating the bacterial spoilage in aging beef.[86] The results of this and other studies suggest that individuals using MAOI drugs should store fresh whole meat for 2 or fewer days at refrigerator temperature or else freeze the meat for less than 20 days.[72,77] The high tyramine levels found in fresh ground pork and beef reported by Mosnaim et al., however, raise the issue of being certain that ground beef comes from very fresh cuts and not meat that has begun to lose quality.[12] Amines in fresh beef of normal pH and the role of bacteria in changes in concentration were observed during storage in vacuum packs at chill temperatures.[24–26,77] Even fresh vacuum packaged beef had a significant level of tyramine (15 µg/g) when stored at 20 d at 2°C (35°F) or when frozen at –2°C (28°F) for 40 d.[77] For individuals at risk for MAOI crisis, this type of packaged meat should be used well before the expiration date. It is also advisable to rinse well under tap water before proceeding to season and cook such meats.

Cooked cured shoulder ham either minced or sliced and wrapped in aluminum foil had no detectable levels of histamine or tyramine after 8 d of storage at 6–8°C (42–46°F) if the initial quality of the meat was high.[86] A biogenic amine index (BAI) calculated from the sum of cadaverine, putrescine, tyramine, and histamine seemed to be a useful indicator of meat freshness. The authors of this study concluded that high levels of tyramine and histamine in cooked pork shoulder would be indicative of poor quality of meat or poor hygiene.[86]

Fresh beef liver and chicken livers can be safely consumed in modest amounts and within the 24–48 h cook or freeze rule as outlined in Food Safety Guidelines in Appendix C.1.

If sanitation, preparation, and storage guidelines have been maintained, fresh meat may be safely consumed within conservative storage time.[3,32–34]

Fermented Meat Products

Whereas biogenic amines in cooked products were, in general, no higher than 10 µg/g, ripened (fermented) products reached levels above 300 µg/g in samples taken from Spanish retail stores [87] Several of these types of Spanish fermented meat products can be found in Hispanic grocery stores and restaurants in the U.S. (e.g., chorizo and salchichon).[99] See Appendix D.1 for specific amounts and types.

Trevino et al. found low levels of histamine (4–7 µg/g) and tyramine (3–12 µg/g) in German minisalami and a range of 0.5–1.1 µg/g for histamine and 0.58–1.19 µg/g for tyramine in cervelat sausage, a raw meat product.[88,89] Thus, several studies suggest that fermented meat products such as some salami, mortadella, air dried sausage, and others have been identified from many countries including Canada and the U.S. Dry fermented sausages have been analyzed from Finland, Spain, southern Italy, and Turkey.[65,100–104] The addition of sulfite to sausage processing actually stimulated tyramine production and, thus, products made with sulfite should be avoided.[104] In general, ham, smoked meats, pepperoni sausage, some corned beef, and some deli-style meats have been found to have acceptably low levels of tyramine, if fresh and stored properly.[3,4,12] See Appendix D.1 for more specific information on tyramine content of various meat products.

Fermented and Nonfermented Vegetables

The vegetable most frequently found to contain tyramine is sauerkraut, but some samples have low levels while others have a potentially dangerous amount. Mosnaim[12] found low levels in a refrigerated-style sauerkraut, but Shulman et al. documented 13.87 mg per serving (easily exceeding the 6 mg adverse level).[3,4] Stratton et al. conclude that sauerkraut routinely falls well below the toxic level of histamine, and a previous study of theirs based on 50 samples reported an average of only 5 mg/100 g.[34] A shorter fermentation period may produce less tyramine.[34] More recent analysis of sauerkraut in Europe confirmed little or no histamine content but potentially high levels of tyramine by the end of 12 months of storage.[105–107]

Fermented vegetables such as Japanese pickled vegetables (urume-zuke) and Korean fermented cabbage (kim chee) were found to have very low levels of histamine.[32,108–109]

Homemade samples have higher level than commercial counterparts.[84] Tyramine levels are given in Appendix D.1. Other brine products such as olives may contain low levels of biogenic amines but are not likely to present a risk if high quality and not stored after opening for any extended period.[110,111]

Mushrooms, another food used as a vegetable, have been tested for tyramine and histamine formation. Yen noted increases in biogenic amines in straw mushrooms during storages at 25°C. over 4°C.[112] Kalac and Krizek found, however, only safe levels of biogenic amines in four edible European mushroom species stored at both temperatures.[70] Nevertheless, mushrooms need to be stored at low temperatures and consumed as soon as possible after harvesting or purchasing.

Although quite safe when fresh, the biogenic amines in prepackaged salad mixtures and leafy vegetables can increase threefold to eightfold over a 6-day storage at an appropriate temperature.[69] By the fourth day, color changes were noted in some but not all products. Safety cannot be judged by sensory or visual changes.[69] Buying fresh by date and consuming quickly after purchase are the best assurances of safe prepackaged foods.

Kalac et al., assessed the biogenic content of frozen spinach puree, ketchup, concentrated tomato paste, and frozen green peas and found little or no biogenic amines.[113] Good storage temperature and use well in advance of the maximum storage time are, however, necessary to be certain of maintaining low or no levels.

Soy Products and Other Asian Foods

Fermented soy products displayed varying amounts of histamine and tyramine.[3,4,12,32–34] Soy sauce varied widely. Whereas some brands might be safe to use in small amounts, others are known to be potentially dangerous even in small amounts. Soy sauce made from black soybeans is generally higher in such compounds than other varieties of soy sauce. Fermented black soybean and soybean curd have been reported to contain high amounts of biogenic amines.[32] Mower et al. analyzed 20 Asian and Pacific foods for tyramine, finding high levels in fermented salted black beans and shrimp sauce.[108] The other dishes, including pickled fruits and vegetables, had low to moderate levels.[108] The authors note that storage under refrigeration still allows further development of tyramine. A case report involving miso soup was published in which the miso base had been stored in the refrigerator for several months, a clinical confirmation of this observation.[14] Soy milk has been found to have a low level of tyramine.[109] Tofu purchased in Switzerland had non-detectable tyramine, while Walker et al. reported a low level for tofu in Canada.[3,109] More recently, Shulman and Walker tested fresh tofu at purchase in Canada and then after 7 days of refrigeration.[4] The level at point of purchase was clinically acceptable in a 300-g portion, but the tyramine content increased to a potentially dangerous level after a week of storage. Their recommendation is that all tofu and soy sauce be avoided.[4] Given the fact that tofu is so often consumed with soy sauce and fermented condiments, this appears to be wise advice. The total tyramine content of a meal should be kept below 6 mg or 6000 µg to prevent adverse events.

A recent analysis of biogenic amines in germinating legume seeds (e.g., broad beans, chick peas, and lupine) showed wide variation in tyramine content by the end of 5 days of germination.[114] Lupine seeds had the highest content.

Fruits

Fruits identified as potential sources of tyramine include avocado, banana, figs, raisins, and raspberries. Later analysis found no or very low detectable levels of biogenic amines except for banana peel that contains several biogenic amines. Moderate-size servings are safe to consume.[3,4,12]

Chocolate

Analysis of various chocolate bars, baking chocolate, hot chocolate, and cocoa powder has found none to very low levels of tyramine and phenylethylamine.[3,115] Methylxanthines were present in significant amounts according to Walker et al., and these stimulants might induce headaches attributed to pressor amines such as tyramine.[3] In modest amounts, chocolate products appear to be safe. Appendix D.12 lists food content of methylxanthines.

Miscellaneous

The adverse reports involving yeast extracts have been with extracts (brand name Marmite™) actually derived the brewing process. Dietary supplements sold as brewer's yeast and baker's yeast have been found to contain very low or no tyramine.[4,12] There is no reason to restrict other food products containing regular yeast or bouillon. Shalaby has noted that brewer's yeast seems to lack the ability to produce amines during fermentation; this suggests that biogenic amines in beers can be related to the raw materials or contamination during brewing.[32]

Meat bases or extracts that are slurries of meat, made by long cooking, have been noted to contain nondetectable to low levels of tyramine.[3,4] Soup bases, on the other hand, are largely salt and spices and negative for tyramine when analyzed. Chicken and vegetable bouillons had none, while beef bouillon mix and cube were found to contain small amounts.[4] Currently available data suggest that soups made with meat bases that are kept for short times and at appropriate temperatures are safe if consumed fresh.

Alcoholic Beverages

Beer

American and Canadian beers appear to contain small amounts of tyramine, while European beers have varied greatly in their levels.[12,14,80,85,116–119] Tap beer in Canada, however, has been involved in two case reports, and a subsequent appraisal suggested that tap beer can contain significant amounts of tyramine.[14] Ale varies significantly in tyramine content from nondetectable to potentially dangerous levels. Dealcoholized beers may contain high amounts.[14]

Distilled Spirits

Biogenic amines have not been detected in gin, vodka, and scotch whiskeys. Liqueurs and after-dinner drinks may have low levels of amines.[4,12,14]

Wines

Of all the alcoholic beverages, wine varies the most in tyramine content.[4,12,20,28,29,64–66,120] After an early case report identified an aged Chianti wine in Italy as the cause of a hypertensive crisis, Chianti has been proscribed on most tyramine-restricted diets. Walker et al. found no tyramine in a sample of an Italian Chianti as others had done previously.[3,4] As a general rule, white wines are lower in biogenic amines. Wine containing as little as 8 mg per liter has been described as causing headaches if consumed in large quantities.[20,79] There appears to be some potentiation of the effects of biogenic amines when consumed with alcohol. Thus, the recommendation must be made to consume any wine in small amounts.

SUMMARY

Beyond the avoidance of aged cheeses, the single most important aspect in avoiding the cheese reaction is to follow the adage "buy fresh, cook fresh, eat fresh." Any food containing protein is capable of causing a reaction *if* contaminated by certain strains of bacteria and stored under conditions favorable to bacterial growth. Appendix C.1 contains guidelines for freshness.

REFERENCES

1. McCabe, B.J. and Tsuang, M.T., Dietary consideration in MAO inhibitor regimens, *J. Clin. Psych.*, 43, 78–81, 1982.

2. Sullivan, E.A. and Shulman, K.I., Diet and monoamine oxidase inhibitors: a reexamination, *Can. J. Psychiatry,* 29, 707–711, 1984.
3. Walker, S.E. et al., Tyramine content of previously restricted foods in monoamine oxidase inhibitor diets, *J. Clin. Psychopharmacol.,* 16, 383–388, 1996.
4. Shulman, K.I. et al., Dietary restriction, tyramine, and the use of monoamine oxidase inhibitors, *J. Clin. Psychopharmacol.,* 9, 397–402, 1989.
5. McCabe, B.J., Dietary tyramine and other pressor amines in MAOI regimens: a review, *J. Am. Diet. Assoc.,* 86, 1059–1064, 1986.
6. Generali, J.A. et al., Hypertensive crisis resulting from avocados and a monoamine oxidase inhibitor, *Drug Intelligence Clin. Pharm.,* 15, 904–906, 1981
7. Nutrition Abstracts and Review, CABI, CAB International Publishers.
8. Food Science and Technology Abstracts (FSTA), Silver Platter.
9. Boulton, A.A., Cookson, B., and Paulton, R., Hypertensive crisis in a patient on MAOI antidepressants following a meal of beef liver, *Can. Med. Assoc. J.,* 102, 1394–1395, 1970.
10. Hedberg, D.L., Gordon, M.W., and Glueck, B.C., Six cases of hypertensive crisis in patients on tranylcypromine after eating chicken livers, *Am. J. Psychiatry,* 122, 933–937, 1966.
11. Pohl, R., Balon, R., and Berchou, R., Reaction to chicken nuggets in a patient taking an MAOI, *Am. J. Psychiatry,* 145, 651, 1989.
12. Mosnaim, A.D. et al., Apparent lack of correlation between tyramine and phenylethylamine content and the occurrence of food-precipitated migraine: re-examination of a variety of food products frequently consumed in the United States and commonly restricted in tyramine-free diets, *Headache Q.,* 7, 239–249, 1996.
13. Mesmer, R.E., Don't mix miso with MAOIs, *J. Am. Med. Assoc.,* 258, 3515, 1987.
14. Tailor, S.A.N. et al., Hypertensive episode associated with phenelzine and tap beer, *J. Clin. Psychopharmacol.,* 14, 5–14, 1994.
15. Da Prada, M. et al., On tyramine, food, beverages and the reversible MAO inhibitor moclobemide, *J. Neural. Transm.,* Suppl. 26, 31–56, 1988.
16. National Library of Medicine, National Institutes of Health, Medline, Pubmed, and Loansome Doc, www.nal.nih.gov.
17. Agricola, www.nalusda.gov/fnic/foodcomp, April, 2000.
18. Moret, S. and Conte, L.S., High performance liquid chromatographic evaluation of biogenic amines in foods: an analysis of different methods of sample preparation in relation to food characteristics, *J. Chromatogr. Assoc.,* 729, 363–369, 1996.
19. Ordonez, A.L. et al., Formation of biogenic amines in Idiazabal ewe's milk cheese: effect of ripening, pasteurization and storage, *J. Food Prot.,* 60, 1372–1375, 1997.
20. Vidal-Caruo, M.C., Codony-Salcedo, R., and Marine-Font, A., Histamine and tyramine in Spanish wines: relationship with total sulfur dioxide level, volatile activity and malo-lactic fermentation intensity, *Food Chem.,* 35, 217–227, 1990.
21. Ben-Guirey, B. et al., Changes in biogenic amines and microbiological analysis in albacore (*Thunnus alalunga*) muscle during frozen storage, *J. Food Prot.,* 61, 608–615, 1998.
22. Crapo, C. and Himelbloom, B., Spoilage and histamine in whole Pacific herring (*Clupea Harengus Pallasi*) and pink salmon (*Oncorhynchus gorbuscha*) fillets, *J. Food Safety,* 19, 45–55, 1999.
23. Sivertsvik, M., Jeksrud, W.K., and Rosnes, J.T., A review of modified atmosphere packaging of fish and fishery products—significance of microbial growth, activities, and safety, *J. Int. Food Sci. Technol.,* 37, 107–127, 2002.

24. Nadon, C.A., Ismond, M.A.H., and Holley, R. Biogenic amines in vacuum-packaged and carbon dioxide-controlled atmosphere-packaged fresh pork stored at −1.5°C, *J. Food Prot.,* 64, 220–227, 2001.

25. Blixt, Y. and Borch, E., Comparison of shelf-life of vacuum-packed pork and beef, *Meat Sci.,* 60, 371–378, 2002.

26. Kaniou, I. et al., Determination of biogenic amines in fresh unpacked and vacuum-packed beef during storage at 4°C, *Food Chem.,* 74, 515–519, 2001.

27. Pennington, J.A. and Schoen, S.A., Total diet study: estimated dietary intakes of nutritional elements, 1982–1991, *Int. J. Vit. Nutr. Res.,* 66, 350–362, 1996.

28. Pennington, J.A. et al., History of the Food and Drug Administration's Total Diet Study (Part II), 1987–93, *J. AOAC Int.,* 79, 163–170, 1996.

29. Subar, A.F. et al., Dietary sources of nutrients among U.S. adults, 1989–1991, *J. Am. Diet Assoc.,* 98, 537–547, 1998.

30. United States Department of Agriculture, Standard Reference No. 17, Food and Nutrition Information Service, Food Composition, http://www.nal.usda.gov/fnic/foodcomp.

31. Continuing Survey of Food Intake by Individuals (CSFII) 1994–96, CD-ROM, Agriculture Research Service, United States Department of Agriculture, 1998.

32. Shalaby, A.R., Significance of biogenic amines to food safety and human health, *Food Res. Int.,* 29, 675–690, 1996.

33. Gardner, D.M. et al., The making of a user-friendly MAOI diet, *J. Clin. Psychiatry,* 57, 99–104, 1996.

34. Stratton, E.J., Hutkins, W.R., and Taylor, L.S., Biogenic amines in cheeses and other fermented foods. A review, *J. Food Prot.,* 54, 640–670, 1991.

35. Sweet, R.A. et al., Monoamine oxidase inhibitor dietary restrictions: what are we asking patients to give up? *J. Clin. Psychiatry,* 56, 196–200, 1995.

36. Neal, L.J., Functional assessment of the home health client, *Home Healthcare Nurse,* 16, 670–677, 1998.

37. McCabe, B.J., Tyramine-restricted diets, in *Arkansas Diet Manual,* Arkansas Dietetic Association, Little Rock, AR, 1987.

38. Taormina, P.J., Beuchat, L.R., and Slutsker, L., Infections associated with eating seed sprouts: An international concern, *CDC Emerging Infectious Diseases,* 5, 1–14, 1999, www.cdc.gov, accessed December 1999.

39. Snetsalaar, L.G., *Nutrition Counseling Skills: Assessment, Treatment and Evaluation,* 2nd ed., Aspen Publishers, Rockville, MD, 1989, pp. 7–8.

40. Ma, J. et al., The importance of decisional balance and self-efficacy in relation to stages of change for fruit and vegetable intakes by young adults, *Am. J. Health Promot.,* 16, 157–166, 2002.

41. Stevens, V.J. et al., Randomized trial of a brief dietary intervention to decrease consumption of fat and increase consumption of fruits and vegetables, *Am. J. Health Promot.,* 16, 129–134, 2002.

42. Van Duyn, M.A. et al., Association of awareness, intrapersonal and interpersonal factors, and stage of dietary change with fruits and vegetables consumption: a national survey, *Am. J. Health Promot.,* 16, 69–78, 2001.

43. Ma, J., Betts, N.M., and Horacek, T., Measuring stage of change for assessing readiness to increase fruit and vegetable intake among 18- to 24-year-olds: Methods, issues and results in evaluation and research: nutrition, *Am. J. Health Promot.,* 16, 88–97, 2001.

44. Lien, N., Lyle, L.A., and Komro, K.A., Applying theory of planned behavior to fruit and vegetable consumption of young adolescents, *Am. J. Health Promot.,* 16, 189–197, 2002.

45. 22nd National Nutrient Databank Conference, Emerging issues for the next generation of databases. http://warp.nal.usda.gov.
46. 23rd National Nutrient Databank Conference, Keeping pace with a changing food supply, http://www.nal.usda.gov.
47. Snetsalaar, L.G., *Nutrition Counseling Skills: Assessment, Treatment, and Evaluation,* 2nd ed., Aspen Publishers, Rockville, MD, 1989, pp. 96–97.
48. Dickey, L.E. and Weihrauch, C. *Composition of Foods: Fast Foods: Raw, Processed, Prepared*, 1 Ag84 Ah no. 8–21, USDA, Washington, D.C., 1988.
49. Florman, M. and Florman, M., Food foods: eating in and eating out, *Consumer Rep.,* 10, 326, 1990.
50. Kennedy, E., Meyers, L., and Layden, W., The 1995 diet guidelines for Americans: an overview, *J. Am. Diet. Assoc.,* 96, 234–237, 1996.
51. Frankel, E., personal communication, 2000.
52. Skaar, D.J., Drug-nutrient interactions: implications for pharmaceutical care, *Partners Pharmaceutical Care,* 91, 11–18, 1991.
53. Yamreudeewong, W. et al., Drug-food interactions in clinical practice, *J. Fam. Pract.,* 40, 376–384, 1995.
54. *Facts and Comparisons,* January 2000, Antidepressants: monoamine oxidase inhibitors, Drug Facts and Comparisons, 2000, pp. 929–932.
55. Lippman, S.B. and Nash, K., Monoamine oxidase inhibitor update: potential adverse food and drug interactions, *Drug Safety,* 5, 195–204, 1990.
56. Volz, H.D. and Gleiter, C.H., Monoamine oxidase inhibitors: a perspective on their use in the elderly, *Drugs Aging,* 13, 341–355, 1998.
57. Antidepressants 28:16.04, Monoamine oxidase inhibitors, *Am. Soc. Health-System Pharmacists,* 2002, pp. 1–15, accessed May 2002.
58. Geornaras, I., Dyes, G.A., and von Holy, A., Biogenic amine formation by poultry-associated spoilage and pathogenic bacteria, *Lett. Appl. Microbiol.,* 21, 164–166, 1995.
59. Shalaby, A.R., Separation, identification and estimation of biogenic amines in foods by thin-layer chromatography, *Food Chem.,* 49, 305–310, 1994.
60. Lovenberg, W., Some vaso- and psychoactive substances in foods: amines, stimulants, depressants and hallucinogens, in *Toxicants Occurring Nationally in Foods,* National Academy of Sciences, Washington, D.C., 1973.
61. Mafra, I. et al., Evaluation of biogenic amines in some Portuguese quality wines by HPLC fluorescence detection of OPA derivatives, *Am. J. Enol. Vitic.,* 50, 128–132, 1999.
62. Nassar, A.M. and Emam, W.H., Biogenic amines in chicken meat products in relation to bacterial load, pH value, and sodium chloride content, *Nahrung/Food,* 46, 197–199, 2002.
63. Lasekan, O.O. and Lasehan, W.O., Biogenic amines in traditional alcoholic beverages produced in Nigeria, *Food Chem.,* 69, 267–271, 2000.
64. Ansorena, D. et al., Analysis of biogenic amines in northern and southern European sausages and role of flora amine production, *Meat Sci.,* 61, 141–147, 2002.
65. Mello, L.D. and Kubota, L.T., Review of the use of biosensors as analytical tools in the food and drink industries, *Food Chem.,* 77, 237–256, 2002.
66. Nout, M.J.R., Fermented foods and food safety, *Food Res. Intern.,* 27, 291–298, 1994.
67. Nout, M.J.R., Ruikes, M.M.W., and Boumeester, H.M., Effect of processing conditions on the formation of biogenic amines and ethyl carbamate in soybean tempe, *J. Food Safety,* 13, 293–303, 1993.

68. Hornero-Mendez, D. and Garraido-Fernandez, A., Rapid high-performance liquid chromatography analysis of biogenic amines in fermented vegetable brines, *J. Food Prot.*, 60, 414–419, 1997.

69. Simon-Sarkadi, L., Holzapfel, W.H., and Halasz A., Biogenic amine content and microbial contamination of leafy vegetables during storage at 5°C, *J. Food Biochem.*, 17, 407–418, 1994.

70. Kalac, P. and Krizek, M., Formation of biogenic amines in four edible mushroom species stored under different conditions, *Food Chem.*, 58, 233–236, 1997.

71. Soufleros, E., Barrios, M.-L., and Bertrand, A., Correlation between the content of biogenic amines and other wine compounds, *Am. J. Enol. Vitic.*, 49, 266–278, 1998.

72. Edwards, R.A. et al., Amines in fresh beef of normal pH and the role of bacteria in changes in concentration observed during storage in vacuum packs at chill temperatures, *J. Appl. Bacteriol.*, 63, 427–434, 1987.

73. Vidal-Carou, M.C. et al., Histamine and tyramine in meat products: relationship with meat spoilage, *Food Chem.*, 37, 239–249, 1990.

74. Veciana-Nogues, M.T., Vidal-Carou, M.C., and Marine-Font, A., Histamine and tyramine during storage and spoilage of anchovies, *Engraulis encrasicholus*, relationship with other fish spoilage indicators, *J. Food Sci.*, 55, 1192–1194, 1990.

75. Serrar, D. et al., The development of a monoclonal antibody-based ELISA for the determination of histamine in food: application to fishery products and comparisons with the HPLC assay, *Food Chem.*, 54, 985–911, 1995.

76. Alur, M.D. et al., Biochemical methods for determination of spoilage of foods of animal origin: a critical evaluation, *J. Food Sci. Technol.*, 32, 181–188, 1995.

77. Krizek, A.R., Smith, J.S., and Phebus, R.K., Biogenic amine formation in fresh vacuum-packaged beef stored at –2 degrees C and 2 degrees C for 100 days, *J. Food Prot.*, 58, 284–288, 1995.

78. Gloria, M.B.A. et al., A survey of biogenic amines in Oregon pinot noir and cabernet sauvignon, *Am. J. Enol. Vitic.*, 49, 279–282, 1998.

79. Ough, C.S., Measurement of histamine in California wines, *J. Agric. Food Chem.*, 19, 241–244, 1971.

80. Vazquez-Lasa, M.B. et al., Biogenic amines in Rioja wines, *Am. J. Enol. Vitic.*, 49, 229, 1998.

81. Edgar, R. and Aidoo, K.E., Microflora of blanched minimally processed fresh vegetables as components of commercially chilled ready-to-eat meals, *Int. J. Food Sci. Technol.*, 36, 107–110, 2001.

82. Baranowski, J.D. et al., Decomposition and histamine in mahimahi (*Coryphaena Hippurus*), *J. Food Prot.*, 53, 217–222, 1990.

83. Kerr, G.W. and Parke, T.R.J., Scombroid poisoning—a pseudoallergic syndrome, *J. Royal Soc. Med.*, 91, 83–84, 1998.

84. DiMaiten, A., Isoniazid, tricyclics, and the "cheese reaction," *Int. Clin. Psychopharmacol.*, 10, 197–198, 1995.

85. Leuschner, R.G. and Hammes, W.P., Degradation of histamine and tyramine by *Brevibacterium linen* during surface ripening of Muenster cheese, *J. Food Prot.*, 61, 874–878, 1998.

86. Yano, Y. et al., Changes in the concentration of biogenic amines and application of tyramine sensor during storage of beef, *Food Chem.*, 54, 155–159, 1995.

87. Hernandez-Jover, T. et al., Biogenic amine sources in cooked cured shoulder pork, *J. Agric. Food Chem.*, 44, 3097–3101, 1996.

88. Trevino, E., Beil, D., and Steinhart, H., Determination of biogenic amines in mini-salami during long-term storage, *Food Chem.*, 58, 385–390, 1996.

89. Trevino, E., Beil, D., and Steinhart, H., Formation of biogenic amines during the maturity process of raw meat products, for example, cervelat sausage, *Food Chem.,* 60, 521–526, 1997.

90. Kahana, L.M. and Todd, E., Histamine intoxication in a tuberculosis patient on isoniazoid, *Can. Dis. Weekly Rep.,* 7, 79–80, 1981.

91. ten Brink, B., Damink, C., and Joosten, H.M., Occurrence and formation of biological active amines in foods, *Int. J. Food Neurobiol.,* 11, 73–84, 1990.

92. Golwyn, D.H. and Sevlie, C.P., Monoamine oxidase inhibitor hypertensive crisis headache: prevention and treatment, *Headache Q.,* 7, 207–214, 1996.

93. Murphy, D.L. et al., Differential trace amine alterations in individual receiving acetylenic inhibitors of MAO-A (clorgyline) or MAO-B (selegiline and pargyline), *J. Neural. Transm.,* Suppl. 52, 39–48, 1998.

94. Callingham, B.A., Drug interactions with reversible MAO-A inhibitors, *Clin. Neuropharmacol.,* 16, Suppl. 2, S42–S50, 1993.

95. Joosten, H.M.L.J., Gaya, P., and Nunez, M., Isolation of tyrosine decarboxylases mutants of a bacteriocin-producing *Enterococcus faecalis* strain and their appearance in cheese, *J. Food Prot.,* 58, 1222–1226, 1995.

96. Galgano, F. et al., Biogenic amines during ripening in Semicotto Caprino cheese: role of enterococci, *Int. J. Food Sci. Technol.,* 36, 153–160, 2001.

97. Valsamaki, K., Michaelidou, A., and Polychroniadou, A., Biogenic amine production in the feta cheese, *Food Chem.,* 71, 259–266, 2000.

98. Shulman, K.I. and Walker, S.E., Refining the MAOI diet: tyramine content of pizza and soy products, *J. Clin. Psychiatry,* 60, 191–193, 1999.

99. Rodriquez, J., personal communication, 2000.

100. Eerola, H.D., Roig Sauges, A.X., and Hirvi, T.K., Biogenic amines in Finnish dry sausages, *J. Food Safety,* 18, 127–138, 1998.

101. Ayhan, K. Kolsarici, N., and Ozkan, G.A., The effects of a starter culture on the formation of biogenic amines in Turkish soudjoucks, *Meat Sci.,* 53, 183–188, 1999.

102. Parente, E. et al., Evolution of microbial populations and biogenic amine production in dry sausages produced in southern Italy, *J. Appl. Microbiol.,* 90, 882–891, 2001.

103. Komprda, T. et al., Effect of starter culture and storage temperature on the content of biogenic amines in dry fermented sausage polican, *Meat Sci.,* 59, 267–272, 2001.

104. Bover-Cid, S., Miguelez-Arrizado, M.J., and Vidal-Carou, M.C., Biogenic amine accumulation in ripened sausages affected by the addition of sodium sulphite, *Meat Sci.,* 59, 391–396, 2001.

105. Kalac, P. et al., Concentrations of seven biogenic amines in sauerkraut, *Food Chem.,* 67, 275–280, 1999.

106. Kalac, P. et al., Changes in biogenic amine concentrations during sauerkraut storage, *Food Chem.,* 69, 309–314, 2000.

107. Kalac, P. et al., The effects of lactic acid bacteria inoculants on biogenic amines formation in sauerkraut, *Food Chem.,* 70, 355–359, 2000.

108. Mower, H.F. et al., Tyramine content of Asian and Pacific foods determined by high performance liquid chromatography, *Food Chem.,* 31, 251–257, 1989.

109. Da Prada, M., and Zurcher, G., Tyramine content of preserved and fermented foods or condiments of Far Eastern cuisine, *Psychopharmacology,* 106, 532–534, 1992.

110. Garcia-Garcia, P. et al., Content of biogenic amines in table olives, *J. Food Prot.,* 63, 111–116, 2000.

111. Cobo, M. and Silva, S., LC analysis of biogenic polyamines in table olives using online dansylation and peroxyoxalate chemiluminescence, *Chromato grahia,* 51, 706–711, 2000.

112. Yen, G.-Ch., Effects of heat treatment and storage temperature on the biogenic amine contents of straw mushrooms (*Volvariella volvacea*), *J. Sci. Agric.,* 58, 59–61, 1992.
113. Kalac, P., Svecova, S., and Pelikanova, T., Levels of biogenic amines in typical vegetable products, *Food Chem.,* 77, 349–351, 2002.
114. Shalaby, A.R.R., Changes in biogenic amines in mature and germinating legume seeds and their behavior during cooking, *Nahrung,* 44, S23–S27, 2000.
115. Baker, G.B. et al., Simultaneous extraction and quantitation of several bioactive amines in cheese and chocolate, *J. Chromatogr.,* 392, 317–331, 1987.
116. Izquierdo-Pulido, M. et al., Biogenic amines in European beers, *J. Agric. Food Chem.,* 44, 3159–3163, 1996.
117. Gloria, M.B.A. and Izquierdo-Pulido, M., Levels and significance of biogenic amines in Brazilian beers, *J. Food Composition Anal.,* 12, 129–136, 1999.
118. Izquierdo-Pulido, M., Marine-Font, A., and Vidal-Carou, M.C., Effect of tyrosine on tyramine formation during beer fermentation, *Food Chem.,* 70, 329–332, 2000.
119. Fernandos, J. O. et al., A GC–MC method for quantitation of histamine and other biogenic amines in beer, *Chromatographia,* 53, S327–S331, 2001.
120. Moreno-Arribas, V. et al., Isolation, properties and behavior of tyramine-producing lactic acid bacteria from wine. *J. Appl. Microbiol.,* 88, 589–593, 2000.

CHAPTER **15**

Prevention of Food–Drug Interactions

Jonathan J. Wolfe and Jan K. Hastings

CONTENTS

Preventing therapeutic interactions presents all members of interdisciplinary care teams with an ongoing challenge. Many drug–drug interactions occur in limited times and settings. This is because much drug therapy is short-term for acute conditions. The concern about drug–drug interactions will be greatest when a short-term therapy may expose the patient to immediate harm.[1] It will be similarly great when a long-term therapy has the potential to expose the patient to serious harm that emerges slowly over time. Nutrition therapy is necessarily long-term treatment because patients do not swiftly replete nutrient stores or produce somatic proteins when a proper diet is instituted. Both short-term and long-term drug interactions may pose risks to long-term nutritional care.[2]

The first principle for avoiding foreseeable harm is to emphasize patient and care-giver education. This is fundamental because patients and lay caregivers will play the chief immediate roles in implementing good nutrition practices in the outpatient setting where most care is delivered. For inpatient care of persons with deficits in activities of daily living (ADL), skilled caregivers with appropriate education and licensure will act in the patient's behalf. The second principle for patient protection is continual vigilance to detect and plan for mitigation of known and predictable drug–food interactions. Planning education and surveillance are the focus of this chapter.[3]

CONSIDERATIONS BEFORE DISPENSING

Dispensing legend (prescription only) drugs and medical equipment is the first practical step toward implementing an overall patient care plan encompassing medications and foods. Such items as test kits for blood sugar determination and urinalysis, although dispensed and used without a prescription, require education nevertheless. Patient education remains very much a concern; it is fundamental to protecting the patient and to ensuring economical use of expensive products.[4] The same principle holds for equipment needed for nutrition care. Equipment may be as simple as a 60-mL irrigation syringe for bolus feeding. It may extend to enteral feeding pumps that are to be used continuously or cyclically. Access may be by nasogastric tube or by a surgically placed percutaneous enterogastric device (PEG). The surgeon may choose a tube or a button access device. The tip may be placed not only gastrically but duodenally. In each case, misuse of equipment subjects the patient to hazard and guarantees that resources allotted to treatment will be wasted. Caregivers can design their planning to guard against such negative outcomes.[5]

The patient who will infuse fixed formula nutritional products requires the same level of concern about education as the patient who injects parenteral drugs (e.g., insulin, anticoagulants, antinauseants, hematopoietic factors). Teaching how to perform self-care is only the first step. The patient must provide proof of knowledge and competence to perform these invasive procedures before any prescription may be filled. The sole appropriate test of knowledge and skill is the reverse demonstration. A professional caregiver will observe the patient or lay caregiver performing the process at issue. The patient will unwrap the packaging, assemble supplies and equipment, and infuse a dose from start to finish. The patient will also dispose of sharp and other hazardous waste appropriately. Until a patient or caregiver can perform the process successfully, dispensing cannot proceed.[6,7]

Drugs and foods provide other challenges. They must be given at proper times and administered by safe routes and at safe rates. Another common problematic element of drug and nutritional therapy involves storage and preparation. The team caring for a patient will be concerned about the availability of controlled room temperatures and refrigeration, potable water, and electric power. These concerns about drugs run in parallel with those related to safe food handling and cooking. Pharmacists and dietitians will both want to know about the home environment before making the decision to undertake outpatient care. Environmental conditions for patients in long-term care can be assessed by reference to official inspection reports. Those in the private home may be assessed only by visiting. The team concept works well here because pharmacists, nurses, dietitians, and social workers may all determine whether conditions are proper for care. On a continuing basis, delivery drivers and other home visitors can provide updates to confirm that the environment remains appropriate and that the patient is safe there.[8]

The acronym SELF may be used to sum up the four interconnected components of long-term self-care with drugs, foods, or a combination of the two. It stands for selection, education, logistics, and follow-up. Each element carries implications for the patient and for the caregivers in the interdisciplinary team. Each element also offers opportunities for all co-workers to assert their professional roles in a complementary manner. The patient unifies the SELF process. Success in treatment is measured by the outcome that the individual patient achieves. The physician will bear ultimate legal responsibility for prescribed treatments, but the work of leadership may properly shift among team members, according to the degree that each has the information and skills most effective in care management.

AVERTING DRUG–FOOD INTERACTIONS

A rich variety of publications document established drug–drug interactions. Chapter 3 of this text offers a representative sample for consideration. Knowledge of proved interactions allows their mechanisms to be understood, thereby arming the caregiver with some ability to predict problems with classes of drugs similar to those known to interact. It is axiomatic that the lists can never be exhaustive. The appearance of new drugs, reformulation of existing dosage forms, and continuing experience with patient care all guarantee that new interactions will regularly be recognized and documented. Care planners can also use summaries of known drug–food interactions and extrapolate from that experience whether a proposed regimen offers any likelihood of problems.

The causes of interactions spring from common scientific bases in pharmacology and pharmacokinetics. Professionals constantly seek to apply this theoretical framework to practical challenges in designing and monitoring care regimens. This can prove particularly valuable in cases where foods exhibit drug-like effects, as in the case of phytoestrogens and other pharmacologically active foods and nutraceuticals. The scientific basis of understanding remains central to cases where a foodstuff alters absorption or disposition of a drug. The chapters dealing with interactions between various drugs (prescription and over-the-counter [OTC]) and nutrients, as well as that dealing with herbal product–nutrient interactions offer apposite examples of problems and of mechanisms for interaction.[9]

WEAVING THE SAFETY NET

The concept of a safety net accepts that problems will occur in any system designed by the human mind or operated by fallible human beings. The process seeks to plan and to put in place safeguards so that when a problem occurs, the system fails safe. This means in practice that a dose cannot be given, or that a nutrient cannot be administered, by a route or in a dose that is likely to harm the patient.

Doses may be missed. Calories or other nutrients may be omitted for a time, but the patient does not suffer from an overdose or a harmful interaction.

Selection

Patient selection stands as the appropriate first step in weaving the safety net. The physician determines that a person is an appropriate candidate for care involving both drug treatment and nutritional modification. In all likelihood, this will be chronic care for an extended time period. All members of the care team must be involved from the first stage of planning forward to discharge from treatment. The pharmacist and the dietitian properly share in patient selection, the first step in planning. Together they can assess what education the patient (or lay caregiver) requires for successful treatment. If a potential patient cannot safely self-treat, it is appropriate to choose not to dispense but instead to refer the patient for continued care in an institutional setting. Only when the patient's known deficits in knowledge and performance are remedied can self-care be approved.

Specialists in drug and nutritional treatment also share a common interest, once the patient is identified. Both will review orders for accuracy, clarity, and consistency with treatment aims. Each applies a complementary professional perspective to screening orders for potential adverse elements. The mutual process of screening for problems documented in the scientific literature, or reasonably predicted by known principles, establishes important safeguards for the patient. Drug–drug and drug–nutrient interactions are best remedied by detection before any product is dispensed. Prevention is always preferable to remediation.

Fundamental questions for reviewing the regimen suggest themselves. Does the pharmacy have the resources and the equipment to compound required drug doses? Are these doses reasonable for the particular patient and for the environment where treatment is to occur? The pharmacist provides important elements of the safety net by making certain of these basic issues before making the informed decision to dispense. The dietitian's process will be similar. Will the intended nutritional regimen serve the patient's needs? Does the nutrient plan complement drug therapy? Will the patient purchase nutritional products in the open market, or will these be dispensed on prescription? Can the patient afford to purchase particular foods? The planning step provides an appropriate time to reflect on patient selection and to make certain that the treatment fits the person.[10]

Education

Education forms the logical next step for safe therapy. Once the patient has been selected, safety is the paramount concern. The risks of home care are justified by the clear safety advantage over care in organized healthcare institutions. The patient at home is removed from exposure to nosocomial infections. The patient also stands to benefit from gaining the skills needed for self-care. The ideal caregiver is the patient. When the patient is diminished in capacity by disease or other processes, a lay caregiver may substitute. Intermittent visits by professional caregivers (visiting nurse, home care aide, etc.) can only supplement self-care.

Therefore, the patient and the lay caregiver will require thorough education in advance of discharge to autonomous drug–nutrient care. Education needs to cover the practical parameters of care. This will run the gamut from identifying each drug and each dietary element through to daily handling and preparation of drugs and foods. Finally, education will concern itself with monitoring. The patient or the lay caregiver will not exercise the same standards of monitoring as would a licensed professional. There is no time, nor is there need, for teaching about pharmacology, pathology, or physiology; however, education must include instruction about significant signs that drugs or diet is not working or that the patient's condition is significantly worsening. The patient or caregiver must know the signs and understand the seriousness of any interactions if their presence or likelihood is uncovered during the process of planning.[11]

Scientific education and clinical training set in place strong and complementary educational foundations for pharmacists and dietitians. Their continuing professional education adds to that an important resource for patient protection. These paired pillars uphold safety above every other concern, for therapeutic benefit can only emerge from an environment where patient protection is the first priority. Education does not end when treatment is planned and commenced. Patients and lay caregivers may appropriately receive continuing instruction, as well as periodic assessment of competence to perform therapy. Routine assessments by repeated reverse demonstration are appropriate, as are inquiries whenever an unexpected event occurs during treatment. All members of the care team may educate or test. At a minimum, each teacher will document permanently that the patient or lay caregiver has demonstrated learning consistent with safe and adequate therapy. Many teaching techniques exist, but the teacher must match teaching to learner, then evaluate and attest the result.[12]

Logistics

Logistics is a mundane concern. Nonetheless, it is imperative for food–nutrient therapy. The patient, regardless of education and willingness to comply with treatment plans, is helpless without regular and reliable access to drugs, foods, and supplies. Social work consultation will be invaluable in making certain that logistical support is secure. The cost of treatment will be a primary issue. The indigent patient will require guidance through the process of application and certification for public assistance through such programs as Medicaid. The disabled patient will need to work with the Social Security Administration in order to establish benefits. The patient with private insurance needs to define precisely what the carrier will cover and what out-of-pocket costs will be. In any case, the patient will need assistance to fit the price of treatment into a realistic budget.

Transportation may also affect logistics. Adequate public transportation simply does not exist in many parts of America. This is particularly true of sparsely peopled rural states. In urban locales with efficient public transportation, access for handicapped patrons is mandated by law. Even this consideration, however, does not make the bus or the subway a convenient or reasonable means for a recuperating patient to transport medical supplies. In some cases, reliable transportation can be arranged within the patient's family, church, or circle of friends. Where this is not possible, or where large parcels are involved, the providers (principally the pharmacy) will need to deliver directly to the residence.

Caregivers will also have concerns about the suitability of the patient's living quarters. It is important to determine in advance of initiating therapy that the home setting meets minimal hygienic needs. Properly working and accessible toilet and bathing facilities, supported with adequate water and electric utilities, represent a minimum acceptable standard. The patient will require protection against discontinuation of these services. In some cases, this will mean insuring payment of utility bills; in other cases, it will require that utility services be quickly restored in the event of storms and other interruptions. Food and drug storage, in particular, demand adequate refrigerated or frozen storage. The battery life of an infusion pump pretty well defines the number of hours that a patient may safely wait for electricity to be restored after a storm. The patient who requires air conditioning because of comorbidities such as chronic obstructive pulmonary disease (COPD) will similarly require these considerations. Where utilities cannot be restored in a timely fashion, the patient needs a definite agreement to be moved temporarily to a suitable environment.

The team planning and supporting drug and nutrient therapy will require evidence that these logistic needs have been met. The best proof, a visit to the proposed residence, rests on the same logic as the reverse demonstration. A visit is often not practicable. The patient may plan to reside at some distance from the original site of care and teaching. If the patient's training is incomplete, particularly if there is reason to surmise that the patient may not be able to learn all the skills needed for safe and effective treatment, the cost of a home visit may be wasted. In such cases, the team can interview the patient and proposed lay caregivers who are familiar with the home environment. Social workers located in the patient's own community may also visit the home and provide a professional assessment of the living facilities.

Follow-Up

Follow-up closes the loop. The concept is certainly familiar to all caregivers because it is the essential last step in quality assurance activities mandated by accrediting authorities such as the Joint Commission on Accreditation of Healthcare Organizations (JCAHO). In the case of drug–nutrient therapy, the entire team must take steps to ensure that adequate information flows back from the patient to document the outcomes of care. The data will vary with the patient and the treatment undertaken. It will include drawing blood specimens and reporting appropriate laboratory values. Different clinical laboratories will supplement the reports with information about their own normal ranges of values and precision of measurement. The patient's weight and hydration status are fundamental to assessing the efficacy of nutritional intervention. Where the patient has an underlying disease such as congestive heart failure, weighing every morning and reporting the results can be life saving.

The patient requires a communication lifeline as part of the follow-up process. Access to a telephone is fundamental. The patient who does not have a telephone in the residence needs the protection of regular visits by a person who does have one. The care team, on its part, needs to supply the patient with a number that allows access to professional staff on a 24-hour daily basis. The patient will need instruction and reminders to report emerging abnormal signs and symptoms. These will be individualized according to the particular drugs and foods involved. At a minimum, however, they will include reports of nausea, vomiting, bleeding, and any irregularities in circulation and respiration.

Professional members of the care team will investigate all out-of-range reports. More often, the team will simply document receipt of expected reports that indicate appropriate progress. At the end of treatment, when the patient is discharged entirely to self-care, these reports form the substance of a proper summary. Where treatment does not end in the desired outcome, the causes of variance will have been properly documented.

THE PROFESSIONAL CAREGIVER'S ROLE IN COORDINATING THERAPY

Each professional caregiver involved in chronic therapies, particularly those involving drug–nutrient therapy, can contribute significantly to good patient outcomes at points throughout the treatment process. These opportunities begin with treatment planning. The pharmacist and the dietitian will be involved in product selection, including preparing and adapting products for various routes of administration. Designing the regimen will often involve inpatient care, where changes can be effected quickly and complications can be dealt with.

In most cases, the patient will be discharged for self-care, often assisted by the lay caregiver such as a family member. This reality places a premium on using time for education to maximum benefit. Where the patient will be in a home care setting, the protections of a licensed care facility must be replaced with those of a suitable living environment. Discussion of the SELF process indicates particular concerns and suggests strategies to meet them. One aspect of self-care that cannot so easily be met is overcoming physical and behavioral limitations.

The review of patient status and disease state will necessarily require each member of the care team to identify issues that will hinder effective drug–nutrient therapy. Matters of access, utilities, home equipment, and the like can be resolved on the patient's behalf by others; however, the patient must prove to be personally able to cooperate in the proposed treatment. Behavioral deficits such as illiteracy may preclude self-care, particularly in cases where the patient must read labeling and follow detailed instructions for preparation of drugs, foods, or equipment. Physical disabilities such as blindness, deafness, paralysis, and even arthritis and similar musculoskeletal disorders may render the patient unable to lift, open, and measure. Some assistive devices may bridge the gaps in hearing and seeing. Devices to aid in jar opening and lifting may help the patient with diminished range of motion or limited grip strength. In all such cases, the care team will need documentation of reverse demonstration that the patient can perform the tasks. It will also be critical to determine that the patient is willing to do so on a routine, long-term basis. Once the patient (or lay caregiver), physician, pharmacist, dietitian, and other providers agree that satisfactory means are in place to deal with the impediment identified in planning, self-care can begin.

Coordination of therapy affords an excellent opportunity to mold drug regimen and dietary intervention into a model system. Each party to the interchange of planning, dispensing, and monitoring brings unique perspectives and skills to the shared task. The caregivers will naturally seek among themselves a problem solver with the best insight into overcoming each difficulty in chronic care. It will not matter which of them takes the lead in surmounting a current problem. What will matter is that the team—on a continuing basis—met the patient's needs. The professional discretion to apply experience and knowledge to patient care knows no preconceived limits. In a truly interdisciplinary setting, each caregiver will daily meet new opportunities to use his or her particular professional faculties.[13]

CONCLUSION

Termination of therapy offers a model for summing up a broad strategy for avoiding food–drug interactions. When treatment ends, the team members have a last opportunity to contribute to patient care. One of several outcomes will have been reached. In the limited sense, food–drug interactions will have been avoided. If they have not been entirely avoided, then any negative effect on the patient will have been minimized or mitigated as completely as possible. The patient will have recovered, experienced some improvement, achieved no change at all, worsened in condition, or died. The range of possibilities is limited. Even optimal treatment will at times be in vain.

The caregivers will close their own circles of surveillance by seeking to account for the effect that their treatment produced. If the goal was reached, it is recorded in terms of therapeutic end points. These will include parameters such as weight, laboratory values, results of testing, remission of symptoms, and such others as fit the individual cases. Reports of medication and diet practices will be matched to the results to see if cause can reasonably be inferred. If the goal was not reached, this too is stated in terms of therapeutic end points missed. Scrutinizing the record of drug and food use may enable the team to identify flaws in the treatment, as well as variances on the part of the patient or lay caregiver in applying the plan. Where failure occurs, it is necessary to state as clearly as possible the reason for the undesired outcome. Treatment of future patients may improve through identification of present inadequacies.

Drug–food interaction is a constantly evolving area of study and concern. Data to improve current knowledge about avoiding and mitigating these effects will continue to emerge from experience in clinical trials and in direct patient care. Attention to documentation and clear statements of treatment endpoints are vital to producing reports that hold value for others involved in patient care. Proper education and good dispensing are the foundation courses of effective therapy. Careful documentation is the sole means to demonstrate the quality of the treatment process. Teams of caregivers will find themselves continuously engaged in a reciprocal process when seeking to avoid food–drug interactions. They will both draw from and contribute to the literature that protects the patient.[14]

SUGGESTED READING

1. Church, R.M., Pharmacy practice in the Indian Health Service, *Am. J. Hosp. Pharm.,* 44, 771–775, 1987.
   Article describes the status of pharmaceutical care in the Indian Health Service (IHS), services provided as well as plans for expansion of the pharmacist's role in the health care of IHS patients. This represents a foundational level of service and a clear appreciation of how to accomplish the tasks fundamental to pharmaceutical care.
2. Grant, E., Improved patient consultation, *Pharmacy Times,* 56, 78, 80, 82, 84, 1990.
   Article describes a short course given to pharmacists within the IHS to ensure that pharmacy officers possess a consistent level of patient counseling skills and interview skills. The skills described are supportive of the IHS mission and its practice.
3. Herrier, R.N. and Boyce, R.W., Establishing an active patient partnership, *Am. Pharm. NS,* 35, 48–57, 1995.
   Article discusses the role of changes taking place within overall medical practice and how this affects pharmacy practice. It provides an excellent perspective for considering present pharmaceutical care initiatives.
4. The IHS Web site (http://www.ihs.gov) offers convenient access to updates of this model educational system.
5. The *United States Pharmacopeia—Drug Information,* Vol. II (USP-DI-II) offers an authoritative source of information in layman's language about drugs and their possible side effects and interactions. It is invaluable in preparing educational interventions for patients, whether beginning acute or chronic drug–nutrient therapy.

REFERENCES

1. Fleisher, D. et al., Drug, meal and formulation interactions influencing drug absorption after oral administration, *Clin. Pharmacokinet.,* 36, 233–249, 1999.
2. Hussar, D., Drug Interactions, in *Remington's Pharmaceutical Sciences,* Gennaro, A.R., Ed., Mack Publishing, Eaton, PA, 1995, pp. 1822–1836.
3. ASHP Guidelines on the Pharmacist's Role in Home Care, *Am. J. Hosp. Pharm.,* 50, 1940–1944, 1993.
4. Nykamp, D. and Miyahara, R., Home medical diagnostic products, in *Home Health Care Practice,* Catania, P. and Rosner, M., Eds., Health Markets Research, Palo Alto, CA, pp. 139–161, 1994.
5. Catania, P., Introduction to home health care, in *Home Health Care Practice,* Catania, P. and Rosner, M., Eds., Health Markets Research, Palo Alto, CA, pp. 1–11, 1994.
6. Conte, R.R., Concepts of Parenteral and Enteral Nutrition, in *Home Health Care Practice,* Catania, P. and Rosner, M., Eds., Health Markets Research, Palo Alto, CA, pp. 265–284, 1994.
7. Moentner, R., Patient teaching: home parenteral/enteral therapy, *Cal. J. Hosp. Pharm.,* 4, 8, 1992.
8. Bemus, A. et al., Task analysis of home care pharmacy, *Am. J. Health-Syst. Pharm.,* 53, 2831–2839, 1996.

9. More potent OTCs emphasize need to counsel patients, *Wholesale Drugs Mag.,* 40, 8, 1988.

10. Feinberg, M. and Zuckerman, I., Assisting caregivers in home health care settings, in *Home Health Care Practice,* Catania, P. and Rosner, M., Eds., Health Markets Research, Palo Alto, CA, pp. 67–75, 1994.

11. Bartlom, P. and Ramsey, R., Evaluation of Drug Information Needs for Caregivers of the Dependent Elderly, paper presented at the ASHP Midyear Clinical Meeting 24, FFF-5, December 1989.

12. Church, R., Pharmacy practice in the Indian Health Service, *Am. J. Hosp. Pharm.,* 44, 771–775, 1987.

13. Blumberg, J. and Couris, R., Pharmacology, nutrition, and the elderly: interactions and implications, in *Geriatrics Nutrition,* Chernoff, R., Ed., Aspen Publishers, Gaithersburg, MD, 1999.

14. Hussar, D., Drug interactions, in *Remington's Pharmaceutical Sciences,* Gennaro, A.R., Ed., Mack Publishing, Eaton, PA, 1995, pp. 1835–1836.

CHAPTER 16

Drug–Nutrient Interactions and JCAHO Standards

Dorothy W. Hagan and Beverly J. McCabe

CONTENTS

Monitoring and measuring quality of care in health systems is the focus of a number of independent, nonprofit organizations. The National Committee for Quality Assurance (NCQA) was formed in 1979 to review and accredit health maintenance organizations.[1] NCQA developed the health plan employer data and information set (HEDIS) to standardize the calculation and reporting of performance information. An example of HEDIS is a standardized question on nutrition/patient service satisfaction on surveys of discharged hospital patients. The Joint Commission on Accreditation of Healthcare Organizations (JCAHO) is another major accrediting body. JCAHO's focus is on performance. A new initiative of JCAHO is ORYX®, which is intended to incorporate outcomes and performance measurement into the accreditation process.[2] Similar to NCQA, JCAHO has its own indicator-based performance measuring system called IMSystem.[1] A third organization is the Foundation for Accountability (FACCT) developed in Portland, Oregon, in 1995. It is a consumer-oriented system developed to measure quality of care through the human experience.[1] The oldest and most influential organization, however, remains JCAHO.

JCAHO was founded in 1951 as an independent, nonprofit organization that set performance standards for hospitals.[3,4] Standards for both dietetic and pharmacy departments have been included for accreditation evaluation since this voluntary service was offered to hospitals. The original focus was only on hospitals (Joint Commission on Accreditation of Hospitals or JCAH), but by the early 1990s, focus was expanded to provide quality assurance guidelines for long-term care facilities and ambulatory care settings.[3] With expansion into healthcare settings other than hospitals and an increased emphasis on quality management services, professional organizations such as the American Dietetic Association formed quality management committees that worked with JCAHO staff to influence and guide appropriate quality assurance standards for their discipline.[3] Likewise, JCAHO sought input into standards from professional organizations.

The original focus of JCAH was process oriented. How and what one did was measured, rather than the outcome of the process. With a major revision of JCAHO thinking and publication of the *Comprehensive Accreditation Manual for Hospitals* in 1996, outcomes of care became paramount.[4] The focus shifted to competency based process and outcomes. Currently, more emphasis is being placed on improving safety for patients and residents in healthcare organizations.[5] Each of these changes in focus has influenced the way facilities and departments do business in a very competitive healthcare marketplace. The value, however, is improved quality of patient care and services. Specific information about the standards is available at the JCAHO web site (www.jcaho.org).[6] Rich[7] describes a framework for improving organization performance, how it relates to continuous quality improvement, and how JCAHO standards are met by implementing such a process. This six-step process includes setting objectives, designing the data collecting process, collecting data, evaluating the data collected, deciding upon improvement priorities, and redesigning existing functions or processes.[7]

About half of JCAHO standards are directly related to safety, and the remainder are indirectly related.[5,6] JCAHO is planning to establish annual patient safety goals.[8] The safety standards require coordination and integration of many existing safety processes. Medication use and management are important components covered by safety standards.[5,6]

The JCAHO standard specifically addressing drug–food interactions is PF.1.5, which states: "Patients are educated about drug–food interactions and provided counseling on nutrition and modified diets."[4,6] Because standards are not department specific, but rather facility specific, each facility can determine the role of various healthcare providers in meeting the standards. Logically, the two departments primarily implicated in fulfilling this JCAHO standard are pharmacy (drug) and dietetics (food). Likewise, both dietetics[9] and pharmacy[10] are required by JCAHO standards to provide a plan of care for patients that identifies drug–food interactions.[11] In 1992, before JCAHO requirements for drug–food patient education, 51% of dietitians and pharmacists did not consider their drug–nutrient programs formal. Some reported no formal program, but 59% reported that a patient counseling program for food–drug interactions would still exist in their facilities, even if not required by JCAHO.[9]

RESPONSIBILITY

Dietetic and pharmacy departments share many common service features that are influenced by Joint Commission standards. Among these are production facilities, safety and sanitation systems, monitoring programs, patient education programs, acute care, and ambulatory patient care services. These similarities offer the reader a point of reference in understanding the systems performed by two departments that offer dissimilar products. Owing to the similarities, however, there are inevitable overlaps in discipline-specific knowledge, patient care responsibilities, and approaches to provision of assigned patient care responsibilities.

Nursing is often brought into this mix of disciplines responsible for patient education. This administrative alignment of patient care responsibilities may vary among the dietetic, pharmacy, and nursing departments from facility to facility, but each facility and each department must show that standards are being met. This overlapping responsibility has led to multidisciplinary approaches to quality patient care outcomes, but can also lead to duplicated programs in dietetics, pharmacy, and nursing or collaborative services among departments. Waltrous et al.[12] propose a computerized system-wide approach where patient education materials are linked to a database of patient information and educational materials provided are automatically recorded in the patient's medical record. Thus, the materials and information are available to other healthcare disciplines.[12] This system creates an easy mechanism for timely follow-up education and auditing of patient education provided.

The reader is referred to chapters on counseling on drug–food interactions for specific information on knowledge and skills required for competent counseling. The nutrition practitioner, however, may stop and ask how the time can be found to effectively counsel patients on food and drug interactions if this much time and effort is required. The answer lies in two important planning components: (1) assigning a priority to food–drug counseling and (2) preparing a library of materials and approaches to be readily available. The November 2001 update of the JCAHO Manual suggests that the pharmacist prepare patient medication profiles as illustrated in Table 16.1.[13] These profiles are then ideally available for use by various care providers at all times.[13] Another suggestion is to review the standards for assessment by dietitians and identify the most critical points to integrate into the daily routine of assessment by dietitians.[13] Examples are compiled in Table 16.2 from the JCAHO standards and criteria using food–drug interaction potentials from other chapters in this book.

High Priority for Food–Drug Counseling

Certain food–drug counseling must be done before the patient is placed on the drug regimen outside the hospital setting. This relates to interactions that may cause

Table 16.1 Patient Medication Profile

Basic Information

Patient's name, birthday, and sex
Problems or diagnosis(es)
Current medication therapy:
  Prescription drugs
  Nonprescription drugs
  Dietary supplements
  Herbal supplements

Optional Information as Appropriate

Patient's use of illegal drugs
Misuse of prescription medications
Use of investigational drugs
Creatinine clearance values for patients 65+ years
Height and weight for dosage calculation
Body surface area, especially for patients undergoing chemotherapy

Storage/Retrieval

Card files
Integrated electronic database

Source: JCAHO Manual, 04/02/02 http://www.jcaho.org/index.htm.

Table 16.2 Assessment Standards for Nutrition Care and Examples of Criteria and Conditions Indicative of Potential Drug and Food Interactions

Standard PE 1.2:

"Nutritional status is assessed when warranted by the patient's needs or conditions."[13]

Examples

Dietitian's Follow-Up Assessment:[13]	Conditions in Food–Drug Interactions[21]
Adequacy of nutrient intake: current, previous, and required	Energy essential to drug metabolism, Appetite affected by drugs
Anthropometric evaluations: weight and weight history	Weight changes may mean dosage changes
Nutritional implications of selected laboratory tests or results	Electrolyte disturbances in face of poor intake or long-term or high dosage
Physical examination for manifest nutrient deficiency	Anemia secondary to drug interference with folate, beriberi due to alcoholism, riboflavin deficiency due to tricyclic antidepressant
Medications that may affect nutrient status	High risk drug regimens (e.g., anticonvulsants, NSAIDs)
Conditions that may affect ingestion, digestion, absorption, or use of nutrients	Alcohol or drug abuse, GI distress, GI surgeries, OTC antacids abuse
Food intolerances or allergies	Gliadin or lactose containing drugs
Religious, cultural, ethnic, and personal food preferences	Fasting religious holidays, vegan
Diet prescriptions	Low tyramine diet for MAOIs

Source: Automated CAMH, *Comprehensive Accreditation Manual for Hospitals*, JCAHO, Oakbrook Terrace, IL, 2001. With permission.

potentially serious illness or problems over a short period of time. The hypertensive crisis that biogenic amines may induce in those on monoamine oxidase inhibitor (MAOI) regimens is clearly one such interaction. Sudden large drops in the dietary intake of sodium may result in lithium toxicity. Another is the loss of potential drug action due to diet. Examples of this include warfarin and vitamin K, and taking mineral rich foods or medications at the same time as tetracycline or other antibiotics. Simultaneous intake of alcohol and medication may reduce or drastically enhance the effectiveness of different drugs. A sample of a vitamin K food frequency questionnaire for assessing a warfarin/Coumadin® regimen is found in Appendix E.4.

Moderate Priority for Food–Drug Counseling

Less critical in the short term but very serious in the long term is the chronic use of certain drugs interfering with nutrient status. Drugs that interfere with folate status can lead to serious and often unrecognized nutrient deficiencies. Examples of these are phenytoin, nonsteroidal antiinflammatory drugs (NSAIDs), and methotrexate. A history of use of such drugs should be part of the routine medical and nutritional assessment of all hospital and clinic patients.

Lower Priority for Special Food–Drug Counseling

A third group of food–drug interactions requires specialized nutrition practitioners to monitor, as part of daily care, patients in specialty areas such as diabetes, cardiovascular disease, hypertension, and kidney diseases. Monitoring is especially important when patients have been on long-term drug regimens. Thiamin status may be negatively affected in the elderly taking loop diuretics such as furosemide, for example. These reactions are less likely to lead to life-threatening crisis, but may increase nutrient or drug requirements over the long term. For example, a high-sodium diet may increase the level of antihypertensive drug required for blood pressure control (with greater side effects and costs) than would be the case using a moderate sodium restriction and a lower drug dose. Critical pathways or protocols can be used to monitor and to identify the need for additional food–drug counseling.

Inman-Felton[9] notes the ten most problematic standards cited in the 1995 comprehensive manual for hospitals. Three of the standards mentioned appear to be applicable to both dietetic and pharmacy departments in relation to drug–nutrient interactions. HR.4 relates to competency assessment.[4] Regardless of the setting, both dietitians and pharmacists must be competent in knowing and understanding the drug–nutrient or drug–food interactions appropriate to the population and setting in which they are working. JACHO defines competency as practitioners' capacities to perform their job functions. This standard remains a problem in the 2000 Briefings on JCAHO.[14] PF.2.1.1[4] education assessment addresses "cultural and religious practices, emotional barriers, desire and motivation to learn, physical and cognitive limitations, language barriers, and financial implications." Patient education issues about drug–food interactions are addressed in PF2.2.3.[4] Thus, knowing and understanding drug–nutrient interactions is only one piece of the puzzle in meeting JCAHO requirements for accreditation. Healthcare facilities must also have in place patient education programs that are sensitive to the population(s) served.

Which healthcare practitioner should have the knowledge, skills, and attitudes to accept responsibility for a patient education on drug–nutrient interactions? Lasswell et al.[15] surveyed family practice residents and found no formal training in drug–nutrient interaction in medical school (83%) or residency (80%), but 79% of family physicians still felt that it was their responsibility. Some family practice residents believed it was a joint responsibility with pharmacists (75%) and dietitians (66%). Residents scored only 61% correct answers on the knowledge component of the survey, which indicates additional education on drug–nutrient interactions is needed before competent patient education by family practice physicians can occur.[15] Thus, it appears that pharmacists and dietitians must accept primary responsibility for patient education on drug–nutrient education.

APPROACHES TO IMPLEMENTATION

Patient education programs have been approached by healthcare facilities in a number of different ways. Gauthier and Malone[16] describe the use of hospital newsletters, educational in-service training, and computerized drug interaction screening and warning systems to inform healthcare providers about potential drug–nutrient interactions. Label systems, written and verbal patient counseling, and standard drug administration schedules have been implemented in some healthcare facilities.[14] Kassel and Lookinland.[17] describe using a project management format to develop a patient family education system. The project management format consists of six steps: (1) creation of problem/outcome statements; (2) describing the current system using a flow chart, (3) brainstorming, (4) options design and selection, (5) implementation, and (6) evaluation.[17] Storyboard presentations have been used to demonstrate interdisciplinary activities to JCAHO surveyors.[18]

Development of a Food–Drug Counseling Center, Library, or Committee

Table 14.2 in Chapter 14 provides a potential model for a food–drug counseling library and center. The model proposes an interdisciplinary resource that could be used by all healthcare professionals. If a hospital already has a poison control center or patient health education center, this might be adapted to serve as the central clearinghouse. An interdisciplinary committee could serve to conduct needs assessment, identify existing educational resources, develop or purchase needed resources, evaluate food–drug counseling techniques and procedures, and review adverse events for future directions.

SETTINGS FOR IMPLEMENTATION

The three primary settings of patient care where dietetics and pharmacy services must be coordinated for optimal outcomes are admission, in-patient care, and ambulatory care.

Admission

Gathering data on food and drug intakes can often be obtained upon admission to a healthcare facility. Early data collection aids in the best drug choices throughout the patient's stay. In addition to current medication use, information on herbs and botanicals, dietary supplements, food allergies, and food likes and dislikes could be collected. Good screening data can assist healthcare practitioners in providing appropriate services immediately upon admission and thus avoid potential complications to medical treatment. Communication of data collected from such screening programs is becoming more feasible with increased use of computerized data-gathering programs and easy access to information collected by appropriate healthcare providers. Currently, however, data frequently have to be manually reentered since drug and nutrient software are not integrated. In addition to notification of potential drug–food interactions, herb–drug interactions and dietary supplement–drug interactions can be noted and explored further by the dietitians and pharmacists. Such initial data collection systems can save the dietitian and pharmacist valuable time and set the stage for complying with JCAHO standards.

In-Patient Care

The in-patient setting can vary from long-term care facilities such as nursing homes, assisted living facilities, and hospice, to acute care hospitals.[19] Avoiding food–drug, herb–drug interactions while a resident, client, or patient, however, remains. Formal in-house systems must be in place to avoid potential interactions. Communication between dietetics and pharmacy becomes critical. Standard drug medication schedules can be implemented to avoid potential interactions.[10,11] Diet and tray modifications by dietary personnel also can be used to avoid interactions. Such systems can be formal notifications between departments or part of the general admission screening system. It appears that formal notification between departments, so that modifications to trays and schedules can be coordinated, would be optimum for patient or resident client care. Coordination of services is paramount.

Patient education programs that include food–drug information should be initiated while the patient is hospitalized. Again, there should be a formal system in place with assigned responsibilities. The methods used for delivery of this information may vary as discussed previously.[11,16,17] Pharmacists and dietitians, however, should consider the clinical significance of a food–drug interaction in establishing such a formal system because monitoring in-patient drugs and food intake is cumbersome in a busy operation, may not make a significant impact on care outcomes, and may be easier dealt with through increased/decreased drug dosage or other means.

A hospital may have a policy of educating patients only on those drugs in which a severe food–drug interaction has a high probability and strong consequences; some hospitals may have a list of only four such drugs: warfarin, MAOIs, phenytoin, and theophylline. Others may have a list that outlines 30 or 40 drugs. Added to the current food–drug patient education system should be a parallel program on herb–drug interactions. Initiation of such a patient education program while the patient is hospitalized is optimum, but may not be in compliance with patient wishes and desires.

Patients rely on healthcare providers to manage and monitor their drug regimens, allowing the professionals to assume responsibility for this aspect of care during hospitalization.[16] Because hospitalized patients may not be interested in learning about food–drug interactions, discharge patient education programs become more important. Research shows that dietitians assume responsibility for identifying and counseling patients on food–drug interactions more frequently than pharmacists.[11] This is likely because patient education and counseling on diet and nutrition is within the normal services provided to patients upon discharge and while hospitalized. Pharmacists, however, were more likely to be involved in providing reference material on potential interactions.[11] Collaboration is thus important.

Ambulatory Care

Ambulatory care patient education takes on a new dimension in service provided and the service environment. Dietitians often see patients in an office or clinic setting and, therefore, have the opportunity to further instruct clients on food–drug or herb–drug interactions. In this setting, enhanced information on food intake and eating patterns and evaluation of potential interactions can be established. Another form of ambulatory care may be the hospital-based home infusion service in which collaboration and teamwork of pharmacist, dietitian, and nurse are essential to ensure JCAHO standards are met.

Prescriptions filled at pharmacies provide another opportunity to address food–drug interactions and medication administration. Formalized written and verbal information systems can be put in place to avoid harmful or potential drug–food interactions. This formal system is required in some states to avoid adverse drug reactions.[11] The local pharmacist may rely on a computer software program that has limitations as described in Chapter 17. Software programs may simply provide package insert materials created when the drug first went on the market; such materials may not have been updated as newer information becomes available. Another limitation may be the presentation of too much information without assigning priority or importance. Presentation of too much or irrelevant information may lead the patient to simply ignore all information.

Falling outside the purview of either pharmacists or dietitians is the frequently used system of providing drug samples to clients by physicians and clinic staff.[20] This service appears to be more common with low-income clients. Such healthcare providers should also be knowledgeable about food–drug interactions and relay such information when giving the sample drugs.[15,20]

FUTURE IMPLICATIONS

With the increasing number of medications coming into the marketplace; the current enthusiasm for herbs, botanicals, and dietary supplements; and the increase in functional food availability, the potential for food–drug interactions will only increase. The potential complexity of these interactions is overwhelming, particularly if one relies on scientific data to provide the healthcare practitioner with the information and guidance needed to adequately advise individuals and meet JCAHO standards. This challenge will test the dietitian's and pharmacist's information databases and demand a formal evaluation system to anticipate potential interactions before experimental testing can be completed. Enhanced use of developing technology discussed in Chapter 17 may assist in meeting this challenge.

The sentinel event policy requires organizations to conduct an intensive assessment of all serious adverse events.[5] The JCAHO sentinel event alert newsletter available online is a means by which organizations can share information on such events and provide recommendations to prevent future adverse events. This could be an extremely valuable tool in recognizing drug–supplement interactions not previously identified and reducing the risk of future sentinel event occurrences.[2,5,6]

The introduction of standardized measurement data into the accreditation process occurred in 2002 through the implementation of the ORYX® initiative.[2] Standardized core performance measures will permit rigorous comparison of the actual care across hospitals. These performance measures will represent a continuous stream of performance information providing statistically valid, data-driven mechanisms to facilities to support claims of quality, to verify the effectiveness of corrective actions, and to compare performance with that of peer organizations using the same measures. These data may be released to external stakeholders who may use the data to make value-based decisions when they seek quality healthcare.[2]

A major reassessment of JCAHO standards is being planned for 2003. Data from performance measurements and sentinel events are expected to provide significant insight, and coalitions that include 17 health professional associations are developing principles for "constructing patient safety reporting programs."[5] New standards that seek continuous improvement in risk reduction and compliance with such standards are intended to reduce the risk of adverse outcomes for both patients and facilities.[2,5,6,8]

REFERENCES

1. O'Malley, C., Quality measurement for health systems: accreditation and report cards, *Am. J. Health-Syst. Pharm.,* 54, 1528–1535, 1997.
2. Escott-Stump, S. et al., Joint Commission on Accreditation of Healthcare Organizations: friend, not foe, *J. Am. Diet. Assoc.,* 100, 839–844, 2000.
3. Automated CAMH, *Comprehensive Accreditation Manual for Hospitals,* JACHO, Oakbrook Terrace, IL, 1999.
4. www.jcaho.org, Standards, accessed July 2002.
5. www.jcaho.org, Facts about Patient Safety, accessed July 2002.
6. www.jcaho.org, Performance Measurement, accessed July 2002.
7. Rich, D.S. Improving organizational performance, *Hosp. Pharm.,* 29, 390–394, 1994.
8. Anon., JCAHO to establish annual patient safety goals, *Joint Commission Perspectives,* 22, 1–2, 2002.
9. Inman-Felton, A.E. and Ward, D.C., Clarifying problematic JCAHO standards: solutions for hospital practitioners, *J. Am. Diet. Assoc.,* 96, 1193–1196, 1996.
10. Rich, D.S., JCAHO's pharmaceutical care plan requirements, *Hosp. Pharm.,* 30, 315–319, 1995.

11. Wix, A.R., Doering, P.L., and Hatton, R.C., Drug–food interaction counseling programs in teaching hospitals, *Am. J. Hosp. Pharm.,* 49, 855–860, 1992.
12. Watrous, J. et al., A theoretical model for coordinating and documenting patient education, *J. Healthcare Qual.,* 18, 22–25, 1996.
13. Automated CAMH, *Comprehensive Accreditation Manual for Hospitals,* JCAHO, Oakbrook Terrace, IL, 2001.
14. Briefings on JCAHO, *Executive Briefings,* 11, 10–11, 2000.
15. Lasswell, A.B. et al., Family medicine residents' knowledge and attitudes about drug-nutrient interactions, *J. Am. Coll. Nutr.,* 14, 137–143, 1995.
16. Gauthier, I. and Malone, M., Drug–food interactions in hospitalized patients: methods of prevention, *Drug Safety,* 18, 383–393, 1998.
17. Kassel, D.G. and Lookinland, S., Patient/family education program: making the project management process operational, *J. Nursing Staff Dev.,* 13, 303–308, 1997.
18. Lampner, B., Storyboard presentation for surveyors, *Am. J. Health-Syst. Pharm.,* 53, 2578–2579, 1996.
19. Cote, L.K., Joint commission hospice survey for pharmaceutical services, *Am. J. Health-Syst. Pharm.,* 57, 174–176, 2000.
20. Rich, D.S., Pharmacy-related standards in the 1994 AMH; drug samples; and adverse drug reaction requirements, *Hosp. Pharm.,* 29, 73–75, 1994.
21. McCabe, B.J., Frankel, E.H., and Wolfe, J.J., Monitoring nutritional status in drug regimens in *Handbook of Food–Drug Interactions,* McCabe, B.J., Frankel, E.H., and Wolfe, J.J., Eds., CRC Press, Boca Raton, FL, 2003, 74–79, 87–98.

CHAPTER 17

Computers in Nutrient–Drug Interaction Management: Understanding the Past and the Present, Building a Framework for the Future

Pete Tanguay and Howell Foster

CONTENTS

0-8493-1531-X/03/$0.00+$1.50

Computer technology can aid in the identification and understanding of drug–nutrient interactions. Excellent sources of data and information accessed by software programs that provide powerful search and analysis capabilities can aid the clinician in the patient care process. Many different systems are possible, ranging from handheld units with local databases to fully integrated hospital information systems that automatically change diet orders when a particular medication is ordered. New technologies are expanding the possibilities for more sophisticated nutrient–drug interaction monitoring, as well as improving the access by medical professionals and individuals.

As technology advances, computer systems are able to go beyond the boundaries of a single discipline or department. Managing nutrient–drug interactions is an interdisciplinary process and therefore dependent on these advances in technology. Technologies that enable the advancement in this field include improved standardization of data, standardization of communication protocols that allow dissimilar devices to communicate, increased processing power of computers, increased access to data through remote and handheld devices, and the penetration of technology to all levels of society.

This chapter begins with a background view of computers and their role in pharmacy and nutrition. Using this as a foundation, it outlines the primary challenges to improving the management of nutrient–drug interactions and presents a framework to understand new technologies that address these challenges. Next, the chapter reviews various levels of computerization that assist in the management of nutrient–drug interactions.

One of the great benefits from advances in technology is that computers are available to everyone, everywhere. Now that computer issues are not solely the concern of computer professionals, it is important for everyone to take the responsibility to understand the basic building blocks of computers applications. This is especially true when using computer technology to assist in interdisciplinary problems like managing nutrient–drug interactions. The chapter closes with a challenge to every member of the clinical team to be committed to computer literacy and leadership for the sake of the overall quality and efficiency of healthcare in the 21st century.

BACKGROUND VIEW

Bill Gates said in his book, *The Road Ahead,* that we always overestimate the change that will occur in the next two years and underestimate the change that will occur in the next ten.[1] In another book, *Business at the Speed of Thought,* he also said that business will change more in the next 10 years than in the last 50.[2] An understanding of how computers have changed in the last 50 years provides an important basis for working with current technologies and preparing for the dramatic changes just ahead. More important, it helps us take a leadership role in developing and implementing technology to further the goal of preventing or correcting negative nutrient–drug interactions and promoting better communication and efficiency in healthcare.

BACKGROUND VIEW OF COMPUTERS

Computers have infiltrated every area of our society. Although computing devices date back to ancient times when the abacus was used for calculations, the history of computers as we know them today began in the mid 1940s. The following outlines the advancements divided into six phases with each phase beginning with the introduction of a major change in technology.

Phase I—Hard-Wired Automation of Repetitive Tasks

The development of computers was driven by the need to accomplish repetitive tasks, primarily by the U.S. government and military. In this phase, a computer was built to perform one task and the instructions were hard wired into the computer using a machine specific language. The earliest machines were very large and powered by vacuum tubes that required a controlled environment to avoid overheating. Their initial uses were the development of military equipment and decennial services in the U.S. Census Bureau. The significant advances of this phase were the introduction of the central processing unit (CPU), stored memory techniques, and conditional control transfer that allowed a computer to stop and resume.[3]

Phase II—Introduction of the Transistor

The introduction of the transistor in 1956 began the process of reducing the size and cost of the processing portion of computers. As a result, the size of electronic machinery has been shrinking ever since. The transistor was much more reliable and energy efficient than the vacuum tube. This advancement made computer technology available and affordable for large businesses. Computer advancements continued to be led by the U.S. government and military, although many businesses began to take advantage of the computer for the automation of repetitive tasks required to process large amounts of data. These tasks related primarily to engineering and accounting functions. By 1965, most large businesses routinely processed financial information using second-generation computers.

Also, during this period, the first computer languages were developed and introduced. The ability to store and execute programs meant the use of the computer could be customized to a specific business. One minute the computer could be performing engineering calculations, and the next it could be calculating a company's payroll. This revolutionized the use of computers and the software industry was born.[4]

Phase III—Introduction of the Integrated Circuit and Operating Systems

The integrated circuit, developed by Texas Instruments in 1958, is the technology that developed into what we know as computer chips. With the improved processing power, reduction in size, and elimination of many environmental restrictions, the industry advanced through the development of operating systems. Operating systems allowed machines to run many different programs at once with a central program (the operating systems) to monitor and coordinate the computer's memory. This advancement, coupled with the reduction in cost, propelled the software industry to expand the applications for which software was developed.

Chip technology and the wide use of operating systems were becoming widespread in the middle to late 1960s. The reduction in the size of computer chips (known as very large-scale integration or VLSI) expanded the use of computers to everyday devices such as automobiles and appliances.[5]

Phase IV—Introduction of the Personal Computer and Local Area Networks

One of the most significant results of the introduction of the personal computer (PC) is the ability for non–computer professionals to program and use computers on their own. Although IBM was not the first computer company to introduce a personal computer, its entrance into the market validated the technology and propelled the personal computer industry. Microsoft entered the industry with the operating system for the IBM personal computer (IBM PC-DOS 1.0). The success of personal computer manufacturers often depended on whether they were IBM-compatible or not. A whole new type of software known as shrink-wrapped software was introduced to provide the software to all of the non–computer professionals learning to use their computers for both business and personal uses.

Computing power in the hands of end users began to decentralize computing power in businesses, including healthcare institutions. Although the computer departments resisted this change, once people had a taste of technology they found a way to access it independently. In the mid-1980s, most hospital department managers wanted to purchase personal computers for use in their departments, often to have their budget requests rejected because the computer department was responsible for the purchase and control of all computers. This began the back-door process of getting a personal computer into the hospital through incentives from medical equipment and other vendors. Vendors would provide a free computer to use as a diagnostic device with their own proprietary equipment or as an outright purchasing incentive to departments that bought product from them. This led to the development of many clinical and administrative solutions by healthcare professionals who used tools such as Visi-Calc®, Lotus 1-2-3®, and dBase II®. Decentralized computing was born and the users gained control of their destinies.

With the proliferation of the personal computers, something had to be done to address the uncontrolled proliferation of business data. Once again, the computer industry responded with the introduction of local area networks to network PCs back together into a shared server that could be managed by the central data-processing function within a business. The two vendors who dominated the local area network market were 3Com and Novell.

Phase V—Is IBM Building a MAC?

In the late 1980s, the personal computer industry was divided into two camps: the Macintosh camp and the IBM camp. IBM's operating system was open so anyone could build a computer that worked like an IBM. Apple's Macintosh (Mac™) computer was closed in that only Apple Computer had the specifications required to build a computer that could operate software built for it. The advantage of the Mac was that it was very easy to use and came with a point-and-click device called a mouse. The advantages of the IBM-compatible computer included its abundance of available software and its lower cost. Both of these advantages were due to the open architecture strategy of IBM and Microsoft. When Microsoft began work on the Windows™ operating system, the joke in the industry was that IBM stood for "I'm building a Mac."

The Windows™ operating system was late in its development and took a number of releases to perfect, but it has become the standard for desktop computers. Microsoft released its networking software product called Windows NT (which stands for new technology), established a strong foothold in the programming language industry, and completely dominated the office automation market through the introduction and refinement of Microsoft Office™. The result is the state of the computer industry we carried into the new millennium.

Phase VI—The Digital Economy Is Born

The world in which we now live is based as much or more on digital bits of information than on atoms.[6] A newspaper is based on atoms, whereas news content on the Internet is based on bits. The scope of this chapter does not include a full explanation of the impact of the digital economy. The following are some of the characteristics of the digital economy:

- The Internet and associated technologies
- Plug-and-play devices
- Fiber optic bandwidth (While data transmission using copper wire has a capacity of about 6 million bits per second, fiber optics can deliver at speeds estimated to be close to 1000 billion bits per second.[6])
- Integration of various types of media
- Kids cannot imagine life without computers or the Internet
- Object-oriented technologies that allow dissimilar data, software, and devices to communicate
- Shift in power from the machine to the user through flexible user preferences

As the preceding list suggests, digital technologies are certainly able to automatically manage nutrient–drug interactions with technology available to the clinician and the patient.

SOFTWARE, THE KEY TO MANIPULATING AND MANAGING DATA

Software brings life to the computer. It is helpful to know the key developments in the software industry to understand how computers today are able to provide functionality that was only dreamed of 20 years ago. Bear with the technical terms and we will apply it to the field of nutrient–drug interactions at the end.

Procedural Programming

The beginning software languages such as COBOL and FORTRAN were procedural and tightly connected to the data they accessed. Data definitions, and often the specific location of the data, were a part of the program itself. As we saw in the background of computers described previously, this was a tremendous advancement over a computer that was hard wired for a single function. Software programs were compiled to create executable modules of machine instructions specific to a machine. The development of a software program consisted of identifying inputs, processes (procedures), and outputs. Programmers in the 1970s who were bored with their jobs joked about their programs having ESP—extract, sort, and print.

Procedural development is powerful, yet very dependent on the data formats and processes identified in the design phase of the application. Efficiencies arose through the development of common subroutines and libraries of common program code, but procedural languages remained dependent on specific data structures and operating environments. These dependencies limit the complexity of the functions they could perform and their ability to be quickly changed.

Object-Oriented Programming

In object-oriented programming, the application developer thinks in terms of objects rather than procedures. Although a full understanding of object-oriented programming is beyond the scope of this chapter, an introduction to the basic concepts provides tremendous insight to the applications we use on a daily basis.

Object-oriented programming is an approach to programming that emphasizes building applications as a group of objects. These objects represent key pieces of the application and contain all the business rules and processing logic related to that piece. Object-oriented programming allows developers to reduce complexity by hiding complicated processing inside objects and then providing a simplified means of invoking that processing. Objects also help make source code more modular and reusable by packaging both the data and the routines that operate on that data inside a single object that can be used anywhere. Object programming reduces the testing time necessary when enhancements are made to applications because all the objects in the application do not have to be tested as extensively.[7]

In the object-oriented world, everything is made up of the following:

- Objects—objects are code-based abstractions of a person, place, thing, or other real world concept that model their characteristics from a software development standpoint. We can therefore define a drug or nutrient object.
- Behaviors—behaviors are how the object interacts with other objects. These are implemented as properties, methods, and events.
- Properties—properties are the attributes that describe an object. Think of the desktop object on your computer and how you set its properties in the control panel or the printer you have connected to your computer and how you set its properties.
- Methods—methods are what provide the services with which other objects can interact. Absorption is a method of the drug object and digestion is a method of a nutrient object.
- Events—events initiate response from objects (see the next section on "Event-Driven Programming").

First DataBank's transition to an object view in their programming tools is a good example of how software and knowledge base vendors are adopting these technologies. In the initial releases of the data, the *Programmers Reference Guide* for accessing First DataBank knowledge bases was a book of file structures and access algorithms, aimed at providing tools for programmers to integrate their data into their procedural applications. Their new Drug Information Framework™ product for application developers provides the objects necessary for developers to deploy applications on a variety of platforms, including the Internet.[8] The 100-page *Programmers Reference Guide* of data structures and algorithms has been replaced with an 882-page documentation manual that includes 350 pages of object, method, and property documentation as well as 500 pages of quality assurance testing instructions. First DataBank's promise is to provide the data and tools necessary for application developers to deliver Internet applications in Internet time.[8] A promise to deliver in Internet time requires object-oriented thinking!

It is important to begin to think about our world in an object-oriented manner in order to eliminate the limitations of the procedural view and take advantage of new technology. When we see everything as an object with properties and methods, we find new possibilities for solving our business and clinical problems. It takes time, but it is worth it.

Event-Driven Programming

Event-driven programming is one of the central constructs of all Windows™ software. Understanding event-driven software makes you a better user of your computer because you understand why things are happening rather than just how to do things. In an event-driven application everything that happens is a response to a detected event. This is not difficult to grasp and is very important. The phone rings, so we answer it. Our temperature goes up, so we take aspirin. An infection is found, so we administer antibiotics. Thus, the three components of event-driven applications are: an event occurs, an event is detected, and the application responds to the event.[9]

As you use your computer, thousands of events are happening, and Windows, as well as the applications you are running, is detecting them and issuing responses. The mouse moving, the pointer going over an image, the paper status of the printer, and a request for data are all events. Self-contained object methods are executing, changing object properties, and interacting with other objects. When new technologies are introduced, the appropriate objects are changed and the applications that use them are easily enhanced.

Why is this important to the study of nutrient–drug interactions? Patient health and nutritional status is a complex problem that consists of many interrelated events happening in different places simultaneously. Using software written with these technologies, we are able to define what we want to happen for each event, independent of a specific instance of the event and communicate it wherever and whenever it needs to be communicated. The result is much more sophisticated software, solving more complex problems in an environment where events are changing constantly. Procedural processes cannot do this because it is near impossible to predict all of the possibilities for each procedure to handle.

Multitier Applications Development

Traditionally, applications operated on a single machine, even if they were accessed from a variety of devices connected to the machine. The presentation layer (user interface), application logic, and data definitions were all contained in the application. These are easy to build and deploy, but are difficult to maintain. Further, there are significant limitations to sharing and processing data from a broad range of applications.

Two-tier applications began in the 1980s with the proliferation of personal computers and networks. In this setting, the presentation layer is on the client machine and the data reside on a server. The application logic can either be on the client or the server. If the application logic is on the client machine, we have what is referred to as a fat, thick, or rich client. If the application logic is on the server, we have a thin client. Microsoft Office and most pharmacy and nutrition software programs are good examples of fat client applications. When you are using your PALM-pilot to get maps from a database server, you are running a thin client program.

Three-tier applications rely on the object model to deliver applications that access the presentation, application logic, and data layers on separate machines (at the risk of becoming confusing, they do not have to be separate physical machines). The Internet is a great example of a three-tier application environment (sometimes called *n*-tier because there can be more than three physical machines). The presentation layer executes in the client browser, the application logic is maintained on a business or Web server, and the data is maintained on a database or Web server. Here is the key: the application software objects can respond to events independent of the location and definition of the specific data sources and required objects.[10]

Why is this important to the study of nutrient–drug interactions? Multitier applications unleash the power of a connected world at the point an application is processing. This means that applications development is no longer constrained by physical location or definition.

Summary

The preceding discussion is a very, very broad presentation of the changes in software technology. These advancements unleash the power of technology to provide a solution to complex problems that require the processing of large amounts of data by a dispersed group of users. A good example of this type of problem is managing the pharmaceutical and nutritional needs of the patient. The purpose in presenting this information is to unleash your creativity as you imagine the systems you will need to solve the complex nature of nutrient–drug interaction management. The technology is ready, waiting for us to catch up to it.

BACKGROUND VIEW OF COMPUTERS IN PHARMACY AND NUTRITION

The use of computers in healthcare follows the general history of computers. It started out with the automation of financial functions, followed by the automation of operations tasks, the integration of information across the health system, and finally access to information by the patient and all members of the clinical care team. Systems started out as department-based systems and have become more integrated with other systems as technology has advanced. Individually, pharmacy and nutrition software are quite advanced. The challenge, however, is to integrate the information in these systems into a seamless patient care system. A review of the primary functions in pharmacy, nutrition, and nursing software precedes addressing the challenges of integrated nutrient–drug interaction systems.

Primary Functions Provided by Pharmacy Software

Pharmacy systems for both retail and hospital pharmacies have been around for many years. They either exist as a complete, stand-alone, system for patient entry, dispensing, and billing (such as in a retail pharmacy) or are integrated with other patient management systems (such as in a hospital pharmacy) to provide the pharmacy component of a larger system. In the latter case, patient and clinical information is transferred in from the inpatient system, and billing information is transferred out from the pharmacy system to the system-wide billing systems. The following are the most common functions found in pharmacy systems:

- Patient directory (admission, discharge, transfer, changes, hospital billing, patient accounts)
- Drug formulary database
- IV calculations and nutritional regimen
- Clinical information (dose range, kinetics, monographs)
- Formulary database (PDS/FDB, diet info, consultations, interactions)
- Inventory and purchasing (PO, online ordering, real-time inventory)
- General (security, bar code, employee prescriptions, personnel)
- Regulatory (narcotics, prescription management, Health Insurance Portability and Accountability Act (HIPPA), Joint Commission for Accreditation of Healthcare Organizations (JCAHO), pharmacy board)
- Financial functions such as budgeting, cost accounting, etc.
- Drug- and patient-specific pharmacy care plan or plan of treatment
- Integration with medical devices such as total parenteral nutrition (TPN) compounding machines and infusion pumps
- Interfaces to integrate information in pharmacy system with other systems in use such as laboratory, nutritional/dietary, or nursing systems

Improvements in technology, which liberate pharmacists from repetitive, time-consuming tasks, release more time to apply cognitive skills to improve the quality of drug therapy and patient care in a multidisciplinary setting. Many leading software companies provide decision support systems for pharmacists. These are discussed in detail in the "Computer Applications for Nutrient–Drug Interaction Management" section later in this chapter.

Primary Functions Provided by Nutrition Software

Modern nutrition software offers greater accuracy and efficiency, more comprehensive and flexible ways of presenting nutritional information, and the ability to analyze and calculate nutritional information related to patients.[11] The following are the most common functions provided by nutrition software:

- Nutrition database
- Database access and analysis
- Intake management
- Recipe management
- Meals and meal planning
- Client information management (basic data, goals, logs, etc.)
- Nutritional analysis
- Exercise management
- Reporting, alarms
- Progress and clinical notes

For the most part, nutrient–drug interaction information is provided by pharmacy systems. Nutrition software often provides information about potential nutrient–drug interactions, but because it does not maintain a medical profile for the patient, it is unable to perform automatic nutrient–drug interaction checking.

Primary Functions Provided by Nursing Software

In order to fully automate the nutrient–drug interaction monitoring process, the information system must involve all clinicians working with the patient. The following is a list of important features that a hospital information system provides its nursing staff.

- Order entry
- Care plan integration with charting functions
- Prepared patient care plans
- Medication administration tracking
- Discharge planning
- Patient acuity level (severity of patient's condition) determination
- Customized patient reports
- Nursing assessment preparation
- Patient education
- Quality assurance
- Access to information in many departments of the hospital
- Graphical display of patient data
- Automated medical records
- Case management of critical pathways

Clinical and Communication Issues in Home Healthcare

One of the fastest growing areas of healthcare is the home healthcare industry. Processes established in hospital settings to care for patients are also important in home care; however, a number of additional challenges exist in this setting. These include the following:

- Broader geographical coverage by the staff and, therefore, increased need for communication
- A less controlled environment and, therefore, less reliable information related to nutrient and drugs
- Reduced direct involvement of the physicians because they may not see the patient in the home environment
- Importance of teaching the patient and the lay caregiver, if available, increases because medication administration and diet are under the control of someone who is not on the clinical staff.
- Medical records and charts required during visits in the home are not available to staff in the office unless they are computerized or additional copies are made.
- The nutrition, pharmacy, and nursing needs of a patient are often performed by different organizations.

These challenges expand the opportunities for the use of technology.

Summary

Everything in the computer field is moving faster, getting smaller, and becoming more accessible. Much of the technology available today would have been considered science fiction 20 years ago. New innovations in the clinical management of patients, including the management of nutrient–drug interactions, are not necessarily waiting for technology that addresses the issues. In many cases, these challenges wait only for the imagination, creativity, and leadership of healthcare professionals to take advantage of technology that already exists. A good understanding and appreciation of how far we have come in such a short time should encourage every clinician to apply insight, intelligence, and creativity to this healthcare challenge. Looking more specifically at the key components of computer technology helps to understand how these systems can guide management of nutrient–drug interactions.

COMPUTERS IN NUTRIENT–DRUG INTERACTION MANAGEMENT

This section begins by considering some challenges related to providing an integrated mechanism for managing nutrient–drug interactions. With this in mind, we will examine in detail the data, software, hardware, and connectivity solutions that address these challenges.

Challenges to the Management of Nutrient–Drug Interactions

Five challenges must be overcome when analyzing data to identify potential nutrient–drug interactions:

1. The problem is complex. The clinical effects of any interaction, no matter how well documented, do not occur in every patient or at the same degree of intensity. The incidence and degree of severity of an interaction depend on both patient-related factors and information about the effects of the interaction (e.g., dose-dependency, route). Patient-related factors (e.g., disease process, genetics, impairment of organ function) must be individually assessed.[12]
2. The sheer amount of information available is overwhelming to clinicians. Although drug interactions may be immediate, effects on the nutritional status may not appear for months after the completion of drug therapy. In addition, with so many variables involved in the patient's biomedical condition, the presentation of all potential interactions can result in reams of paper.
3. Some conditions cannot be measured. Although laboratory tests may measure many nutrient or drug levels, some important biomedical values, such as vitamin K, defy accurate measurement through a diagnostic test.
4. Manual assessment and documentation systems. Many systems used in the patient care process, especially those that gather key data required for nutrient–drug interactions, are still manual. Any system where the data are less than 100% available in machine-readable format is unacceptable when one depends on data in a digital form for automated nutrient–drug interaction systems.
5. Data collection and communication systems are not integrated.

Fortunately, technology is at its best when the problem is complex, when it involves large amounts of data, and when data are provided in a standard format that can be processed using predefined rules. This is what software is all about and what we will look at next.

Data, the Building Blocks of Information

Many of us have heard the phrase garbage in/garbage out. This phrase expresses the essence of how important data is in all types of computer applications. Gathering and storing data in a usable format is the first step toward building an information system. Data must be timely, accurate, accessible, standardized, and represented at the appropriate level of detail. Data put together in a meaningful format comprises information. Software applications can provide very useful information when data with the above qualities are available. Here, we will look at data issues as they apply to healthcare in general and to pharmacy and nutrition in particular.

Healthcare Data Standards

The ability to cross-reference data across applications to create healthcare requires data stored in a uniform format, independent of the application using the data. The following are some of the standardized data formats used in healthcare systems.

- ICD-9—standard coding for diagnoses
- NDC—national drug code assigned to drugs by the Food and Drug Administration (FDA)
- HCPCS—Medicare procedure code for services covered by Medicare
- DRG—diagnosis-related group to categorize a patient diagnosis
- CPT—current procedural terminology codes used to identify procedures for billing
- UPIN—universal provider identification number
- NDB number—nutrient data bank number assigned by the U.S. Department of Agriculture (USDA)
- USDA food group—food group designators assigned by the Nutrient Data Laboratory
- IFDA number—a number assigned by the International Food Distributors Association to each nutrient

The existence and use of these and other codes provides standardized data necessary to create meaningful, interdisciplinary healthcare information. Information systems depend on standardized codes to provide quick access (through the use of indexes) and produce accurate information. The important point to understand is that, without standardized data, we are unable to take advantage of the powerful processing capabilities of computer technology.

National Drug Code (NDC)

The NDC code is the primary piece of data used to identify drug data and create drug information, including nutrient–drug interaction reports. The NDC system was originally established as an essential part of an out-of-hospital drug reimbursement program under Medicare. The NDC serves as a universal product identifier for human drugs.

The Drug Listing Act of 1972, amending the Federal Food, Drug, and Cosmetic Act, became effective February 1, 1973. Its purpose is to provide the commissioner of the FDA a current list of all drugs manufactured, prepared, propagated, compounded, or processed by a drug establishment registered under the Federal Food, Drug, and Cosmetic Act. The Act requires submission of information on commercially marketed drugs and is used in the enforcement of the Federal Food, Drug, and Cosmetic Act.[13] Complete information and files are available in the Center for Drug Evaluation and Research section of the U.S. FDA Web site (www.fda.gov).

Components of the NDC

Each drug product listed under Section 510 of the Federal Food, Drug, and Cosmetic Act is assigned a unique ten-digit, three-segment number. This number, known as the NDC, identifies the labeler/vendor, product, and package size. The following are the meanings for each part of the code:

- The first segment, the labeler code, is assigned by the FDA. A labeler is any firm that manufactures, repacks, or distributes a drug product.
- The second segment, the product code, identifies a specific strength, dosage form, and formulation for a particular firm.
- The third segment, the package code, identifies package sizes. Both the product and package codes are assigned by the firm.

The NDC will be in one of the following configurations: 4-4-2, 5-3-2, or 5-4-1. For consistency, other government agencies may display the NDC in an 11-digit format. For example, the Healthcare Financing Administration (HCFA) displays the labeler code as five digits with leading zeros; the product code as four digits with leading zeros; the package size as two characters with leading zeros.[14]

In addition to the NDC code, a number of other data fields are important to understand when using drug data. These are as follows:

- Product trade name or catalog name
- Dosage form—tablet, gel, powder, lipstick, spray, lotion, etc.
- Routes of administration—oral, nasal, respiratory, enteral, subcutaneous, etc.
- Active ingredient(s)—ingredients that constitute an NDC, linked to an ingredient file
- Strength—strength of the ingredient or combined ingredients
- Unit—milligram, ounce, milliequivalent, tablespoon, etc.
- Package size and type—box, vial, bottle, syringe, etc.
- Major drug class—the major drug class is a general therapeutic or pharmacological classification scheme for drug products reported to the FDA under the provisions of the drug listing act.

These and other fields of raw data about each drug provide the building blocks to build pharmaceutical information. The NDC code is the primary standard for nutrient–drug interactions, just as the UPC product code is the primary standard for purchasing and scanning systems for the products we buy in stores.

Clinical Knowledge Bases

Scholars and pharmaceutical research companies compile information from primary biomedical literature, critically evaluate the studies, and provide an authoritative consensus as to the clinical relevance of the published information. This information is assembled into information products referred to as knowledge bases. These knowledge bases, accessed by NDC code, are integrated into pharmacy systems to provide drug interaction information reports.

Five providers of electronic drug information as described previously are as follows:

- Micromedex—www.micromedex.com
- First DataBank—www.firstdatabank.com
- Facts and Comparisons—www.factsandcomparisons.com and www.drugfacts.com
- Gold Standard Multimedia—www.gsm.com
- Multum Information Services—www.multum.com

A tremendous amount of information can be found on these sites (and the sites linked to these sites) that is useful in understanding drug therapy. Time spent studying the information on these Internet sites, in the context of the information in this book, will provide a deeper understanding and appreciation for clinical knowledge bases and their importance to the management of nutrient–drug interactions.

Sources of Nutrition Data

Most nutrition software developers use one of the three USDA data sets as their primary sources of data.[15] These databases, along with information about them, are available at the USDA Web site, www.usda.gov. The database names are as follows:

- The Nutrient Database for Standard Reference
- The Nutritive Value of Foods
- The Survey Nutrient Database

Nutrition databases do not contain drug information, although nutrition information compiled from them may contain warnings or precautions regarding the interaction of certain drugs and nutrients. The primary source of data and information used for automated nutrient–drug interaction checking are the pharmacy databases and knowledge bases.

COMPUTER APPLICATIONS FOR NUTRIENT–DRUG INTERACTION MANAGEMENT

In this section, we will look at how drug interaction checking is performed in traditional pharmacy software, followed by a discussion and examples of decision support systems that extend these capabilities. Finally, we will look at information and systems available to the patient via the Internet.

Drug Interaction Checking in Traditional Pharmacy Software

Drug interaction checking functionality has been an essential part of pharmacy systems for quite some time. Most programs have been developed using procedural development languages. From a technical perspective, it is a very simple process, and it is readily examined by looking at the inputs, processes, and outputs in the interaction checking process.

The following are the inputs required for drug interaction checking:

- Basic patient data captured during the intake and assessment process including the sex, height, weight, birth date, etc.
- Prior adverse drug reaction and allergy information for the patient
- System setup parameters that dictate user selections such as the significance level (see below) of interactions to be included in reporting, location of files, security, etc.
- Drug formulary containing the individual drug items that are available to the pharmacist when entering prescription orders
- Clinical knowledge base from companies such as First DataBank, as mentioned previously
- Prescription orders, including the drugs and the associated NDC code
- Medication profile of all other drugs the patient is on or has been on in the recent past; typically, this is gathered through the nursing assessment process

With the preceding information, you can perform a drug interaction check. The software program processes the preceding data according to the logic defined by the company that established the knowledge base. It is important to note that no nutritional data or information is used in the drug interaction process. The nutrient–drug interaction information is provided as part of the outputs as discussed below. The drug interaction checking process is usually executed automatically when a prescription is entered or filled by a pharmacist. In addition, most systems allow the pharmacist to check for drug interactions on demand.

The drug interaction checking process found in most pharmacy systems produces the following outputs:

- Patient education monograph for the drugs being dispensed. The monograph provides the drug name, generic drug name, approved indications for the drug, how to use the medication, side effects, and precautions. The information on the drug monograph is not specific to the patient. It may include nutrition-related information such as whether to take it with food and a list of foods that should not be taken with the medication.
- Drug interaction monograph based on the patient information and the medication profile. A drug interaction monograph typically contains the following information:
  - The drugs, drug classes, and nutrients that will interact; known and potentially interacting drugs are listed; common trade names are given for ease of reference
  - A significance level that is assigned based on the severity and documentation
  - Whether the onset is rapid (within 24 h) or delayed

- Whether the severity is major (life-threatening or permanent damage, moderate (deterioration of patient's status) or minor (bothersome or little effect)
- The confidence that an interaction can occur—This evaluation is based on supporting biomedical literature. The discussion in each monograph provides specific comments on the data reviewed. The documentation is either established (proved to occur in well controlled studies), probable (very likely, but not proved clinically), suspected (may occur, some good data, but needs more study), possible (could occur, but data are very limited), or unlikely (doubtful, no good evidence of a clinical effect).
- Discussion—brief review of published data and selected primary references
- The pharmacological effects and clinical manifestations
- The mechanism or how the interaction occurs
- How to manage the interaction or the appropriate action to prevent or respond to an interaction
- Discussion and references that support the clinical information[16]
- In addition to the above reports, patient medication files are generally updated to indicate that a drug interaction check was performed.

Outputs from the preceding process can be extremely lengthy if the patient is seriously ill or takes many medications. The drug interaction checking process produces information that the clinical team must then apply to support important decisions. This information must be received on a timely basis and analyzed along with the data and information from the dietary, nursing, and diagnostic systems. When specific conditions (events) exist, action (behaviors—methods and properties) must be taken to prevent undesirable results (events). If the system is set to include all severity levels (the last two levels being possible and unlikely), filling a prescription for a patient taking many different medications may easily generate 20 or more drug interaction reports. At the volume of prescription processing in most pharmacies, this is a tremendous amount of information to go through to find the one possible interaction that is significant to the patient.

Sophisticated systems enable users to specify these conditions (events) based on specific criteria (rules or event properties) and specify what action (actions or behaviors) needs to be taken. These are appropriately called decisions support or alert systems and are the logical extension of our traditional pharmacy systems using the new technology described earlier.

Decision Support and Clinical Alert Systems

Two types of systems have the potential to address challenges to nutrient–drug interaction checking identified previously. These are decision support systems and clinical alert systems. These are available as healthcare-specific products as well as generic software tools:

- Decision support systems are interactive, computer-based systems intended to help decision makers use data and models to identify and solve problems and make decisions. Alert- or event-based systems automatically communicate data or information electronically, based on specific criteria and destination addresses (text pagers, telephone, e-mail, print, fax, etc.). Four powerful systems for the pharmacy industry are listed next. Keep in mind, the application of these tools extends far beyond the pharmacy area of the healthcare system and, by design, these are ideal for addressing the interdisciplinary challenges of patient care. The products undergo continual development, and their inclusion here is not intended to represent an inclusive list or to imply any endorsement of any product as superior to any others in the marketplace.

- The Siemens Pharmacy System™: decision assistance[17]
- Sunquest Information Systems™: clinical event manager[18]
- McKessonHBOC™: horizon alert system[19]
- Cerner Corporation™: discern expert[20]

Time spent studying the information on these Internet sites, in the context of the information in this book, will provide a deeper understanding and appreciation for the way new technologies are addressing the complexities of nutrient–drug interaction management. The following is a summary of information about these systems, which illustrates the power of decision support and alert systems for the management of nutrient–drug interactions:

- These systems provide the ability to interact with a variety of databases to perform complex calculations and generate user-defined alerts.
- They provide the ability to make medication recommendations based on changes in dietary status. For example, by including dietary status as a part of an antibiotic rule clinicians can be prompted to consider the cost savings of switching from an intravenous medication to an oral dosage form when the patient's status warrants.
- They provide diagnostic results, such as laboratory and radiology results, and trigger clinical messages based on user-defined rules. Messages are sent to clinicians based on filters that exclude messages unrelated to their patient load.
- They provide information to wireless and mobile devices integrated with scheduling and staff assignment systems to ensure the message gets to the appropriate person.
- They can provide information directly to the patient.
- They provide alerts and messages specific to user-defined protocols. For example, an alert could be set up for a specific drug such as Coumadin® or the existence of a text string in the education monograph such as "diabetic," "vitamin K" or "grapefruit juice."

Systems like these are possible, in part, because application development has moved away from single system, procedural applications to multitier, object-oriented and event-driven applications. With these technologies, decision support systems can be developed that process data based on user-defined rules, present information in the form of alerts and exception reports, and deliver the information to a variety of devices (objects) that are set up to receive them. In fact, the beauty of object orientation is that the object that creates the alert is not concerned with the object that requests or sends the information. Furthermore, the object that presents the information can be updated to handle a variety of devices capable of receiving it. This is very important to understand.

The good news is that technology is here and solutions are coming. The bad news is that these systems require the involvement of the entire health system, including risk taking and leadership in each department. As clinicians, we must change our way of thinking and lead the process of changing our institutions to accept and implement these new systems.

Computerized Prescription Ordering and Handheld Systems

In November 1999, the Institute of Medicine (IOM) of the National Academy of Sciences published a report, *To Err Is Human,* which highlights the prevalence and consequences of medical errors. "Avoidable medical mistakes kill anywhere from 44,000 to 98,000 people a year—more than breast cancer, highway accidents, or AIDS." The report also states that more than 7,000 deaths are caused by medication errors.[21] The IOM study found that 50% of hospital medication errors stem from the prescription-ordering process. Still, hospitals have been slow to adopt technology that supersedes systems for handwritten treatment orders. According to Arnold Milstein, a San Francisco physician and national healthcare leader, "Of the one-third of hospitals nationwide that have installed computerized order-entry systems, only 1 percent require physicians to use them."[22]

AdvancePCS (www.advancepcsrx.com) and ePocrates (www.epocrates.com) reported the results of a study where the ePocrates software product was used on a Palm Vx (www.palm.com) handheld device at the point of care in order to provide drug reference and formulary information to the patient. Of more than 100 physicians who participated in the project, over 80% said the program was valuable or very valuable. The project provided the ability to use a handheld device to access drug information and write prescription orders. The physicians who participated in the project reported the following:

- The handheld solution improved quality of care because it helped the physician offer lower copays, prescribe correctly the first time, and increase prescription accuracy.
- Pharmacy call volume related to prescribing choices declined after physicians began using the handheld devices.
- Seventy-five percent of the physicians believe the technology is likely to influence their choices of prescription medications to more appropriate, cost-effective drugs.
- The information at the point of care can reduce errors, help doctors choose the appropriate medication, and reduce patients' out-of-pocket expenses.[23]

Applications like these, as well as the decision support system applications discussed previously, use technology to improve the quality of care provided to patients.

Internet-Based Systems Available to the Patient

No one cares as much about patient health as patients themselves. An individual's health is the shared responsibility of the patient, the social support system (usually the family), and the clinician. The role of the clinician should be the use of knowledge and professional status to guide the patient through the day-to-day management of personal health, with the patient assuming a participative, cooperative role. The Internet provides a tremendous new set of resources for patients to apply to these responsibilities. The following lists some of the functions of Internet-based software and technology that the patient can use when exercising personal responsibility for nutrient–drug interaction monitoring:[24]

- Drug information and search capabilities available from healthcare providers such as Johns Hopkins (www.intellihealth.com) and drug knowledge base distributors (www.gsm.com)
- Advancements in secure access and encryption technology address the privacy needs of patients
- Secured access to a patient's medication profile and e-mail access to pharmacists and dieticians
- Disease-related support groups available through the Internet
- An online method for consumers to report adverse drug reactions as well as any other matter the FDA regulates

A tremendous amount of information residing on the Internet is readily available to the patient; however, great care should be taken to understand and validate the sources of information before making medical decisions. Some sources are outdated or poorly updated or simply incorrect. This content is inherently dangerous. Some others contain hidden endorsements for products or biased viewpoints. Every user—lay or professional—will best proceed by being properly critical of each site, source, and recommendation. Bad information is often worse than no information at all.

Promises of the Integrated Healthcare Systems

The consolidation of hospitals into integrated healthcare systems creates economies of scale for the implementation of technology across the patient care continuum. This will have a significant impact on the coordination of systems that address interdisciplinary patient care challenges. Today, over 250 integrated delivery networks (IDNs) exist in the U.S.

According to a recent study by the U.S. Senate Labor and Human Resources Committee, of the current $1 trillion spent on healthcare, slightly less than one-half is spent on required care. Of the remainder, avoidable care consumes $330 billion, including an estimated $100 billion to resolve medication errors. Administrative costs consume another $180 billion, including an estimated $18 billion in logistics and supply-related waste.[26]

Integrated delivery networks and large computer software vendors are working on the following initiatives that will have an impact on the nutrient–drug interactions management problem in healthcare:

- Provide a lifetime clinical record (LCR) for all medical information for a patient, regardless of the provider.
- Automate labor processes using robots and dispensing devices to eliminate errors and free up more time for patient care.
- Optimize the use of pharmaceuticals and supplies to provide the right product and the right quantity for the patient.
- Computerize physician ordering and care management.
- Provide advanced decision support software that is rules-based and has access to all of the data across the integrated delivery network.

- Provide clinician productivity tools to improve the productivity of physicians, pharmacists, and nurses to enable them to spend more time in direct patient care.
- Provide standardized data exchange using protocols such as HL-7.

Summary

Healthcare hardware and software vendors are developing and releasing a variety of technological devices to assist in the order entry and dispensing process. These include physician-based order-entry systems, prescription dispensing robots, scanning devices that match the bar code on a prescription label to the bar code on the patient wristband, TPN compounding machines, and handheld devices to access clinical information and receive clinical alerts. Physicians and other healthcare executives are learning the value of using information technology (IT) to keep things from slipping through the cracks and are adopting such technologies at an increasing rate.

CLINICAL RESPONSIBILITY

As we move forward into the 21st century, challenges and solutions abound. Computer technology has advanced past our ability to fully use it, and this technology continues to advance at an increasing rate. We have reviewed the nature of the nutrient–drug interaction problem as complex, overwhelming, difficult to measure at times, too often manual, and divided along functional lines of the clinical team. We have also demonstrated the power of technology available to address each of these challenges, as well as some examples of systems already making an impact.

The key to the implementation of technology that addresses challenges described in this chapter rests with the software development professionals who develop the applications, the IT professionals who implement them and the clinicians who use them on a daily basis. This includes the physician, nurse, pharmacist, clinical dietitian, diagnostic technicians, patients, and caregivers. Each person listed is a part of the clinical care process and therefore responsible for understanding and supporting the systems necessary to provide safe, efficient, and effective healthcare.

With this in mind, the following are ten things you can do to become a responsible user of technology in an interdisciplinary patient care setting:

1. Integrate technology into daily life. Integrate all messaging systems (e-mail, cell phone, calendar, address book, etc.) into a single system. Constantly find ways to access information digitally and use them. Using new technology to convert the way one communicates, invests, manages money, and plans each day brings a deeper understanding of technology. This will impact the ability to understand and use technology in clinical situations.
2. Think about systems from a data perspective. Often we take the data for granted when receiving information. Think about where and how data is stored and how it is standardized. Find new applications for this data. Apply this to personal and professional life.
3. Become comfortable with establishing rules, setting properties, and organizing information electronically. A good place to begin is with the e-mail system. Most e-mail systems have rules-based processors that allow a user to automatically

process incoming messages based on sophisticated rules. Locate sources on the Internet that allow you to establish rules and alerts, such as investment Web sites that provide stock market alerts and reminder services, which remind users to do important things such as sending birthday cards.

4. Become an e-learner. New technology is having a profound impact on the way we learn and how we collaborate with others through the learning process. There is so much we must learn and the old methods of teaching through books and conventions are not sufficient. Many of the things we must know are too new to have been published in a book. Many of the facts published in books are no longer accurate.

5. Take time to learn the systems used by the other members of the clinical team. Time spent by nurses, physicians, and nutritionists learning how a pharmacist receives a prescription order, enters it into the system, dispenses it, and documents the information in the patient chart is time very well spent. Remember, each provider forms part of an interdisciplinary care team.

6. Support the IT efforts within the organization to increase the level of systems integration between departments. There is a saying in IT that the first step is to do the first 90% of the integration and the second step is to do the second 90% of the integration. This is because the last 10% is often as hard as the first 90%.

7. Be willing to change. Change is hard and requires leaders. Be willing to throw away the three-ring binder that has been used for scheduling on-call staff for the past 20 years. Wipe off and take down the white board that lists the patients who have special needs. Realize the role as part of an interdisciplinary team and that this information is vital to the rest of the teammates. Use technology to integrate and share information.

8. Be an expert at the basic features of the technology in daily life. Learn to type and use a mouse. Be able to connect a three-way phone call when called upon to do so. Learn the advanced features and settings of the cell phone. Be able to set up a distribution list in the fax machine or e-mail system.

9. Learn a query language and data presentation tool such as the tools in Microsoft Office (Word, Excel, Powerpoint, and Access) or one of the other tools available through your present employer. Work with the IT department to learn to access corporate data when using these tools, rather than maintaining private data that only the compiler can access. Most clinicians focus on the operational functions of their systems and miss the power and flexibility provided by tools that easily access the data stored from these operations.

10. Think of ten more things like these to do, and become disciplined in doing them while learning more. Ask children for help if necessary. They do not know which answers are wrong or which pathways are impossible.

The challenges are great, the possibilities are endless, the technology is here, and the responsibility is yours. Apply the understanding of computer technology and clinical systems to make a difference.

INTERNET RESOURCES

1. Micromedex—www.Micromedex.com. The Drugdex System™, one of many systems provided by Micromedex, is a comprehensive drug information source that provides some drug–food interaction capabilities.

2. First DataBank—www.firstdatabank.com. First DataBank also provides a comprehensive drug information platform and healthcare knowledge databases. Nutritionist Pro is a knowledge database that provides thorough nutrient analysis of diets, menus, and recipes.

3. Facts and Comparisons—www.factsandcomparisons.com or www.drugfacts.com. Facts and Comparisons is a standard reference found in most pharmacies. It provides easy-to-use basic drug information. When combined with the other online references, such as Drug Interaction Facts, The Review of Natural Products, and Med Facts, a fairly comprehensive review can be conducted. Nutrition is not the focus, but relevant nutrition information can be found.

4. Gold Standard Multimedia—www.gsm.com. Gold Standard Multimedia provides numerous software options for healthcare professionals. Clinical pharmacology is a well-rounded, clinically relevant database with information on herbals, nutritional products, over-the-counter medications, and prescription medications. The database can be queried to create a patient-specific therapeutic regimen detailing potential adverse reactions, interactions, contraindications, and allergies.

5. Multum Information Services—www.multum.com. Multum offers critical point-of-care information services. The drug interaction portion of the database provides drug–food interactions that include the potential severity and recommended course of action and provides information on discontinued medications if they are still active based on half-life.

6. American Society for Nutritional Sciences (ASNS)—www.asns.org. The ASNS Web page is geared toward members, but a few recent articles from the *Journal of Nutrition* can be found. Position statements are also available.

7. American Dietetic Association—www.eatright.org. The American Dietetic Association Web site provides reams of consumer related dietary information. Access to the *Journal of the American Dietetic Association* full text articles requires membership.

8. American Society for Parenteral and Enteral Nutrition (ASPEN)—www.clinnutr.org or www.nutritioncare.org. The ASPEN Web site is geared toward parenteral and enteral nutrition. For best use of the site, membership is required; however, useful information can be gleaned from this site. Unlike the previous five sites, this site has little point of contact use.

9. MedicineNet—www.medicinenet.com. MedicineNet.com is a consumer-oriented Web site; however, physicians write the healthcare information that is available. A featured area is weight management, and it provides very useful information for the consumer and the professional.

10. American Diabetes Association—www.diabetes.org. Diabetes is a disease with pervasive dietary considerations. This site provides extremely useful nutritional information. This information has utility for the both the diabetic and the nondiabetic.

11. National Institutes of Health (NIH) Clinical Center Nutrition Department—www.nih.gov or www.cc.nih.gov. This site provides clinical and research-oriented services as well as drug–nutrient interaction for patient education on a limited number of drugs.

12. Food and Drug Administration Center for Food Safety and Applied Nutrition—www.fda.gov or www.cfsan.fda.gov. The CFSAN is responsible for ensuring that the nation's food supply is safe, sanitary, wholesome, and honestly labeled. They are also charged with ensuring the safety and proper labeling of cosmetics.

The site is very useful for questions regarding contamination from pathogens, pesticides, or tampering.

REFERENCES

1. Gates, Bill. *The Road Ahead.* Penguin USA, East Rutherford, N.J., 1996.
2. Gates, Bill. *Business at the Speed of Thought.* Time Warner Co., Atlanta, 1999.
3. http://www.digitalcentury.com/encyclo/update/comp_hd.html, Christopher LaMorte with John Lilly, today, Jones Technology and Multimedia Encyclopedia. *Computers: History and Development; First Generation (1945-1956).*
4. http://www.digitalcentury.com/encyclo/update/comp_hd.html, Christopher LaMorte with John Lilly, today, Jones Technology and Multimedia Encyclopedia. *Computers: History and Development; Second Generation Computers (1956-1963).*
5. http://www.digitalcentury.com/encyclo/update/comp_hd.html, Christopher LaMorte with John Lilly, today, Jones Technology and Multimedia Encyclopedia. *Computers: History and Development; Third Generation Computers (1964-1971).*
6. Negroponte, Nicholas. *Being Digital.* Random House, New York, 1995, p. 32.
7. Blackburn, Ian et al. *Professional Access 2000 Programming*, Wrox Publishing, Chicago, 2000, p. 297.
8. *Drug Information Framework Foundation Classes version 1.0 Developers Reference Guide.* First DataBank, San Bruno, CA, 2001.
9. Smith, Robert and Sussman, David, *Beginning Access 2000 Visual Basic Assistant,* Wrox Publishing, Chicago, 2000.
10. Blackburn, Ian et al., *Professional Access 2000 Programming*, Wrox Publishing, Chicago, 2000, p. 297.
11. *Today's Dietitian: The Magazine for Nutrition Professionals*, v. 2, no. 1, Great Valley Publishing, Co., Spring City, PA, February, 2000.
12. *Clinisphere 2.0 database,* Facts and Comparisons, Inc., August, 2000.
13. http://www.fda.gov/cder/ndc/preface.htm
14. http://www.fda.gov/cder/ndc/faq.htm
15. Stumbo, Phyllis et al. *Computer applications in controlled diet studies*, In Dennis, B.H. et al., *Well-Controlled Diet Studies in Humans: A Practical Guide to Design and Management*, American Dietetic Association, Chicago, 1999.
16. *Clinisphere 2.0 database.* Facts and Comparisons, Inc. August 2000.
17. http://www.smed.com/solutions/products/pharmacy/pharmacy-decision.php, *The Siemens Pharmacy System: Decision Assistance Product Information, 2001.*
18. http://www.sunquest.com. *Clinical Event Manager Product Information*, 2001.
19. http://www.hboc.com, *McKessonHBOC's Horizon Alert System*, 2001.
20. http://www.cerner.com, *Cerner Discern Expert System*, 2001.
21. Institute of Medicine, *To Err Is Human,* National Academy Press, Washington, D.C., 2000, pp. 1-16.
22. Rx Files—Health-Care I.T., *CIO Magazine,* November 1, 2000, www.cio.com/archive/110100_rx_content.html.
23. *Advance PCS, ePocrates Handheld Technology Drives Physician Office Efficiency.* January 9, 2001, http://www.epocrates.com/headlines/story.cfm?story=10057
24. McKee, J., *Pharmacy Week*, 2/13/2000: 6; 19. p.1.
25. http://www.fda.gov/./opacom/backgrounders/problem.html, U.S. Food and Drug Administration problem reporting web site.
26. *McKessonHBOC Annual Report*, 1999.

Drug Side Effects

The following list of adverse effects — and the drugs that could cause them — focuses on those reactions affecting nutrition and metabolism. Oftentimes, these types of actions are overlooked, causing medical professionals to perform unnecessary tests to determine the problem. Therefore, it is important that the health professionals who deal with nutritional and drug concerns have knowledge of the potential effects of drugs on metabolism. Intervention by a dietitian or pharmacist who sees a potential interaction is vital in correcting and improving a patient's medication regimen to avoid adverse effects on the patient's nutritional status. Please be aware that this list is by no means complete. It was designed to provide examples of some of the most common or significant adverse effects related to nutrition.

Owing to the proliferation of antineoplastic medications, only representative agents are included in this table. For any patient being actively treated for cancer, caregivers must review the agents individually. When reviewing an individual patient's medication regimen, a drug-by-drug review is warranted and strongly recommended by the authors. Several resources are available on the World Wide Web. An example of such a site is www.rxlist.com. Another Internet site that lists newly approved drug therapies and searchable information on the drugs is at http://www.centerwatch.com. Local drug information services should be the primary source for data.

Side Effect	Brand Name	Generic Name of Example Drug	Drug Class
Abdominal pain	Mevacor®	Lovastatin	Antihyperlipidemic agent
	Pravachol®	Pravastatin	Antihyperlipidemic agent
	Prinivil®	Lisinopril	Antihypertensive agent (ace inhibitor)
	Retrovir®	Zidovudine	HIV therapy (narti)
	Zerit®	Stavudine	Anti-HIV agent (narti)
	Zometa®	Zoledronic	Bisphosphanate
Altered taste	Videx®	Didanosine	Anti-HIV agent (narti)
Altered taste acuity	Imuran®	Azathioprine	Immunosuppressant
Anabolism	Deca-Durabolin®	Nandrolone	Anabolic steroids
	Oxandrin®	Oxandroline	Anabolic steroid
	Winstrol®	Stanozol	Anabolic steroid
Anorexia	Focalin®	Dexmethylphenidate	Central nervous system (CNS) stimulant
	Reminyl®	Galantamine	Alzheimer's dementia
	Retrovir®	Zidovudine	HIV therapy (narti)
	Ritalin®	Methylphenidate	CNS stimulant
	Ziagen®	Abacavir	Anti-HIV agent (narti)
Constipation	Amphogel®	Aluminum hydroxide	Antacid (aluminum and calcium containing)
	Arixtra®	Fonaparinux	Anticoagulant
	Artane®	Trihexyphenidyl	Anti-Parkinson's agent
	Benadryl®	Diphenhydramine	Antihistamine (H1 blocker)
	Catapres®	Clonidine	Antihypertensive (alpha 2 adrenergic agonist)
	Chlor-Trimeton®	Chlorpheniramine	Antihistamine (H1 blocker)
	Citrate 600®	Calcium carbonate	Calcium salt
	Cogentin®	Benztropine	Anti-Parkinson's agent
	Demerol®	Meperidine	Analgesic agent (opioid)
	Femiron®	Ferrous fumarate	Iron salt
	Feosol®	Ferrous sulfate	Iron salt
	Fergon®	Ferrous gluconate	Iron salt
	FiberCon®	Calcium polycarbophil	Antidiarrheal
	HydroDiuril®	Hydrochlorthiazide	Diuretic (thiazide, non-potassium sparing)
	Imodium A-D®	Loperamide	Antidiarrheal
	Kalcinate®	Calcium gluconate	Calcium salt

Kaopectate II®	Loperamide	Antidiarrheal
Kytril®	Granisetron	Antiemetic (5HT3 antagonist)
Lasix®	Furosemide	Diuretic (loop, non–potassium sparing)
Lomotil®	Diphenoxalate/atropine	Antidiarrheal
Lortab®	Hydrocodone	Analgesic agent (opioid)
Mevacor®	Lovastatin	Antihyperlipidemic agent
MSContin®	Morphine	Analgesic agents (opioids)
MSIR®	Morphine	Analgesic agents (opioids)
Neo-Calglucon®	Calcium glubionate	Calcium salt
Niferex®	Polysaccharide-iron complex	Iron salt
OxyContin®	Oxycodone	Analgesic agent (opioid)
OxyIR®	Oxycodone	Analgesic agent (opioid)
Pepto-Bismol®	Bismuth subsalicylate	Antidiarrheal
Periactin®	Cyproheptadine	Antihistamine (H1 blocker)
Permax®	Pergolide	Anti-Parkinson's agent
Phenergan®	Promethazine	Antiemetic
PhosLo®	Calcium acetate	Calcium salt
Pravachol®	Pravastatin	Antihyperlipidemic agent
Roxanol®	Morphine	Analgesic agent (opioid)
Sandostatin®	Octreotide	Antisecretory
Sinemet®	Levodopa and carbidopa	Anti-Parkinson's agent
Tavist®	Clemastine	Antihistamine (H1 blocker)
Transderm-Scop®	Scopalamine	Antiemetic
Tums®	Calcium carbonate	Calcium salt
Zofran®	Ondasteron	Antiemetic (5HT3 antagonist)

Decreased appetite

Acutrim®	Phenylpropanolamine	Anorexiant
Adderall®	Amphetamine mixture	Amphetamine
Adiphex-P®	Phenteramine	Anorexiant
Desoxyn®	Methamphetamine	Amphetamine
Dexedrine®	Dextroamphetamine	Amphetamine
Ionamin®	Phenteramine	Anorexiant
Meridia®	Sibutramine	Anorexiant
Pondimin®	Fenfluramine	Anorexiant

Side Effect	Brand Name	Generic Name of Example Drug	Drug Class
Diarrhea	Actonel®	Risedronate	Bisphosphonate
	Agenerase®	Amprenavir	Anti-HIV (protease inhibitors)
	Aldomet®	Methyldopa	Antihypertensive agent (alpha adrenergic blocking)
	Amoxil®	Amoxicillin	Antibiotic
	Aricept®	Donepezim	Alzheimer's agents
	Avelox®	Moxifloxacin	Antibiotic
	Bactrim®	Co-trimoxazole	Antibiotic
	Ceftin Suspension®	Cefuroxime	Sorbitol containing suspensions
	CellCept®	Mycophenolate	Immunosuppressant
	Chronulac®	Lactulose	Laxative
	Chronulac®	Lactulose	Laxative (abuse)
	Cipro®	Ciprofloxacin	Antibiotic
	Cleocin®	Clindamycin	Antibiotic
	Cognex®	Tacrine	Alzheimer's agents
	Colace®	Docusate sodium	Stool softener
	Combivir®	Zidovudine, lamivudine	Anti-HIV agent (narti)
	Dulcolax®	Bisacodyl	Laxative
	Dulcolax®	Bisacodyl	Laxative (abuse)
	EES®	Erythromycin	Antibiotic and off-label motility agent
	E-Mycin®	Erythromycin	Antibiotic and off-label motility agent
	Epivir®	Lamivudine	Anti-HIV agent
	Fortovase®	Saqunavir	Anti-HIV agent (protease inhibitors)
	GoLytely®	Polyethylene glycol	Laxative
	Imuran®	Azathioprine	Immunosuppressant
	Kytril®	Granisetron	Antiemetic (5HT3 antagonist)
	Lanoxin®	Digoxin	Cardiac agent
	MagOx®	Magnesium oxide	Magnesium supplement
	Mestinon®	Pyridostgmine	Myasthenia gravis agent
	Metamucil®	Psyllium	Laxative
	Phillips™ milk of magnesia	Magnesium hydroxide	Antacid (magnesium containing)

Brand	Generic	Class
Prinivil®	Lisinopril	Antihypertensive agent (ace inhibitor)
Prostigmin®	Neostigmine	Myasthenia gravis agents
Quinaglute®	Quinidine	Cardiac agent
Reglan®	Metoclopramide	Motility agent
Reminyl®	Galantamine	Alzheimer's dementia
Riopan®	Magaldrate	Antacid (magnesium containing)
Rocephin®	Ceftriaxone	Antibiotic
Senokot®	Senna	Laxative
Senokot®	Senna	Laxative (abuse)
Septra®	Co-trimoxazole	Antibiotic
Sorbitol-containing suspensions	Sorbitol may not be listed on label	Sorbitol-containing suspensions
Surfak®	Docusate calcium	Stool softener
Sustiva®	Efavirenz	Anti-HIV agent (nnrti)
Tagamet Suspension®	Cimetidine	Sorbitol containing suspension
Topamax®	Topiramate	Anticonvulsant
Trimox Suspension®	Amoxicillin	Sorbitol containing suspension
Trizivir®	Zidovudine, lamivudine, abacavir	Anti-HIV agent
Tylenol Children's Suspension®	Acetaminophen	Sorbitol containing suspension
Videx®	Didanosine	Anti-HIV agent (narti)
Viracept®	Nelfinavir	Anti-HIV agent (protease inhibitor)
Viread®	Tenofovir disoproxil fumarate	Anti-HIV agent (narti)
Zerit®	Stavudine	Anti-HIV agent (narti)
Ziagen®	Abacavir	Anti-HIV agent (narti)
Zithromax Suspension®	Azithromycin	Sorbitol containing suspension
Zofran®	Ondasteron	Antiemetic (5HT3 antagonist)
Zometa®	Zoledronic	Bisphosphanate
Retrovir®	Zidovudine	HIV therapy (narti)
Desyrel®	Trazodone	Antidepressant
Remeron®	Mirtazapine	Antidepressant (atypical)
Arixtra®	Fonaparinux	Anticoagulant
Actonel®	Risedronate	Bisphosphonate

Dry mouth

Edema

Epigastric pain

Side Effect	Brand Name	Generic Name of Example Drug	Drug Class
Flatulence	Viread®	Tenofovir disoproxil fumarate	Anti-HIV agent (narti)
Fluid depletion	Aldactone®	Spironolactone	Diuretic (potassium sparing)
	Diamox®	Acetazolamide	Diuretic
	HydroDiuril®	Hydrochlorthiazide	Diuretic (thiazide, non–potassium sparing)
	Lasix®	Furosemide	Diuretic (loop, non–potassium sparing)
	Zaroxylin®	Metolazone	Diuretic
Fluid retention	Advil®	Ibuprofen	Nonsteroidal antiinflammatory agent (all)
	Aldomet®	Methyldopa	Antihypertensive agent (alpha adrenergic blocking)
	Aleve®	Naproxen	Nonsteroidal antiinflammatory agent (all)
	Celestone®	Betamethasone	Steroid (corticosteroid)
	Cortef®	Hydrocortisone	Steroid (corticosteroid)
	Cortone®	Cortisone	Steroid (corticosteroid)
	Decadron®	Dexamethasone	Steroid (corticosteroid)
	Delta-Cortef®	Prednisolone	Steroid (corticosteroid)
	Deltasone®	Prednisone	Steroid (corticosteroid)
	Florinef®	Fludrocortisone	Steroid (mineralocorticoid)
	Hytrin®	Terazosin	Antihypertensive (alpha adrenergic blocking agent)
	Indocin®	Indomethacin	Nonsteroidal antiinflammatory agent
	Loniten®	Minoxidil	Vasodilator
	Minipress®	Prazosin	Antihypertensive (alpha adrenergic blocking agent)
	Motrin®	Ibuprofen	Nonsteroidal antiinflammatory agent (all)
	Naprosyn®	Naproxen	Nonsteroidal antiinflammatory agent (all)
	Orasone®	Prednisone	Steroid (corticosteroid)
	Prelone®	Prednisolone	Steroid (corticosteroid)
	Premarin®	Estrogen	Estrogen
	Solu-Cortef®	Methylprednisolone	Steroid (corticosteroid)
Hypercalcemia		Calcium chloride parenteral solution	Calcium salt
		Calcium gluceptate parenteral solution	Calcium salt
		Calcium gluconate parenteral solution	Calcium salt
		Vitamin A and D combination products	Vitamin A and D (toxic)
	Aquasol A®	Vitamin A	Vitamin A (toxic)

	Calciferol®	Vitamin D	Vitamin D (toxic)
	Citrate 600®	Calcium carbonate	Calcium salt
	Dyazide®	Hydrochlorthiazide and triamterene	Diuretic (potassium sparing, contains thiazide as well)
	HydroDiuril®	Hydrochlorthiazide	Diuretic (thiazide, non–potassium sparing)
	Kalcinate®	Calcium gluconate	Calcium salt
	Lithane®	Lithium	CNS agent (lithium) (toxic)
	Lithonate®	Lithium	CNS agent (lithium) (toxic)
	Maxzide®	Hydrochlorthiazide and triamterene	Diuretic (potassium sparing, contains thiazide as well)
	PhosLo®	Calcium acetate	Calcium salt
	SloBid®	Theophylline	Bronchodilator (toxic)
	TheoDur®	Theophylline	Bronchodilator (toxic)
	Tums®	Calcium carbonate	Calcium salt
Hyperchloremia	Topamax®	Topiramate	Anticonvulsant
Hyperglycemia	Adrenalin®	Epinephrine	Bronchodilator
	Agenerase®	Amprenavir	Anti-HIV (protease inhibitors)
	Celestone®	Betamethasone	Steroid (corticosteroid)
	Cortef®	Hydrocortisone	Steroid (corticosteroid)
	Cortone®	Cortisone	Steroid (corticosteroid)
	Decadron®	Dexamethasone	Steroid (corticosteroid)
	Delta-Cortef®	Prednisolone	Steroid (corticosteroid)
	Deltasone®	Prednisone	Steroid (corticosteroid)
	Dilantin®	Phenytoin	Anticonvulsant (hydantoin)
	Dyazide®	Hydrochlorthiazide and triamterene	Diuretic (potassium sparing contains thiazide as well)
	Elspar®	Asparginase	Antineoplastic agent
	Florinef®	Fludrocortisone	Steroid (mineralocorticoid)
	Hivid®	Zalcitabine	Anti-HIV agent (narti)
	HydroDiuril®	Hydrochlorthiazide	Diuretic (thiazide, non–potassium sparing)
	Lasix®	Furosemide	Diuretic (loop, non–potassium sparing)
	Lithane®	Lithium	CNS agent
	Lithonate®	Lithium	CNS agent
	Luminal®	Phenobarbital	Anticonvulsant (barbiturate)
	Maxzide®	Hydrochlorthiazide and triamterene	Diuretic (potassium sparing contains thiazide as well)
	Miacalcin®, Cibacalcin®	Calcitonin	Calcitonin

Side Effect	Brand Name	Generic Name of Example Drug	Drug Class
Hyperglycemia (continued)	Orasone®	Prednisone	Steroid (corticosteroid)
	Prelone®	Prednisolone	Steroid (corticosteroid)
	Prograf®	Tacrolimus	immunosuppressant
	Rifadin®	Rifampin	Antitubercular agent
	Sandimmune®	Cyclosporine	Immunosuppressant agent
	Solu-Cortef®	Methylprednisolone	Steroid (corticosteroid)
	Ziagen®	Abacavir	Anti-HIV agent (narti)
Hyperkalemia	Advil®	Ibuprofen	Nonsteroidal antiinflammatory agent (all)
	Aldactone®	Spironolactone	Diuretic (potassium sparing)
	Aleve®	Naproxen	Nonsteroidal antiinflammatory agent (all)
	Altace®	Ramipril	Antihypertensive agent (ace inhibitors)
	Capoten®	Captopril	Antihypertensive agent (beta-1 blockers and ace inhibitors)
	Dyazide®	Hydrochlorthiazide and triamterene	Diuretic (potassium sparing contains thiazide as well)
	Inderal®	Propranolol	Antihypertensive agent (beta-1 blockers)
	Indocin®	Indomethacin	Nonsteroidal antiinflammatory agent
	K-Dur®	Potassium chloride	Potassium supplements
	K-Lyte®	Potassium bicarbonate and potassium citrate	Potassium supplements
	K-Phos®	Potassium phosphate/sodium phosphate	Potassium supplements
	Lanoxin®	Digoxin	Cardiac agent (toxic)
	Lopressor®	Metoprolol	Antihypertensive agent (beta-1 blocker)
	Lotensin®	Benazepril	Antihypertensive agent (ace inhibitor)
	Maxzide®	Hydrochlorthiazide and triamterene	Diuretic (potassium sparing contains thiazide as well)
	Micro-K®	Potassium chloride	Potassium supplement
	Midamor®	Amiloride	Diuretic (potassium sparing)
	Motrin®	Ibuprofen	Nonsteroidal antiinflammatory agent (all)
	Naprosyn®	Naproxen	Nonsteroidal antiinflammatory agent (all)
	NeutraPhos®	Potassium phosphate/sodium phosphate	Potassium supplement

Condition	Drug	Brand	Class
	Tacrolimus	Prograf®	Immunosuppressant
	Cyclosporine	Sandimmune®	Immunosuppressant agent
	Potassium chloride	Slow K®	Potassium supplement
	Atenolol	Tenormin®	Antihypertensive agent (beta-1 blocker)
	Metoprolol	Toprol XL®	Antihypertensive agent (beta-1 blocker)
	Enalapril	Vasotec®	Antihypertensive agents (beta-1 blockers and ace inhibitors)
Hyperlipidemia	Cyclosporine	Sandimmune®	Immunosuppressant agent
Hypermagnesemia	Magnesium citrate	Citrate of Magnesia®	Laxative (magnesium containing)
	Magnesium citrate	Evac-Q-Mag®	Laxative (magnesium containing)
	Magnesium oxide	MagOx®	Magnesium supplement
	Magnesium hydroxide	MOM®	Antacid (magnesium containing)
	Magaldrate	Riopan®	Antacid (magnesium containing)
Hypernatremia	3% sodium chloride parenteral solution		Hypertonic sodium fluid
	5% sodium chloride parenteral solution		Hypertonic sodium fluid
	Bumetanide	Bumex®	Diuretic (loop)
	Torsemide	Demadex®	Diuretics (loop)
	Ethacrynic acid	Edecrin®	Diuretic (loop)
	Furosemide	Lasix®	Diuretic (loop, non–potassium sparing)
Hyperphosphatemia	Potassium phosphate parenteral solution		Phosphorus salt
	Sodium phosphate parenteral solution		Phosphorus salt
	Sodium phosphate	Fleets Enema®	Laxative (phosphate containing)
	Sodium phosphate	Fleets Phospho-soda®	Laxative (phosphate containing)
Hypertriglyceridemia	Efavirenz	Sustiva®	Anti-HIV agent (nnrti)
	Amprenavir	Agenerase®	Anti-HIV (protease inhibitors)
	Indinavir	Crixivan®	Anti-HIV agent (protease inhibitor)
	Saquanavir	Fortovase®	Anti-HIV agent (protease inhibitors)
	Zalcitabine	Hivid®	Anti-HIV agent (narti)
	Didanosine	Videx®	Anti-HIV agent (narti)
	Nelfinavir	Viracept®	Anti-HIV agent (protease inhibitor)
	Abacavir	Ziagen®	Anti-HIV agent (narti)

Side Effect	Brand Name	Generic Name of Example Drug	Drug Class
Hypocalcemia	Didronel®	Etidronate	Bisphosphonate
		Potassium phosphate parenteral solution	Phosphorus salt
		Sodium phosphate parenteral solution	Phosphorus salt
	Aredia®	Pamidronate	Bisphosphonate
	Bumex®	Bumetanide	Diuretic (loop)
	Demadex®	Torsemide	Diuretics (loop)
	Dilantin®	Phenytoin	Anticonvulsant (hydantoin)
	Edecrin®	Ethacrynic acid	Diuretic (loop)
	Fleets Enema®	Sodium phosphate	Laxative (phosphate containing)
	Fleets Phospho-soda®	Sodium phosphate	Laxative (phosphate containing)
	Fosamax®	Alendronate	Bisphosphonate
	Lasix®	Furosemide	Diuretic (loop, non–potassium sparing)
	Luminal®	Phenobarbital	Anticonvulsant (barbiturate)
	Miacalcin®, Cibacalcin®	Calcitonin	Calcitonin
	Mithramycin®	Plicamycin	Antineoplastic agent
	Paraplatin®	Carboplatin	Antineoplastic agent
	Platinol®	Cisplatin	Antineoplastic agents
	Rifadin®	Rifampin	Antitubercular agent
Hypocapnia	Topamax®	Topiramate	Anticonvulsant
Hypoglycemia	Actos®	Pioglitazone	Hypoglycemic agent
	Atromid-S®	Clofibrate	Lipid lowering agent
	Avandia®	Rosiglitazone	Hypoglycemic agent
	Depo-Testosterone®	Cypionate	Anabolic steroid
	Diabeta®	Glyburide	Hypoglycemic agent
	Dianabol®	Methandrostenolone	Anabolic steroid
	Elavil®	Amitriptyline	Antidepressant
	Glucophage®	Metformin	Hypoglycemic agent
	Glucotrol®	Glipizide	Hypoglycemic agent
	Glyset®	Miglitol	Hypoglycemic agent
	Humulin N, R, L, U, 70/30®	Insulin	Insulin

Brand name	Generic name	Category
Humulin N, R, L, U, 70/30®	Insulin	Insulin (excessive)
Humalog®	Insulin lispro	Insulin
Humalog®	Insulin lispro	Insulin (excessive)
Inderal®	Propranolol	Antihypertensive agent (beta-1 blockers)
Lantos®	Insulin glargine	Insulin
Lantos®	Insulin glargine	Insulin (excessive)
Lopressor®	Metoprolol	Antihypertensive agent (beta-1 blocker)
Micronase®	Glyburide	Hypoglycemic agent
Nardil®	Phenelzine	CNS agent (monoamine oxidase inhibitor)
Novolin R, N, L, 70/30®	Insulin, all types	Insulin
Novolog®	Insulin aspart	Insulin
Orinase®	Tolbutamide	Hypoglycemic agent
Oxandrin®	Oxandroline	Anabolic steroid
Pamelor®	Nortriptyline	Antidepressant (tricyclic)
Parnate®	Tranylcypromine	Antidepressant (monoamine oxidase inhibitor)
Prandin®	Repaglinide	Hypoglycemic agent
Precose®	Acarbose	Hypoglycemic agent
Sinequin®	Doxepin	Antidepressant (tricyclic)
Tenormin®	Atenolol	Antihypertensive agent (beta-1 blocker)
Tofranil®	Imipramine	Antidepressant
Toprol XL®	Metoprolol	Antihypertensive agent (beta-1 blocker)
Winstrol®	Stanozol	Anabolic steroid

Hypokalemia

Brand name	Generic name	Category
Abelcet®	Amphotericin B	Antibiotic
Amikin®	Amikacin	Antibiotic
Celestone®	Betamethasone	Steroid (corticosteroid)
Chronulac®	Lactulose	Laxative (abuse)
Cortef®	Hydrocortisone	Steroid (corticosteroid)
Cortone®	Cortisone	Steroid (corticosteroid)
Decadron®	Dexamethasone	Steroid (corticosteroid)
Delta-Cortef®	Prednisolone	Steroid (corticosteroid)
Deltasone®	Prednisone	Steroid (corticosteroid)
Dulcolax®	Bisacodyl	Laxative (abuse)
Florinef®	Fludrocortisone	Steroid (mineralocorticoid)

Side Effect	Brand Name	Generic Name of Example Drug	Drug Class
Hypokalemia (*continued*)	Fungizone®	Amphotericin B	Antibiotic
	Garamycin®	Gentamicin	Antibiotic
	GoLytely®	Polyethylene glycol	Laxative (abuse)
	Humulin N, R, L, U, 70/30®	Insulin	Insulin (excessive)
	Humalog®	Insulin lispro	Insulin (excessive)
	HydroDiuril®	Hydrochlorthiazide	Diuretic (thiazide, non–potassium sparing)
	Lantos®	Insulin glargine	Insulin (excessive)
	Lasix®	Furosemide	Diuretic (loop, non–potassium sparing)
	MagOx®	Magnesium oxide	Magnesium supplement
	Nebcin®	Tobramycin	Antibiotics
	Novolin R®	Insulin, regular	Insulin (excessive)
	Novolog®	Insulin aspart	Insulin (excessive)
	PenTids®	Penicillins (high dose)	Antibiotic
	PenVK®	Penicillins (high dose)	Antibiotic
	Senokot®	Senna	Laxative (abuse)
	Timentin®	Ticarcillin and clavulanate acid	Antibiotics
	Zosyn®	Pipercillin and tazobactam	Antibiotic
Hypomagnesemia	Didronel®	Etidronate	Bisphosphonate
		Alcohol	Alcohol
	Abelcet®	Amphotericin B	Antibiotic
	Aldactone®	Spironolactone	Diuretic (potassium sparing)
	Amikin®	Amikacin	Antibiotic
	Aredia®	Pamidronate	Bisphosphonate
	Diamox®	Acetazolamide	Diuretic
	Fosamax®	Alendronate	Bisphosphonate
	Fungizone®	Amphotericin B	Antibiotic
	Garamycin®	Gentamicin	Antibiotic
	Humulin N, R, L, U, 70/30®	Insulin	Insulin (excessive)
	Humalog®	Insulin lispro	Insulin (excessive)
	HydroDiuril®	Hydrochlorthiazide	Diuretic (thiazide, non–potassium sparing)
	Lanoxin®	Digoxin	Cardiac agent (toxic)

Lantos®	Insulin glargine	Insulin (excessive)
Lasix®	Furosemide	Diuretic (loop, non–potassium sparing)
Nebcin®	Tobramycin	Antibiotics
Neoral®	Cyclosporine	Immunosuppressant agent
Novolin R®	Insulin, regular	Insulin (excessive)
Novolog®	Insulin aspart	Insulin (excessive)
Paraplatin®	Carboplatin	Antineoplastic agent
Platinol®	Cisplatin	Antineoplastic agents
Sandimmune®	Cyclosporine	Immunosuppressant agent
Zaroxylin®	Metolazone	Diuretic

Hyponatremia

Aldactone®	Spironolactone	Diuretic (potassium sparing)
Cytoxan®	Cyclophosphamide	Cytotoxic chemotherapy (alkylating agent)
Diabenase®	Chlorpropamide	Hypoglycemic agent
Diamox®	Acetazolamide	Diuretic
HydroDiuril®	Hydrochlorthiazide	Diuretic (thiazide, non–potassium sparing)
Lasix®	Furosemide	Diuretic (loop, non–potassium sparing)
Neosar®	Cyclophosphamide	Cytotoxic chemotherapy (alkylating agent)
Pitocin®	Oxytoxin	Hormone (oxytocic)
Zaroxylin®	Metolazone	Diuretic

Hypophosphatemia

Aldactone®	Calcium chloride parenteral solution	Calcium salt
Aredia®	Calcium gluceptate parenteral solution	Calcium salt
Ascriptin®	Calcium gluconate parenteral solution	Calcium salt
Bufferin®	Spironolactone	Diuretic (potassium sparing)
Carafate®	Pamidronate	Bisphosphonate
Celestone®	Aspirin	Salicylate (toxic)
Citrate 600®	Aspirin	Salicylate (toxic)
Cortef®	Sucralfate	Gastrointestinal agent
Cortone®	Betamethasone	Steroid (corticosteroid)
Decadron®	Calcium carbonate	Calcium salt
Delta-Cortef®	Hydrocortisone	Steroid (corticosteroid)
	Cortisone	Steroid (corticosteroid)
	Dexamethasone	Steroid (corticosteroid)
	Prednisolone	Steroid (corticosteroid)

Side Effect	Brand Name	Generic Name of Example Drug	Drug Class
Hypophosphatemia (*continued*)	Deltasone®	Prednisone	Steroid (corticosteroid)
	Diamox®	Acetazolamide	Diuretic
	Didronel®	Etidronate	Bisphosphonate
	Ecotrin®	Aspirin	Salicylate (toxic)
	Florinef®	Fludrocortisone	Steroid (mineralocorticoid)
	Fosamax®	Alendronate	Bisphosphonate
	Humulin N, R, L, U, 70/30®	Insulin	Insulin (excessive)
	Humalog®	Insulin lispro	Insulin (excessive)
	HydroDiuril®	Hydrochlorthiazide	Diuretic (thiazide, non–potassium sparing)
	Kalcinate®	Calcium gluconate	Calcium salt
	Lantos®	Insulin glargine	Insulin (excessive)
	Lasix®	Furosemide	Diuretic (loop, non–potassium sparing)
	Neo-Calglucon®	Calcium glubionate	Calcium salt
	Novolin R®	Insulin, regular	Insulin (excessive)
	Novolog®	Insulin aspart	Insulin (excessive)
	Orasone®	Prednisone	Steroid (corticosteroid)
	PhosLo®	Calcium acetate	Calcium salt
	Prelone®	Prednisolone	Steroid (corticosteroid)
	SloBid®	Theophylline	Bronchodilator (toxic)
	Solu-Cortef®	Methylprednisolone	Steroid (corticosteroid)
	TheoDur®	Theophylline	Bronchodilator (toxic)
	Tums®	Calcium carbonate	Calcium salt
	Zaroxylin®	Metolazone	Diuretic
Increased appetite	Celestone®	Betamethasone	Steroid (corticosteroid)
	Clozapine®	Clozaril	Antipsychotic
	Cortef®	Hydrocortisone	Steroid (corticosteroid)
	Cortone®	Cortisone	Steroid (corticosteroid)
	Decadron®	Dexamethasone	Steroid (corticosteroid)
	Delta-Cortef®	Prednisolone	Steroid (corticosteroid)
	Deltasone®	Prednisone	Steroid (corticosteroid)
	Depo-Provera®	Medroxyprogesterone	Hormone

Desyrel®	Trazodone	Antidepressant
Elavil®	Amitriptyline	Antidepressant
Florinef®	Fludrocortisone	Steroid (mineralocorticoid)
Marinol®	Dronabinol	Cannabinoid
Megace®	Megesterol	Steroid (antineoplastic hormonal)
Nardil®	Phenelzine	CNS agent (monoamine oxidase inhibitor)
Norpramin®	Desipramine	Antidepressant
Olanzapine®	Thienbenzodiazepine	Antipsychotic
Orasone®	Prednisone	Steroid (corticosteroid)
Oxandrin®	Oxandroline	Anabolic steroid
Parnate®	Tranylcypromine	Antidepressant (monoamine oxidase inhibitor)
Paxil®	Paroxetine	Antidepressant (SSRI)
Periactin®	Cyproheptadine	Antihistamine (H1 blocker)
Prelone®	Prednisolone	Steroid (corticosteroid)
Quetiapine®	Dibenzothiazepine	Antipsychotic
Remeron®	Mirtazapine	Antidepressant (atypical)
Risperidone®	Benzisoxazole	Antipsychotic
Solu-Cortef®	Methylprednisolone	Steroid (corticosteroid)
Tofranil®	Imipramine	Antidepressant
Abelcet®	Amphotericin B	Antibiotic
Agenerase®	Amprenavir	Anti-HIV (protease inhibitors)
Amaryl®	Glimepiride	Hypoglycemic agent
Amoxil®	Amoxicillin	Antibiotic
Arixtra®	Fonaparinux	Anticoagulant
Avelox®	Moxifloxacin	Antibiotic
Cleocin®	Clindamycin	Antibiotic
Combivir®	Zidovudine, lamivudine	Anti-HIV agent (narti)
Crixivan®	Indinavir	Anti-HIV agent (protease inhibitor)
Demerol®	Meperidine	Analgesic agent (opiates)
Desyrel®	Trazodone	Antidepressant
Dilantin®	Phenytoin	Anticonvulsant (toxic)
EES®	Erythromycin	Antibiotic and off-label motility agent
E-Mycin®	Erythromycin	Antibiotic and off-label motility agent

Nausea

Side Effect	Brand Name	Generic Name of Example Drug	Drug Class
Nausea (*continued*)	Epivir®	Lamivudine	Anti-HIV agent
	Focalin®	Dexmethylphenidate	CNS stimulant
	Fungizone®	Amphotericin B	Antibiotic
	Ifex®	Ifosfamide	Antineoplastic agent
	Imuran®	Azathioprine	Immunosuppressant
	Lanoxin®	Digoxin	Cardiac agent (toxic)
	Lortab®	Hydrocodone	Analgesic agent (opioid)
	Mevacor®	Lovastatin	Antihyperlipidemic agent
	MSContin®	Morphine	Analgesic agents (opioids)
	MSIR®	Morphine	Analgesic agents (opioids)
	Mutamycin®	Mitomycin	Antineoplastic agent
	Oncovin®	Vincristine	Antineoplastic agent
	OxyContin®	Oxycodone	Analgesic agent (opioid)
	OxyIR®	Oxycodone	Analgesic agent (opioid)
	Paraplatin®	Carboplatin	Antineoplastic agent
	Platinol®	Cisplatin	Antineoplastic agents
	Pravachol®	Pravastatin	Antihyperlipidemic agent
	Prograf®	Tacrolimus	Immunosuppressant
	Reminyl®	Galantamine	Alzheimer's dementia
	Rescriptor	Delavirdine	Anti-HIV agent (nnrti)
	Retrovir®	Zidovudine	HIV therapy (narti)
	Ritalin®	Methylphenidate	CNS stimulant
	Roxanol®	Morphine	Analgesic agent (opioid)
	SloBid®	Theophylline	Bronchodilator
	SloBid®	Theophylline	Bronchodilator (toxic)
	Sumycin®	Tetracycline	Antibiotic
	Sustiva®	Efavirenz	Anti-HIV agent (nnrti)
	Tegretol®	Carbamazepine	Anticonvulsant (toxic)
	TheoDur®	Theophylline	Bronchodilator
	TheoDur®	Theophylline	Bronchodilator (toxic)
	Trizivir®	Zidovudine, Lamivudine, Abacavir	Anti-HIV agent

Category	Brand	Generic	Class
Oral ulcers	Velban®	Vinblastine	Antineoplastic agents
	Videx®	Didanosine	Anti-HIV agent (nrti)
	Viramune®	Nevirapine	Anti-HIV agent (nnrti)
	Viread®	Tenofovir disoproxil fumarate	Anti-HIV agent (nrti)
	Zerit®	Stavudine	Anti-HIV agent (nrti)
	Ziagen®	Abacavir	Anti-HIV agent (nrti)
	Zometa®	Zoledronic	Bisphosphanate
	Hivid®	Zalcitabine	Anti-HIV agent (nrti)
pH changes	Aldactone®	Spironolactone	Diuretic (potassium sparing)
	Ascriptin®	Aspirin	Salicylate (toxic)
	Bufferin®	Aspirin	Salicylate (toxic)
	Chronulac®	Lactulose	Laxative (abuse)
	Diamox®	Acetazolamide	Diuretic
	Dulcolax®	Bisacodyl	Laxative (abuse)
	Ecotrin®	Aspirin	Salicylate (toxic)
	GoLytely®	Polyethylene glycol	Laxative (abuse)
	HydroDiuril®	Hydrochlorthiazide	Diuretic (thiazide, non–potassium sparing)
	Lasix®	Furosemide	Diuretic (loop, non–potassium sparing)
	Senokot®	Senna	Laxative (abuse)
	Zaroxylin®	Metolazone	Diuretic
	Amoxil®	Amoxicillin	Antibiotic
Pseudomembranous colitis	Augmentin®	Amoxicillin and clavulanate	Antibiotic
	Cleocin®	Clindamycin	Antibiotic
	EES®	Erythromycin	Antibiotic and off-label motility agent
	E-Mycin®	Erythromycin	Antibiotic and off-label motility agent
	Fortaz®	Ceftazadime	Antibiotic
	Rocephin®	Ceftriaxone	Antibiotic
	Sumycin®	Tetracycline	Antibiotic
	Zosyn®	Pipercillin and tazobactam	Antibiotic
Sore throat	Imuran®	Azathioprine	Immunosuppressant
Ulcers	Advil®	Ibuprofen	Nonsteroidal antiinflammatory agent (all)
	Aleve®	Naproxen	Nonsteroidal antiinflammatory agent (all)

Side Effect	Brand Name	Generic Name of Example Drug	Drug Class
Ulcers (*continued*)	Ascriptin®	Aspirin	Salicylate
	Celestone®	Betamethasone	Steroid (corticosteroid)
	Cortef®	Hydrocortisone	Steroid (corticosteroid)
	Cortone®	Cortisone	Steroid (corticosteroid)
	Decadron®	Dexamethasone	Steroid (corticosteroid)
	Delta-Cortef®	Prednisolone	Steroid (corticosteroid)
	Deltasone®	Prednisone	Steroid (corticosteroid)
	Fosamax®	Alendronate	Bisphosphonate
	Ifex®	Ifosfamide	Antineoplastic agent
	Indocin®	Indomethacin	Nonsteroidal antiinflammatory agent
	Motrin®	Ibuprofen	Nonsteroidal antiinflammatory agent (all)
	Mutamycin®	Mitomycin	Antineoplastic agent
	Naprosyn®	Naproxen	Nonsteroidal antiinflammatory agent (all)
	Oncovin®	Vincristine	Antineoplastic agent
	Orasone®	Prednisone	Steroid (corticosteroid)
	Paraplatin®	Carboplatin	Antineoplastic agent
	Platinol®	Cisplatin	Antineoplastic agents
	Prelone®	Prednisolone	Steroid (corticosteroid)
	Solu-Cortef®	Methylprednisolone	Steroid (corticosteroid)
	Velban®	Vinblastine	Antineoplastic agents
Vomiting	Agenerase®	Amprenavir	Anti-HIV (protease inhibitors)
	Combivir®	Zidovudine, lamivudine	Anti-HIV agent (narti)
	Desyrel®	Trazodone	Antidepressant
	Focalin®	Dexmethylphenidate	CNS stimulant
	Imuran®	Azathioprine	Immunosuppressant
	Mevacor®	Lovastatin	Antihyperlipidemic agent
	Pravachol®	Pravastatin	Antihyperlipidemic agent
	Prograf®	Tacrolimus	immunosuppressant
	Reminyl®	Galantamine	Alzheimer's dementia
	Trizivir®	Zidovudine, lamivudine, abacavir	Anti-HIV agent
	Viread®	Tenofovir disoproxil fumarate	Anti-HIV agent (narti)

Weight gain	Zerit®	Stavudine	Anti-HIV agent (narti)
	Ziagen®	Abacavir	Anti-HIV agent (narti)
	Zometa®	Zoledronic	Bisphosphanate
	Celexa®	Citalopram	Antidepressant (SSRI)
	Effexor®	Venlafaxine	Antidepressant (SSRI)
	Luvox®	Fluvoxamine	Antidepressant (SSRI)
	Paxil®	Paroxetine	Antidepressant (SSRI)
	Prozac®, Sarafem®	Fluoxetine	Antidepressant (SSRI)
	Remeron®	Mirtazapine	Antidepressant (atypical)
	Zoloft®	Sertraline	Antidepressant (SSRI)
Weight loss	Celexa®	Citalopram	Antidepressant (SSRI)
	Effexor®	Venlafaxine	Antidepressant (SSRI)
	Luvox®	Fluvoxamine	Antidepressant (SSRI)
	Paxil®	Paroxetine	Antidepressant (SSRI)
	Prozac®, Sarafem®	Fluoxetine	Antidepressant (SSRI)
	Reminyl®	Galantamine	Alzheimer's dementia
	Topamax®	Topiramate	Anticonvulsant
	Zoloft®	Sertraline	Antidepressant (SSRI)

Brand Name Medications and Side Effects

The following list of medications is arranged by brand name and includes adverse effects, among which may be side effects of the drugs. This list focuses on those adverse effects that potentially affect nutrition and metabolism. Oftentimes, these types of actions are overlooked, causing medical professionals to perform unnecessary tests to determine the problem. Therefore, it is important that the health professionals who deal with nutritional and drug concerns have knowledge of the potential effects of drugs on metabolism. Intervention by a dietitian or pharmacist who sees a potential interaction is vital in correcting and improving a patient's medication regimen to avoid adverse effects on the patient's nutritional status. Please be aware that this list is by no means complete. It was designed to provide examples of some of the most common or significant adverse effects related to nutrition.

Owing to the proliferation of antineoplastic medications, only representative agents are included in this table. For any patient being actively treated for cancer, caregivers must review the agents individually. When reviewing an individual patient's medication regimen, a drug-by-drug review is warranted and strongly recommended by the authors. Several resources are available on the World Wide Web. An example of such a site is www.rxlist.com. Another Internet site that lists newly approved drug therapies and searchable information on the drugs is at http://www.centerwatch.com. Local drug information services should be the primary source for data.

Brand Name	Generic Name of Example Drug	Drug Class	Side Effect
	3% sodium chloride parenteral solution	Hypertonic sodium fluid	Hyponatremia
	5% sodium chloride parenteral solution	Hypertonic sodium fluid	Hypernatremia
	Alcohol	Alcohol	Hypomagnesemia
	Calcium chloride parenteral solution	Calcium salt	Hypercalcemia, hypophosphatemia
	Calcium gluceptate parenteral solution	Calcium salt	Hypercalcemia, hypophosphatemia
	Calcium gluconate parenteral solution	Calcium salt	Hypercalcemia, hypophosphatemia
	Potassium phosphate parenteral solution	Phosphorus salt	Hyperphosphatemia, hypocalcemia
	Sodium phosphate parenteral solution	Phosphorus salt	Hyperphosphatemia, hypocalcemia
	Vitamin A and D combination products	Vitamin A and D (toxic)	Hypercalcemia
Abelcet®	Amphotericin B	Antibiotic	Hypokalemia, hypomagnesemia, nausea
Actonel®	Risedronate	Biphosphonate	Diarrhea, epigastric pain
Actos®	Pioglitazone	Hypoglycemic agent	Hypoglycemia
Acutrim®	Phenylpropanolamine	Anorexiant	Decreased appetite
Adderall®	Amphetamine mixture	Amphetamine	Decreased appetite
Adiphex-P®	Phentermine	Anorexiant	Decreased appetite
Adrenalin®	Epinephrine	Bronchodilator	Hyperglycemia
Advil®	Ibuprofen	Nonsteroidal antiinflammatory agent (all)	Fluid retention, hyperkalemia, ulcers
Agenerase®	Amprenavir	Anti-HIV (protease inhibitors)	Diarrhea, hyperglycemia, hypertriglyceridemia, nausea, vomiting
Aldactone®	Spironolactone	Diuretic (potassium-sparing)	Fluid depletion, hyperkalemia, hypomagnesemia, hyponatremia, hypophosphatemia, pH changes
Aldomet®	Methyldopa	Antihypertensive agent (alpha adrenergic blocking)	Diarrhea, fluid retention
Aleve®	Naproxen	Nonsteroidal antiinflammatory agent (all)	Fluid retention, hyperkalemia, ulcers
Altace®	Ramipril	Antihypertensive agent (ace inhibitors)	Hyperkalemia
Amaryl®	Glimepiride	Hypoglycemic agent	Nausea
Amikin®	Amikacin	Antibiotic	Hypokalemia, hypomagnesemia
Amoxil®	Amoxicillin	Antibiotic	Diarrhea, nausea, pseudomembranous colitis
Amphogel®	Aluminum hydroxide	Antacid (aluminum and calcium containing)	Constipation

Brand name	Generic	Class	Side effects
Aquasol A®	Vitamin A	Vitamin A (toxic)	Hypercalcemia
Aredia®	Pamidronate	Bisphosphonate	Hypocalcemia, hypomagnesemia, hypophosphatemia
Aricept®	Donepezim	Alzheimer's agents	Diarrhea
Arixtra®	Fonaparinux	Anticoagulant	Constipation, edema, nausea
Artane®	Trihexyphenidyl	Anti-Parkinson's agent	Constipation
Ascriptin®	Aspirin	Salicylate	Ulcers
Ascriptin®	Aspirin	Salicylate (toxic)	Hypophosphatemia, pH changes
Atromid-S®	Clofibrate	Lipid-lowering agent	Hypoglycemia
Augmentin®	Amoxicillin and clavulanate	Antibiotic	Pseudomembranous colitis
Avandia®	Rosiglitazone	Hypoglycemic agent	Hypoglycemia
Avelox®	Moxifloxacin	Antibiotic	Diarrhea, nausea
Bactrim®	Co-trimoxazole	Antibiotic	Diarrhea
Benadryl®	Diphenhydramine	Antihistamine (H1 blocker)	Constipation
Bufferin®	Aspirin	Salicylate	Ulcers
Bufferin®	Aspirin	Salicylate (toxic)	Hypophosphatemia, pH changes
Bumex®	Bumetanide	Diuretic (loop)	Hypernatremia, hypocalcemia
Calciferol®	Vitamin D	Vitamin D (toxic)	Hypercalcemia
Capoten®	Captopril	Antihypertensive agent (beta-1 blockers and ace inhibitors)	Hyperkalemia
Carafate®	Sucralfate	Gastrointestinal agent	Hypophosphatemia
Catapres®	Clonidine	Antihypertensive (alpha 2 adrenergic agonist)	Constipation
Celexa®	Citalopram	Antidepressant (SSRI)	Weight gain, weight loss
Ceftin Suspension®	Cefuroxime	Sorbitol-containing suspensions	Diarrhea
Celestone®	Betamethasone	Steroid (corticosteroid)	Fluid retention, hyperglycemia, hypokalemia, hypophosphatemia, increased appetite, ulcers
CellCept®	Mycophenolate	Immunosuppressant	Diarrhea
Chlor-Trimeton®	Chlorpheniramine	Antihistamine (H1 blocker)	Constipation
Chronulac®	Lactulose	Laxative	Diarrhea
Chronulac®	Lactulose	Laxative (abuse)	Diarrhea, hypokalemia, pH changes
Cipro®	Ciprofloxacin	Antibiotic	Diarrhea

Brand Name	Generic Name of Example Drug	Drug Class	Side Effect
Citrate 600®	Calcium carbonate	Calcium salt	Constipation, hypercalcemia, hypophosphatemia
Citrate of Magnesia®	Magnesium citrate	Laxative (magnesium containing)	Hypermagnesemia
Cleocin®	Clindamycin	Antibiotic	Diarrhea, nausea, pseudomembranous colitis
Clozapine®	Clozaril	Antipsychotic	Increased appetite
Cogentin®	Benztropine	Anti-Parkinson's agent	Constipation
Cognex®	Tacrine	Alzheimer's agents	Diarrhea
Colace®	Docusate sodium	Stool softener	Diarrhea
Combivir®	Zidovudine, lamivudine	Anti-HIV agent (narti)	Diarrhea, nausea, vomiting
Cortef®	Hydrocortisone	Steroid (corticosteroid)	Fluid retention, hyperglycemia, hypokalemia, hypophosphatemia, increased appetite, ulcers
Cortone®	Cortisone	Steroid (corticosteroid)	Fluid retention, hyperglycemia, hypokalemia, hypophosphatemia, increased appetite, ulcers
Crixivan®	Indinavir	Anti-HIV agent (protease inhibitor)	Hypertriglyceridemia, nausea, hypertriglyceridemia
Cytoxan®	Cyclophosphamide	Cytotoxic chemotherapy (alkylating agent)	Hyponatremia
Decadron®	Dexamethasone	Steroid (corticosteroid)	Fluid retention, hyperglycemia, hypokalemia, hypophosphatemia, increased appetite, ulcers
Deca-Durabolin®	Nandrolone	Anabolic steroids	Anabolism
Delta-Cortef®	Prednisolone	Steroid (corticosteroid)	Fluid retention, hyperglycemia, hypophosphatemia, increased appetite, ulcers
Deltasone®	Prednisone	Steroid (corticosteroid)	Fluid retention, hyperglycemia, hypophosphatemia, increased appetite, ulcers
Demadex®	Torsemide	Diuretics (loop)	Hypernatremia, hypocalcemia
Demerol®	Meperidine	Analgesic agent (opiates)	Constipation, nausea
Depo-Provera®	Medroxyprogesterone	Hormone	Increased appetite

Brand	Generic	Class	Side effects
Depo-Testosterone®	Cypionate	Anabolic steroid	Hypoglycemia
Desoxyn®	Methamphetamine	Amphetamine	Decreased appetite
Desyrel®	Trazodone	Antidepressant	Dry mouth, increased appetite, nausea, vomiting
Dexedrine®	Dextroamphetamine	Amphetamine	Decreased appetite
Diabenase®	Chlorpropamide	Hypoglycemic agent	Hyponatremia
Diabeta®	Glyburide	Hypoglycemic agent	Hypoglycemia
Diamox®	Acetazolamide	Diuretic	Fluid depletion, hypomagnesemia, hyponatremia, hypophosphatemia, pH changes
Dianabol®	Methandrostenolone	Anabolic steroid	Hypoglycemia
Didronel®	Etidronate	Bisphosphonate	Hypocalcemia, hypomagnesemia, hypophosphatemia
Dilantin®	Phenytoin	Anticonvulsant (hydantoin)	Hyperglycemia, hypocalcemia, nausea
Dulcolax®	Bisacodyl	Laxative	Diarrhea
Dulcolax®	Bisacodyl	Laxative (abuse)	Diarrhea, hypokalemia, pH changes
Dyazide®	Hydrochlorthiazide, Triameterene	Diuretic (potassium sparing contains thiazide as well)	Hypercalcemia, hyperglycemia, hyperkalemia
Ecotrin®	Aspirin	Salicylate (toxic)	Hypophosphatemia, pH changes
Edecrin®	Ethacrynic acid	Diuretic (loop)	Hypernatremia, hypocalcemia
EES®	Erythromycin	Antibiotic and off-label motility agent	Diarrhea, nausea, pseudomembranous colitis
Effexor®	Venlafaxine	Antidepressant (SSRI)	Weight gain, weight loss
Elavil®	Amitriptyline	Antidepressant	Hypoglycemia, increased appetite
Elspar®	Asparaginase	Antineoplastic agent	Hyperglycemia
E-Mycin®	Erythromycin	Antibiotic and off-label motility agent	Diarrhea, nausea, pseudomembranous colitis
Epivir®	Lamivudine	Anti-HIV agent	Diarrhea, nausea
Evac-Q-Mag®	Magnesium citrate	Laxative (magnesium containing)	Hypermagnesemia
Femiron®	Ferrous fumarate	Iron salt	Constipation
Feosol®	Ferrous sulfate	Iron salt	Constipation
Fergon®	Ferrous gluconate	Iron salt	Constipation
FiberCon®	Calcium polycarbophil	Antidiarrheal	Constipation

Brand Name	Generic Name of Example Drug	Drug Class	Side Effect
Fleets enema®	Sodium phosphate	Laxative (phosphate containing)	Hyperphosphatemia, hypocalcemia
Fleets phospho-soda®	Sodium phosphate	Laxative (phosphate containing)	Hyperphosphatemia, hypocalcemia
Florinef®	Fludrocortisone	Steroid (mineralocorticoid)	Fluid retention, hyperglycemia, hypokalemia, hypophosphatemia, increased appetite
Focalin®	Dexmethylphenidate	Central nervous system stimulant	Anorexia, nausea, vomiting
Fortaz®	Ceftazadime	Antibiotic	Pseudomembranous colitis
Fortovase®	Saqunavir	Anti-HIV agent (protease inhibitors)	Hypertriglyceridemia, diarrhea
Fosamax®	Alendronate	Bisphosphonate	Hypocalcemia, hypomagnesemia, hypophosphatemia, ulcers
Fungizone®	Amphotericin B	Antibiotic	Hypokalemia, hypomagnesemia, nausea
Garamycin®	Gentamicin	Antibiotic	Hypokalemia, hypomagnesemia
Glucophage®	Metformin	Hypoglycemic agent	Hypoglycemia
Glucotrol®	Glipizide	Hypoglycemic agent	Hypoglycemia
Glyset®	Miglitol	Hypoglycemic agent	Hypoglycemia
GoLytely®	Polyethylene glycol	Laxative	Diarrhea
GoLytely®	Polyethylene glycol	Laxative (abuse)	Hypokalemia, pH changes
Hivid®	Zalcitabine	Anti-HIV agent (narti)	Hyperglycemia, hypertriglyceridemia, oral ulcers
Humulin N, R, L, U, 70/30®	Insulin	Insulin	Hypoglycemia
Humulin N, R, L, U, 70/30®	Insulin	Insulin (excessive)	Hypoglycemia, hypokalemia, hypomagnesemia, hypophosphatemia
Humalog®	Insulin lispro	Insulin	Hypoglycemia
Humalog®	Insulin lispro	Insulin (excessive)	Hypoglycemia, hypokalemia, hypomagnesemia, hypophosphatemia
HydroDiuril®	Hydrochlorthiazide	Diuretic (thiazide, non-potassium sparing)	Constipation, fluid depletion, hypercalcemia, hyperglycemia, hypokalemia, hypomagnesemia, hyponatremia, hypophosphatemia, pH changes

Brand	Type	Side effects
Hytrin®	Terazosin	Antihypertensive (alpha adrenergic blocking agent)	Fluid retention
Ifex®	Ifosfamide	Antineoplastic agent	Nausea, ulcers
Imuran®	Azathioprine	Immunosuppressant	Diarrhea, nausea, vomiting, altered taste acuity, sore throat
Imodium A-D®	Loperamide	Antidiarrheal	Constipation
Inderal®	Propranolol	Antihypertensive agent (beta-1 blockers)	Hypoglycemia, hyperkalemia
Indocin®	Indomethacin	Nonsteroidal antiinflammatory agent	Ulcers, fluid retention, hyperkalemia
Ionamin®	Phentermine	Anorexiant	Decreased appetite
Kalcinate®	Calcium gluconate	Calcium salt	Constipation, hypophosphatemia, hypercalcemia
Kaopectate II®	Loperamide	Antidiarrheal	Constipation
K-Dur®	Potassium chloride	Potassium supplements	Hyperkalemia
K-Lyte®	Potassium bicarbonate, Potassium citrate	Potassium supplements	Hyperkalemia
K-Phos®	Potassium phosphate, Sodium phosphate	Potassium supplements	Hyperkalemia
Kytril®	Granisetron	Antiemetic (5HT3 antagonist)	Constipation, diarrhea
Lanoxin®	Digoxin	Cardiac agent	Diarrhea
Lanoxin®	Digoxin	Cardiac agent (toxic)	Nausea, hyperkalemia, hypomagnesemia
Lantos®	Insulin glargine	Insulin	Hypoglycemia
Lantos®	Insulin glargine	Insulin (excessive)	Hypophosphatemia, hypomagnesemia, hypokalemia, hypoglycemia
Lasix®	Furosemide	Diuretic (loop, non-potassium sparing)	Constipation, fluid depletion, hypokalemia, hypernatremia, hyponatremia, hypophosphatemia, hypocalcemia, hypomagnesemia, pH changes
Lithane®	Lithium	Central nervous system agent	Hyperglycemia
Lithane®	Lithium	Central nervous system agent (lithium) (toxic)	Hypercalcemia
Lithonate®	Lithium	Central nervous system agent	Hyperglycemia
Lithonate®	Lithium	Central nervous system agent (lithium) (toxic)	Hypercalcemia
Lomotil®	Diphenoxalate/atropine	Antidiarrheal	Constipation
Loniten®	Minoxidil	Vasodilator	Fluid retention

Brand Name	Generic Name of Example Drug	Drug Class	Side Effect
Lopressor®	Metoprolol	Antihypertensive agent (beta-1 blocker)	Hypoglycemia, hyperkalemia
Lortab®	Hydrocodone	Analgesic agent (opiate)	Nausea, constipation
Lotensin®	Benazepril	Antihypertensive agent (ace inhibitor)	Hyperkalemia
Luminal®	Phenobarbital	Anticonvulsant (barbiturate)	Hypocalcemia, hyperglycemia
Luvox®	Fluvoxamine	Antidepressant (SSRI)	Weight gain, weight loss
MagOx®	Magnesium oxide	Magnesium supplement	Hypokalemia, hypermagnesemia, diarrhea
Marinol®	Dronabinol	Cannabinoid	Increased appetite
Maxzide®	Hydrochlorthiazide, Triameterene	Diuretic (potassium sparing, contains thiazide as well)	Hyperkalemia, hyperglycemia, hypercalcemia
Megace®	Megesterol	Steroid (antineoplastic hormonal)	Increased appetite
Meridia®	Sibutramine	Anorexiant	Decreased appetite
Mestinon®	Pyridostgmine	Myasthenia gravis agent	Diarrhea
Metamucil®	Psyllium	Laxative	Diarrhea
Mevacor®	Lovastatin	Antihyperlipidemic agent	Nausea, vomiting, abdominal pain, constipation
Miacalcin®, Cibacalcin®	Calcitonin	Calcitonin	Hyperglycemia, hypocalcemia
Micro-K®	Potassium chloride	Potassium supplement	Hyperkalemia
Micronase®	Glyburide	Hypoglycemic agent	Hypoglycemia
Midamor®	Amiloride	Diuretic (potassium sparing)	Hyperkalemia
Phillips™ milk of magnesia	Magnesium hydroxide	Antacid (magnesium containing)	Diarrhea
Minipress®	Prazosin	Antihypertensive (alpha adrenergic blocking agent)	Fluid retention
Mithramycin®	Plicamycin	Antineoplastic agent	Hypocalcemia
MOM®	Magnesium hydroxide	Antacid (magnesium containing)	Hypermagnesemia
Motrin®	Ibuprofen	Nonsteroidal antiinflammatory agent (all)	Ulcers, fluid retention, hyperkalemia
MSContin®	Morphine	Analgesic agents (opioids)	Nausea, constipation
MSIR®	Morphine	Analgesic agents (opioids)	Nausea, constipation
Mutamycin®	Mitomycin	Antineoplastic agent	Nausea, ulcers
Naprosyn®	Naproxen	Nonsteroidal antiinflammatory agent (all)	Ulcers, fluid retention, hyperkalemia

Nardil®	Phenelzine	Central nervous system agent (monoamine oxidase inhibitor)	Hypoglycemia, increased appetite
Nebcin®	Tobramycin	Antibiotics	Hypokalemia, hypomagnesemia
Neo-Calglucon®	Calcium glubionate	Calcium salt	Constipation, hypophosphatemia
Neoral®	Cyclosporine	Immunosuppressant agent	Hypomagnesemia
Neosar®	Cyclophosphamide	Cytotoxic chemotherapy (alkylating agent)	Hyponatremia
NeutraPhos®	Potassium phosphate/sodium phosphate	Potassium supplement	Hyperkalemia
Niferex®	Polysaccharide-iron complex	Iron salt	Constipation
Norpramin®	Desipramine	Antidepressant	Increased appetite
Novolin R, N, L, 70/30®	Insulin, all types	Insulin	Hypoglycemia
Novolin R®	Insulin, regular	Insulin (excessive)	Hypophosphatemia, hypomagnesemia, hypokalemia
Novolog®	Insulin aspart	Insulin	Hypoglycemia
Novolog®	Insulin aspart	Insulin (excessive)	Hypophosphatemia, hypomagnesemia, hypokalemia
Olanzapine®	Thienbenzodiazepine	Antipsychotic	Increased appetite
Oncovin®	Vincristine	Antineoplastic agent	Nausea ulcers
Orasone®	Prednisone	Steroid (corticosteroid)	Increased appetite, ulcers, fluid retention, hyperglycemia, hypophosphatemia
Orinase®	Tolbutamide	Hypoglycemic agent	Hypoglycemia
Oxandrin®	Oxandroline	Anabolic steroid	Hypoglycemia, increased appetite, anabolism
OxyContin®	Oxycodone	Analgesic agent (opioid)	Constipation, nausea
OxyIR®	Oxycodone	Analgesic agent (opioid)	Constipation, nausea
Pamelor®	Nortriptyline	Antidepressant (tricyclic)	Hypoglycemia
Paraplatin®	Carboplatin	Antineoplastic agent	Nausea, ulcers, hypocalcemia, hypomagnesemia
Parnate®	Tranylcypromine	Antidepressant (monoamine oxidase inhibitor)	Increased appetite, hypoglycemia
Paxil®	Paroxetine	Antidepressant (SSRI)	Increased appetite, weight gain, weight loss
PenTids®	Penicillins (high dose)	Antibiotic	Hypokalemia
PenVK®	Penicillins (high dose)	Antibiotic	Hypokalemia

Brand Name	Generic Name of Example Drug	Drug Class	Side Effect
Pepto-Bismol®	Bismuth subsalicylate	Antidiarrheal	Constipation
Periactin®	Cyproheptadine	Antihistamine (H1 blocker)	Increased appetite, constipation
Permax®	Pergolide	Anti-Parkinson's agent	Constipation
Phenergan®	Promethazine	Antiemetic	Constipation
PhosLo®	Calcium acetate	Calcium salt	Constipation, hypophosphatemia, hypercalcemia
Pitocin®	Oxytoxin	Hormone (oxytocic)	Hyponatremia
Platinol®	Cisplatin	Antineoplastic agents	Nausea, ulcers, hypocalcemia, hypomagnesemia
Pondimin®	Fenfluramine	Anorexiant	Decreased appetite
Prandin®	Repaglinide	Hypoglycemic agent	Hypoglycemia
Pravachol®	Pravastatin	Antihyperlipidemic agent	Nausea, vomiting, abdominal pain, constipation
Precose®	Acarbose	Hypoglycemic agent	Hypoglycemia
Prelone®	Prednisolone	Steroid (corticosteroid)	Increased appetite, ulcers, hyperglycemia, hypophosphatemia, fluid retention
Premarin®	Estrogen	Estrogen	Fluid retention
Prinivil®	Lisinopril	Antihypertensive agent (ace inhibitor)	Diarrhea, abdominal pain
Prograf®	Tacrolimus		Hyperglycemia, hyperkalemia, nausea, vomiting
Prostigmin®	Neostigmine	Myasthenia gravis agents	Diarrhea
Prozac®, Sarafem®	Fluoxetine	Antidepressant (SSRI)	Weight gain, weight loss
Quetiapine®	Dibenzothiazepine	Antipsychotic	Increased appetite
Quinaglute®	Quinidine	Cardiac agent	Diarrhea
Reglan®	Metoclopramide	Motility agent	Diarrhea
Remeron®	Mirtazapine	Antidepressant (atypical)	Dry mouth, increased appetite, weight gain
Reminyl®	Galantamine	Alzheimer's dementia	Nausea, vomiting, diarrhea, anorexia, weight loss
Rescriptor®	Delavirdine	Anti-HIV agent (nnrti)	Nausea

Brand	Generic	Category	Side Effects
Retrovir®	Zidovudine	HIV therapy (narti)	Nausea, abdominal pain, anorexia, diarrhea,
Rifadin®	Rifampin	Antitubercular agent	Hyperglycemia, hypocalcemia
Riopan®	Magaldrate	Antacid (magnesium containing)	Diarrhea, hypermagnesemia
Risperidone®	Benzisoxazole	Antipsychotic	Increased appetite
Ritalin®	Methylphenidate		Anorexia, nausea
Rocephin®	Ceftriaxone	Antibiotic	Diarrhea, pseudomembranous colitis
Roxanol®	Morphine	Analgesic agent (opiate)	Nausea, constipation
Sandimmune®	Cyclosporine	Immunosuppressant agent	Hypomagnesemia, hyperglycemia, hyperlipidemia, hyperkalemia
Sandostatin®	Octreotide	Antisecretory	Constipation
Senokot®	Senna	Laxative	Diarrhea
Senokot®	Senna	Laxative (abuse)	Hypokalemia, pH changes, diarrhea
Septra®	Co-trimoxazole	Antibiotic	Diarrhea
Sinemet®	Levodopa, Carbidopa	Anti-Parkinson's agent	Constipation
Sinequin®	Doxepin	Antidepressant (tricyclic)	Hypoglycemia
SloBid®	Theophylline	Bronchodilator	Nausea
SloBid®	Theophylline	Bronchodilator (toxic)	Hypophosphatemia, hypercalcemia, nausea
Slow K®	Potassium chloride	Potassium supplement	Hyperkalemia
Solu-Cortef®	Methylprednisolone	Steroid (corticosteroid)	Ulcers, fluid retention, hyperglycemia, hypophosphatemia, increased appetite
Sorbitol-containing suspensions	May not have sorbitol listed on label	Sorbitol-containing suspensions	Diarrhea
Sumycin®	Tetracycline	Antibiotic	Nausea, pseudomembranous colitis
Surfak®	Docusate calcium	Stool softener	Diarrhea
Sustiva®	Efavirenz	Anti-HIV agent (nnrti)	Nausea, hypertriglyceridemia, diarrhea
Tagamet Suspension®	Cimetidine	Sorbitol-containing suspension	Diarrhea
Tavist®	Clemastine	Antihistamine (H1 blocker)	Constipation
Tegretol®	Carbamazepine	Anticonvulsant (toxic)	Nausea
Tenormin®	Atenolol	Antihypertensive agent (beta-1 blocker)	Hypoglycemia, hyperkalemia
TheoDur®	Theophylline	Bronchodilator	Nausea

Brand Name	Generic Name of Example Drug	Drug Class	Side Effect
TheoDur®	Theophylline	Bronchodilator (toxic)	Hypophosphatemia, hypercalcemia, nausea
Timentin®	Ticarcillin, Clavulanate acid	Antibiotics	Hypokalemia
Tofranil®	Imipramine	Antidepressant	Increased appetite, hypoglycemia
Topamax®	Topiramate	Anticonvulsant	Diarrhea, weight loss, hyperchloremia, hypocapnia
Toprol XL®	Metoprolol	Antihypertensive agent (beta-1 blocker)	Hypoglycemia, hyperkalemia
Transderm-Scop®	Scopalamine	Antiemetic	Constipation
Trimox Suspension®	Amoxicillin	Sorbitol-containing suspension	Diarrhea
Trizivir®	Zidovudine, lamivudine, abacavir	Anti-HIV agent	Nausea, vomiting, diarrhea
Tums®	Calcium carbonate	Calcium salt	Constipation, hypophosphatemia, hypercalcemia
Tylenol Children's Suspension®	Acetaminophen	Sorbitol-containing suspension	Diarrhea
Vasotec®	Enalapril	Antihypertensive agents (beta-1 blockers and ace inhibitors)	Hyperkalemia
Velban®	Vinblastine	Antineoplastic agents	Nausea, ulcers
Videx®	Didanosine	Anti-HIV agent (narti)	Hypertriglyceridemia, altered taste, diarrhea, nausea
Viracept®	Nelfinavir	Anti-HIV agent (protease inhibitor)	Hypertriglyceridemia, diarrhea
Viramune®	Nevirapine	Anti-HIV agent (nnrti)	Nausea
Viread®			Flatulence, vomiting, diarrhea, nausea
Winstrol®	Stanozol	Anabolic steroid	Anabolism, hypoglycemia
Zaroxyln®	Metolazone	Diuretic	Hyponatremia, fluid depletion, hypophosphatemia, hypomagnesemia, pH changes
Zerit®	Stavudine	Anti-HIV agent (narti)	Abdominal pain, diarrhea, nausea, vomiting

Ziagen®	Abacavir	Anti-HIV agent (narti)	Hyperglycemia, hypertriglyceridemia, anorexia, diarrhea, nausea, vomiting
Zithromax Suspension®	Azithromycin	Sorbitol-containing suspension	Diarrhea
Zofran®	Ondasteron	Antiemetic (5HT3 antagonist)	Constipation, diarrhea
Zoloft®	Sertraline	Antidepressant (SSRI)	Weight gain, weight loss
Zometa®	Zoledronic	Bisphosphanate	Nausea, diarrhea, vomiting, abdominal pain
Zosyn®	Pipercillin, Tazobactam	Antibiotic	Pseudomembranous colitis, hypokalemia

APPENDIX **A.3**

Generic Name Medications and Side Effects

The following list of medications is arranged by generic name and includes adverse effects, among which may be side effects of the drugs. This list focuses on those reactions that potentially affect nutrition and metabolism. Oftentimes, these types of actions are overlooked, causing medical professionals to perform unnecessary tests to determine the problem. Therefore, it is important that health professionals who deal with nutritional and drug concerns have knowledge of the potential effects of drugs on metabolism. Intervention by a dietitian or pharmacist who sees a potential interaction is vital in correcting and improving a medication regimen to avoid adverse effects on the patient's nutritional status. Please be aware that this list is by no means complete. It was designed to provide examples of some of the most common or significant adverse effects related to nutrition.

Owing to the proliferation of antineoplastic medications, only representative agents are included in this table. For any patient being actively treated for cancer, caregivers must review the agents individually. When reviewing an individual patient's medication regimen, a drug-by-drug review is warranted and strongly recommended by the authors. Several resources are available on the World Wide Web. An example of such a site is www.rxlist.com. Another Internet site that lists newly approved drug therapies and searchable information on the drugs is at http://www.centerwatch.com. Local drug information services should be the primary source for data.

Generic Name of Example Drug	Brand Name	Drug Class	Side Effect
3% sodium chloride parenteral solution		Hypertonic sodium fluid	Hyponatremia
5% sodium chloride parenteral solution		Hypertonic sodium fluid	Hypernatremia
Abacavir	Ziagen®	Anti-HIV agent (narti)	Hyperglycemia, hypertriglyceridemia, anorexia, diarrhea, nausea, vomiting
Acarbose	Precose®	Hypoglycemic agent	Hypoglycemia
Acetaminophen	Tylenol Children's Suspension®	Sorbitol-containing suspension	Diarrhea
Acetazolamide	Diamox®	Diuretic	Fluid depletion, hypomagnesemia, hyponatremia, hypophosphatemia, pH changes
Alcohol		Alcohol	Hypomagnesemia
Alendronate	Fosamax®	Bisphosphonate	Hypocalcemia, hypomagnesemia, hypophosphatemia, ulcers
Aluminum hydroxide	Amphogel®	Antacid (aluminum and calcium containing)	Constipation
Amikacin	Amikin®	Antibiotic	Hypokalemia, hypomagnesemia
Amiloride	Midamor®	Diuretic (potassium sparing)	Hyperkalemia
Amitriptyline	Elavil®	Antidepressant	Hypoglycemia, increased appetite
Amoxicillin	Amoxil®	Antibiotic	Diarrhea, nausea, pseudomembranous colitis
Amoxicillin	Trimox Suspension®	Sorbitol containing suspension	Diarrhea
Amoxicillin and clavulanate	Augmentin®	Antibiotic	Pseudomembranous colitis
Amphetamine mixture	Adderall®	Amphetamine	Decreased appetite
Amphotericin B	Abelcet®	Antibiotic	Hypokalemia, hypomagnesemia, nausea
Amphotericin B	Fungizone®	Antibiotic	Hypokalemia, hypomagnesemia, nausea
Amprenavir	Agenerase®	Anti-HIV (protease inhibitors)	Diarrhea, hyperglycemia, hypertriglyceridemia, nausea, vomiting
Asparginase	Elspar®	Antineoplastic agent	Hyperglycemia
Aspirin	Ascriptin®	Salicylate	Ulcers
Aspirin	Ascriptin®	Salicylate (toxic)	Hypophosphatemia, pH changes
Aspirin	Bufferin®	Salicylate	Ulcers
Aspirin	Bufferin®	Salicylate (toxic)	Hypophosphatemia, pH changes

Generic Name	Brand Name	Class	Side Effects
Aspirin	Ecotrin®	Salicylate (toxic)	Hypophosphatemia, pH changes
Atenolol	Tenormin®	Antihypertensive agent (beta-1 blocker)	Hypoglycemia, hyperkalemia
Azathioprine	Imuran®	Immunosuppressant	Diarrhea, nausea, vomiting, altered taste acuity, sore throat
Azithromycin	Zithromax suspension®	Sorbitol containing suspension	Diarrhea
Benazepril	Lotensin®	Antihypertensive agent (ace inhibitor)	Hyperkalemia
Benzisoxazole	Risperidone®	Antipsychotic	Increased appetite
Benztropine	Cogentin®	Anti-Parkinson's agent	Constipation
Betamethasone	Celestone®	Steroid (corticosteroid)	Fluid retention, hyperglycemia, hypokalemia, hypophosphatemia, increased appetite, ulcers
Bisacodyl	Dulcolax®	Laxative	Diarrhea
Bisacodyl	Dulcolax®	Laxative (abuse)	Diarrhea, hypokalemia, pH changes
Bismuth subsalicylate	Pepto-Bismol®	Antidiarrheal	Constipation
Bumetanide	Bumex®	Diuretic (loop)	Hypernatremia, hypocalcemia
Calcitonin	Miacalcin®, Cibacalcin®	Calcitonin	Hyperglycemia, hypocalcemia
Calcium acetate	PhosLo®	Calcium salt	Constipation, hypophosphatemia, hypercalcemia
Calcium carbonate	Citrate 600®	Calcium salt	Constipation, hypercalcemia, hypophosphatemia
Calcium carbonate	Tums®	Calcium salt	Constipation, hypophosphatemia, hypercalcemia
Calcium chloride parenteral solution		Calcium salt	Hypercalcemia, hypophosphatemia
Calcium glubionate	Neo-Calglucon®	Calcium salt	Constipation, hypophosphatemia
Calcium gluceptate parenteral solution		Calcium salt	Hypercalcemia, hypophosphatemia
Calcium gluconate	Kalcinate®	Calcium salt	Constipation, hypophosphatemia, hypercalcemia
Calcium gluconate parenteral solution		Calcium salt	Hypercalcemia, hypophosphatemia
Calcium polycarbophil	FiberCon®	Antidiarrheal	Constipation
Captopril	Capoten®	Antihypertensive agent (beta-1 blockers and ace inhibitors)	Hyperkalemia
Carbamazepine	Tegretol®	Anticonvulsant (toxic)	Nausea

Generic Name of Example Drug	Brand Name	Drug Class	Side Effect
Carboplatin	Paraplatin®	Antineoplastic agent	Nausea, ulcers, hypocalcemia, hypomagnesemia
Ceftazadime	Fortaz®	Antibiotic	Pseudomembranous colitis
Ceftriaxone	Rocephin®	Antibiotic	Diarrhea, pseudomembranous colitis
Cefuroxime	Ceftin Suspension®	Sorbitol-containing suspensions	Diarrhea
Chlorpheniramine	Chlor-Trimeton®	Antihistamine, (H1 blocker)	Constipation
Chlorpropamide	Diabenase®	Hypogylcemic agent	Hyponatremia
Cimetidine	Tagamet Suspension®	Sorbitol-containing suspension	Diarrhea
Ciprofloxacin	Cipro®	Antibiotic	Diarrhea
Cisplatin	Platinol®	Antineoplastic agents	Nausea, ulcers, hypocalcemia, hypomagnesemia
Citalopram	Celexa®	Antidepressant (SSRI)	Weight gain, weight loss
Clemastine	Tavist®	Antihistamine, (H1 blocker)	Constipation
Clindamycin	Cleocin®	Antibiotic	Diarrhea, nausea, pseudomembranous colitis
Clofibrate	Atromid-S®	Lipid-lowering agent	Hypoglycemia
Clonidine	Catapres®	Antihypertensive (alpha-2 adrenergic agonist)	Constipation
Clozaril	Clozapine®	Antipsychotic	Increased appetite
Cortisone	Cortone®	Steroid (corticosteroid)	Fluid retention, hyperglycemia, hypokalemia, hypophosphatemia, increased appetite, ulcers
Co-trimoxazole	Bactrim®	Antibiotic	Diarrhea
Co-trimoxazole	Septra®	Antibiotic	Diarrhea
Cyclophosphamide	Cytoxan®	Cytotoxic chemotherapy (alkylating agent)	Hyponatremia
Cyclophosphamide	Neosar®	Cytotoxic chemotherapy (alkylating agent)	Hyponatremia
Cyclosporine	Neoral®	Immunosuppressant agent	Hypomagnesemia
Cyclosporine	Sandimmune®	Immunosuppressant agent	Hypomagnesemia, hyperglycemia, hyperlipidemia, hyperkalemia
Cypionate	Depo-testosterone®	Anabolic steroid	Hypoglycemia
Cyproheptadine	Periactin®	Antihistamine, (H1 blocker)	Increased appetite, constipation
Delavirdine	Rescriptor	Ant-HIV agent (nnrti)	Nausea
Desipramine	Norpramin®	Antidepressant	Increased appetite

Generic name	Brand name	Class	Side effects
Dexamethasone	Decadron®	Steroid (corticosteroid)	Fluid retention, hyperglycemia, hypokalemia, hypophosphatemia, increased appetite, ulcers
Dexmethylphenidate	Focalin®	Central nervous system (CNS) stimulant	Anorexia, nausea, vomiting
Dextroamphetamine	Dexedrine®	Amphetamine	Decreased appetite
Dibenzothiazepine	Quetiapine®	Antipsychotic	Increased appetite
Didanosine	Videx®	Anti-HIV agent (narti)	Hypertriglyceridemia, altered taste, diarrhea, nausea
Digoxin	Lanoxin®	Cardiac agent	Diarrhea
Digoxin	Lanoxin®	Cardiac agent (toxic)	Nausea, hyperkalemia, hypomagnesemia
Diphenhydramine	Benadryl®	Antihistamine, (H1 blocker)	Constipation
Diphenoxalate/atropine	Lomotil®	Antidiarrheal	Constipation
Docusate calcium	Surfak®	Stool softener	Diarrhea
Docusate sodium	Colace®	Stool softener	Diarrhea
Donepezim	Aricept®	Alzheimer's agents	Diarrhea
Doxepin	Sinequin®	Antidepressant (tricyclic)	Hypoglycemia
Dronabinol	Marinol®	Cannabinoid	Increased appetite
Efavirenz	Sustiva®	Anti-HIV agent (nnrti)	Nausea, hypertriglyceridemia, diarrhea
Enalapril	Vasotec®	Antihypertensive agents (beta-1 blockers and ace inhibitors)	Hyperkalemia
Epinephrine	Adrenalin®	Bronchodilator	Hyperglycemia
Erythromycin	EES®	Antibiotic and off-label motility agent	Diarrhea, nausea, pseudomembranous colitis
Erythromycin	E-Mycin®	Antibiotic and off-label motility agent	Diarrhea, nausea, pseudomembranous colitis
Estrogen	Premarin®	Estrogen	Fluid retention
Ethacrynic acid	Edecrin®	Diuretic (loop)	Hypernatremia, hypocalcemia
Etidronate	Didronel®	Bisphosphonate	Hypocalcemia, hypomagnesemia, hypophosphatemia
Fenfluramine	Pondimin®	Anorexiant	Decreased appetite
Ferrous fumarate	Femiron®	Iron salt	Constipation
Ferrous gluconate	Fergon®	Iron salt	Constipation
Ferrous sulfate	Feosol®	Iron salt	Constipation
Fludrocortisone	Florinef®	Steroid (mineralocorticoid)	Fluid retention, hyperglycemia, hypokalemia, hypophosphatemia, increased appetite

Generic Name of Example Drug	Brand Name	Drug Class	Side Effect
Fluoxetine	Prozac®, Sarafem®	Antidepressant (SSRI)	Weight gain, weight loss
Fluvoxamine	Luvox®	Antidepressant (SSRI)	Weight gain, weight loss
Fonaparinux	Arixtra®	Anticoagulant	Constipation, edema, nausea
Furosemide	Lasix®	Diuretic (loop, non-potassium sparing)	Constipation, fluid depletion, hypokalemia, hypernatremia, hyponatremia, hypophosphatemia, hypocalcemia, hypomagnesemia, pH changes
Galantamine	Reminyl®	Alzheimer's dementia	Nausea, vomiting, diarrhea, anorexia, weight loss
Gentamicin	Garamycin®	Antibiotic	Hypokalemia, hypomagnesemia
Glimepiride	Amaryl®	Hypoglycemic agent	Nausea
Glipizide	Glucotrol®	Hypoglycemic agent	Hypoglycemia
Glyburide	Diabeta®	Hypoglycemic agent	Hypoglycemia
Glyburide	Micronase®	Hypoglycemic agent	Hypoglycemia
Granisetron	Kytril®	Antiemetic (5HT3 antagonist)	Constipation, diarrhea
Hydrochlorthiazide	HydroDiuril®	Diuretic (thiazide, non-potassium sparing)	Constipation, fluid depletion, hypercalcemia, hyperglycemia, hypokalemia, hypomagnesemia, hyponatremia, hypophosphatemia, pH changes
Hydrochlorthiazide, Triamterene	Dyazide®	Diuretic (potassium sparing, contains thiazide as well)	Hypercalcemia, hyperglycemia, hyperkalemia
Hydrochlorthiazide, Triamterene	Maxzide®	Diuretic (potassium sparing, contains thiazide as well)	Hyperkalemia, hyperglycemia, hypercalcemia
Hydrocodone	Lortab®	Analgesic agent (opiate)	Nausea, constipation
Hydrocortisone	Cortef®	Steroid (corticosteroid)	Fluid retention, hyperglycemia, hypokalemia, hypophosphatemia, increased appetite, ulcers
Ibuprofen	Advil®	Nonsteroidal antiinflammatory agent (all)	Fluid retention, hyperkalemia, ulcers
Ibuprofen	Motrin®	Nonsteroidal antiinflammatory agent (all)	Ulcers, fluid retention, hyperkalemia
Ifosfamide	Ifex®	Antineoplastic agent	Nausea, ulcers
Imipramine	Tofranil®	Antidepressant	Increased appetite, hypoglycemia
Indinavir	Crixivan®	Anti-HIV agent (protease inhibitor)	Hypertriglyceridemia, nausea, hypertriglyceridemia
Indomethacin	Indocin®	Nonsteroidal antiinflammatory agent	Ulcers, fluid retention, hyperkalemia

Insulin	Humulin N, R, L, U, 70/30®	Insulin	Hypoglycemia
Insulin	Humulin N, R, L, U, 70/30®	Insulin (excessive)	Hypoglycemia, hypokalemia, hypomagnesemia, hypophosphatemia
Insulin aspart	Novolog®	Insulin	Hypoglycemia
Insulin aspart	Novolog®	Insulin (excessive)	Hypophosphatemia, hypomagnesemia, hypokalemia
Insulin glargine	Lantos®	Insulin	Hypoglycemia
Insulin glargine	Lantos®	Insulin (excessive)	Hypophosphatemia, hypomagnesemia, hypokalemia, hypoglycemia
Insulin lispro	Humalog®	Insulin	Hypoglycemia
Insulin lispro	Humalog®	Insulin (excessive)	Hypoglycemia, hypokalemia, hypomagnesemia, hypophosphatemia
Insulin, all types	Novolin R, N, L, 70/30®	Insulin	Hypoglycemia
Insulin, regular	Novolin R®	Insulin (excessive)	Hypophosphatemia, hypomagnesemia, hypokalemia
Lactulose	Chronulac®	Laxative	Diarrhea
Lactulose	Chronulac®	Laxative (abuse)	Diarrhea, hypokalemia, pH changes
Lamivudine	Epivil®	Anti-HIV agent	Diarrhea, nausea
Levodopa and carbidopa	Sinemet®	Anti-Parkinson's agent	Constipation
Lisinopril	Prinivil®	Antihypertensive agent (ace inhibitor)	Diarrhea, abdominal pain
Lithium	Lithane®	CNS agent	Hyperglycemia
Lithium	Lithane®	CNS agent (lithium) (toxic)	Hypercalcemia
Lithium	Lithonate®	CNS agent	Hyperglycemia
Lithium	Lithonate®	CNS agent (lithium) (toxic)	Hypercalcemia
Loperamide	Imodium A-D®	Antidiarrheal	Constipation
Loperamide	Kaopectate II®	Antidiarrheal	Constipation
Lovastatin	Mevacor®	Antihyperlipidemic agent	Nausea, vomiting, abdominal pain, constipation
Magaldrate	Riopan®	Antacid (magnesium containing)	Diarrhea, hypermagnesemia
Magnesium citrate	Citrate of Magnesia®	Laxative (magnesium containing)	Hypermagnesemia
Magnesium citrate	Evac-Q-Mag®	Laxative (magnesium containing)	Hypermagnesemia
Magnesium hydroxide	Phillips'™ milk of magnesia	Antacid (magnesium containing)	Diarrhea
Magnesium hydroxide	MOM®	Antacid (magnesium containing)	Hypermagnesemia

Generic Name of Example Drug	Brand Name	Drug Class	Side Effect
Magnesium oxide	MagOx®	Magnesium supplement	Hypokalemia, hypermagnesemia, diarrhea
May not have sorbitol listed on label		Sorbitol-containing suspensions	Diarrhea
Medroxyprogesterone	Depo-Provera®	Hormone	Increased appetite
Megesterol	Megace®	Steroid (antineoplastic hormonal)	Increased appetite
Meperidine	Demerol®	Analgesic agent (opioids)	Constipation, nausea
Metformin	Glucophage®	Hypoglycemic agent	Hypoglycemia
Methamphetamine	Desoxyn®	Amphetamine	Decreased appetite
Methandrostenolone	Dianabol®	Anabolic steroid	Hypoglycemia
Methyldopa	Aldomet®	Antihypertensive agent (alpha adrenergic blocking)	Diarrhea, fluid retention
Methylphenidate	Ritalin®		Anorexia, nausea
Methylprednisolone	Solu-Cortef®	Steroid (corticosteroid)	Ulcers, fluid retention, hyperglycemia, hypophosphatemia, increased appetite
Metoclopramide	Reglan®	Motility agent	Diarrhea
Metolazone	Zaroxlyn®	Diuretic	Hyponatremia, fluid depletion, hypophosphatemia, hypomagnesemia, pH changes
Metoprolol	Lopressor®	Antihypertensive agent (beta-1 blocker)	Hypoglycemia, hyperkalemia
Metoprolol	Toprol XL®	Antihypertensive agent (beta-1 blocker)	Hypoglycemia, hyperkalemia
Miglitol	Glyset®	Hypoglycemic agent	Hypoglycemia
Minoxidil	Loniten®	Vasodilator	Fluid retention
Mirtazapine	Remeron®	Antidepressant (atypical)	Dry mouth, increased appetite, weight gain
Mitomycin	Mutamycin®	Antineoplastic agent	Nausea, ulcers
Morphine	MSContin®	Analgesic agents (opioids)	Nausea, constipation
Morphine	MSIR®	Analgesic agents (opioids)	Nausea, constipation
Morphine	Roxanol®	Analgesic agent (opioid)	Nausea, constipation
Moxifloxacin	Avelox®	Antibiotic	Diarrhea, nausea
Mycophenolate	CellCept®	Immunosuppressant	Diarrhea
Nandrolone	Deca-Durabolin®	Anabolic steroids	Anabolic
Naproxen	Aleve®	Nonsteroidal antiinflammatory agent (all)	Fluid retention, hyperkalemia, ulcers

Naproxen	Naprosyn®	Nonsteroidal antiinflammatory agent (all)	Ulcers, fluid retention, hyperkalemia

Generic	Brand	Class	Side Effects
Naproxen	Naprosyn®	Nonsteroidal antiinflammatory agent (all)	Ulcers, fluid retention, hyperkalemia
Nelfinavir	Viracept®	Anti-HIV agent (protease inhibitor)	Hypertriglyceridemia, diarrhea
Neostigmine	Prostigmin®	Myasthenia gravis agents	Diarrhea
Nevirapine	Viramune®	Anti-HIV agent (nnrti)	Nausea
Nortriptyline	Pamelor®	Antidepressant (tricyclic)	Hypoglycemia
Octreotide	Sandostatin®	Antisecretory	Constipation
Ondasteron	Zofran®	Antiemetic (5HT3 antagonist)	Constipation, diarrhea
Oxandrolone	Oxandrin®	Anabolic steroid	Hypoglycemia, increased appetite, anabolic
Oxycodone	OxyContin®	Analgesic agent (opioid)	Constipation, nausea
Oxycodone	OxyIR®	Analgesic agent (opioid)	Constipation, nausea
Oxytoxin	Pitocin®	Hormone (oxytocic)	Hyponatremia
Pamidronate	Aredia®	Bisphosphonate	Hypocalcemia, hypomagnesemia, hypophosphatemia
Paroxetine	Paxil®	Antidepressant (SSRI)	Increased appetite, weight gain, weight loss
Penicillins (high dose)	PenTids®	Antibiotic	Hypokalemia
Penicillins (high dose)	PenVK®	Antibiotic	Hypokalemia
Pergolide	Permax®	Anti-Parkinson's agent	Constipation
Phenelzine	Nardil®	CNS agent (monoamine oxidase inhibitor)	Hypoglycemia, increased appetite
Phenobarbital	Luminal®	Anticonvulsant (barbiturate)	Hypocalcemia, hyperglycemia
Phentermine	Adiphex-P®	Anorexiant	Decreased appetite
Phentermine	Ionamin®	Anorexiant	Decreased appetite
Phenylpropanolamine	Acutrim®	Anorexiant	Decreased appetite
Phenytoin	Dilantin®	Anticonvulsant (hydantoin)	Hyperglycemia, hypocalcemia, nausea
Pioglitazone	Actos®	Hypoglycemic agent	Hypoglycemia
Pipercillin and tazobactam	Zosyn®	Antibiotic	Pseudomembranous colitis, hypokalemia
Plicamycin	Mithramycin®	Antineoplastic agent	Hypocalcemia
Polyethylene glycol	GoLytely®	Laxative	Diarrhea
Polyethylene glycol	GoLytely®	Laxative (abuse)	Hypokalemia, pH changes
Polysaccharide-iron comple	Niferex®	Iron salt	Constipation
Potassium bicarbonate and potassium citrate	K-Lyte®	Potassium supplements	Hyperkalemia
Potassium chloride	K-Dur®	Potassium supplements	Hyperkalemia

Generic Name of Example Drug	Brand Name	Drug Class	Side Effect
Potassium chloride	Micro-K®	Potassium supplement	Hyperkalemia
Potassium chloride	Slow K®	Potassium supplement	Hyperkalemia
Potassium phosphate parenteral solution		Phosphorus salt	Hyperphosphatemia, hypocalcemia
Potassium phosphate, Sodium phosphate	K-Phos®	Potassium supplements	Hyperkalemia
Potassium phosphate, Sodium phosphate	NeutraPhos®	Potassium supplement	Hyperkalemia
Pravastatin	Pravachol®	Antihyperlipidemic agent	Nausea, vomiting, abdominal pain, constipation
Prazosin	Minipress®	Antihypertensive (alpha adrenergic blocking agent)	Fluid retention
Prednisolone	Delta-Cortef®	Steroid (corticosteroid)	Fluid retention, hyperglycemia, hypophosphatemia, increased appetite, ulcers
Prednisolone	Prelone®	Steroid (corticosteroid)	Increased appetite, ulcers, hyperglycemia, hypophosphatemia, fluid retention
Prednisone	Deltasone®	Steroid (corticosteroid)	Fluid retention, hyperglycemia, hypophosphatemia, increased appetite, ulcers
Prednisone	Orasone®	Steroid (corticosteroid)	Increased appetite, ulcers, fluid retention, hyperglycemia, hypophosphatemia
Promethazine	Phenergan®	Antiemetic	Constipation
Propranolol	Inderal®	Antihypertensive agent (beta-1 blockers)	Hypoglycemia, hyperkalemia
Psyllium	Metamucil®	Laxative	Diarrhea
Pyridostgmine	Mestinon®	Myasthenia gravis agent	Diarrhea
Quinidine	Quinaglute®	Cardiac agent	Diarrhea
Ramipril	Altace®	Antihypertensive agent (ace inhibitors)	Hyperkalemia
Repaglinide	Prandin®	Hypoglycemic agent	Hypoglycemia
Rifampin	Rifadin®	Antitubercular agent	Hyperglycemia, hypocalcemia
Risedronate	Actonel®	Biphosphonate	Diarrhea, epigastric pain
Rosiglitazone	Avandia®	Hypoglycemic agent	Hypoglycemia
Saqunavir	Fortovase®	Anti-HIV agent (protease inhibitors)	Hypertriglyceridemia, diarrhea

Generic Name	Trade Name	Classification	Side Effects
Scopalamine	Transderm-Scop®	Antiemetic	Constipation
Senna	Senokot®	Laxative	Diarrhea
Senna	Senokot®	Laxative (abuse)	Hypokalemia, pH changes, diarrhea
Sertraline	Zoloft®	Antidepressant (SSRI)	Weight gain, weight loss
Sibutramine	Meridia®	Anorexiant	Decreased appetite
Sodium phosphate	Fleets Enema®	Laxative (phosphate containing)	Hyperphosphatemia, hypocalcemia
Sodium phosphate	Fleets Phospho-soda®	Laxative (phosphate containing)	Hyperphosphatemia, hypocalcemia
Sodium phosphate parenteral solution		Phosphorus salt	Hyperphosphatemia, hypocalcemia
Spironolactone	Aldactone®	Diuretic (potassium sparing)	Fluid depletion, hyperkalemia, hypomagnesemia, hyponatremia, hypophosphatemia, pH changes
Stanozol	Winstrol®	Anabolic steroid	Anabolism, hypoglycemia
Stavudine	Zerit®	Anti-HIV agent (narti)	Abdominal pain, diarrhea, nausea, vomiting
Sucralfate	Carafate®	Gastrointestinal agent	Hypophosphatemia
Tacrine	Cognex®	Alzheimer's agents	Diarrhea
Tacrolimus	Prograf®		Hyperglycemia, hyperkalemia, nausea, vomiting
Tenofovir disoproxil fumarate	Viread®		Flatulence, vomiting, diarrhea, nausea
Terazosin	Hytrin®	Antihypertensive (alpha adrenergic blocking agent)	Fluid retention
Tetracycline	Sumycin®	Antibiotic	Nausea, pseudomembranous colitis
Theophylline	SloBid®	Bronchodilator	Nausea
Theophylline	SloBid®	Bronchodilator (toxic)	Hypophosphatemia, hypercalcemia, nausea
Theophylline	TheoDur®	Bronchodilator	Nausea
Theophylline	TheoDur®	Bronchodilator (toxic)	Hypophosphatemia, hypercalcemia, nausea
Thienbenzodiazepine	Olanzapine®	Antipsychotic	Increased appetite
Ticarcillin and clavulanate acid	Timentin®	Antibiotics	Hypokalemia
Tobramycin	Nebcin®	Antibiotics	Hypokalemia, hypomagnesemia
Tolbutamide	Orinase®	Hypoglycemic agent	Hypoglycemia
Topiramate	Topamax®	Anticonvulsant	Diarrhea, weight loss, hyperchloremia, hypocapnia
Torsemide	Demadex®	Diuretics (loop)	Hypernatremia, hypocalcemia
Tranylcypromine	Parnate®	Antidepressant (monoamine oxidase inhibitor, MAOI)	Increased appetite, hypoglycemia
Trazodone	Desyrel®	Antidepressant	Dry mouth, increased appetite, nausea, vomiting
Trihexyphenidyl	Artane®	Anti-Parkinson's agent	Constipation

Generic Name of Example Drug	Brand Name	Drug Class	Side Effect
Venlafaxine	Effexor®	Antidepressant (SSRI)	Weight gain, weight loss
Vinblastine	Velban®	Antineoplastic agents	Nausea, ulcers
Vincristine	Oncovin®	Antineoplastic agent	Nausea ulcers
Vitamin A	Aquasol A®	Vitamin A (toxic)	Hypercalcemia
Vitamin A and D combination products		Vitamin A and D (toxic)	Hypercalcemia
Vitamin D	Calciferol®	Vitamin D (toxic)	Hypercalcemia
Zalcitabine	Hivid®	Anti-HIV agent (narti)	Hyperglycemia, hypertriglyceridemia, oral ulcers
Zidovudine	Retrovir®	HIV therapy (narti)	Nausea, abdominal pain, anorexia, diarrhea,
Zidovudine, Lamivudine	Combivir®	Anti-HIV agent (narti)	Diarrhea, nausea, vomiting
Zidovudine, Lamivudine, Abacavir	Trizivir®	Anti-HIV agent	Nausea, vomiting, diarrhea
Zoledronic	Zometa®	Bisphosphanate	Nausea, diarrhea, vomiting, abdominal pain

Most Commonly Prescribed Trade Name Drugs[a]

1. Lipitor
2. Synthroid
3. Premarin Tablets
4. Norvasc
5. Prilosec
6. Zoloft
7. Zithromax Z-Pak
8. Claritin
9. Paxil
10. Celebrex
11. Glucophage
12. Prevacid
13. Vioxx
14. Augmentin
15. Zocor
16. Zestril
17. Ortho Tri-Cyclen
18. Prempro
19. Levoxyl
20. Allegra
21. Ambien
22. Zyrtec
23. Prozac
24. Celexa
25. Toprol XL
26. Viagra
27. Fosamax
28. Cipro
29. Accupril
30. Pravachol
31. Neurontin
32. Lanoxin
33. Wellbutrin SR
34. Prinivil
35. Ultram
36. Flonase
37. Singulair
38. Glucotrol XL
39. Coumadin Tablets
40. Levaquin
41. Amoxil
42. Effexor XR
43. Diflucan
44. Flovent
45. Lotensin
46. Nasonex
47. Zithromax Susp
48. Plavix
49. K-Dur 20
50. Lotrel
51. Cozaar
52. Avendia
53. Depakote
54. Claritin D 24 Hr
55. Diovan
56. Risperdal
57. Claritin D 12 Hr
58. Adderall
59. Humulin N
60. Xalatan
61. Allegra-D
62. OxyContin
63. Klor-Con
64. Altace
65. Actos
66. Serevent
67. Zyprexa
68. Evista
69. Monopril
70. Aciphex
71. Effexor XR
72. Protonix
73. Hyzaar
74. Amaryl
75. Combivent
76. Flomax
77. Ortho-Novum 7/7/7
78. Cefzil
79. Levothyroid
80. Dilantin Kapseals
81. Zestoretic
82. Ceftin
83. Alesse-28
84. Roxicet
85. Diovan HCT
86. Ortho-Cyclen
87. Biaxin
88. Imitrex Oral
89. Humulin70/30
90. Serzone
91. Valtrex
92. Macrobid
93. Digitek
94. Concerta
95. Necon 1/35
96. Claritin RediTabs

97. Glucovance
98. Baycol
99. Avapro
100. Bactroban
101. Glucophage XR
102. Triphasil
103. Mircette
104. Skelaxin
105. Lescol
106. Zyrtec Syrup
107. Remeron
108. Nexium
109. Tricor
110. Tiazac
111. Plendil
112. Trivora-28
113. Advair Diskus
114. Elocon
115. Vicoprofin Non-
     Inj
116. Miacalcin Nasal
117. Nasacort AQ
118. Detrol
119. Endocet
120. Biaxin XL
121. Tequin
122. Loestrin Fe 1/20
123. Relafen
124. Tobradex
125. Seroquel
126. Humalog
127. Atrovent Inh
128. Phenergan
     Supp
129. Adalat CC
130. Proventil HFA
131. Tussionex

132. Loestrin Fe
     1.5/30
133. Aricept
134. Alphagan
135. Zithromax
136. Lo/Ovral 28
137. Patanol
138. Coreg
139. Apri
140. Lotrisone
141. Azmacort
142. Rhinocort Aqua
143. Ditropan XL
144. Pepcid
145. Differin
146. Low-Ogestrel
147. Atacand
148. Prinzide
149. Climara
150. Demadex
151. Ciloxan
152. Estratest Tablet
153. Humulin R
154. Bezamycin
155. Duragesic
156. Lamisil Oral
157. Topamax
158. Cardizem CD
159. Guaifenex PSE
160. Proscar
161. Omnicef
162. Zanaflex
163. Prometrium
164. Mobic
165. Vasotec
166. Desogen
167. Ocuflex

168. Premphase
169. Xenical
170. Niaspan
171. Estratest HS
172. Estrostep Fe
173. Metrogel-
     Vaginal
174. Detrol LA
175. Accolate
176. Actonel
177. Univasc
178. Procardia XL
179. Covera-HS
180. Zantac
181. Lac-Hydrin
182. Thyroid, Armour
183. Asacol
184. Lotensin HCT
185. Claritin Syrup
186. Cardura
187. Femhrt
188. Zaroxolyn
189. Sonata
190. Cosopt
191. Axid
192. Nizoral
     Shampoo
193. Zovia 1/35
194. Terazol 7
195. Avelox
196. Avalide
197. Rhinocort
198. Xanax
199. Accutane
200. Meridia

---

[a] Top 200 trade names by units dispensed in the U.S. during 2001. All drug names are registered trademarks of the respective manufacturers.

Reprinted from *Drug Topics,* March 4, 2002, with approval of Scott-Levin Associates, Newtown, PA.

Most Commonly Prescribed Generic Drugs[a]

1. Hydrocodone/APAP
2. Atenolol
3. Amoxicillin
4. Furosemide Oral
5. Albuterol Oral
6. Alprazolam
7. Hydrochlorothiazide
8. Propoxyphene-N/APAP
9. Cephalexin
10. Triamterene w HCTZ
11. Ibuprofen
12. Acetaminophen w Cod
13. Prednisone Oral
14. Trimox
15. Lorazepam
16. Metoprolol Tartrate
17. Amitriptyline
18. Ranitidine HCl
19. Trimethoprim/Sulfa
20. Naproxen
21. Cyclobenzaprine
22. Clonazepam
23. Trazodone HCl
24. Diazepam
25. Verapamil SR
26. Glyburide
27. Enalapril
28. Potassium Chloride
29. Carisoprodol
30. Doxycycline
31. Warfarin
32. Medroxyprogesterone Tab
33. Isosorbide Mononit
34. Albuterol Neb Soln
35. Methylprednisolone Tab
36. Allopurinol
37. Estradiol Oral
38. Clonidine
39. Fluoxetine
40. Penicillin VK
41. Doxazosin
42. Folic Acid
43. Temazepam
44. Oxycodone w/APAP
45. Hydroxyzine
46. Meclizine HCl
47. Metronidazole Tab
48. Gemfibrozil
49. Promethazine Tab
50. Terazosin
51. Triamcinolone Acet Top
52. Cartia XT
53. Spironolactone
54. Metoclopramide
55. Minocycline
56. Bisoprolol/HCTZ
57. Nifedipine ER
58. Propranolol HCl
59. Promethazine/Codeine
60. Acyclovir
61. Glipizide
62. Captopril
63. Butalbital/APAP/Caf
64. Clindamycin Systemic
65. Diltiazem CD
66. Nortriptyline
67. Tamoxifen
68. Methylphenidate

69. Tetracycline
70. Albuterol Oral Liq
71. Cimetidine
72. Benzonatate
73. Phenobarbital
74. Naproxen Sodium
75. Nitroglycerin
76. Phenazopyridine HCl
77. Ferrous Sulfate
78. Aspirin Enteric-Coat
79. Hyoscamine
80. Guaifenesin/Pseudoeph
81. Buspirone HCl
82. Quinine Sulfate
83. Phentermine
84. Methocarbamol
85. Propranolol LA
86. Diclofenac Sodium
87. Dicyclomine HCl
88. Nitroquick
89. Doxepin
90. Carbamazepine
91. Famotidine
92. Ery-Tab
93. Indomethacin
94. Methotrexate
95. Nystatin, Systemic
96. Indapemide
97. Hydrocortisone Top Rx
98. Imipramine HCl
99. Diltiazem SR
100. Neomycin/Polymx/HC
101. Guaituss AC
102. Acetaminophen
103. Theopyhlline SR
104. Prednisolone Oral
105. Digoxin
106. Benztropine
107. Prochlorperaz Mal
108. Atenolol Chlorthal
109. Chlorhexidine Gluc
110. Levothyroxine
111. Hydroxychloroquine
112. Fluocinonide
113. Nadolol
114. Nystatin Topical
115. Etodolac
116. Lithium Carbonate
117. Oxybutynin Chloride
118. Clobetasol
119. Clindamycin Top
120. Multivits s/Flur Chw
121. Nystatin/Triamcinoln
122. Phenytoin Sodium Ext
123. Ibuprofen Liquid
124. Guaifenesin Rx
125. Diphenoxylate w/Atro
126. Isosorbide Dinitrate
127. Diphenhydramine Tabs
128. Colchicine
129. Promethazine DM
130. Docusate Sodium
131. Cefaclor
132. Hydroxyzine Pamoate
133. Pentoxifylline
134. Labetalol
135. Estropipate
136. Carbidopa/Levodopa
137. Baclofen
138. Ketoconazole Topical
139. Gentamicin Ophth
140. Amiodarone
141. Dexamethasone Oral
142. Glyburide Micronized
143. Prednisolone Acet Oph
144. Clorazepate Dipot
145. Erythromycin Oph
146. Bumetanide Non-Inj
147. Polymyxin B/Trimeth
148. Cardec DM
149. Nitrofurantoin Micronized
150. Ipratroprium Bromide
151. Sodium Fluoride
152. Guiafenesin LA
153. Quintex PSA
154. Clotrimazl/Betamthsn
155. Timolol Maleate GFS
156. Tobramycin Oph
157. Haloperidol
158. Cefadroxil
159. Sulfatrim Pediatric
160. Hydrocortn Valerate
161. Erythromycin Ethylsc
162. Octicair
163. Piroxicam
164. Timolol Maleate Oph
165. Clotrimazole Top
166. Nifedipine
167. Chlordiaz c/Clind
168. Chlordiazepoxide HCl
169. Hycoclear Tuss
170. Prenatal Plus
171. Promethazine VC w/Cod
172. Butalbital Cmpd
173. Triazolam
174. Buproprion
175. Hydralazine
176. Nifedical XL
177. Cyproheptadine
178. Erythromycin Topical

179.	Tretinoin	190.	Guanfacine HCl
180.	Erythromycin Base	191.	Ketorolac Oral
181.	Orphenadrine Citrate	192.	Lactulose
182.	Dipyridamole	193.	Lindane
183.	Sulindac	194.	Sulfasalazine
184.	Butalbital Cmpd w/Cod	195.	Methadone HCl Non Inh
185.	Phenobarb/Bella	196.	Azathioprine
186.	Morphine Sul Non Inj	197.	Promethazine VC
187.	Promethazine Liq	198.	Enulose
188.	Theocron	199.	Hemorrhoidal HC
189.	Lonox	200.	Cheratussin AC

a Top 200 generic drugs by number of prescriptions dispensed in U.S. during 2001.

Reprinted from *Drug Topics,* March 4, 2002, with approval of Scott-Levin Associates, Newtown, PA.

pH of Bodily Fluids

Fluid	pH
Ascites	6.8–7.6
Aqueous humor	7.35–7.45
Bile (gall bladder)	5.4–6.9
Bile (hepatic duct)	7.4–8.5
Cerebrospinal fluid	7.35–7.40
Feces	7.0–7.5
Intestinal secretions	7.0–8.0
Gastric fluid	1.0–2.0
Milk	6.6–6.9
Pancreatic secretions	7.5–8.0
Pericardial fluid	6.8–7.6
Pleural fluid	6.8–7.6
Saliva	6.35–6.85
Semen	7.2–8.0
Serum	7.3–7.5
Skin (intracellular fluid)	6.2–7.5
Synovial fluid	7.3–7.5
Tears	7.4
Urine	4.5–7.5

Weight–Mass Conversions

Metric	Avoirdupois (avd)	Apothecary[a]
60 milligrams (mg)	n/a	1 grain (gr)
1 gram (g)	n/a	16 gr
4 g	n/a	1 dram (dr)
30 g	1 ounce (oz)	n/a
31.1 g	n/a	1 ounce
454 g	16 oz	n/a
454 g	1 pound (lb)	n/a
1000 g (1 kilogram)	2.2 lb	n/a

[a] Apothecary measures are included only for completeness. They are no longer recognized as official for drug orders in the U.S. Avoid all use of the apothecary or avoirdupois (common) systems of measures in orders for drugs or for dietary products.

Approximate Volume Conversions

Metric	Avoirdupois (avd)	Apothecary[a]
1 milliliter (mL)	n/a	16 minims (M)
5 mL	1 teaspoonful (tsp)	1 fluid dram (fl. dr)
15 mL	1 tablespoonful (tbsp)	3 fluid drams (fl. dr)
30 mL	2 tbsp[b]	1 fluid ounce (fl. oz)
240 mL	1 cup	8 fl. oz
500 mL	1 pint (pt)	16 fl. oz
1000 mL	1 quart (qt)	32 fl. oz
4000 mL	1 gallon (gal)	128 fl. oz

[a] Apothecary measures are included only for completeness. They are no longer recognized as official for drug orders in the U.S. Avoid all use of the apothecary or avoirdupois (common) systems of measures in orders for drugs or for dietary products.

[b] It may be necessary to convert to common system measures for patients who cannot conveniently use metric measures. In case of conversions, consult a chart of exact volume conversions because measures of 2 tbsp (1 ounce) and larger actually represent smaller volumes than shown in the metric column of this table (e.g., 1 fl.oz = 28.45 mL).

Electrolyte Content of Common IV Solutions

Table A.9.1 Dextrose Solutions Containing No Electrolytes

Product	g/L Dextrose
$D_{2.5}W$	25
D_5W	50
$D_{10}W$	100
$D_{20}W^a$	200
$D_{30}W$	300
$D_{40}W$	400
$D_{50}W^b$	500
$D_{60}W$	600
$D_{70}W$	700

[a] Solutions greater than 10% Dextrose (i.e., $D_{20}W$ and more concentrated solutions) are not to be infused intravenously through peripheral veins. These are marketed as components of Total Parenteral Nutrition (hyperalimentation) solutions for central venous administration.

[b] Dextrose 50% packaged in a 50 mL syringe for infusion is intended for emergency use in the face of life-threatening hypoglycemia. It is the only hypertonic dextrose product appropriate for peripheral intravenous infusion.

Table A.9.2 Dextrose and Ethanol Solutions Containing No Electrolytes

Product	g/L Dextrose	g/L Ethanol
$D_5Alcohol_5$	50	50
$D_{10}Alcohol_5$	100	50

Table A.9.3 Sodium Chloride Solutions Containing
No Dextrose

Product	Cations mEq/L Na+
Sodium Chloride 0.45% (Half-Normal Saline) (Hypotonic)	77
Sodium Chloride 0.9% (Normal Saline) (Isotonic)	154
Sodium Chloride 3%[a] (Hypertonic)	513
Sodium Chloride 5% (Hypertonic)	855

[a] Hypertonic Sodium Chloride solutions (3% and 5%, as well as the more concentrated solutions for use as additives to parenteral admixtures) are extremely hazardous products. They should not be stocked outside the central pharmacy. They should be dispensed only after verifying that they are correctly ordered for a patient suffering from extreme hyponatremia. They should be infused only with a volumetric infusion pump by experienced personnel in a setting providing appropriate monitoring.

Table A.9.4 Combination Electrolyte Solutions Containing No Dextrose

Product	Cations mEq/L			
	Na+	K+	Ca++	Mg++
Ringer's Injection	147	4	4	—
Lactated Ringer's	130	4	3	—
Plasma-Lyte 65™[a]	40	13	—	3
Plasma-Lyte R™	140	10	5	3
Isolyte- S™[b]	40	5	—	3
Normosol-R™[c]	140	5	—	3
Plasma-Lyte 148™	140	5	—	3
Isolyte-E™	140	10	5	3

[a] Trademark of Baxter Healthcare Corporation
[b] Trademark of McGaw Laboratories
[c] Trademark of Abbott Laboratories

Table A.9.5 Dextrose and Electrolyte Solutions

Product	Cations mEq/L			
	Na^+	K^+	Ca^{++}	Mg^{++}
$D_{2.5\frac{1}{2}}$Normal Saline	77	—	—	—
$D_{5\frac{1}{8}}$Normal Saline	19	—	—	—
$D_{5\frac{1}{4}}$Normal Saline	34–39	—	—	—
$D_{5\frac{1}{3}}$Normal Saline	51–56	—	—	—
$D_{5\frac{1}{2}}$Normal Saline	77	—	—	—
D_5Normal Saline	154	—	—	—
$D_{10\frac{1}{4}}$Normal Saline	34–39	—	—	—
$D_{10\frac{1}{3}}$Normal Saline	51–56	—	—	—
$D_{10\frac{1}{2}}$Normal Saline	77	—	—	—
D_{10}Normal Saline	154	—	—	—
D_5Lactated Ringer's	130	4	3	—
D_{10}Lactated Ringer's	130	4	3	—
D_5Isolyte G	65	17	—	—
D_5E75	40	35	—	—
D_5Isolyte M	38	35	—	—
D_5 in Ringer's Inj.	147	4	4.5	—
$D_{2.5}$ in Half-Strength Ringer's Inj.	66	2	1.5	—
D_5E48	25	20	—	3
D_5Isolyte H	42	13	—	3
D_5Normosol M	40	13	—	3
D_5Plasma-Lyte 56	41	13	—	3
D_5Isolyte P	25	20	—	3
D_5Isolyte S	142	5	—	3
D_5Normosol R	140	5	—	3
D_5Plasmalyte 148	140	5	—	3
D_5Isolyte R	41	16	5	3
D_5Plasma-Lyte M	40	16	5	3
D_5Plasma-Lyte R	140	10	5	3
D_5Isolyte E	141	10	5	3
D_{10}E48	25	20	—	3

Table A.9.6 Dextrose and Electrolyte Base Solutions with Added Potassium Chloride

Product		Cations mEq/L			
		Na$^+$	K$^+$	Ca^{++}	Mg^{++}
D$_5$W with KCl	0.075% (10 mEq/L)	—	10	—	—
D$_5$W with KCl	0.15% (20 mEq/L)	—	20	—	—
D$_5$W with KCl	0.224% (30 mEq/L)	—	30	—	—
D$_5$W with KCl	0.3% (40 mEq/L)	—	40	—	—
D$_{5^{1/4}}$NS with KCl	0.075% (10 mEq/L)	34–39	10	—	—
D$_{5^{1/4}}$NS with KCl	0.15% (20 mEq/L)	34–39	20	—	—
D$_{5^{1/4}}$NS with KCl	0.224% (30 mEq/L)	34–39	30	—	—
D$_{5^{1/4}}$NS with KCl	0.3% (40 mEq/L)	34–39	40	—	—
D$_{5^{1/3}}$NS with KCl	0.15% (20 mEq/L)	51–56	20	—	—
D$_{5^{1/3}}$NS with KCl	0.224% (30 mEq/L)	51–56	30	—	—
D$_{5^{1/3}}$NS with KCl	0.3% (40 mEq/L)	51–56	40	—	—
D$_{5^{1/2}}$NS with KCl	0.075% (10 mEq/L)	77	10	—	—
D$_{5^{1/2}}$NS with KCl	0.15% (20 mEq/L)	77	20	—	—
D$_{5^{1/2}}$NS with KCl	0.224% (30 mEq/L)	77	30	—	—
D$_{5^{1/2}}$NS with KCl	0.3% (40 mEq/L)	77	40	—	—
D$_5$NS with KCl	0.15% (20 mEq/L)	154	20	—	—
D$_5$NS with KCl	0.224% (30 mEq/L)	154	30	—	—
D$_5$NS with KCl	0.3% (40 mEq/L)	154	40	—	—
D$_{10}$NS with KCl	0.15% (20 mEq/L)	154	20	—	—
D$_5$LR with KCl	0.179% (20 mEq/L)	130	24	3	—
D$_5$LR with KCl	0.328% (40 mEq/L)	130	44	3	—

Milliequivalent/Milligram Conversions for Commonly Used Salts

Salt	Common Abbreviation	mg[a]	mEq[b]
Calcium chloride	$(CaCl_2)$	73	1
Calcium gluconate	(CaGluc)	224	1
Magnesium sulfate	$(MgSO_4)$	60	1
Potassium acetate	(Koac)	98	1
Potassium chloride	(KCl)	75	1
Sodium bicarbonate	$(NaHCO_3)$	84	1
Sodium chloride	(NaCl)	58	1
Sodium lactate	(NaLactate)	112	1

[a] Milligram amounts of salts may vary from one product to another, and from this table, because of water of hydration associated with a molecule of the individual salt. Some salts (e.g., magnesium sulfate) may have different numbers of molecules of water of hydration associated with them.

[b] A milliequivalent is the gram weight of a substance that will combine with or replace one milligram (one millimole) of hydrogen. It is therefore 1/1000 of an equivalent weight. The expression relates the mass of a substance to its chemical valence.

MILLIEQUIVALENT/MILLIGRAM CONVERSIONS FOR COMMONLY USED IONS

To determine milliequivalent (mEq) values of each ion listed next, divide the mass in mg of ion present in a product by its mEq mass, as stated.

Ion	mEq[a] mass to use in Equation 1[b]
Sodium (Na⁺)	23.0 mg
Potassium (K⁺)	39.0 mg
Magnesium (Mg⁺⁺)	12.0 mg
Phosphorous (P⁼)	15.5 mg
Calcium (Ca⁺⁺)	20.0 mg
Chloride (Cl⁻)	35.5 mg
Chloride (as NaCl)	58.5 mg

[a] A milliequivalent is the gram weight of a substance that will combine with or replace one milligram (one millimole) of hydrogen. It is therefore 1/1000 of an equivalent weight. The expression relates the mass of a substance to its chemical valence.

[b] A practical formula for computing milliequivalents (mEq) when milligrams (mg) of a product is known may be expressed as follows:

Formula 1:

$$\frac{\text{milligrams (mg)} \times \text{valence}}{\text{atomic weight (in mg)}} = \text{milliequivalents (mEq)}$$

Recombining, the formula may also be expressed as follows:

$$\frac{\text{milliequivalents (mEq)} \times \text{atomic weight}}{\text{valence}} = \text{milligrams (mg)}$$

Another approach is to use previously calculated conversion factors to convert between mg and mEq, as indicated in the formula and the table below:

Formula 2:

milligrams × conversion factor = milliequivalents

Ion	Atomic Weight	Valence	Conversion Factor
Sodium	23	1	0.0435
Potassium	39.1	1	0.02557
Magnesium	24.32	2	0.08141
Phosphorous	31.04	2	0.06443
Calcium	40.07	2	0.05
Chloride	35.46	1	0.0282

APPENDIX **B.2**

Average pH Values of Some Common Beverages and Foods

Food Group	Food	pH Mean or Range	Reference
Dairy Products			
	Acidophilus	4.0	1
	Buttermilk	4.5	1
	Half-and-half	6.6–6.7	2
	Skim milk	6.5–6.7	2
	Whole milk	6.6–6.7	2
Fruits			
	Apples	3.1	1
	Apricots	3.3	1
	Banana	4.6	1
	Blackberries	3.3	1
	Blueberries	3.7	1
	Figs	4.6	1
	Gooseberries	3.0	1
	Grapefruit	3.1	1
	Lemon	2.2	1
	Lime	2.0	1
	Oranges	3.7	1
	Peaches	3.5	1
	Pears	3.9	1
	Plums	2.9	1
	Prunes	3.1	1
	Raspberries	3.6	1
	Rhubarb	3.2	1
	Strawberries	3.4	1
	Sweet cherries	3.8	1

Fruit juices

	Apple juice	3.6	2
	Apricot nectar	3.8	2
	Cranberry juice	2.6–2.7	2
	Grape juice	3.3–3.4	2
	Grapefruit juice	3.5	2
	Orange juice	3.4–3.8	2
	Peach nectar	3.6	2
	Pineapple juice	3.4–3.5	2
	Prune juice	4.2	2
	Tomato juice	4.3	2

Fruit drinks and soda

	Club soda (Shasta®)	3.7	2
	Coca-Cola®, regular	2.8	2
	Coca-Cola®, diet	2.9	2
	Ginger ale	2.7–2.8	2
	Orange drink (HiC®)	2.6	2
	Orange soda (Shasta®)	2.8	2
	7-Up®	3.0–3.1	2

Meat, eggs, poultry, seafood

	Egg albumin	4.6	1
	Egg white	8.0	1
	Egg yolk	6.4	1
	Meat, unripened	7.0	1
	Meat, ripened	5.8	1
	Oysters	6.3	1
	Poultry	5.8	1
	Shrimp	6.9	1
	Tuna	6.0	1

Vegetables, starches

	Asparagus	5.6	1
	Beets	5.3	1
	Bread	5.4	1
	Cabbage	5.2	1
	Carrots	5.0	1
	Cauliflower	5.6	1
	Cucumber	5.1	1
	Dill pickles	3.2	1
	Green beans	5.3	1
	Green peppers	5.3	1
	Hominy (rye)	7.1	1
	Lima beans	5.7	1
	Parsnips	5.3	1
	Peas	6.2	1
	Potatoes	6.1	1
	Pumpkin	5.0	1
	Red kidney beans	5.7	1
	Sauerkraut	3.6	1
	Spinach	5.5	1

	Squash	5.2	1
	Succotash	5.8	1
	Sweet potatoes	5.4	1
	Tomatoes	4.2	1
Miscellaneous			
	Cocoa	6.7–6.8	2
	Coffee, regular	4.9–5.1	2
	Coffee, decaf	5.1–5.2	2
	Tap water	7.6–8.2	2
	Tea	6.9	2
	Vinegar	3.1–3.2	2

Sources: Adapted from Food and nutrition section, *Handbook of Food Preparation,* American Association of Family and Consumer Sciences, 9th ed., Kendall-Hunt, Dubuque, IA, 1993, p. 48, and Flick, A.L., *Digestive Dis.,* 15, 317–320, 1970. With permission.

Commonly Used Electrolyte Additives for Intravenous Therapy

Name	Common Abbreviation	Strength(s)[a]
Calcium chloride	$CaCl_2$	10% (1.36 mEq/mL)
Calcium gluconate	CaGluc	10% (0.46 mEq/mL)
Potassium acetate	KOac	(2 mEq/mL)
Potassium chloride	KCl	(2 mEq/mL)
Potassium phosphates[b]	KPO_4	K^+ (4.4 mEq/mL)
		$PO_4^=$ (3 mMol/mL)
Magnesium sulfate	$MgSO_4$	10% (0.8 mEq/mL)
		12.5% (1 mEq/mL)
		50% (4.08 mEq/mL)
Sodium acetate	NaOac	(2 mEq/mL)
		32.8% (4 mEq/mL)
Sodium chloride	NaCl	14.6% (2.5 mEq/mL)
		23.4% (4 mEq/mL)
Sodium phosphates[b]	$NaPO_4$	Na^+ (4 mEq/mL)
		$PO_4^=$ (3 mMol/mL)

[a] Use extra caution when selecting and measuring all electrolyte additive products. They are hypertonic and must be diluted before intravenous administration. Even when diluted, they will require controlled infusion rates. Where a product is marketed in more than one strength, greater caution is indicated. Note also that the color or vial cap does *not* indicate the drug product in a vial because no standards have been established on cap colors to mark any drug or drug strength. The sole exception is potassium chloride, which must have a black cap with the legend, "Must be diluted before administration."

[b] Phosphate solutions must be ordered in millimoles (m*M*). This is the sole accurate measure because the polyvalent phosphate moiety may be present in variant combining states, dependent on the pH of the solution. Commercially available potassium phosphates and sodium phosphates injection are associated with different milliequivalents of their cations because of the polyvalent properties of phosphate.

Commonly Used Micronutrient Additives for Intravenous Therapy

Name	Abbreviation	Strength(s)[a,b]
Chromium	Cr	(4, 10, 20 μg/mL)
Copper	Cu	(0.4, 1, 2 mg/mL)
Iodine	I	(100 μg/mL)
Manganese	Mn	(0.1, 0.5 mg/mL)
Molybdenum	Mb	(25 μg/mL)
Selenium	Se	(40 μg/mL)
Zinc	Zn	(1, 4, 5 mg/mL)

[a] The presence of multiple concentrations of additives demands extra care in the selection and measurement of trace metal additives. It is necessary to order all individual trace element additives in mass units (μg, mg).

[b] Combination trace element injection products are marketed to meet usual needs for supplementation and to reduce the number of aseptic manipulations with needle and syringe in preparing an order. When products such as MTE® or MTE-6® are ordered, it is appropriate to order a volume of the products (e.g., 1 mL in 24 h TPN solution). These multiple trace element products are packaged in vials of different sizes, so it is never acceptable to order a unit of trace elements injection without stating a volume in mL (e.g., "MTE® 1 vial daily" is a hazardous order because a vial may contain 1 mL or 10 mL).

Food Storage Guidelines for the General Population and for High-Risk Populations

Food	Maximum Storage Periods			
	General Population		High-Risk Population	
	Refrigeration	Freezing	Refrigeration	Freezing
Meat: fresh, uncooked				
Beef				
Ground, strips, or cubed	1–2 days	3–4 months	1 day	1 month
Roasts, steaks	2–5 days	6–9 months	2 days	3 months
Lamb				
Ground	1–2 days	3–5 months	1 day	1.5 months
Roasts, chops	2–5 days	6–9 months	2 days	3 months
Pork				
Ground, strips	1–2 days	2 months	1 day	1 month
Roasts, chops	3–4 days	4–8 months	2–3 days	2 months
Poultry:				
Chicken, turkey, duck, goose				
Chicken, turkey, whole	1–2 days	12 months	1 day	6 months
Chicken, cut up	1–2 days	4 months	1 day	2 months
Stuffing	1 day			
Cooked meat products:				
Ham, frankfurters, luncheon meats				
Ham, whole	7 days	2 weeks	3–4 days	1 week
Ham, half or sliced	3–5 days	NR	3 days	NR
Canned Ham	9 months–1 year	NR	6 months	NR
Frankfurters, Bacon	5–7 days	NR	3–5 days	NR
Luncheon Meats	3–5 days	NR	3 days	NR
Leftover cooked meats	1–2 days	2–3 months	same day	1 month
and gravy, broth	1–2 days	2–3 months	same day	1 month
Fish and shellfish:				
Fresh fish	1–2 days	2–3 months	1 day	6 weeks
Frozen fish	1–2 days	2–3 months	1 day	3 months
Shellfish (lobster, shrimp)	1–2 days	2–3 months	1 day	6–8 weeks

Dairy Products:

Fluid milk (after carton date)	5–7 days	NR[b]	3 days	NR
Hard cheeses (e.g., cheddar, parmesan, romano)	1 month	NR	2 weeks	NR
Soft Cheeses	7 days	NR	3–4 days	NR
Dry milk (nonfat)	1 year unopened	NR	6 months unopened	NR
Reconstituted milk	1 week	NR	3 days	NR
Cooked dishes with eggs, meat, milk, fish, poultry	Serve day prepared	1–2 months	Serve day prepared	2 weeks

NR: Not recommended for freezing.

Source: Adapted with permission from *ServSafe Coursebook, 2nd edition,* copyright 2002 by the National Restaurant Association Educational Foundation, and McCabe, B.J., Chapter 14, this volume.

Guidelines for Drug Approval (U.S. Food and Drug Administration)

Drugs marketed in the U.S. must be approved in advance by the U.S. Food and Drug Administration (FDA). This is required before products may pass in interstate commerce. The power to regulate drug products rests on the Interstate Commerce of the United States Constitution. The law requires all drug products passing in interstate commerce to meet compendial standards (set by the U.S. Pharmacopeial Convention, an independent, science-based nongovernmental corporation founded in 1820). Federal law also requires the products to be safe, and to have proved efficacy in the diagnosis, treatment, or amelioration of disease. Drug products passing in interstate commerce must also be manufactured under defined conditions (current good manufacturing practice), free of contamination, and accurately labeled. Products may also be required to meet certain packaging standards. Finally, products must be accompanied by appropriate information about their safe use. All packaging, labeling, and advertising of drug products are controlled by the FDA; the Administration's explicit approval is required for all printed content.

In order to be approved for marketing, the manufacturer of a proposed new drug entity (NDE) must secure an approved new drug application (ANDA). After that, the sponsor must present to appropriate FDA scientific panels valid data gained from clinical trials. Four phases of clinical trials are defined in federal law:

Phase I   Testing in limited numbers of individuals to determine the characteristics and the adverse effects of a proposed NDE.

Phase II   Testing in larger numbers of human volunteers to determine the efficacy of a drug against a particular disease state that it is intended to treat.

Phase III   Testing in larger numbers of human volunteers to determine the safety in longer-term dosing and the efficacy (including efficacy measured in double-blind trials against drugs medically accepted as effective against particular disease states).

Phase IV   Postmarketing surveillance, in which users of each drug approved for U.S. marketing report to the FDA all adverse experiences related to the use of a drug product. Phase IV trial continues through the reporting requirements as long as a drug remains on the market.

Grapefruit Juice–Drug Interactions and Their Clinical Significance

Drug	Interaction				Clinically Significant		
	Yes	No	Maybe	Unknown	Yes	No	Unknown
Antiarrythmics:							
Amiodarone	+				X^a		
Quinidine			+			X	
Antiasthmatics:							
Montelukast				+			X
Theophylline		+				X	
Antibiotics:							
Clarithromycin		+				X	
Dapsone				+			X
Itraconazole	+				X^b		
Quinine		+				X	
Anticoagulants:							
Warfarin			+		X^a		
Anticonvulsants:							
Carbamazepine	+				**X**		
Phenytoin		+				X	
Antiemetic:							
Ondansetron				+			X
Antihistamines:							
Ebastine	+				**X**		
Terfenadine	+				**X**		
Cetirizine		+				X	
Loratidine		+				X	
Fexofenadine			+				X
Miscellaneous							
Antihypertensives:							
Carvedilol			+				X
Losartan			+				X
Terazosin				+			X

Drug	Interaction				Clinically Significant		
	Yes	No	Maybe	Unknown	Yes	No	Unknown
Antineoplastics:							
Tamoxifen			+				X
Antiulcer:							
Omeprazole	+						X
Benzodiazepines:							
Alprazolam				+			X
Clonazepam				+			X
Diazepam	+				X		
Flurazepam				+			X
Midazolam	+				X		
Triazolam	+				X		
Lorazepam				+			X
Calcium Channel Blockers:							
Amlodipine	+					X	
Felodipine	+				X		
Nifedipine	+					X	
Nimodipine	+				X		
Nisoldipne	+				X		
Nitrendipine	+				X		
Pranidipine	+				X		
Diltiazem		+				X	
Verapamil	+					X	
Corticosteroids/Hormones:							
Ethinyl estradiol	+						X
Progesterone			+				X
Prednisone/Prednisolone		+				X	
Thyroid hormone supplement		+				X	
HIV Protease Inhibitors:							
Indinavir		+				X	
Nelfinavir				+			X
Ritonavir				+			X
Saquinavir	+				X		
HMG-CoA Reductase Inhibitors:							
Atorvastatin	+				X		
Cerivastatin	+				X		
Fluvistatin		+				X	
Lovastatin	+				X		
Pravastatin		+				X	
Simvastatin	+				X		
Immunosuppressants:							
Cyclosporine	+				X		
Tacrolimus	+				X		
Narcotic:							
Methadone				+			X
Miscellaneous Psychiatric Medications:							
Buspirone	+				X		
Clomipramine	+				X		
Haloperidol				+			X
Pimozide			+				X

Drug	Interaction				Clinically Significant		
	Yes	No	Maybe	Unknown	Yes	No	Unknown
Quetiapine			+				X
Sertraline			+			X	
Trazodone				+			X
Zaleplon			+				X
Zolpidem				+		X	
Phosphodiesterase Inhibitors:							
Cilostazol			+				X
Sildenafil			+		X^a		
Miscellaneous Medicines:							
Cisapride	+				**X**		
Donepezil			+				X
Tamsulosin			+				X

[a] Possibly or perhaps clinically significant.
[b] Capsules only.

Note: **bold X** = Consumption of grapefruit juice (GFJ) while taking medicine not safe; X = Consumption of GFJ while taking medicine is safe; *italic X* = Effect not fully known, use caution, avoid consumption of GFJ while taking medicine until the magnitude and timing of this interaction is evaluated further.

Guide to Gliadin in Drugs

Prescription and Nonprescription Drugs Containing Gliadin			
Brand	Generic Name	Form	Amount[a]
Actifed Plus®	Acetaminophen	Caplets	Significant
	Psudoephedrine HCl		Significant
	Triprolidine HCl		Significant
Advil®	Ibuprofen	Tablets	Significant
Aspirin (enteric coated)		Tablets	Significant
Augmentin®	Amoxicillin-clavulanate potassium	Tablets	Trace
Bayer Plus Aspirin®		Tablets	Significant
Benadryl®	Diphenhydramine hydrochloride	Capsules	Significant
Centrum® advanced formula	High-potency multivitamin	Tablets	Significant
Centrum® Silver		Tablets	Significant
Centrum®		Tablets	Significant
Chlortrimeton®	Chlorpheniramine	Tablets	Significant
Cipro®	Ciproflaxacin hydrochloride	Tablets	Trace
Coumadin®	Crystalline warfarin sodium, USP	Tablets	Significant
Dairy Ease®	Natural lactase enzyme digestive aid	Tablets	Significant
Dairy Ease®	Natural lactase enzyme digestive aid	Drops	Significant
Excedrin 1B®	Ibuprofen	Tablets	Significant
Gas-X®	Simethicone	Tablets	Significant
Glucotrol®	Glipizide	Tablets	Significant
Hismanal®	Astemizole	Tablets	Significant
Ibubrofen®	Ibuprofen	Tablets	Significant
Inderal®	Propranolol hydrochloride	Tablets	Significant
Lasix®	Furosemide	Tablets	Trace
Lopid®	Gemfibrosil	Tablets	Trace
Lopressor®	Metoprolol tartarate USP	Tablets	Trace
Naprosyn®	Naproxen	Tablets	Significant
One-a-Day® Extra C formula	Mulitvitamin supplement with high-potency vitamin C	Tablets	Significant
One-a-Day® Maximum Formula	Multimineral supplement for adults and teens	Tablets	Significant
Ortho-Novum® 7/7/7	Norethinorone and ethinyl estradiol	Tablets	Significant

| Prescription and Nonprescription Drugs Containing Gliadin | | | |
Brand	Generic Name	Form	Amount[a]
Pepcid®	Famotidine	Tablets	Significant
Premarin®	Conjugated estrogens, USP	Tablets	Significant
Prednizone	Predisone	Tablets	Trace
Seldane®	Terfendadine	Tablets	Trace
Septra DS®	Trimethoprim and sulfamethoxazole	Caplets	Significant
Tagamet®	Cimetidine	Tablets	Significant
Tenormin®	Atenolol	Tablets	Significant
Triphasil®	Levonorgestrel and ethinyl estradiol	Tablets	Significant
Tylenol Allergy Sinus®	Acetaminophen	Gelcaps	Significant
Tylenol®	Acetaminophen	Tablets	Significant
Tylenol®	Acetaminophen	Gelcaps	Significant
Vasotec®	Enalapril maleate	Tablets	Significant
Voltaren®	Diclofenac sodium	Tablets	Significant
Zestril®	Lisinopril	Tablets	Trace

[a] The lower level of method sensitivity is 0.0115 mg of gliadin/tablet, cap, etc.

Source: Adapted from Miletic, I.D., *J. Pediatr. Gastroenterol. Nutr.,* 19, 29, 1994. With permission

Foods Containing Gliadin

A list of the gliadin content of specific foods has not been developed. Instead references provide lists of foods considered to be gluten-containing, gluten-free, or questionable as to gluten contents. Further confusion in the literature can be created by the use of the same word to denote foods or cooking methods from one geographical region to another, e.g., "corn" used as a generic term for "cereal crops" or "maize." Gluten may be used as a generic word for a cereal protein and not be limited to the definition of gluten as "a water-soluble protein consisting of an insoluble fraction, glutenin, and a soluble fraction containing a series of gliadins (∂, β, γ, and ω)."[1] The gliadins are the toxic fractions of gluten and are also soluble in alcohol yielding gliadin from alcoholic beverages including distilled spirits made from the offending cereal grains. [2] Extremes may be reached by advocates who try to eliminate all possible sources of gliadin, however minute. An overzealous elimination of all foods containing any flavoring agents with a alcohol base, e.g., vanilla-flavored ice cream, is not needed for gluten-sensitive enteropathy due to the extremely small amounts of gliadin content in the alcohol base of the flavoring that is further reduced by the small amount of flavoring added to the food itself.

Certain Gliadin Containing Foods:	Likely Gliadin-Free Foods:
Barley	Corn flour or meal
Rye	Cornstarch
Wheat	Potato or potato flour
Foods made with these grains	Oats or oatmeal
e.g., Carob-soy flour mixed with wheat	Rice or rice flour
	Soy or soy flour

Uncertain Gliadin Containing Foods:*
Amaranth
Buckwheat, groats, or kasha
"Gluten-free" wheat starch

Uncertain Gliadin Containing Foods*

Quinoa
Spelt
Teff

* Uncertainty arises from a high risk for cross-contamination by gluten-containing grains in milling process.

Source: Garrow, J.S. and James, W.P.T., Eds., *Human Nutrition and Dietetics,* 9th ed., Churchill Livingstone, Edinburgh, 1993, p. 490 and Shils, M.E. et al., Eds., *Modern Nutrition in Health and Disease,* 9th ed., 1998, p. 1164.

Food Carbohydrate Replacements for Illness or Hypoglycemia

For insulin-dependent diabetic patients, hypoglycemia is treated by the Rule of 15. Give 15 g of carbohydrate in readily absorbable form.

Wait 15 min and retest serum glucose. Repeat process as needed.

If serum glucose is still low, give 15 g of carbohydrates again. If longer than 30 min to next meal or snack, give a snack with 15 g of carbohydrates and 7 g of protein (e.g., 1 cup milk, 8 oz yogurt, 1 oz cheese, and 6 crackers).

For illness in which regular intake cannot be maintained, replace carbohydrates approximately in the following foods by the groups as indicated:

Group I: (1/2 c. = 4 fl. oz)   Orange or grapefruit juice, Coca-Cola®, 7-Up®, Sprite®, apple juice, pineapple juice; applesauce (unsweetened); generic cola beverages; flavored gelatin; ice cream; frozen fruit bar; custard

Group II: (1 c. = 8 fl. oz)   Gatorade™, milk, sugar-free pudding, cream soup, yogurt (plain)

Group III: (1/3 c. = 2.7 fl. oz) Grape, prune, or regular cranberry juice; flavored low-fat yogurt

Group IV: (1/4 c. = 2 fl. oz)   Sherbet, pudding

Usual Food Standard Serving Size	CHO (g)	Approximate Replacement (in cups/fl. oz)			
		Group I	Group II	Group III	Group IV
Milk, 1 cup	12	1/2 cup	1/2 cup	1/3 cup	1/4 cup
Fruits (1/2 cup)	15	1/2 cup	1/2 cup	1/3 cup	1/4 cup
Breads, Starches (1 or 1/2 c)	15	1/2 cup	1/2 cup	1/3 cup	1/4 cup
Vegetables, Starchy (1/2 c)	15	1/2 cup	1/2 cup	1/3 cup	1/4 cup

Source: Adapted from Dietary Department, *Recent Advances in Therapeutic Diets,* 3rd ed., The Iowa State University Press, Ames, IA, 1980, p. 85. With permission.

Tyramine Content of Foods and Beverages in μg/g or μg/mL

Alcoholic Beverages

Food	Sample Size	μg/g	Serving Size	μg/Serving	Reference
Distilled Spirits					
Dubonnet	N = 1	1.6	120 g	190.0	Shulman 1989
Harvey's® Bristol Cream	N = 1	2.7	120 g	320.0	Shulman 1989
London distilled dry gin (Beefeater®)	N = 1	ND	120 g	ND	Shulman 1989
Rare blended scotch whiskies	N = 1	ND	120 g	ND	Shulman 1989
Vodka	N = 1	ND	120 g	ND	Shulman 1989
Beer—Bottled or Canned					
Amstel®	N = 1	4.5	341 mL	1,541.3	Shulman 1989
Blue	N = 1	1.8	341 mL	613.8	Shulman 1989
Blue Light	N = 1	3.4	341 mL	1,166.2	Shulman 1989
Canadian	N = 1	3.0	341 mL	1,026.4	Shulman 1989
Carlsberg Light®	N = 1	1.2	341 mL	392.2	Shulman 1989
Coors Light®	N = 1	1.5	341 mL	494.5	Shulman 1989
Coors Light beer 4% alc/vol, Canadian can 1	N = 1	0.6	341 mL	218.2	Tailor 1994
Coors Light beer 4% alc/vol, Canadian can 2	N = 1	0.8	341 mL	255.8	Tailor 1994
Coors Light beer 4% alc/vol, bottle 1	N = 1	1.7	341 mL	583.1	Tailor 1994
Coors Light beer 4% alc/vol, bottle 2	N = 1	0.5	341 mL	177.3	Tailor 1994
Coors Light beer 4% alc/vol, U.S. can 1	N = 1	1.1	341 mL	371.7	Tailor 1994
Export	N = 1	2.8	341 mL	948.0	Shulman 1989
Export Draft	N = 1	3.8	341 mL	1,292.4	Shulman 1989
Genesee® Cream	N = 1	0.9	341 mL	293.3	Shulman 1989
Guinness® Extra Stout®	N = 1	3.4	341 mL	1,149.2	Shulman 1989
Guinness® Extra Stout 5% alc/vol., bottle 1	N = 1	3.2	341 mL	1,077.6	Tailor 1994
Guinness® Extra Stout 5% alc/vol., bottle 2	N = 1	2.9	341 mL	1,002.5	Tailor 1994
Heineken®	N = 1	1.8	341 mL	617.2	Shulman 1989
Labatt® Genuine Draft, bottle 1	N = 1	0.5	341 mL	180.7	Tailor 1994

Labatt Genuine Draft® , bottle 2	N = 1	2.3	341 mL	787.7	Tailor 1994
Labatt's Blue Light Pilsener® 4% alc/vol.	N = 1	0.9	341 mL	300.1	Tailor 1994
Labatt's Blue Pilsener® 4% alc/vol.	N = 1	2.3	341 mL	794.5	Tailor 1994
Michelob®	N = 1	1.0	341 mL	334.2	Shulman 1989
Miller® Genuine Draft Cold Filt. 5% alc/vol.	N = 1	0.6	341 mL	191.0	Tailor 1994
Miller Light®	N = 1	2.9	341 mL	992.3	Shulman 1989
Molson® Export 5% alc/vol	N = 1	0.8	341 mL	269.4	Tailor 1994
Molson® Golden	N = 1	0.5	341 mL	170.5	Tailor 1994
Molson® Special Dry, can 1	N = 1	2.0	341 mL	692.2	Tailor 1994
Molson® Special Dry, can 2	N = 1	0.5	341 mL	180.7	Tailor 1994
Molson® Canadian Lager 5% alc/vol.	N = 1	0.7	341 mL	245.5	Tailor 1994
Northern Extra Light	N = 1	0.8	341 mL	272.8	Tailor 1994
Old Milwaukee®	N = 1	0.3	341 mL	115.9	Tailor 1994
Old Vienna®	N = 1	3.3	341 mL	1,132.1	Shulman 1989
Stroh's®	N = 1	0.8	341 mL	266.0	Shulman 1989
Stroh's® (fire brewed) 4.4% alc/vol., Canadian	N = 1	0.7	341 mL	228.5	Tailor 1994
Stroh's®, U.S. brand	N = 1	0.7	341 mL	235.3	Tailor 1994
Toby	N = 1	0.8	341 mL	269.4	Tailor 1994
Upper Canada® Colonial Stout	N = 1	2.0	341 mL	665.0	Tailor 1994
Upper Canada® Dark Ale	N = 1	0.0	341 mL	0.0	Tailor 1994
Upper Canada® Lager	N = 1	0.0	341 mL	0.0	Tailor 1994
Upper Canada® Natural Light Lager	N = 1	0.0	341 mL	0.0	Tailor 1994
Upper Canada® Rebellion Malt Lager	N = 1	0.0	341 mL	0.0	Tailor 1994
Upper Canada® Wheat	N = 1	0.0	341 mL	0.0	Tailor 1994

Beer—Tap

Amstel®, Molson	N = 1	0.5	341 mL	156.9	Tailor 1994
Carlsberg®, Carling	N = 1	0.8	341 mL	269.4	Tailor 1994
Coor's Light®, Coors	N = 1	0.4	341 mL	122.8	Tailor 1994
Criemone Spurgs Lager	N = 1	1.7–2.5	341 mL	579.7–852.5	Tailor 1994
Labatt's® Blue	N = 1	1.8	341 mL	607.0	Tailor 1994
Molson® Canadian, Molson	N = 1	0.6	341 mL	218.2	Tailor 1994
Molson®, Export Draft, Molson	N = 1	0.9	341 mL	313.7	Tailor 1994

Food	Sample Size	µg/g	Serving Size	µg/Serving	Reference
Olde Jacke Bitter Strong Ale®, Niagara Falls	N = 1	0.0	341 mL	0.0	Tailor 1994
Pacific Real Draft®, Pacific Western	N = 1	1.1	341 mL	368.3	Tailor 1994
Rickard's Red Draft®, Molson	N = 1	0.0	341 mL	0.0	Tailor 1994
Rotterdam's Irish Stout®, Rotterdam	**N = 1**	**1.3**	**341 mL**	**456.9**	**Tailor 1994**
Rotterdam's Lager®, Rotterdam	**N = 1**	**0.6**	**341 mL**	**204.6**	**Tailor 1994**
Rotterdam's® Pilsener beer[a]	N = 1	29.5	341 mL	10,042.5	Tailor 1994
Rotterdam's® Scotch Ale[a]	N = 1	9.1	341 mL	3,103.1	Tailor 1994
Sleeman Cream Ale®, Sleeman	N = 1	3.4	341 mL	1,149.2	Tailor 1994
Sleeman Lager®, Sleeman	N = 1	0.0	341 mL	0.0	Tailor 1994
Toby, Molson	N = 1	1.0	341 mL	341.0	Tailor 1994
Upper Canada® Lager, Sleeman[a]	**N = 1**	**112.9**	**341 mL**	**38,502.3**	**Tailor 1994**
Upper Canada® Natural Light Lager, Sleeman	N = 1	0.0	341 mL	0.0	Tailor 1994
Upper Canada® True Boch, Sleeman	N = 1	3.1	341 mL	1,067.3	Tailor 1994
Wellington® Best Bitter, Wellington	N = 1	1.9	341 mL	637.7	Tailor 1994
Wellington® County Ale, Wellington	N = 1	3.3	341 mL	1,111.7	Tailor 1994
Wellington® Imperial Stout, Wellington	N = 1	6.2	341 mL	2,114.2	Tailor 1994
France					
Kronenbourg®, Kronenbourg[a]	**N = 1**	**37.9**	**341 mL**	**12,906.9**	**Tailor 1994**
Scotland					Tailor 1994
McEwan's® Lager, Scottish and Newcastle	N = 1	0.7	341 mL	248.9	Tailor 1994
Tennents® Lager, Tennents	N = 1	0.5	341 mL	180.7	Tailor 1994
United Kingdom					
New Castle® Brown ale, Scottish and Newcastle	N = 1	1.0	341 mL	337.6	Tailor 1994
Stones® Best Bitter, William Stones	N = 1	0.5	341 mL	156.9	Tailor 1994
Germany					
DAB Premium, Dortmunder Actien	N = 1	1.5	341 mL	525.1	Tailor 1994
Ireland					
Smithwick's Ale®, Irish Ale	N = 1	1.3	341 mL	436.5	Tailor 1994
Guinness, Arthur Guinness	N = 1	1.0	341 mL	344.4	Tailor 1994
Murphy's Irish Stout	N = 1	0.5	341 mL	184.1	Tailor 1994

Holland					
Heineken®	N = 1	0.6	341 mL	194.4	Tailor 1994
Dealcoholized Beers					
Labatt® 0.5% alc/vol.	N = 1	1.2	341 mL	402.4	Tailor 1994
Holland					
Buckler® 0.5% alc/vol Bottle #1	N = 1	1.1	341 mL	368.3	Tailor 1994
Buckler® 0.5% alc/vol Bottle #2	N = 1	0.4	341 mL	126.2	Tailor 1994
France					
Kronenbourg®	N = 1	1.5	341 mL	511.5	Tailor 1994
Switzerland					
Beer	N = 1	0.0	341 mL	3.4	DaPrada 1992
Beer—Heineken®	N = 1	0.0	341 mL	3.4	DaPrada 1992
Beer—Thai Singhai®	N = 1	0.0	341 mL	3.3	DaPrada 1992
Korean beer	N = 1	0.4	341 mL	136.4	DaPrada 1992
Wine (Color/Type)					
U.S.					
Cabernet Sauvignon		ND–7.53	103 mL		Gloria 1998
Cabernet Sauvignon		1.6	103 mL	166.9	Gloria 1998
Pinot Noir		ND–2.5	103 mL		Gloria 1998
Pinot Noir			103 mL		
Spain					
Crianza red wines	N = 26	5.8	103 mL	595.3	Vazquez-Lasa 1998
Gran reserva red wines	N = 10	6.0	103 mL	615.9	Vazquez-Lasa 1998
Reserva red wines	N = 17	4.0	103 mL	412.0	Vazquez-Lasa 1998
Rioja (Siglo)	N = 1	4.4	103 mL	454.2	Shulman 1989
Rosé wines	N = 10	1.0	103 mL	97.9	Vazquez-Lasa 1998
Spanish wines	N = 111	3.0	103 mL	312.1	Vidal-Carou 1990
White wines	N = 10	0.9	103 mL	91.7	Vazquez-Lasa 1998
Young red wines	N = 36	5.0	103 mL	512.9	Vazquez-Lasa 1998
Portugal					
Dao (red) wine	N = 6	0.8	103 mL	83.4	Mafra 1999
Range	N = 6	ND–2.01			Mafra 1999
Vinho Verde (white) wine	N = 6	0.5	103 mL	55.6	Mafra 1999

Food	Sample Size	µg/g	Serving Size	µg/Serving	Reference
Range	N = 6	ND–0.78			Mafra 1999
Moscatel	N = 2	0.3	103 mL	29.9	Mafra 1999
Range	N = 2	0.27–0.032			Mafra 1999
Porto (Tawny)	N = 2	0.1	103 mL	14.4	Mafra 1999
Porto (aged 20–40 yr)	N = 2	0.09–0.19			Mafra 1999
Madeira	N = 12	1.7	103 mL	179.2	Mafra 1999
Range	N = 12	0.74–3.10			Mafra 1999
Italy					
Brolio, red Chianti	N = 1	0.4	103 mL	45.3	Shulman 1989
Cinzano, red Vermouth,	N = 1	ND	103 mL	ND	Shulman 1989
La Colombaia, red Chianti	N = 1	0.6	103 mL	64.9	Shulman 1989
Le Piazze, red Chianti	N = 1	ND	103 mL	ND	Shulman 1989
Ruffino, red Chianti	N = 1	3.0	103 mL	313.1	Shulman 1989
Germany					
Blue Nun®, white	N = 1	2.7	103 mL	278.1	Shulman 1989
Greece					
Retsina, white	N = 1	1.8	103 mL	184.4	Shulman 1989
France					
Beau-Rivage® red Bordeaux	N = 1	0.4	103 mL	36.1	Shulman 1989
Beau-Rivage®, white Bordeaux	N = 1	0.4	103 mL	40.2	Shulman 1989
Canada					
Maria Christina®, red	N = 1	0.2	103 mL	20.6	Shulman 1989
Asian Foods					
Pickled eggplant (Honolulu—first day)	N = 1	0.0	48 g	0.0	Mower 1989
Pickled eggplant (Honolulu—stored 3 weeks)	N = 1	2.3	48 g	110.4	Mower 1989
Salted black beans (Hong Kong—first day)	N = 1	450.0	172 g	77,400.0	Mower 1989
Salted black beans (Hong Kong—stored 3 weeks)	N = 1	563.0	172 g	96,836.0	Mower 1989
Soy milk	N = 1	2.0	250 mL	500.0	Walker 1996
Soybean curd, veggie, 9-d refrigerated	N = 1	6.0	100 g	600.0	Shulman 1999

Food	N		Serving		Reference
Soybean curd, veggie patty, 7-d refrigerated	N = 1	0.6	100 g	60.0	Shulman 1999
Tamari garlic marinade	N = 1	15.3	15 mL	229.5	Shulman 1999
Teriyaki marinade (soybean oil)—Golden Dipt® ginger	N = 1	0.0	15 mL	0.0	Shulman 1999
Teriyaki marinade (soybean oil)—Golden Dipt® ginger	N = 1	0.0	15 mL	0.0	Shulman 1999
Teriyaki marinade (soybean oil)—Golden Dipt® low fat honey	N = 1	3.1	15 mL	46.5	Shulman 1999
Tofu	N = 1	8.0	100 g	800.0	Walker 1996
Tofu, 7-d refrigerated	**N = 1**	**16.0**	**300 g**	**4,800.0**	**Shulman 1999**
Tofu, fresh	N = 1	0.8	300 g	228.0	Shulman 1999
Vita® tofu, 7-d refrigerated	**N = 1**	**16.0**	**300 g**	**4,800.0**	**Shulman 1999**
Vita® tofu, fresh	N = 1	0.8	300 g	240.0	Shulman 1999
Switzerland					
Bean flour, to thicken sauces, etc. (Thailand)	N = 1	0.1	85 g	8.5	DaPrada 1992
Duck, dried breast	**N = 1**	**35.3**	**100 g**	**3530.0**	**DaPrada 1992**
Duck, dried rib	N = 1	2.3	100 g	1990.0	DaPrada 1992
Duck, dried shank	N = 1	19.9	100 g	1,990.0	DaPrada 1992
Sausages	N = 1	30.6	23 g	703.8	DaPrada 1992
Soya bean drink (Singapore)	N = 1	ND	240 g	ND	DaPrada 1992
Soya bean drink (Swiss)	N = 1	ND	240 g	ND	DaPrada 1992
Soya bean drink, dehydrated (P.R. China)	N = 1	0.2	124 g	28.5	DaPrada 1992
Soya bean fermented, Miso Soup (Japan)	N = 1	1.8	138 g	251.2	DaPrada 1992
Soya bean paste, fermented (Korea)	**N = 1**	**206.0**	**50 g**	**10,300.0**	**DaPrada 1992**
Soya bean soup, concentrate (Japan)	N = 1	2.2	50 g	111.0	DaPrada 1992
Soya bean soup, prepared (Korea)	N = 1	0.2	50 g	11.0	DaPrada 1992
Soya bean, condiment (Formosa)	**N = 1**	**939.0**	**20 g**	**18,780.0**	**DaPrada 1992**
Soya beans, fermented (Singapore)	**N = 1**	**713.0**	**50 g**	**35,650.0**	**DaPrada 1992**
Tempe, 2 weeks storage at 5°C[a]	**N = 1**	**733.0**	**50 g**	**36,650.0**	**Nout 1993**
Tempe, fresh	**N = 1**	**575.0**	**50 g**	**28,750.0**	**Nout 1993**
Tempe, fresh, fried	**N = 1**	**632.0**	**50 g**	**31,600.0**	**Nout 1993**
Tempe, fresh, stewed	**N = 1**	**500.0**	**50 g**	**25,000.0**	**Nout 1993**
Tofu (Japan)	N = 1	ND	124 g	ND	DaPrada 1992
Tofu baked (Japan)	N = 1	0.0		0.0	DaPrada 1992
Tofu fried (Hong Kong)	N = 1	0.7	13 g	8.6	DaPrada 1992

Food	Sample Size	µg/g	Serving Size	µg/Serving	Reference
Cheese/Dairy					
3-yr-old white	**N = 1**	**779.7**	**30 g**	**23,392.2**	**Shulman 1989**
Black Diamond Hickory Smoked Cheese	N = 3–6	26.0	30 g	780.0	Baker 1987
Bleu cheese 1	N = 1	38.7	30 g	1,161.3	Mosnaim 1996
Bleu cheese 2	N = 1	37.2	30 g	1,115.4	Mosnaim 1996
Blue cheese	**N = 1**	**997.8**	**30 g**	**29,933.7**	**Shulman 1989**
Blue cheese dressing	N = 1	39.2	30 g	1,176.0	Shulman 1989
Bonbel	N = 1	ND	30 g	ND	Shulman 1989
Boursin	N = 1	0.9	30 g	27.9	Shulman 1989
Brie 1	N = 1	0.1	30 g	2.1	Mosnaim 1996
Brie 2	N = 1	0.1	30 g	2.4	Mosnaim 1996
Cambozola blue vein (germ)	N = 1	18.3	30 g	549.3	Shulman 1989
Camembert 1	N = 1	0.1	30 g	2.9	Mosnaim 1996
Camembert 2	N = 1	0.1	30 g	4.1	Mosnaim 1996
Cheddar Bruch	N = 1	0.1	30 g	2.3	Mosnaim 1996
Cheddar Bruch	N = 1	6.5	30 g	196.0	Mosnaim 1996
Cheddar cheese—old (Kraft®)	N = 3–6	62.2	30 g	1,866.0	Baker 1987
Cheese spread (Handi-snack®)	**N = 1**	**133.8**	**30 g**	**4,014.3**	**Shulman 1989**
Cheez Whiz®	N = 1	8.5	30 g	253.8	Shulman 1989
Cream cheese	N = 1	9.0	30 g	271.2	Shulman 1989
Cream cheese (Philadelphia)	N = 1	ND	30 g	ND	Shulman 1989
Extra old[a]	**N = 1**	**608.2**	**30 g**	**18,245.7**	**Shulman 1989**
Farmers, plain	N = 1	11.1	30 g	331.5	Shulman 1989
Feta	N = 1	75.8	30 g	2,273.4	Shulman 1989
Feta 1	N = 1	0.0	30 g	0.4	Mosnaim 1996
Feta 2	N = 1	0.0	30 g	0.0	Mosnaim 1996
Feta with sun-dried tomatoes and oregano	N = 1	5.8	30 g	173.4	Shulman 1999
Generic medium cheddar cheese (7 d refrigerated)	**N = 1**	**337.4**	**30 g**	**10,122.0**	**Shulman 1999**
Generic medium cheddar cheese (8 d refrigerated)	**N = 1**	**359.7**	**30 g**	**10,791.0**	**Shulman 1999**

Generic medium cheddar cheese (fresh)	**N = 1**	**218.0**	**30 g**	**6,540.0**	**Shulman 1999**
Goat cheese 1	N = 1	0.0	30 g	1.3	Mosnaim 1996
Goat cheese 2	N = 1	0.1	30 g	3.4	Mosnaim 1996
Havarti	N = 1	ND	30 g	ND	Shulman 1989
Havarti w/dill 1	N = 1	58.9	30 g	1,767.3	Mosnaim 1996
Havarti w/dill 2	**N = 1**	**166.9**	**30 g**	**5,006.1**	**Mosnaim 1996**
Jack Colby 1	N = 1	45.7	30 g	1,371.9	Mosnaim 1996
Jack Colby 2	N = 1	24.5	30 g	734.4	Mosnaim 1996
Light Italian cheese, Sargeto	N = 1	8.2	30 g	246.0	Shulman 1999
Medium (black diamond)	N = 1	40.0	30 g	1,200.0	Shulman 1989
Mild (black diamond)	N = 1	33.3	30 g	1,000.0	Shulman 1989
Mozarella	**N = 1**	**158.1**	**30 g**	**4,740**	**Shulman 1989**
Mozarella 1	N = 1	0.1	30 g	2.3	Mosnaim 1996
Mozarella 2	N = 1	0.3	30 g	7.5	Mosnaim 1996
Mozzarella cheese	N = 1	17.1	30 g	513.0	Shulman 1999
Muenster[a]	**N = 1**	**101.7**	**30 g**	**3,051.0**	**Shulman 1989**
Old cheddar	**N = 1**	**497.9**	**30 g**	**14,937.0**	**Shulman 1989**
Old coloured	N = 1	77.5	30 g	2,324.1	Shulman 1989
Parmesan	N = 1	74.6	30 g	2,237.1	Shulman 1989
Pizza cheese 1	N = 1	2.2	30 g	66.9	Mosnaim 1996
Pizza cheese 2	N = 1	2.1	30 g	63.9	Mosnaim 1996
Processed cheese slice	N = 1	ND	30 g	ND	Shulman 1989
Ricotta	N = 1	ND	30 g	ND	Shulman 1989
Romano cheese, aged	N = 1	4.1	30 g	123.0	Shulman 1999
Sour cream	N = 1	1.2	30 g	36.9	Shulman 1989
Swiss Emmenthal	N = 1	24.0	30 g	719.7	Shulman 1989
Swiss Gruyere[a]	**N = 1**	**125.2**	**30 g**	**3,755.1**	**Shulman 1989**
Woodward's® Cheshire cheese	**N = 3–6**	**144.0**	**30 g**	**4,320.0**	**Baker 1987**
Woodward's® Stilton cheese	**N = 3–6**	**115.0**	**30 g**	**3,450.0**	**Baker 1987**
Yogurt	N = 1	ND	30 g	ND	Schulman 1989
Brazil					
Parmesan	N = 1	17.0	30 g	510.0	Vale and Gloria 1997

Food	Sample Size	µg/g	Serving Size	µg/Serving	Reference
Holland					
Cheese		138.0	30 g	4,140.0	**ten Brink 1990**
Denmark					
Danish blue	***N = 1***	**294.7**	**30 g**	**8,840.1**	**Shulman 1989**
Danish blue	***N = 1***	**369.5**	**30 g**	**11,084.1**	**Shulman 1989**
Italian					
Brie 1	*N = 1*	0.0	30 g	0.9	Mosnaim 1996
Brie 2	*N = 1*	0.1	30 g	1.9	Mosnaim 1996
Brie (d'OKA) with rind	*N = 1*	5.7	30 g	171.3	Shulman 1989
Brie (d'OKA) without rind	*N = 1*	14.7	30 g	439.5	Shulman 1989
Brie (M-C) with rind	*N = 1*	21.2	30 g	635.7	Shulman 1989
Brie (M-C) without rind	*N = 1*	2.8	30 g	84.6	Shulman 1989
Gorgonzola	*N = 1*	55.9	30 g	1,678.2	Shulman 1989
Parmesan	*N = 1*	74.6	30 g	2,237.1	Shulman 1989
England					
English Stilton	***N = 1***	**1,156.9**	**30 g**	**34,707.3**	**Shulman 1989**

Cheese/Dairy Dishes (Serving Weight without Crust)

Food	Sample Size	µg/g	Serving Size	µg/Serving	Reference
Pizza Pizza®					
Half medium double pizza	*N = 1*	1.3	133 g	172.4	Shulman 1999
Half medium double cheese, double pepperoni pizza	*N = 1*	0.0	314 g	0.0	Shulman 1999
Pizza Hut®					
Half medium double cheese, double pepperoni pizza	*N = 1*	0.5	137 g	68.3	Shulman 1999
McDonald's®					
1 single slice McDonald's deluxe pizza	*N = 1*	0.5	83 g	41.6	Shulman 1999
1 single slice McDonald's pepperoni pizza	*N = 1*	8.6	76 g	653.6	Shulman 1999

Domino's®

Half medium double cheese, double pepperoni pizza	N = 1	3.6	104 g	375.1	Shulman 1999

Chocolate

Baker's® Semi-Sweet Chocolate	N = 3–6	0.8	28 g	21.0	Baker 1987
Cadbury's® hot chocolate	N = 3–6	0.6	28 g	17.9	Baker 1987
Chocolate bar (Toblerone®)	N = 1	0.0	35 g	0.0	Walker 1996
Chocolate Hershey® bar	N = 1	0.1	14 g	1.4	Mosnaim 1996
Fry's® cocoa	N = 3–6	3.5	28 g	98.0	Baker 1987
Rowntree's® Aero bar	N = 3–6	0.2	28 g	6.2	Baker 1987

Fish

Chopped herring 1	N = 1	0.2	85 g	16.7	Mosnaim 1996
Chopped herring 2	N = 1	0.3	85 g	22.9	Mosnaim 1996
Cod filet—fresh 1	N = 1	0.2	85 g	13.9	Mosnaim 1996
Cod filet—fresh 2	N = 1	0.3	85 g	24.2	Mosnaim 1996
Fresh catfish filet—farm 1	N = 1	0.7	85 g	55.3	Mosnaim 1996
Fresh catfish filet—farm 2	N = 1	0.5	85 g	45.8	Mosnaim 1996
Gelfilte fish 1	N = 1	1.2	42 g	50.4	Mosnaim 1996
Gelfilte fish 2	N = 1	10.3	42 g	434.3	Mosnaim 1996
Lump fish roe	N = 1	4.4	50 g	220.0	Shulman 1989
Mahi mahi filet 1	N = 1	1.2	85 g	104.6	Mosnaim 1996
Mahi mahi filet 2	N = 1	3.9	85 g	331.3	Mosnaim 1996
Ocean perch filet 1	N = 1	0.0	85 g	0.2	Mosnaim 1996
Ocean perch filet 2	N = 1	0.1	85 g	9.7	Mosnaim 1996
Pickled herring 1	N = 1	81.7	30 g	2,450.1	Walker 1996
Pickled herring 2	N = 1	ND	30 g	ND	Shulman 1989
Pickled herring juice	N = 1	8.0	30 mL	240.0	Walker 1996
Salmon steak 1	N = 1	0.3	85 g	24.1	Mosnaim 1996
Salmon steak 2	N = 1	0.6	85 g	52.0	Mosnaim 1996
Sliced schmaltz herring in oil	N = 1	4.0	50 g	200.0	Shulman 1989

Food	Sample Size	µg/g	Serving Size	µg/Serving	Reference
Smoked carp	N = 1	ND	85 g	ND	Shulman 1989
Smoked salmon	N = 1	ND	85 g	ND	Shulman 1989
Smoked trout 1	N = 1	0.1	85 g	4.9	Mosnaim 1996
Smoked trout 2	N = 1	0.1	85 g	10.6	Mosnaim 1996
Smoked whitefish	N = 1	ND	85 g	ND	Shulman 1989
Smoked whitefish 1	N = 1	20.9	85 g	1,776.5	Mosnaim 1996
Smoked whitefish 2	N = 1	20.0	85 g	1,695.8	Mosnaim 1996
Sole filet 1	N = 1	0.6	85 g	48.7	Mosnaim 1996
Sole filet 2	N = 1	1.2	85 g	106.2	Mosnaim 1996
Talapia skinless	N = 1	3.2	85 g	272.0	Mosnaim 1996
Talapia skinless	N = 1	15.5	85 g	1,315.8	Mosnaim 1996
Walleye pike 1	N = 1	10.8	85 g	917.4	Mosnaim 1996
Walleye pike 2	N = 1	17.4	85 g	1,480.6	Mosnaim 1996
Fruit					
Avocado	N = 1	ND	173 g	ND	Shulman 1989
Banana	N = 1	ND	114 g	ND	Shulman 1989
Banana peel	N = 1	51.7	1 peel	1,424.0	Shulman 1989
Banana pulp (overripe)	N = 1	13.0	100 g	1,300.0	Walker 1996
Banana skin (overripe)	N = 1	86.0	30 g	2,580.0	Walker 1996
Cranberry juice	N = 1	0.0	250 g	0.0	Walker 1996
Figs (California, blue ribbon)	N = 1	ND	50 g	ND	Shulman 1989
Raisins (California, seedless)	N = 1	ND	100 g	ND	Shulman 1989
Raspberries fresh (Chile)	N = 1	0.0	100 g	0.0	Walker 1996
Raspberries frozen	N = 1	21.0	100 g	2,100.0	Walker 1996
Ripe avocado	N = 1	ND	173 g	ND	Shulman 1989
Meat					
Beef ground chuck (80%) 1	**N = 1**	**40.0**	**100 g**	**3,997.0**	**Mosnaim 1996**

Beef ground chuck (80%) 2	*N* = 1	47.7	100 g	4,767.0	**Mosnaim 1996**
Chicken liver, day 1	*N* = 1	ND	30 g	ND	Shulman 1989
Chicken liver, day 5	*N* = 1	ND	30 g	ND	Walker 1996
Chicken liver, day 9	*N* = 1	2,128.0	30 g	63,840.0	**Walker 1996**
Chicken liver, fresh	*N* = 1	6.4	200 g	1,270.0	Walker 1996
Fresh beef—ground sirloin 1	*N* = 1	37.9	100 g	3,786.0	**Mosnaim 1996**
Fresh beef—ground sirloin 2	*N* = 1	49.0	100 g	4,900.0	**Mosnaim 1996**
Fresh ground pork 1	*N* = 1	34.1	100 g	3,406.8	**Mosnaim 1996**
Fresh ground pork 2	*N* = 1	39.4	100 g	3,936.8	**Mosnaim 1996**
Ham, smoked 1	*N* = 1	1.1	100 g	107.2	Mosnaim 1996
Ham, smoked 2	*N* = 1	1.3	100 g	125.1	Mosnaim 1996
Kielbasa sausage	*N* = 1	6.0	30 g	180.0	Shulman 1989
Liverwurst	*N* = 1	2.0	30 g	60.0	Shulman 1989
Pork country sausage 1	*N* = 1	0.4	30 g	10.5	Mosnaim 1996
Pork country sausage 2	*N* = 1	0.5	30 g	15.6	Mosnaim 1996
Smoked meat	*N* = 1	18.0	30 g	540.0	Shulman 1989
Pate					
Country style	*N* = 1	3.0	30 g	90.0	Shulman 1989
Peppercorn	*N* = 1	2.0	30 g	60.0	Shulman 1989
Salmon mousse	*N* = 1	22.0	30 g	660.0	Shulman 1989
Luncheon Meats and Meat Products					
Aged sausage	*N* = 1	29.0	30 g	870.0	Shulman 1989
Air dried sausage	*N* = 1	125.0	30 g	3,750.0	**Shulman 1989**
Bacon	*N* = 1	25.0	30 g	750.0	Walker 1996
Cacciatore	*N* = 1	252.3	30 g	7,569.9	**Walker 1996**
Cacciatore sausage mild	*N* = 1	150.0	30 g	4,500.0	**Walker 1996**
Chicken smoked, sliced 1	*N* = 1	201.9	30 g	6,056.9	**Mosnaim 1996**
Chicken smoked, sliced 2	*N* = 1	503.6	30 g	15,108.9	**Mosnaim 1996**
Cooked sliced ham	*N* = 1	4.3	30 g	129.9	Walker 1996
Corned beef	*N* = 1	11.0	30 g	330.0	Shulman 1989

Food	Sample Size	µg/g	Serving Size	µg/Serving	Reference
Corned beef 1	N = 1	2.5	30 g	73.7	Mosnaim 1996
Corned beef 2	N = 1	2.5	30 g	74.1	Mosnaim 1996
Jumbo franks 1	N = 1	0.1	57 g	7.8	Mosnaim 1996
Jumbo franks 2	N = 1	0.2	57 g	8.6	Mosnaim 1996
Lasagna (Chef Boyardee®)	N = 1	0.0	212 g	0.0	Walker 1996
Mini pepperoni (Piller® sausages)	N = 1	3.7	30 g	110.1	Walker 1996
Mixed Meat Dishes (Canned)					
Mortadella	**N = 1**	**184.0**	**30 g**	**5,520.0**	**Shulman 1989**
Nostrano chub (Venetian®) inside	**N = 1**	**238.7**	**30 g**	**7,160.1**	**Walker 1996**
Nostrano chub (Venetian®) skin	N = 1	33.0	30 g	990.0	Walker 1996
Pastrami (Shopsy's®)	N = 1	10.0	30 g	300.0	Walker 1996
Pastrami (Ziggy's®)	N = 1	69.3	30 g	2,079.9	Walker 1996
Pepperettes (Springer®)	N = 1	6.3	30 g	189.9	Walker 1996
Pepperoni (Fortinos®) inside	N = 1	13.7	30 g	410.1	Walker 1996
Pepperoni (Fortinos®) skin	N = 1	62.7	30 g	1,880.1	Walker 1996
Pepperoni (Mastro®)	N = 1	26.0	30 g	780.0	Walker 1996
Pepperoni sausage	N = 1	ND	30 g	ND	Shulman 1989
Ravioli (Chef Boyardee®)	N = 1	1.0	212 g	209.9	Walker 1996
Salami	**N = 1**	**188.0**	**30 g**	**5,640.0**	**Shulman 1989**
Salami 1	N = 1	0.2	30 g	5.4	Mosnaim 1996
Salami 2	N = 1	2.2	30 g	65.1	Mosnaim 1996
Salami calabrese	N = 1	52.7	30 g	1,580.1	Walker 1996
Salami calabrese (Mastro®)	N = 1	52.7	30 g	1,580.1	Walker 1996
Salami Cacciatore (Mastro®) inside	**N = 1**	**152.7**	**30 g**	**4,580.1**	**Walker 1996**
Salami Cacciatore (Mastro®) skin	**N = 1**	**180.0**	**30 g**	**5,400.0**	**Walker 1996**
Salami genoa (Mastro®) inside	N = 1	38.7	30 g	1,160.1	Walker 1996
Salami genoa (Mastro®) skin	N = 1	73.3	30 g	2,199.9	Walker 1996
Sausage 1	N = 1	2.0	30 g	61.2	Mosnaim 1996
Sausage 2	N = 1	5.2	30 g	154.7	Mosnaim 1996

Food	N	μg/g or μg/mL	Serving size	per serving	Reference
Sausage fermented[a]	**N = 14**	**110.0**	**30 g**	**3,300.0**	**ten Brink 1990**
Sliced chicken	N = 1	8.3	30 g	249.9	Walker 1996
Smoked sausage	N = 1	1.0	30 g	30.0	Shulman 1989
Spaghetti and meatballs (Chef Boyardee®)	N = 1	2.6	212 g	540.6	Walker 1996
Sweet Italian sausage	N = 1	1.0	30 g	30.0	Shulman 1989
Turkey smoked 1	N = 1	0.2	30 g	7.0	Mosnaim 1996
Turkey smoked 2	N = 1	0.2	30 g	7.1	Mosnaim 1996
Waxed bologna	N = 1	3.7	30 g	110.1	Walker 1996
Weiners	N = 1	8.0	45 g	360.0	Walker 1996
Weiners 1	N = 1	0.0	45 g	0.9	Mosnaim 1996
Weiners 2	N = 1	0.2	45 g	8.6	Mosnaim 1996
Spain					
Chorizo	**N = 5**	**324.6**	**60 g**	**19,476.0**	**Hernandez-Jover 1996**
Cooked ham	N = 5	2.7	100 g	270.0	Hernandez-Jover 1996
Cooked Mortadella	N = 5	18.8	30 g	564.0	Hernandez-Jover 1996
Fresh beef	N = 5	ND	100 g	ND	Hernandez-Jover 1996
Fresh pork	N = 5	0.7	100 g	70.0	Hernandez-Jover 1996
Salchicon[a]	**N = 5**	**300.1**	**30 g**	**9,003.0**	**Hernandez-Jover 1996**

Sauces and Gravies

Food	N	μg/g or μg/mL	Serving size	per serving	Reference
Beef gravy (Franco-American®)	N = 1	0.9	57 mL	49.0	Shulman 1989
Chicken bouillon mix	N = 1	ND	6 g	ND	Shulman 1989
Chicken gravy (Franco-American®)	N = 1	0.5	57 mL	26.2	Shulman 1989
Vegetable bouillon mix	N = 1	ND	12 g	ND	Shulman 1989
Diane sauce (BBQ)	N = 1	0.0	15 mL	0.0	Shulman 1999
Fish sauce (Thailand—first day)	N = 1	23.8	113 g	2,689.4	Mower 1989
Fish sauce (Thailand-stored 3 weeks)	N = 1	19.7	113 g	2,226.1	Mower 1989
Shrimp sauce (Hong Kong—first day)[a]	**N = 1**	**245.5**	**100 g**	**24,550.0**	**Mower 1989**
Shrimp sauce (Hong Kong—stored 3 weeks)[a]	**N = 1**	**307.2**	**100 g**	**30,720.0**	**Mower 1989**
Soy sauce (Kikkoman®)	N = 1	29.0	15 mL	435.0	Shulman 1999
Soy sauce (Kimlan®)	N = 1	36.6	15 mL	549.0	Shulman 1999
Soy sauce (Kimlan®)	**N = 1**	**941.0**	**15 mL**	**14,115.0**	**Walker 1996**
Soy sauce (Ozeki Sachimi®)	N = 1	83.4	15 mL	1,251.0	Shulman 1999

Food	Sample Size	µg/g	Serving Size	µg/Serving	Reference
Soy sauce (Pearl River Bridge®)	**N = 1**	**224.4**	**15 mL**	**3,366.0**	**Shulman 1999**
Soy sauce (Wing's®)	N = 1	9.9	15 mL	148.5	Shulman 1999
Soya sauce	N = 1	18.7	58 mL	1,085.8	Shulman 1989
Soya sauce (Swiss)	N = 1	195.3	15 mL	2,930.0	DaPrada 1992
Soya sauce (Taiwan)	**N = 1**	**585.3**	**15 mL**	**8,780.0**	**DaPrada 1992**
Worchestershire sauce (Generic brand)	N = 1	4.3	15 mL	64.5	Shulman 1999
Worchestershire sauce (Lea and Perrins®)	N = 1	8.3	15 mL	124.5	Shulman 1999
Worchestershire sauce (Sharwood's®)	N = 1	0.5	15 mL	7.5	Shulman 1999
Seafood					
Bay scallops 1	N = 1	0.1	85 g	8.9	Mosnaim 1996
Bay scallops 2	N = 1	0.1	85 g	10.0	Mosnaim 1996
Bluepoint oysters 1	N = 1	1.9	84 g	156.3	Mosnaim 1996
Bluepoint oysters 2	N = 1	3.9	84 g	327.6	Mosnaim 1996
Sea scallops 1	N = 1	0.4	85 g	31.3	Mosnaim 1996
Sea scallops 2	N = 1	0.4	85 g	32.8	Mosnaim 1996
Shrimp (40–50/lb) 1	N = 1	1.1	85 g	93.8	Mosnaim 1996
Shrimp (40–50/lb) 2	N = 1	1.5	85 g	125.7	Mosnaim 1996
Shrimp jumbo (16–20/lb) 1	N = 1	0.1	85 g	7.3	Mosnaim 1996
Shrimp jumbo (16–20/lb) 2	N = 1	1.4	85 g	117.9	Mosnaim 1996
Vegetables					
American sauerkraut (refrigerated style)	N = 2	0.1	250 g	18.5	Mosnaim 1996
Sauerkraut	**N = 1**	**55.5**	**250 g**	**13,867.5**	**Shulman1989**
Sauerkraut (Canada)	N = 1	3.1	250 g	775.0	Walker 1996
Beans	N = 1	0.0	172 g	1.4	Mosnaim 1996
Black 1	N = 1	0.0	172 g	1.9	Mosnaim 1996
Black 2	N = 1	ND	170 g	ND	Mosnaim 1996
Fava beans	N = 1	0.0	172 g	1.0	Mosnaim 1996
Pinto 1	N = 1	0.0	172 g	1.9	Mosnaim 1996

Food	N	µg/g	Serving	µg	Reference
Pinto 2	N = 1	0.0	172 g	2.4	Mosnaim 1996
Red 1	N = 1	0.0	172 g	2.6	Mosnaim 1996
Red 2	N = 1	0.0	179 g	1.6	Mosnaim 1996
Small white 1	N = 1	0.0	179 g	2.7	Mosnaim 1996
Small white 2					
Taiwan					
Straw mushroom (boiled in water)	N = 1	4.1	78 g	319.8	Yen 1992
Straw mushroom (commercially canned)	N = 1	3.3	78 g	257.4	Yen 1992
Straw mushroom (raw)	N = 1	65.5	35 g	2,292.5	Yen 1992
Straw mushroom (day 0–4°C)	**N = 1**	**49.4**	**78 g**	**3,853.2**	**Yen 1992**
Straw mushroom (day 0–25°C)	**N = 1**	**49.4**	**78 g**	**3,853.2**	**Yen 1992**
Straw mushroom (day 1–4°C)	**N = 1**	**195.7**	**78 g**	**15,264.6**	**Yen 1992**
Straw mushroom (day 1–25°C)	**N = 1**	**104.2**	**78 g**	**8,127.6**	**Yen 1992**
Straw mushroom (day 3–4°C)	**N = 1**	**356.5**	**78 g**	**27,807.0**	**Yen 1992**
Straw mushroom (day 3–25°C)	**N = 1**	**295.4**	**78 g**	**23,041.2**	**Yen 1992**
Straw mushroom (day 5–4°C)	**N = 1**	**359.0**	**78 g**	**28,002.0**	**Yen 1992**
Straw mushroom (day 5–25°C)	**N = 1**	**431.2**	**78 g**	**33,633.6**	**Yen 1992**
Czech Republic					
Agaricus bisporus	N = 1	ND	35 g	ND	Kalac 1997
Boletus badius mushroom	N = 1	ND	35 g	ND	Kalac 1997
Boletus variegatus mushroom	N = 1	ND	35 g	ND	Kalac 1997
Botetus chrysentereon mushroom	N = 1	ND	35 g	ND	Kalac 1997
Yeast Extracts					
Brewer's yeast debittered—maximum nutrition	N = 1	ND	15 g	ND	Shulman 1989
Brewer's yeast flakes	N = 1	0.6	15 g	9.4	Shulman 1989
Brewer's yeast tablets—drug trade company	N = 1	0.5	400 mg	191.3	Shulman 1989
Brewer's yeast tablets—Jamieson	N = 1	0.2	400 mg	66.7	Shulman 1989
Marmite® concentrated yeast extract[a]	**N = 1**	**645.0**	**10 g**	**6,450.0**	**Shulman 1989**

ND = Nondetectable.

Note: Food is of Canada/U.S. origin unless otherwise noted.

Boldfaced words indicate adverse levels in a single or double serving.

[a] Adverse level (6000 µg).

APPENDIX **D.2**

Histamine Content of Foods and Beverages in μg/g or μg/mL

Food	Sample Size	µg/g or µg/mL	Serving Size g or mL	µg/Serving	Reference
Asian Food					
Soy sauce	N = 1	7.8–64.0	15 mL	117–960	**Fardiaz 1979**
Taiwan					
Inyu (soy sauce from black soybeans)	N = 1	80.0–462.0	15 mL	1,200–6,930	**Yen 1986**
Toushi (fermented black soybean)	N = 1	22.4–133.7	100 g	2,240–13,370	Yen 1986
Switzerland					
Tempe, fresh	N = 1	100.0	50 g	5,000.0	Nout 1993
Tempe, fresh, fried	N = 1	<10	50 g	<500	Nout 1993
Tempe, fresh, stewed	N = 1	<5	50 g	<250	Nout 1993
Cheese/Dairy					
Black diamond hickory smoked cheese	N=3–6	5.5	30 g	165.0	Baker 1987
Cheddar cheese—old (Kraft®)	N=3–6	4.4	30 g	132.0	Baker 1987
Netherlands	**N = 6**	**250–1,300**	**30 g**	**7,500–39,000**	**ten Brink 1990**
Woodward's® Cheshire cheese	N=3–6	209.0	30 g	6,270.0	Baker 1987
Woodward's® Stilton cheese	N=3–6	39.0	30 g	1,170.0	Baker 1987
Brazil					
Parmesan	N = 2	107.0	30 g	3,210.0	Vale and Gloria 1997
Chocolate					
Baker's® semisweet chocolate	N=3–6	0.4	28 g	12.0	Baker 1987
Cadbury's® hot chocolate	N=3–6	0.4	28 g	11.5	Baker 1987
Fry's® cocoa	N=3–6	1.3	21 g	27.3	Baker 1987
Rowntree's® Aero Bar	N=3–6	0.6	28 g	15.4	Baker 1987
Fish					
Fish paste	N = 1	7.8–64.0	7 g	54.6–448	Fardiaz 1979

Netherlands					
Herring	**N = 3**	**300–1,300**	**85 g**	**25,500–110,500**	**ten Brink 1990**
Mackerel	**N = 8**	**100–3,000**	**85 g**	**8,500–25,5000**	**ten Brink 1990**
Tuna	**N = 3**	**500–8,000**	**85 g**	**42,500–680,000**	**ten Brink 1990**
Scotland					
Mackerel muscle—1 d stored in ice	**N = 3**	**3,862.0**	**85 g**	**328,270.0**	**Mackie 1997**
Spain					
Albacore tuna—after 9 months of frozen storage	N = 32	5.0	85 g	425.0	Ben-Guirey 1998
Anchovies packed in brine	N = 16	1.4	20 g	27.0	Veciana-Nogues 1996
Anchovies packed in oil	N = 16	13.9	20 g	278.0	Veciana-Nogues 1996
Meat					
Dry sausage	N = 1	Trace–55.0	30 g	Trace–1,650	Taylor 1978; Vandekerckhove 1977
Spain					
Bacon for fuet sausage, raw	N = 2	ND	30 g	ND[b]	Hernandez-Jover 1996
Chorizo 1	N = 5	ND	60 g	ND	Hernandez-Jover 1996
Chorizo 2	N = 5	34.8	60 g	2,088.0	Hernandez-Jover 1996
Cooked ham 1	N = 5	ND	100 g	ND	Hernandez-Jover 1996
Cooked ham 2	N = 20	0.9	100 g	90.0	Hernandez-Jover 1996
Fresh beef	N = 5	0.4	100 g	40.0	Hernandez-Jover 1996
Fresh pork	N = 5	ND	100 g	ND	Hernandez-Jover 1996
Mortadella 1	N = 5	ND	30 g	ND	Hernandez-Jover 1996
Mortadella 2	N = 20	0.0	30 g	0.0	Hernandez-Jover 1996
Pork meat for fuet sausage, raw	N = 2	ND	30 g	ND	Hernandez-Jover 1996
Salchicon 1	N = 5	2.4	30 g	70.5	Hernandez-Jover 1996
Salchicon 2	N = 5	0.0	30 g	0.0	Hernandez-Jover 1996
Vegetables					
Mixed vegetables	N = 1	ND–0.1	91 g	ND–9.1	Anderson 1988
Sauerkraut	N = 1	0.7–20.0	250 g	175–5,000	Mayer 1972; Taylor 1978
Germany					
Chinese cabbage-vacuum packed (0 d storage)	N = 2	1.1	35 g	38.5	Simon-Sarkadi 1994

Food	Sample Size	µg/g or µg/mL	Serving Size g or mL	µg/Serving	Reference
Chinese cabbage-vacuum packed (1 d storage)	N = 2	0.8	35 g	28.0	Simon-Sarkadi 1994
Chinese cabbage-vacuum packed (2 d storage)	N = 2	0.9	35 g	31.5	Simon-Sarkadi 1994
Chinese cabbage-vacuum packed (5 d storage)	N = 2	0.9	35 g	31.5	Simon-Sarkadi 1994
Endive-vacuum packed (0 d storage)	N = 2	ND	25 g	ND	Simon-Sarkadi 1994
Endive-vacuum packed (5 d storage)	N = 2	ND	25 g	ND	Simon-Sarkadi 1994
Iceberg lettuce-vacuum packed (0 d storage)	N = 2	ND	28 g	ND	Simon-Sarkadi 1994
Iceberg lettuce-vacuum packed (5 d storage)	N = 2	ND	28 g	ND	Simon-Sarkadi 1994
Radicchio—vacuum packed (0 d storage)	N = 2	ND	20 g	ND	Simon-Sarkadi 1994
Radicchio—vacuum packed (5 d storage)	N = 2	ND	20 g	ND	Simon-Sarkadi 1994
Taiwan (Mushrooms)					
Straw mushroom (boiled in water)	N = 1	0.7	78 g	53.0	Yen 1992
Straw mushroom (commercially canned)	N = 1	ND	78 g	ND	Yen 1992
Straw mushroom (raw)	N = 1	1.8	35 g	63.0	Yen 1992
Straw mushroom (day 0–4°C OR 25°C)	N = 1	0.7	78 g	54.6	Yen 1992
Straw mushroom (day 5–4°C)	N = 1	8.3	78 g	647.4	Yen 1992
Straw mushroom (day 5–25°C)	N = 1	244.4	78 g	19,063.2	Yen 1992
Alcoholic Beverages					
Beer					
Canadian beer	N = 1	4.8–5.4	341 mL	1,636.8–1,841.4	Zee 1981
European beer	N = 1	2.6–20.0	341 mL	886.6–6,820	Granerus 1969; Zee 1981
Distilled Spirits					
Scotch whiskey	N = 1	ND	28 mL	ND	Granerus 1969
Whiskey	N = 1	ND	28 mL	ND	Granerus 1969
Wine					
American red wine	N = 1	0.2–15.5	103 mL	20.6–1,596.5	Baucom 1986; Ough 1971

	N				Reference
American white wine	N = 1	0.2–11.4	103 mL	20.6–1,174.2	Baucom 1986; Ough 1971
Brandy	N = 1	ND	60 mL	ND	Granerus 1969
Cabernet Sauvignon	N = 5	2.7	103 mL	279.1	Gloria 1998
Cabernet Sauvignon	N = 5	ND–10.1	103 mL		Granerus 1969
Cognac	N = 1	ND	60 mL	ND	Granerus 1969
European red	N = 1	ND–30	103 mL	ND–3,090	Granerus 1968; Ough 1971; Pechanek 1983
European white	N = 1	ND–20	103 mL	ND–2,060	Granerus 1968; Ough 1971
Pinot Noir	N = 18	7.2	103 mL	741.6	Gloria 1998
Pinot Noir	N = 18	ND–23.98	103 mL		Gloria 1998
Spain					
Young Red	N = 36	8.7	103 mL	898.2	Vazquez-Lasa 1998
Gran Reserva red	N = 10	5.1	103 mL	527.4	Vazquez-Lasa 1998
Reserva red	N = 17	6.9	103 mL	710.7	Vazquez-Lasa 1998
Crianza red	N = 26	6.7	103 mL	687.0	Vazquez-Lasa 1998
Rose	N = 10	1.2	103 mL	124.6	Vazquez-Lasa 1998
White	N = 10	0.8	103 mL	86.5	Vazquez-Lasa 1998
Portugal					
Aged Porto (fortified, 20–40 yr)	N = 2	0.3	103 mL	29.9	Vazquez-Lasa 1998
Aged Porto (fortified, 20–40 yr)	N = 2	0.25–0.32	103 mL		Vazquez-Lasa 1998
Dao red	N = 7	1.2	103 mL	124.6	Vazquez-Lasa 1998
Dao red	N = 7	0.39–1.66	103 mL		Vazquez-Lasa 1998
Madeira (fortified)	N = 12	0.5	103 mL	51.5	Vazquez-Lasa 1998
Madeira (fortified)	N = 12	ND–0.88	103 mL		Vazquez-Lasa 1998
Moscatel	N = 2	0.9	103 mL	92.7	Vazquez-Lasa 1998
Moscatel	N = 2	0.81–0.99	103 mL		Vazquez-Lasa 1998
Tawny Porto (fortified)	N = 2	0.5	103 mL	54.6	Vazquez-Lasa 1998
Tawny Porto (fortified)	N = 2	0.41–0.64	103 mL		Vazquez-Lasa 1998
Vinko Verde white	N = 6	1.2	103 mL	123.6	Vazquez-Lasa 1998
Vinko Verde white	N = 6	0.84–1.70	103 mL		Vazquez-Lasa 1998

Note: ND = Nondetectable; boldfaced words indicate adverse event level >400 μg/g (400 ppm); Food is of Canada/U.S. origin unless otherwise noted.

Calcium Content of Selected Foods

Food Description	Ca (mg)/Serving	Serving Size (g)
Milk		
Whole milk	291	240
2% milk	297	240
1% milk	313	240
Nonfat milk	316	240
Cultured Dairy Foods		
Yogurt, plain, whole	296	227
Yogurt, plain, nonfat	488	227
Buttermilk, lowfat	285	240
Cheeses		
Cheese sandwich	375	90
American cheese	317	30
Gruyere	303	30
Swiss cheese	300	30
Cheddar	284	30
Mozzarella	265	30
Monterey	234	30
Provolone	227	30
Gouda/Edam	215	30
Muenster	215	30
Colby Jack	215	30
Imitation cheese	212	30
Processed American	205	30
Processed cheddar	188	30
Processed cheese, can	169	30
Limburger	149	30
Feta cheese	133	30

Food Description	Ca (mg)/Serving	Serving Size (g)
Fish		
Sardines	325	85
Cereals		
Multigrain Raisin Bran	277	55
Total®	258	30
Total® Raisin Bran	238	55
Total® Corn Flakes	237	30
Basic Four®	169	30
Sauces		
Sesame sauce	198	60
Nuts and Seeds		
Almonds	85	30
Miscellaneous		
Hush puppy	56	20
Waffle	104	35
Corn-based snacks	107	30
Cheese biscuit	107	35
Pancake	118	40
Special Supplements		
Power bar	185	40
Meal-replacement powders	173	30
Breakfast bar	118	40

Vitamin K1 (Phylloquinone) Content of Foods in μg/100 g and μg/serving (in g or mL)

Food item	μg/100 g	Serving Size	μg/Serving	References
Alcoholic Beverage				
Beer	<0.01	341 mL	<0.01	3
Martini	<0.01	70 mL	<0.01	3
Whiskey	<0.01	28 mL	<0.01	3
Wine, dry table	<0.01	103 mL	<0.01	3
Wine, table	Trace	103 mL	Trace	1
Beverages				
Cola, carbonated beverage	0.02	246 mL	0.05	3
Cola, diet	Trace	240 mL	Trace	1
Cola, low-calorie carbonated beverage	<0.01	237 mL	<0.01	3
Cola, regular	Trace	240 mL	Trace	1
Cranberry juice cocktail	Trace	240 mL	Trace	1
Fruit drink, canned	0.02	248 mL	0.05	3
Fruit drink, from powder	<0.01	262 mL	<0.01	3
Ginger ale, diet	Trace	240 mL	Trace	1
Ginger ale, regular	0.01	240 mL	0.02	1
Lemonade, frozen concentrate	0.03	240 mL	0.07	1
Lemonade, frozen concentrate	0.06	248 mL	0.15	3
Sake	Trace	240 mL	Trace	1
Tap water	<0.01	237 mL	<0.01	3
Dried Tea Leaves		***1 serving = 1 teabag***		
Black currant	1,019.00	2 g	23.44	2

Food item	µg/100 g	Serving Size	µg/Serving	References
Black Tea 1	945.00	2 g	21.74	2
Black Tea 2	312.00	2 g	7.18	2
Blackberry	1,056.00	2 g	24.29	2
China black	1,174.00	2 g	27.00	2
Darjeeling	976.00	2 g	22.45	2
Earl Grey	979.00	2 g	22.52	2
Green tea 1	1,654.00	2 g	38.04	2
Green tea 2	482.00	2 g	11.09	2
Herbal Tea	568.00	2 g	13.06	2
Honey and Cinnamon	517.00	2 g	11.89	2
Irish Tea	981.00	2 g	22.56	2
Jasmine	1,300.00	2 g	29.90	2
Mint Tea	804.00	2 g	18.49	2
Oolong	713.00	2 g	16.40	2
Orange pekoe	827.00	2 g	19.02	2
Brewed Tea		**6 oz cup**	**6 oz cup**	
Black tea	0.02	180 mL	0.04	2
Green tea	0.03	180 mL	0.05	2
Tea, brewed	0.05	180 mL	0.09	1
Tea, from tea bag	0.08	180 mL	0.14	3
Black tea	0.02	240 mL	0.05	2
Green tea	0.03	240 mL	0.07	2
Tea, brewed	0.05	240 mL	0.12	1
Tea, from tea bag	0.08	240 mL	0.19	3
Brewed Coffee				
Coffee, brewed	10.00	180 mL	18.00	1
Coffee, decaffeinated, from instant	0.02	180 mL	0.04	3
Coffee, decaffeinated	Trace	Trace	Trace	2
Coffee, from ground beans	<0.01	180 mL	<0.01	3
Coffee, instant, decaffeinated	0.03	180 mL	0.05	2
Coffee, instant, regular	0.02	180 mL	0.04	2
Coffee, regular	0.02	180 mL	0.04	2
Coffee, brewed	10.00	240 mL	24.00	1
Coffee, decaffeinated, from instant	0.02	240 mL	0.05	3
Coffee, decaffeinated	Trace	Trace	Trace	2
Coffee, from ground beans	<0.01	240 mL	<0.01	3
Coffee, instant, decaffeinated	0.03	240 mL	0.07	2
Coffee, instant, regular	0.02	240 mL	0.05	2
Coffee, regular	0.02	240 mL	0.05	2
Bread/Cereals/Pasta				
Bagel, plain	0.40	71 g	0.28	3
Barley flour	1.00	30 g	0.30	1
Biscuit, from refrigerated dough, baked	4.60	70 g	3.22	3
Blueberry muffin, commercial	25.00	57 g	14.25	3
Bran flakes	2.00	28 g	0.56	1

Food item	μg/100 g	Serving Size	μg/Serving	References
Bread, assorted types	3.00	50 g	1.50	1
Buckwheat flour, whole groats, cooked	7.00	120 g	8.40	1
Butter-type crackers	13.10	30 g	3.93	3
Corn bread, (H)	7.40	65 g	4.81	3
Corn flakes	0.04	28 g	0.01	1
Corn grits, regular, cooked	<.01	242 g	<0.01	3
Cornflakes	0.03	25 g	0.01	3
Cracked wheat bread	3.50	50 g	1.75	3
Crackers, graham	0.50	30 g	0.15	1
Crackers, saltines	2.00	30 g	0.60	1
Crisped rice cereal	<.01	28 g	<0.01	3
Egg noodles, boiled	0.09	160 g	0.14	3
English muffin, plain, toasted	0.30	57 g	0.17	3
Fruit-flavored, sweetened cereal	0.20	35 g	0.07	3
Graham crackers	8.90	28 g	2.49	3
Granola cereal	1.80	56 g	1.01	3
Macaroni, boiled	0.05	140 g	0.07	3
Millet, uncooked	0.90	30 g	0.27	1
Oat ring cereal	0.80	25 g	0.20	3
Oatmeal, instant, dry, plain	3.00	40 g	1.20	1
Oatmeal, quick (1–3 min), cooked	0.40	234 g	0.94	3
Pancakes from mix	6.50	114 g	7.41	3
Puffed rice	0.08	14 g	0.01	1
Puffed wheat, plain	2.00	14 g	0.28	1
Raisin bran cereal	1.60	56 g	0.90	3
Rice, flour	0.04	163 g	0.07	1
Rice, white, uncooked	1.00	45 g	0.45	1
Rye bread	3.00	62 g	1.86	3
Saltine crackers	3.60	30 g	1.08	3
Shredded wheat cereal	1.50	47 g	0.71	3
Shredded wheat	0.70	55 g	0.39	1
Spaghetti, dry	0.20	55 g	0.11	1
Tortilla, flour	3.10	70 g	2.17	3
Total cereal	0.70	28 g	0.20	1
Wheat cereal, farina, quick (1–3 min), cooked	0.06	233 g	0.14	3
Wheat flour, all-purpose	0.60	30 g	0.18	1
White bread	1.90	50 g	0.95	3
White rice, cooked	<.01	102 g	<0.01	3
White roll	2.10	57 g	1.20	3
Whole wheat bread	3.40	57 g	1.94	3

Cheese/Dairy

Food item	μg/100 g	Serving Size	μg/Serving	References
American, processed cheese	1.60	28 g	0.45	3
Butter	0.40	250 g	1.00	1
Cheddar cheese	2.10	28 g	0.59	3
Cheese, cheddar	7.00	15 g	1.05	1
Chocolate milk, fluid	0.20	250 mL	0.50	3
Chocolate milk, low fat	3.00	30 g	0.90	1
Cottage cheese, 4% milk fat	0.40	113 g	0.45	3

Food item	µg/100 g	Serving Size	µg/Serving	References
Cream cheese	2.90	28 g	0.81	3
Egg white, raw	0.01	33 g	0.00	1
Egg yolk, raw	2.00	17 g	0.34	1
Eggs, boiled	0.30	50 g	0.15	3
Eggs, fried	6.90	46 g	3.17	3
Eggs, scrambled	12.00	64 g	7.68	3
Evaporated milk, canned	1.60	32 g	0.51	3
Fruit-flavored yogurt, low fat (fruit mixed)	3.00	227 g	6.81	3
Lowfat (2% fat) milk, fluid	0.20	244 mL	0.49	3
Milk, skim	0.02	245 mL	0.05	1
Milk, whole	0.30	245 g	0.74	1
Plain yogurt, low fat	0.10	227 g	0.23	3
Skim milk, fluid	0.01	245 mL	0.02	3
Sour cream, cultured	1.00	12 g	0.12	1
Soy milk	3.00	240 mL	7.20	1
Swiss cheese	2.80	28 g	0.78	3
Whole milk, fluid	0.30	244 g	0.73	3
Yogurt, low fat, plain	0.30	225 g	0.68	1
Desserts				
Apple pie, fresh frozen, commercial	11.00	125 g	13.75	3
Brownies, commercial	14.00	57 g	7.98	3
Cake doughnuts with icing, any flavor	9.80	47 g	4.61	3
Caramel candy	1.70	40 g	0.68	3
Chocolate cake with chocolate icing, commercial	13.00	64 g	8.32	3
Chocolate chip cookies, commercial	10.00	30 g	3.00	3
Chocolate milkshake, fast food	0.20	283 g	0.57	3
Chocolate pudding, from instant mix	0.40	17 g	0.07	3
Chocolate snack cake with chocolate icing	5.70	50 g	2.85	3
Fruit flavor sherbet	0.30	87 g	0.26	3
Gelatin dessert, any flavor	0.02	120 g	0.02	3
Milk chocolate candy bar, plain	0.40	40 g	0.16	3
Popsicle™, any flavor	<0.01	75 g	<0.01	3
Pumpkin pie, fresh/frozen, commercial	10.00	109 g	10.90	3
Sandwich cookies with crème filling, commercial	8.70	30 g	2.61	3
Suckers, any flavor	<0.01	15 g	<0.01	3
Sugar cookies, commercial	11.00	30 g	3.30	3
Sweet roll/Danish, commercial	11.00	65 g	7.15	3
Vanilla ice cream	0.30	66 g	0.20	3
Yellow cake with white icing	8.50	64 g	5.44	3
Fish/Seafood				
Mackerel, Atlantic, raw	5.00	110 g	5.50	1

Food item	µg/100 g	Serving Size	µg/Serving	References
Octopus, common, raw	0.07	85 g	0.06	1
Oyster, eastern, wild, raw	0.10	84 g	0.08	1
Salmon, pink, raw	0.40	110 g	0.44	1
Sardine, raw	0.09	24 g	0.02	1
Shrimp, mixed species, raw	0.03	85 g	0.03	1
Squid, mixed species, raw	0.02	85 g	0.02	1
Tuna, bluefin, raw	0.03	85 g	0.03	1
Yellowtail, mixed species, raw	0.08	85 g	0.07	1
Fruit				
Apple juice, bottled	<0.01	244 g	<0.01	3
Apple juice, canned or bottled	0.10	240 mL	0.24	1
Apple sauce, canned	0.50	122 g	0.61	1
Apple, red, raw	1.80	154 g	2.77	3
Apples, w/o skin, raw	0.50	128 g	0.64	1
Applesauce, bottled	0.60	128 g	0.77	3
Apricot, raw	3.30	141 g	4.65	3
Apricots, canned w/ water, skin	5.00	90 g	4.50	1
Avocado, raw	14.00	30 g	4.20	3
Avocados, raw	40.00	173 g	69.20	1
Banana, raw	0.20	126 g	0.25	3
Bananas, raw	0.50	114 g	0.57	1
Blueberries, canned w/heavy syrup	6.00	128 g	7.68	1
Cantaloupe, raw	0.40	134 g	0.54	3
Cranberry sauce, canned, sweet	1.00	70 g	0.70	1
Fruit cocktail, canned in heavy syrup	2.60	128 g	3.33	3
Fruit cocktail, canned w/water pack	0.80	140 g	1.12	1
Grape juice, canned or bottled	0.20	253 mL	0.51	1
Grape juice, from frozen concentrate	0.40	250 g	1.00	3
Grapefruit juice, canned	0.20	240 mL	0.48	1
Grapefruit juice, from frozen concentrate	0.05	247 g	0.12	3
Grapefruit, raw	0.02	118 g	0.02	1
Grapefruit, raw	<0.01	154 g	<0.01	3
Grapes, European-type, raw	3.00	160 g	4.80	1
Grapes, red/green, seedless, raw	8.30	138 g	11.45	3
Melon, raw	1.00	140 g	1.40	1
Orange juice, from frozen concentrate	<0.01	249 g	<0.01	3
Orange juice, raw	0.10	248 mL	0.25	1
Orange, raw	<0.01	154 g	<0.01	3
Oranges, raw	0.10	131 g	0.13	1
Peach, raw	2.10	112 g	2.35	3
Peaches, raw	3.00	87 g	2.61	1
Pear, canned in light syrup	0.20	158 g	0.32	3
Pear, raw	4.90	166 g	8.13	3
Pears, canned w/water pack	0.50	244 g	1.22	1
Pineapple juice, canned	0.70	240 mL	1.68	1

Food item	μg/100 g	Serving Size	μg/Serving	References
Pineapple juice, from frozen concentrate	0.30	250 g	0.75	3
Pineapple, canned in juice	0.30	116 g	0.35	3
Pineapple, raw	0.10	155 g	0.16	1
Plums, raw	12.00	66 g	7.92	1
Plums, raw	8.20	132 g	10.82	3
Prune juice, bottled	3.40	256 g	8.70	3
Prunes, dried	1.40	42 g	0.59	3
Raisins, dried	1.70	36 g	0.61	3
Strawberries, raw	1.50	147 g	2.21	3
Sweet cherries, raw	1.50	140 g	2.10	3
Watermelon, raw	0.20	280 g	0.56	3
Infant and Junior Foods				
Apple juice, strained	0.01	124 mL	0.01	3
Applesauce, strained/jr.	1.30	113 g	1.47	3
Banana with tapioca, strained/jr.	0.10	113 g	0.11	3
Beef, strained/jr.	1.70	113 g	1.92	3
Beets, strained/jr.	0.10	113 g	0.11	3
Carrots, strained/jr.	5.80	113 g	6.55	3
Chicken and noodle dinner, strained/jr.	0.90	113 g	1.02	3
Chicken, strained/jr.	<0.01	113 g	<0.01	3
Creamed corn, strained/jr.	0.05	113 g	0.06	3
Creamed spinach, strained/jr.	292.00	113 g	329.96	3
Custard pudding, strained/jr.	<0.01	113 g	<0.01	3
Egg yolk, strained/jr.	0.40	113 g	0.45	3
Fruit dessert/pudding, strained/jr.	0.50	113 g	0.57	3
Green beans, strained/jr.	26.00	113 g	29.38	3
Macaroni, tomatoes, and beef, strained/jr.	1.70	113 g	1.92	3
Milk-based infant formula, high iron, ready-to-feed	12.00	30 mL	3.60	3
Milk-based infant formula, low iron, ready-to-feed	13.00	30 mL	3.90	3
Mixed vegetables, strained/jr.	7.40	113 g	8.36	3
Orange juice, strained	<0.01	124 mL	<0.01	3
Peaches, strained/jr.	4.90	113 g	5.54	3
Pears, strained/jr.	4.30	113 g	4.86	3
Peas, strained/jr.	17.00	113 g	19.21	3
Rice cereal, strained/jr.	0.30	113 g	0.34	3
Rice infant cereal, instant, whole milk	0.30	113 g	0.34	3
Soy-based infant formula, ready-to-feed	16.00	30 mL	4.80	3
Split peas with vegetables and ham/bacon, strained/jr.	3.00	113 g	3.39	3
Sweet potatoes, strained/jr.	1.00	113 g	1.13	3
Teething biscuits	4.50	11 g	0.50	3
Turkey and rice, strained/jr.	4.20	113 g	4.75	3
Vegetables and beef, strained/jr.	4.10	113 g	4.63	3

Food item	µg/100 g	Serving Size	µg/Serving	References
Vegetables and chicken, strained/jr.	3.50	113 g	3.96	3
Vegetables and ham, strained/jr.	1.60	113 g	1.81	3

Legumes and Nuts

Food item	µg/100 g	Serving Size	µg/Serving	References
Kidney beans, dry, boiled	8.40	88 g	7.39	3
Mixed nuts, no peanuts, dry roasted	13.00	28 g	3.64	3
Peanut, dry, roasted	0.30	28 g	0.08	3
Peanuts, raw	0.20	30 g	0.06	1
Peas, mature, dry, boiled	5.00	98 g	4.90	3
Pinto beans, dry, boiled	3.70	86 g	3.18	3
Pistachio nuts, dried	70.00	28 g	19.60	1
Pork and beans, canned	1.10	126 g	1.39	3
Sesame seeds, dried	8.00	9 g	0.72	1

Meat, Poultry, and Fish

Food item	µg/100 g	Serving Size	µg/Serving	References
Beef chuck roast, baked	0.70	85 g	0.60	3
Beef steak, loin, pan-cooked	1.80	85 g	1.53	3
Beef, ground, regular, raw	6.00	99 g	5.94	1
Bologna, sliced	0.30	56 g	0.17	3
Chicken breast, roasted	<.01	85 g	<0.01	3
Chicken meat, raw	0.10	100 g	0.10	1
Chicken nuggets, fast food	1.50	109 g	1.64	3
Chicken, fried (breast, leg, and thigh) (H)	4.50	85 g	3.83	3
Chicken, fried (breast, leg, and thigh) fast food	1.30	85 g	1.11	3
Fish sticks, frozen, heated	6.80	85 g	5.78	3
Frankfurters, beef, boiled	1.80	57 g	1.03	3
Ground beef, pan-cooked	2.40	85 g	2.04	3
Haddock, pan-cooked	5.20	85 g	4.42	3
Ham, baked	<.01	85 g	<.01	3
Ham, luncheon meat, sliced	<.01	56 g	<0.01	3
Lamb chop, pan-cooked	4.60	85 g	3.91	3
Liver, beef, fried	2.70	85 g	2.30	3
Pork bacon, pan-cooked	0.10	19 g	0.02	3
Pork chop, pan-cooked	3.10	85 g	2.64	3
Pork roast, baked	<.01	85 g	<.01	3
Pork sausage, pan-cooked	3.40	56 g	1.90	3
Pork, fresh, raw	0.07	100 g	0.07	1
Salami, sliced	1.30	56 g	0.73	3
Shrimp, boiled	<.01	85 g	<0.01	3
Tuna, canned in oil, drained	24.00	56 g	13.44	3
Turkey breast, roasted	<.01	85 g	<0.01	3
Turkey meat, raw	0.02	100 g	0.02	1
Veal cutlet, pan-cooked	6.60	85 g	5.61	3

Mixed Dishes and Meals

Food item	µg/100 g	Serving Size	µg/Serving	References
Bean with bacon/pork soup, canned, condensed	0.90	253 g	2.28	3

Food item	µg/100 g	Serving Size	µg/Serving	References
Beef chow mein, from Chinese carryout	31.00	250 g	77.50	3
Beef stew with potatoes, carrots, and onion (H)	4.80	245 g	11.76	3
Beef stroganoff (H)	1.70	198 g	3.37	3
Cheese and pepperoni pizza, regular crust, carryout	3.80	130 g	4.94	3
Cheese pizza, regular crust, carryout	4.20	130 g	5.46	3
Chicken noodle soup, canned, condensed	0.10	241 g	0.24	3
Chicken potpie, frozen, heated	2.70	277 g	7.48	3
Chili con carne with beans (H)	4.70	255 g	11.99	3
Clam chowder, New England, canned, condensed	0.30	248 g	0.74	3
Egg, cheese, and ham on English muffin, fast food	3.70	16 g	0.59	3
Fish sandwich on bun, fast food	17.00	158 g	26.86	3
Frankfurter on bun, fast food	4.40	98 g	4.31	3
Frozen meal—Salisbury steak with gravy	2.30	312 g	7.18	3
Frozen meal—turkey with gravy	5.30	312 g	16.54	3
Green peppers stuffed with beef and rice (H)	7.40	198 g	14.65	3
Lasagna with meat (H)	5.30	198 g	10.49	3
Macaroni and cheese, from box mix	5.30	200 g	10.60	3
Meatloaf (H)	12.00	85 g	10.20	3
Mushroom soup, canned, condensed	2.00	248 g	4.96	3
Quarter-pound cheeseburger on bun, fast food	4.10	219 g	8.98	3
Quarter-pound hamburger on bun, fast food	3.80	218 g	8.28	3
Spaghetti with tomato sauce and meatballs (H)	5.70	248 g	14.14	3
Spaghetti with tomato sauce, canned	0.70	250 g	1.75	3
Taco/tostada, carryout	16.00	171 g	27.36	3
Tomato soup, canned, condensed	1.50	248 g	3.72	3
Tuna noodle casserole (H)	20.00	240 g	48.00	3
Vegetable beef soup, canned, condensed	0.60	244 g	1.46	3
Vegetables				
Artichokes, raw	14.00	300 g	42.00	1
Asparagus, fresh/frozen, boiled	80.00	90 g	72.00	3
Asparagus, raw	40.00	76 g	30.40	1
Beans, snap, raw	47.00	85 g	39.95	1
Beets, fresh/frozen, boiled	1.20	85 g	1.02	3
Beets, raw	3.00	85 g	2.55	1
Broccoli, cooked	270.00	78 g	210.60	1
Broccoli, fresh/frozen, boiled	113.00	78 g	88.14	3

Food item	µg/100 g	Serving Size	µg/Serving	References
Broccoli, raw	205.00	44 g	90.20	1
Brussels sprouts, fresh/frozen, boiled	289.00	78 g	225.42	3
Cabbage, fresh, boiled	98.00	75 g	73.50	3
Cabbage, raw	145.00	35 g	50.75	1
Cabbage, red, raw	44.00	35 g	15.40	1
Cabbage, turnip, raw	2.00	35 g	0.70	1
Carrot, fresh, boiled	15.00	78 g	11.70	3
Carrots, cooked	18.00	78 g	14.04	1
Carrots, raw	5.00	72 g	3.60	1
Cauliflower, cooked	10.00	78 g	7.80	1
Cauliflower, fresh/frozen, boiled	20.00	62 g	12.40	3
Cauliflower, raw	5.00	50 g	2.50	1
Celery, raw	12.00	40 g	4.80	1
Celery, raw	32.00	55 g	17.60	3
Chayote leaf, cooked	270.00	80 g	216.00	1
Coleslaw with dressing, (H)	100.00	120 g	120.00	3
Collards, fresh/frozen, boiled	440.00	85 g	374.00	3
Corn, fresh/frozen, boiled	0.30	83 g	0.25	3
Cream style corn, canned	0.03	128 g	0.04	3
Cucumber with skin, raw	19.00	52 g	9.88	1
Cucumber, raw	2.20	99 g	2.18	3
Eggplant, fresh, boiled	2.90	96 g	2.78	3
Eggplant, raw	0.50	41 g	0.21	1
Endive, raw	231.00	25 g	57.75	1
French fries, fast food	4.40	68 g	2.99	3
French fries, frozen, heated	7.10	70 g	4.97	3
Green beans, fresh/frozen, boiled	16.00	62 g	9.92	3
Green peas, fresh/frozen, boiled	24.00	80 g	19.20	3
Green pepper, raw	2.50	148 g	3.70	3
Iceberg lettuce, raw	31.00	89 g	27.59	3
Kale, leaf, raw	817	85 g	694.00	1
Leek, raw	14.00	26 g	3.64	1
Lettuce leaf, raw	210.00	28 g	58.80	1
Lettuce, butterhead, raw	122.00	15 g	18.30	1
Lima beans, immature, frozen, boiled	5.10	85 g	4.34	3
Mashed potatoes, from flakes	5.10	105 g	5.36	3
Mixed vegetables, frozen, boiled	19.00	82 g	15.58	3
Mushrooms, raw	0.02	35 g	0.01	1
Mushrooms, raw	0.06	70 g	0.04	3
Mustard greens, raw	170	28 g	47.60	1
Okra, fresh/frozen, boiled	40.00	80 g	32.00	3
Onion, mature, raw	0.30	148 g	0.44	3
Onions, raw	2.00	80 g	1.60	1
Onions, spring	207.00	50 g	103.50	1
Peppers, sweet, raw	17.00	50 g	8.50	1
Pickles, dill cucumber	13.00	28 g	3.64	1
Pickles, sweet cucumber	23.00	28 g	6.44	1
Potato, flesh, raw	0.80	112 g	0.90	1
Potatoes, French fried, prepared	5.00	50 g	2.50	1
Pumpkin, canned	16.00	122 g	19.52	1

Food item	μg/100 g	Serving Size	μg/Serving	References
Purslane, raw	381.00	58 g	220.98	1
Radish, raw	0.40	85 g	0.34	3
Radishes, raw	0.01	45 g	0.00	1
Sauerkraut, canned	25.00	118 g	29.50	1
Sauerkraut, canned	13.00	118 g	15.34	3
Scalloped potatoes, (H)	3.30	122 g	4.03	3
Seaweed, laver, green	4.00	100 g	4.00	1
Seaweed, laver, purple	1,385.00	100 g	1,385.00	1
Spinach leaf, raw	400.00	28 g	112.00	1
Spinach, fresh/frozen, boiled	360.00	90 g	324.00	3
Squash, summer, w/o skin, raw	3.00	65 g	1.95	1
Squash, summer, w/o skin, raw	3.00	65 g	1.95	1
Summer squash, fresh/frozen, boiled	4.40	90 g	3.96	3
Sweet potato, fresh, baked	2.40	114 g	2.74	3
Sweet potatoes, canned	4.00	200 g	8.00	1
Tomato juice, bottled	2.30	244 g	5.61	3
Tomato sauce, plain, bottled	2.90	61 g	1.77	3
Tomato, red, raw	3.00	148 g	4.44	3
Tomato, stewed, canned	2.40	101 g	2.42	3
Tomatoes, ripe, raw	6.00	123 g	7.38	1
Turnip greens, raw	251.00	28 g	70.28	1
Turnip, fresh/frozen, boiled	0.07	78 g	0.05	3
Watercress, raw	250.00	17 g	42.50	1
White potato, baked with skin	1.10	140 g	1.54	3
White potato, boiled without skin	0.30	136 g	0.41	3
Winter squash, fresh/frozen, baked, mashed	1.10	102 g	1.12	3
Oils/Spreads/Fats/Dressings				
Brown gravy (H)	0.30	65 g	0.20	3
Butter, regular, salted	7.00	14 g	0.98	3
Canola oil	141.00	14 g	19.74	1
Chocolate syrup dessert topping	0.20	38 g	0.08	3
Corn oil	3.00	14 g	0.42	1
Cream substitute, frozen	5.70	15 g	0.86	3
French salad dressing, regular	51.00	29 g	14.79	3
Fruit spread, assorted flavors	0.50	20 g	0.10	1
Half and half	1.30	30 g	0.39	3
Honey	0.02	21 g	0.00	1
Honey	<0.01	21 g	<0.01	3
Italian salad dressing, low calorie	2.90	29 g	0.84	3
Jelly, any flavor	12.00	19 g	2.28	3
Margarine, regular, hard stick	51.00	14 g	7.14	1
Margarine, stick, regular	33.00	14 g	4.62	3
Mayonnaise, regular, bottled	41.00	14 g	5.74	3
Mayonnaise	81.00	14 g	11.34	1
Olive oil	49.00	14 g	6.86	1
Olive/safflower oil	28.00	14 g	3.92	3
Pancake syrup	<0.01	80 g	<0.01	3
Peanut butter, smooth style	10.00	32 g	3.20	1

Food item	μg/100 g	Serving Size	μg/Serving	References
Peanut butter, smooth style	0.30	32 g	0.10	3
Peanut oil	0.70	14 g	0.10	1
Safflower oil	11.00	14 g	1.54	1
Sesame oil	10.00	14 g	1.40	1
Sour cream	1.00	30 g	0.30	3
Soybean oil	193.00	14 g	27.02	1
Sunflower oil	9.00	14 g	1.26	1
Tomato catsup	3.60	15 g	0.54	3
Walnut oil	15.00	14 g	2.10	1
White sauce (H)	6.90	66 g	4.55	3
Yellow mustard	2.20	5 g	0.11	3
Miscellaneous				
Corn chips	7.30	28 g	2.04	3
Popcorn, popped in oil	20.00	22 g	4.40	3
Potato chips	10.00	28 g	2.80	1
Potato chips	15.00	28 g	4.20	3
Pretzels, hard, salted, any shape	2.90	28 g	0.81	3
Pretzels, hard	1.00	28 g	0.28	1
Rice cake, brown rice, plain	0.60	18 g	0.11	1
Sugar, white, granulated	<0.01	2 g	<0.01	3
Tofu, regular, raw	2.00	12 g	2.48	1

Note: Dihydro vitamin K1 values are not included in table because this form of vitamin K1 is not involved in coagulation reactions; H = homemade; tea and coffee brews are not dietary sources of vitamin K-1 (phylloquinone).

Source: Adapted from Provisional Table, Vitamin K, USDA; Booth, S.L. et al., Tea and coffee brews are not dietary sources of Vitamin K-1 (phylloquinone), *J. Am. Diet. Assoc.,* 95, 82–83, 1995. With permission; Booth, S.L., Sadowski, J.A., and Pennington, J.A.T., Phylloquinone (Vitamin K1) content of foods in the U.S. Food and Drug Administration's total diet study, *J. Am. Food Chem.,* 43, 1574–1579, 1995. With permission.

APPENDIX **D.5**

Iron Content in Selected Foods

Food Description	Iron (mg) per Serving	Serving Size (g)
Cereals		
Baby food	30	70
Raisin bran	27	55
Bran cereals	9.3	30
Fortified cereals	6.2	30
Fortified cereals	5	30
Infant cereals/finger foods	1.2	2.5
Meat, Poultry, Fish, Eggs		
Beef, lean	2.09–3.79	100
Sausage, bologna	0.35	72
Fish, nonbreaded	1.22	85
Chicken breast, cooked	1.06	90
Egg, whole, boiled	1.04	80
Organ Meats		
Liver	7.0	100
Pork liver	18.0	100
Seafood		
Octopus	0.37	85
Clam	13	85
Supplements		
Algae, dried	27	100
Seaweed, dried	25	100
Protein supplement	13.3	30
Meal-replacement bar	7.4	40

Food Description	Iron (mg) per Serving	Serving Size (g)
Milk drink mixes	6.7	30
Tiger's milk	5.6	30
Vegetables, Cooked		
Broccoli	0.9	80
Spinach	1.4	90
Lentils	6.6	200
Beans, red kidney	3.1	175
Peas	1.2	80
Corn	0.5	80

Magnesium Content in Selected Foods

Food Description	Magnesium (mg)/Serving	Serving Size (g)
Nuts and Seeds		
Pumpkin seeds, dried	155	30
Flax seeds, dried	142	30
Mixed seeds, dried	129	30
Peanut butter	109	30
Sunflower seeds, dry roasted	37	30
Sesame seeds	105	30
Almonds	91	30
Hazelnuts	86	30
Cashews	78	30
Mixed nuts	75	30
Butter nuts	71	30
Pine nuts	70	30
Brazil nuts	68	30
Mixed nuts with dried fruit and seeds	65	45
Peanuts	56	30
Hickory nuts	52	30
Walnuts	51	30
Pistachios	47	30
Soy nuts	44	30
Pecans	38	30
Meats/Poultry		
Beef, lean	17–24	100
Pork, lean	22–30	100
Chicken, breast, roasted	25	100
Cereals/Grains		
Rice bran, dry	235	30

Food Description	Magnesium (mg)/Serving	Serving Size (g)
Wheat bran, dry	168	30
Whole wheat flour, dry	160	120
Fruit and Fibre	101	60
Granola	98	55
Oat bran, dry	94	40
Raisin bran	94	55
Chex®	38	30
Raw oats	60	40
Ethnic Foods		
Papad	209	100
Fish sauce (bagoong)	105	60
Conch	200	85
Cod, dried, salted	113	85
Seaweed, dried	483	100
Algae, dried	340	100
Snails	260	85
Vegetables		
Dried vegetables	102	60
Dried tomatoes	7.5	5
Breads		
Muffin	70	60
Pretzel	14	55
Miscellaneous		
Molasses, medium	48	20
Yeast spread	31	15
Tofu	58	20
Popcorn	7.5	5
Coffee, instant powder	6.5	2
Tea, instant powder	3.6	1

Phosphorus Content in Selected Foods

Food Description	Phosphorus (mg)/Serving	Serving Size (g)
Nuts and Seeds		
Pumpkin seeds	350	30
Sunflower seeds	340	30
Mixed seeds	280	30
Sunflower seeds, unroasted	211	30
Brazil nuts	180	30
Nut mix with dried fruits	167	35
Almonds	165	30
Almond butter	157	30
Peanuts	155	30
Pistachios	150	30
Pine nuts	150	30
Cashews	147	30
Mixed nuts	140	30
Flax seeds	138	30
Sesame seeds	77	30
Milk Products		
Dry milk, low fat	295	30
Buttermilk, dry	280	30
Dry milk, whole	230	30
Dried Fish		
Cod	808	85
Squid	714	85
Octopus	601	85
Carp	551	85
Herring	503	30
Carp, baked or broiled	452	85

Food Description	Phosphorus (mg)/Serving	Serving Size (g)
Sardines, cooked	417	85
Scallops	398	85

Miscellaneous

Gelatin	1099	85
Cocoa	326	20
Yeast	129	10
Textured vegetable protein	101	15
Egg yolk	73	15
Turkey bacon, cooked	46	10

Cheeses

Cheese, processed (American/Cheddar)	280	30
Low sodium, low-fat processed cheese	250	30
Parmesan	242	30
Cheese spread	233	30
Processed Swiss	230	30
Canned w/pressure cheese spread	214	30
Mozzarella	197	30
Low-sodium Swiss	182	30
Low-fat Swiss	182	30
Gouda	161	30
Cheddar	150	30
Provolone	149	30
Cheddar/colby	145	30
Muenster	140	30
Goat cheese	135	30

Special Supplements

Meal-replacement powders	340	30
Protein supplements	265	30
Power Bar	220	40

Cereals

Rice bran	503	30
Raisin bran	380	60
Bran	370	30
Wheat germ	340	30
Fruit and Fibre®	310	60
Oat bran	293	40
Granola	230	50
Total®	211	30
Bran flakes	155	30
Oat bran	152	30
Oats	140	30
Baby cereal	80	15

Meats

Beef, roast	235	100
Pork, roast	215	100
Poultry, chicken roasted	215	100

Potassium Content in Selected Foods

Food Description	Potassium (mg)/Serving	Serving Size (g)
Fruits		
Lychee	1110	100
Raisins	751	100
Papaya, dried	680	40
Prunes, dried	630	85
Dried banana	447	30
Dried peach	398	40
Currants, dried	357	45
Fig, dried	285	40
Orange juice	67	10
Vegetables		
Potato, microwave with skin	212	200
Bamboo shoots	24	120
Dried carrot chips	762	30
Tamarind, raw	754	120
Collard greens	216	70
French fries	402	85
Potato skins	430	85
Palm hearts	106	30
Cabbage, green, shredded, boiled	73	75
Tomato paste	281	30
Onion, dehydrated	243	15
Potato chips	216	30
Dried red tomatoes	171	5
Soy/Nuts		
Soybean meal	3018	120
Soy nuts	1320	90

Food Description	Potassium (mg)/Serving	Serving Size (g)
Natto	620	85
Tofu, okara	130	61
Flax seeds	395	30
Pistachios	290	30
Mixed seeds	261	35
Sunflower seeds	255	30
Mixed nuts with dried fruit and seeds	250	35
Almonds	231	30
Peanut butter, low sodium	224	30
Peanut butter	200	30
Dried/Steamed Fish		
Cod, dried	1240	85
Octopus, dried	1130	85
Fish moochim	754	85
Flounder	741	85
Herring	703	85
Octopus, steamed	530	85
Scallops	530	85
Milk		
Dry milk, low fat	421	25
Dry milk, whole	398	30
Buttermilk, dried	159	10
Special Supplements		
Algae, dried	1300	100
Seaweed, dried	1245	100
Protein powder	1037	100
Cereals/Grains		
Fruit and Fibre®	425	60
Wheat bran	354	30
100% bran	296	30
Wheat germ	284	30
Baby rice cereal	115	15
Miscellaneous		
Mousse	1050	115
Yeast spread	780	30
Cocoa	708	30
Chocolate covered coffee beans	533	40
Chopped, canned, spiced meat	370	60
Molasses	290	30
Processed cheese	220	30
Yeast	200	10
Sorghum	200	20
Carob chips	190	30
Cocoa powder	152	10

Food Description	Potassium (mg)/Serving	Serving Size (g)
Instant coffee	130	13
Onion soup, dry mix	67	10
Tea powder/leaves	66	1
Sugar substitute	45	1
Ethnic foods		
Papad (Indian appetizer bread)	1136	55
Sweet potatoes (Puerto Rican)	666	40
Meat		
Beef, roast	263	100
Pork, roast	363	100
Chicken, roasted	247	100

Sodium Content in Selected Foods

Food Description	Sodium (mg)/Serving	Serving Size (g)
Dried/Pickled Fish		
Pickled jellyfish	5330	55
Cod	3865	55
Mackerel	3782	85
Herring	1445	85
Canned Meats		
Deviled ham	1216	85
Pickled beef	1134	100
Corned beef	1134	100
Potted meats	1096	85
Chipped beef jerky	1041	30
Vienna sausage	685	50
Cured/Smoked Meats		
Ham	1443	100
Smoked pork roast	1385	100
Smoked pork chops	1255	100
Prosciutto	809	30
Pork jerky	575	20
Breakfast Meats/Sausage		
Smoked sausage	450	30
Smoked link sausage	225	15
Sausage	388	30
Pork bacon	239	15
Beef bacon	388	15
Bacon strip, meatless	366	25
Cervelat, soft	248	20

Food Description	Sodium (mg)/Serving	Serving Size (g)
Thuringer	248	20
Pickled sausage	238	15
Mortadella	187	15

Cheeses

Food Description	Sodium (mg)/Serving	Serving Size (g)
Processed American or Cheddar, reduced fat	475	30
Processed American or Cheddar, nonfat	458	30
Processed cheese, American and Swiss blends	429	30
Processed cheese, Swiss, low fat	429	30
Bleu cheese or Roquefort	419	30
Processed cheese, regular	411	30
Cheese spread	404	30
Cheese spread, pressurized	404	30
Imitation cheese	402	30
Processed cheese food	357	30
Feta cheese	335	30
Parmesan, dry, grated	279	15

Luncheon Meats

Food Description	Sodium (mg)/Serving	Serving Size (g)
Salami	837	45
Canadian bacon	773	50
Minced ham	643	45
Hot dog	565	50
Luncheon loaf	435	30
Turkey N cheddar	429	30
Ham and cheese loaf	403	30
Ham loaf	386	30
Head cheese	377	30
Bologna	237	20
Beef salami	235	20
Liverwurst	229	20
Pepperoni	102	5

Pickled/Fermented/Dried Vegetables

Food Description	Sodium (mg)/Serving	Serving Size (g)
Tomato relish	710	30
Pickled eggplant	670	40
Dill pickles	385	30
Pickles	383	30
Olives	360	15
Dried tomato	105	5

Ethnic Dishes and Sauces

Food Description	Sodium (mg)/Serving	Serving Size (g)
Fish moochim (Korean)	2753	55
Stewed codfish (Puerto Rican)	1568	85
Shrimp teriyaki	1313	85
Fish sauce	1158	15
Sweet and sour shrimp	975	85
Soy sauce	857	15
Teriyaki sauce	575	15
Miso	547	15

Food Description	Sodium (mg)/Serving	Serving Size (g)
Hoisin sauce	242	15
Papad	209	10

Supplements

Food Description	Sodium (mg)/Serving	Serving Size (g)
Seaweed prepared with soy sauce	1105	100
Protein Powder	462	60

Salty Snacks

Food Description	Sodium (mg)/Serving	Serving Size (g)
Pretzels, hard	772	55
Pretzels, soft	772	55
Pork rinds	551	30
Package peanut butter and crackers	448	40
Low fat cheese crackers	341	30
Cuca crackers	195	15
Oyster crackers	195	15
Saltines crackers	195	15
Croutons	124	10

Convenience Dishes (Frozen)

Food Description	Sodium (mg)/Serving	Serving Size (g)
Chicken burritos (diet frozen)	4648	300
Linguine with clam sauce	3256	270

Breads

Food Description	Sodium (mg)/Serving	Serving Size (g)
Ham on biscuit	1078	85
Bacon on biscuit	611	55
Biscuit, low fat, refrigerated dough	435	30
Biscuit, refrigerated dough	361	30

Miscellaneous

Food Description	Sodium (mg)/Serving	Serving Size (g)
Fat-free mayonnaise	178	15
Mustard	63	5

Zinc Content in Selected Foods

Food Description	Amount Zn (mg)/Serving	Serving Size (g)
Seafood/Fish		
Oysters, smoked	79.2	30
Oysters, canned	84	100
Oysters, raw	32	84
Oysters, stewed	64	85
Oysters, fried	62.1	85
Oyster pie	29.2	85
Oysters, baked	38	85
Oysters, steamed	36	85
Oysters, fritter	37	85
Oysters Rockefeller	37	100
Oyster sauce	8	30
Dressing with oysters	24	100
Octopus, dried	5.4	100
Cereals/Grains		
Bran flakes	1.0	28
Oatmeal	1.3	40
Total® Cornflakes	4.2	28
Total® Raisin Bran	3.1	28
Shredded Wheat®	1.5	28
Mueslix®	2.8	55
Apple Jacks®	3.8	33
Granola®	1.2	28
Cap'n Crunch®	1.2	28
Oh's®	3.8	30
Fruit rings	1.3	30

Food Description	Amount Zn (mg)/Serving	Serving Size (g)
Special Supplements		
Meal-replacement powders	16	100
Protein powder	2.8	30
Power bar	2.5	36

Oxalate Content by High, Moderate, and Little or No Oxalate Categories

Oxalate Content by Category (mg/100 gram/1/2 cup or standard serving size)		
Little or None	**Moderate**	**High**
Beverages/Juices		
Aloe vera juice	Beer (12 fl. oz.)	Beer (12 fl. oz.)
Apple juice	Budweiser®	Guiness Stout®
Beer (12 fl. oz.)	Draft, NFS[a]	Tuborg Pilsner®
Bottled, NFS[a]	Black currant juice	Juices of berries[b]
Cider	Coffee (8 fl. oz.)	Cocoa drinks
Coca-Cola®	Cranberry juice	Indian tea
Coffee, brewed 4 min	Carnation® cocoa mix	Ovaltine® mix
Cranberry juice, Minute Maid®	Grape juice	Nescafe® powder
Lime/lemon juice	Lipton® Tea (5 min)	
Diet Coke®	Orange squash drink	
Dry Sherry	Tomato juice (4 oz.)	
Ginger Ale, Schwepes®	Tea, rosehip	
Grapefruit juice		
Orange juice		
Lemon/limeade		
Orange soda, Minute Maid®		
Pepsi Cola® (12 fl.oz.)		
Pineapple juice		
Root beer, Barq's®		
Root beer, A&W®		
Tap water		
Wine, red, rose, white		
Milk (2 or more cups)/Milk Products		
Milk, all types		
Yogurt, plain		

Oxalate Content by Category (mg/100 gram/1/2 cup or standard serving size)		
Little or None	**Moderate**	**High**
Yogurt with allowed fruits		
Cheddar cheese		

Vegetables

Little or None	Moderate	High
Avocado	Artichoke	Beans boiled or raw
Broccoli, cooked	Broccoli, raw	green, wax or dried
Brussels sprouts, cooked	Carrots, canned	Beet tops, roots, greens
Cabbage, cooked	Corn, sweet white	Celery
Cauliflower, cooked	Corn, yellow	Chard, Swiss
Chives	Eggplant	Chicory
Cucumber, raw	Endive	Collards
Green peas, cooked/canned	Fennel leaves	Dandelion greens
Potatoes, white, boiled	Green beans, frozen	Eggplant, boiled
Radishes, small	and steamed	Escarole
Water chestnuts, canned	Kohlrabi	Kale, raw
	Lima beans, cooked	Leeks
	Mustard greens	Okra
	Mushrooms	Parsley, raw
	Onions, raw, boiled	Parsnips
	Tomato, fresh	Peppers green, sweet
	Turnips	Peppers, chilies
	Savoy cabbage	Pokeweed/salad
	Red cabbage	Potatoes, sweet
	Peas, ripe, podded	Rutabagas
		Spinach
		Summer squash
		Watercress

Fruits

Little or None	Moderate	High
Avocado	Apple	Berries: black, dew
Banana	Apricots	Blueberries
Cherries, bing/sour	Black currants	Red currants
Cranberries, canned, Ocean	Cherries, sweet	Concord grapes
Spray®		
Grapes, Thompson seedless	Cranberries, dried	Fruit cocktail, canned
Mangoes	Coconut	Gooseberries
Grapes, Red	Grapefruit	Lime peel
Melons: Cantaloupe	Kiwi	Lemon peel
Melon: Honeydew	Orange, raw, navel	Orange peel
Melon: Cassaba	Orange, raw	Plums
Nectarines	Peaches, Alberta	Plums, Damson
Peaches, Hiley® canned	Pears, raw	Raspberries (all)
Peaches, Stokes® canned	Pineapple, Dole®	Rhubarb, cooked/canned
Pineapple canned, cooked	Plums, stewed	Strawberries, cn
Plums, green or gage	Prunes, Italian	Strawberries, raw
Pear, bartlett, raw/canned		Tangerine
Papaya		
Watermelon		

Oxalate Content by Category (mg/100 gram/1/2 cup or standard serving size)		
Little or None	**Moderate**	**High**
Bread/Starches		
Bread, white (1 slice, 1 oz)	Bagel (medium, 2 oz)	Fig Newtons®
Cornflakes (1 cup)	Bread, whole wheat	Fruit cake
Macaroni, cooked (1 cup)	Barley, ck	Grits
Noodles, egg	Brown rice	Graham crackers
Oatmeal, porridge	Cheerios® (1 cup)	Popcorn (4 cups)
Rice, white, boiled	Corn tortilla	Soybean crackers
Spaghetti, cooked	Cornbread	Wheat germ
Wild rice, cooked	Cornmeal, dry	Whole wheat flour
	English muffin	
	Garbanzo beans	
	Spaghetti canned in tomato sauce	
	Split peas, cooked	
	Sponge cake	
Fats and Oils		
Mayonnaise	Bacon	Nuts:
Salad dressings		Peanuts
Vegetable oils		Pecans
Butter and margarine		Sunflower seeds
Miscellaneous		
Apple cider vinegar	Basil, fresh (1 T.)	Chocolate, plain
Chicken noodle soup	Cinnamon ground (1 t.)	Cadbury® milk
Corn syrup, Karo®	Ginger raw (1 T.)	chocolate
Cornstarch (1 T.)	Malt (1 T.)	Cadbury® cocoa
Hard candy	Marmalade (1 T.)	
Honey	Strawberry jam (1 T.)	Pepper (>1 t./d)
Jelly/preserved made with	Tomato soup	
Allowable fruits	Vegetable soup	
Pure maple syrup		
Mustard, Dijon style		
Nutmeg, dry (1 t.)		
Oxtail soup		
Oregano, dried		
Red plum jam (1 T.)		
Salt/pepper (1 t./d)		
Soups with allowed items		
Sugar		
Unflavored gelatin		
Vanilla extract		

[a] NFS = not further specified as to type or brand.
[b] Unallowable fruits/vegetables.

Source: Selected values from Brzezinski, E. et al., *Oxalate Content of Selected Foods,* The General Clinical Research Center, University of California, San Diego Medical Center, San Diego, CA, 1998, 17–29. With permission.

Dietary Caffeine and Other Methylxanthines

Three methylxanthines are important food ingredients: caffeine, theobromine, and theophylline. Although many physiological effects are shared in common, the degree of effect varies with the specific methylxanthine. The following table summarizes the effects and the relative degree of effect.

Table D.12   Relative Effects of Methylxanthines on Physiologic Processes

	Caffeine	Theobromine	Theophylline
CNS, respiratory stimulation	+++	+	++
Smooth muscle relaxant	+	++	+++
Diuresis	+	++	+++
Cardiac stimulation	+	++	+++
Skeletal muscle stimulation	+++	+	++

CNS = central nervous system.

Source: From Linder, M.C., Ed., *Nutritional Biochemistry and Metabolism with Clinical Applications,* Elsevier, New York, 1991, p. 229. With permission.

Caffeine Content of Common Beverages and Foods

Caffeine content in soft drinks and other products vary by brand, but the U.S. Food and Drug Administration limits the maximum amount in carbonated beverages to 6 mg/fluid ounce. Thus, the maximum amount of caffeine in a 12-oz soft drink is 72 mg.

Caffeine-free products are also available in many brands and should be considered to contain less than 1 mg of caffeine per serving.

Beverage/Food Group by Brand or Generic Product

Beverages	Caffeine per 8 fl. oz	Caffeine per 12 fl. oz
Carbonated Beverages		
Coca-Cola® Products		
Barq's® root beer	15	22
Cherry Coca-Cola®	23	34
Diet Cherry Coca-Cola®	23	34
Classic Coke®	23	34
Diet Coke®	31	45
KMX®	31	45
Mello Yello®	35	51
Diet Mello Yello®	35	51
Mr. Pibb®	27	40
Diet Mr. Pibb®	27	40
Red Flash®	27	40
Surge®	35	51
TAB®	31	45
Generic Values		
Generic cola	—	37
Generic cherry cola type	—	37

Beverage/Food Group by Brand or Generic Product

Beverages	Caffeine per 8 fl. oz	Caffeine per 12 fl. oz
Generic diet cola		
Aspartame sweetened	–	50
Sodium saccharin sweetened	—	39
Dr. Pepper® Products		
A&W Crème Soda®	20	29
Diet A&W Crème Soda®	15	22
Dr. Pepper®	28	41
Diet Dr. Pepper®	28	41
IBC® Cherry Soda	16	23
Ruby Red Squirt®	26	39
Diet Ruby Red Squirt®	26	39
Sun Drop® Regular	43	63
Diet Sun Drop®	47	69
Sun Drop® Cherry	43	64
Sunkist®Orange Soda	28	41
Diet Sunkist® Orange Soda	28	42
Tahitian Treat®	Less than 1	Less than 1
Pepsi Cola® Products		
Mountain Dew®	37	55
Diet Mountain Dew®	37	55
Pepsi-Cola®	25	38
Diet Pepsi-Cola®	24	36
Pepsi One®	37	55
Wild Cherry Pepsi®	25	55
Diet Wild Cherry Pepsi®	24	36
Royal Crown (RC)® Products		
Royal Crown Cola®	28.8	43.2
Cherry RC Cola®	28.8	46.2
RC Edge®	46.8	70.2
Royal Crown® Flavors		
Dr. Nehi®	28	42
Kick®	38.4	57.6
Nehi® Flavors		
Nehi Wild Red Soda®	33.4	50.1
Bottled or Canned Teas		
Coca-Cola® Tea Products		
Nestea® lemon iced tea	11	16
Nestea® diet lemon tea	11	16
Nestea® peach iced tea	11	16
Nestea® raspberry iced tea	11	16
Nestea® sweet iced tea	17	26
Nestea® unsweetened iced tea	17	26
Cool from Nestea®	11	16
Diet Cool from Nestea®	7	11

Beverage/Food Group by Brand or Generic Product

Beverages	Caffeine per 8 fl. oz	Caffeine per 12 fl. oz
Mystic® Teas		
Lemon Tea	12	18
Diet Lemon Tea	12	18
Peach Tea	12	18
Pepsi-Cola® Company Teas		
Lipton® Brisk, All Varieties	6	9
Snapple® Teas:		
Green Tea with Lemon	16	24
Ginseng Tea	5	7.5
Lemon Tea	21	31.5
Decaffeinated Lemon Tea	3	13.5
Diet Lemon Tea	21	31.5
Lemonade Iced Tea	9	13.5
Lightning (Black Tea)	14	21
Mint Tea	21	31.5
Moon (Green Tea)	12	18
Peach Tea	21	31.5
Diet Peach Tea	21	31.5
Raspberry Tea	21	31.5
Diet Raspberry Tea	21	31.5
Sun Tea	5	7.5
Diet Sun Tea	5	7.5
Sweet Tea	8	12

Source: Based on manufacturer's data posted on the National Soft Drink Association Web site www.nsda.org/brand/index.html, June 1, 2001 and selected values from Pennington, J.A.T., *Bowes and Church Food Values of Portions Commonly Used,* 17th ed., Lippincott, Philadelphia, 1998, pp. 383–384.

Beverage/Food Group	Serving Description	Caffeine (mg)/Serving
Coffee		
Brewed[a]	6 fl. oz/177 g	103
Ground, Folgers®	1 T./4 g	59
Ground, Folgers,® Decaffeinated	1 T./4 g	1
Instant powder	1 rd t./1.8 g	57
Cappuccino flavor, sugared	2 td t./14 g	73
Decaffeinated	1 rd t./1.8 g	2
French flavor, sugared	2 rd t./12 g	51
Mocha flavor, sugared	2 rd t./12 g	33
With chicory	1 rd t./1.8 g	37
Prepared from instant powder		
Generic	6 fl. oz water and 1 rd t. powder/179g	57
Cappuccino flavor, sugared	6 fl oz water and 2 rd t. powder/192 g	75
Decaffeinated	6 fl. oz water and 1 rd t. powder/179 g	2
French flavor, sugared	6 fl. oz water and 2 rd t. powder/189 g	51
Mocha flavor, sugared	6 fl oz water and 2 rd t. powder/188 g	34
with chicory	6 fl. oz water and 1 rd t. powder/170 g	38

Beverage/Food Group	Serving Description	Caffeine (mg)/Serving
Tea, Hot/Iced		
Brewed, black, 3 min[b]	6 fl. oz/178 g	36
Iced, instant powder	1 t./0.7 g	30
With lemon flavor	1 rd t./1.4 g	25
With lemon flavor and sodium saccharin	2 t./1.6 g	36
With lemon flavor and sugar	3 rd t./23 g	29
Prepared from instant powder	1 t. powder in 8 oz water/237 g	31
With lemon flavor	1 rd t. powder in 8 oz water/238 g	26
With sodium saccharin and lemon flavor	2 t. powder in 8 oz water/238 g	36
With sugar and lemon flavor	3 rd t. powder in 8 oz water/259 g	28
Candy and Gum		
After Eight® Mints	2 mints/8 g	2
Baby Ruth®	2.1 oz bar/60 g	2
Butterfinger®	2.16 oz bar/61 g	2
Chocolate chips, semi-sweet	1 cup/6 oz pkg/168 g	104
Chocolate coated		
Peanuts	10 pieces/40 g	9
Peanuts, Goobers®	1.38 oz pkg/39 g	9
Raisins	10 pieces/10 g	3
Raisins, Raisinets®	1.58 oz pkg/45 g	11
Chocolate, semisweet	1 oz/28 g	18
Chocolate, sweet, dark	1.45 oz bar/41 g	27
Special dark, Hershey®	1.5 oz bar/41 g	31
Chunky	1.4 oz bar/40 g	12
Crunch, Nestle®	1.4 oz bar/40 g	10
Golden Almond, Hershey®		
Hershey®	3.2 oz bar/91 g	16
III, Hershey®	3.2 oz bar/91 g	15
Solitaires® with Almonds	3 oz pkg/85 g	14
Hundred Grand®	1.5 oz bar/43 g	11
Kit Kat ®Wafer, Hershey	1.5 oz bar/42 g	5
Krackel ®Chocolate Bar, Hershey	1.5 oz bar/41 g	7
Milk chocolate	1.55 oz bar/44 g	11
With almonds	1.55 oz bar/44 g	10
With rice cereal	1.45 oz bar/41 g	9
Milk chocolate chips	1 cup chips/168 g	43
Mr. Goodbar®, Hershey	1.75 oz bar/49 g	5
Peanut Butter Cups, Reese's®	2 pieces/1.8 oz/50 g	6
Rolo® caramels with milk chocolate	9 pieces/1.9 oz/53 g	4
Turtles, Demet's®	0.6 oz piece/17 g	1
Twix®, caramel	2 oz pkg/2 pieces/57 g	2
Desserts		
Frozen Desserts		
Ice cream, chocolate	1/2 cup/66 g	2
Granola, Cereal, and Snack Bars		
Peanut butter, sof w/choc coating	1.3 oz bar/37 g	2

Beverage/Food Group	Serving Description	Caffeine (mg)/Serving
Puddings, Custards, and Pie Fillings		
Chocolate, ready-to-eat	5 oz can/142 g	7
Sauces, Syrups, and Toppings for Desserts		
Chocolate fudge topping	1 T./21 g	2
Chocolate syrup	2 T./1 fl. oz/38 g	5
Milk, Milk Beverages, Milk Mixes, and Yogurt		
Milk, cow, Beverages		
Chocolate dairy drink w/aspartame, from mix, prep w/water	1/4 oz pkt. in 4 oz water w/3 ice cubes/204 g	22
Chocolate malted milk, whole milk	3 hp t. powder in 8 fl oz milk/265 g	8
Chocolate malted milk, whole milk with added nutrients	4–5 hp t. powder in 8 fl. oz milk/265 g	5
Chocolate milk, whole milk with chocolate powder	2–3 hp t. powder in 8 fl. oz milk/266 g	8
Chocolate milk, whole milk with chocolate syrup	2 T. syrup in 8 fl oz milk/272 g	6
Cocoa (hot chocolate):		
Prep with water from mix	3–4 hp t. powder in 6 fl. oz milk/206 g	4
Prep with water from mix with added nutrients	1 pkt. in 6 fl oz water/209 g	6
Prep with water from mix, aspartame sweetened	0.53 oz pkt. powder in 6 fl. oz water/192 g	15
Milk Mixes		
Chocolate milk powder	2–3 hp t./22 g	8
Malted	0.75 oz/3 hp t./21 g	8
Malted with added nutrients	0.75 oz/4–5 hp t./21 g	6
Cocoa mix, powder	1 oz pkt/3–4 hp t./28 g	5
Aspartame sweetened	0.53 oz pkt./15 g	16
With added nutrients	1.1 oz pkt./31 g	6
Miscellaneous		
Baking chocolate, unsweetened	1 oz square/28 g	57
Cocoa, unsweetened, dry powder	1 T./5 g	12
Processed with alkali	1 T./5 g	4

Note: A usual coffee cup holds 6 fluid ounces, and a usual coffee mug or glass holds 8 fluid ounces. Other serving sizes may appear in cups and glasses. To determine unknown serving size, fill with water and measure into household measuring cup(s).

[a] Unless noted otherwise, the product is not further specified as to brand and is considered generic. Different varieties of coffee beans and different blends of coffee bean types yield varying amounts of caffeine. Different methods of brewing can also change the amount of caffeine extracted from coffee grounds. The degree of roasting can also influence the amount of caffeine extracted during brewing. Thus, the values presented are approximate estimates and may vary widely.

[b] Unless otherwise noted, the product is not further specified as to brand and is considered a generic value. Values in teas vary between geographical source and processing source. Blending of one or more types of tea leaves also yields different values. Thus, the values presented are approximate estimates.

Source: Selected values from Pennington, J.A.T., *Bowes & Church's Food Values of Portions Commonly Used,* 17th Ed., Lippincott, Philadelphia, 1998, pp. 383–384. With permission.

Theobromine in Foods

Beverage/Food Group	Serving Size	Theobromine (mg)
Beverages		
Tea, Hot/Iced		
Brewed, 3 min	6 fl. oz. (178 g)	3.6
Instant powder	1 t. (0.7 g)	2.1
Prepared with instant powder and water	1 t. (0.7 g) 8 fl. oz.	2.4
Candy		
Milk chocolate, Cadbury®	1 oz. (28 g)	44.0
Milk Beverages		
Chocolate flavor mix in whole milk	2–3 hp t. powder 8 fl. oz. (265 g)	120.0
Chocolate malted milk flavor mix in whole milk	3 hp t powder 8 fl. oz. (265 g)	106.0
Chocolate malted milk flavor mix with added nutrients, milk	4–5 hp t. powder 8 fl. oz. (265 g)	217.0
Chocolate syrup in whole milk	2 T. syrup 8 fl. oz.	90.0
Cocoa/hot chocolate mix, prepared with water	1/4 oz. (3 hp t) 6 fl. oz.	68.0
Milk Beverage Mixes		
Chocolate flavor mix, powder	2–3 hp t (22 g)	123.0
Chocolate malted milk flavor, powder	1/4 oz./3 hp t (21 g)	106.0
Chocolate malted milk flavor mix with added nutrients powder	1/4 oz./4–5 hp t.	217.0
Chocolate syrup	2 T (1 fl. oz.) (38 g)	89.0
Cocoa mix, powder	1 oz. pkt. (3–4 hp t)(28 g)	67.0

Beverage/Food Group	Serving Size	Theobromine (mg)
Special Dietary Formulas, Commercial and Hospital		
Chocolate flavored HN, Ross®	8 fl. oz. (253 g)	45.5
Chocolate flavored Plus, Ross®	8 fl. oz. (259)	62.1

Source: Selected values from Pennington, J.A.T., *Bowes & Church's Food Values of Commonly Used Portions,* 15th ed., Harper & Row, New York, 1989, p. 278. With permission.

Alcohol (Ethanol) Content of Alcoholic Beverages

Beverage Group	Serving Size (fl. oz)	Alcohol (Ethanol)	
		Weight (g)[a]	Volume (%)
Ales, Beers and Malt Liquors (12 fl. oz)			
Ale, Blatz Cream®	12 fl. oz	15.5	
Beer—generic—12 fl. oz (356 g)		12.8	4.5
Anheuser-Busch®.		13.5	
Black Label®		12.6	
Blatz®		13.1	4.6
Coors® Premium		13.2	
Heileman's Old Style®		13.7	
Heileman's Special Export®		15.5	
Heileman's Special Export Dark®		15.5	
Herman Joseph's®		14.2	4.95
Killian's ®		15.6	5.43
Rainier®		13.1	
Schmidt®		13.1	
Stroh's American Lager®		12.0	
Beer, light generic—12 fl. oz (354 g)		11.3 (7.8–15.6)	
Anheuser-Busch®		11.0	
Blatz®		11.9	
Coors®		11.9	4.18
Heileman's Old Style®		10.3	
Heileman's Special Export®		11.9	
Beer, LA (low alcohol)			
Anheuser-Busch®		6.4	
Blatz®		6.5	
Heileman's Old Style®		6.5	
Malt Beverages, nonalcoholic—12 oz (355 g)		0.7	0.30
Kingsbury®		1.0	

| | Serving Size | Alcohol (Ethanol) | |
Beverage Group	(fl. oz)	Weight (g)[a]	Volume (%)
Malt Liquor—12 oz			
Blatz Old Fashioned Private Stock®		13.7	
Colt 45®		15.7	

Cocktails and Cocktail Mixes

Bloody Mary (tomato and lemon juice, vodka)	5 fl. oz	13.9	11.7
Bourbon and soda	4 fl. oz	15.1	16.1
Daiquiri			
Canned	6.8 fl. oz	19.9	11.9
Rum, lime juice and sugar	2 fl. oz	13.9	28.3
Gin and tonic (tonic water, gin and lime juice)	7.5 fl. oz	16.0	8.8
Manhattan (whiskey and vermouth)	2 fl. oz	17.4	36.9
Martini (gin and vermouth)	2.5 fl. oz	22.4	38.4
Pina colada			
Canned	6.8 fl. oz	20.0	11.2
Pineapple juice, rum, coconut cream	4.5 fl. oz	14.0	12.3
Screwdriver (orange juice and vodka)	7 fl. oz	14.1	8.2
Tequila sunrise			
Canned	6.8 fl. oz	19.8	11.7
Orange/lime juice, tequila, grenadine	5.5 fl. oz	18.7	13.5
Tom Collins (club soda, gin, lemon juice, sugar)	7.5 fl. oz	16.0	9.0
Whiskey sour			
Canned	6.8 fl. oz	19.9	11.8
Lemon juice, whiskey, sugar	3.0 fl. oz	15.1	20.6
Prepared from bottled mix and whiskey	2.0 fl. oz		
	1.5 fl. oz	14.9	17.4
Prepared from powdered mix and whiskey	17 grams		
	1.5 fl. oz	15.0	18.0

Distilled Spirits

Gin, 90 proof	1.5 fl. oz	15.9	45.0
Gin/rum/vodka/whiskey, 94 proof	1.5 fl. oz	16.7	47.0
Gin/rum/vodka/whiskey, 100 proof	1.5 fl. oz	17.9	50.0
Rum/vodka 80 proof	1.5 fl. oz	14.0	40.0
Whiskey, 86 proof	1.5 fl. oz	15.1	43.0

Liqueurs

Coffee, 53 proof	1.5 fl. oz	11.3	26.5
Coffee, 63 proof	1.5 fl. oz	13.5	31.5
Coffee with cream, 34 proof	1.5 fl. oz	6.5	17.0
Crème de menthe	1.5 fl. oz	14.9	36.0

Wines and Wine Beverages

Sparkling cooler, citrus, La Croix®	12 fl. oz	12.6	
Sparkling cooler, strawberry, La Croix®	12 fl. oz	12.6	
Wine, dessert, dry	2 fl. oz	9.0	18.8
Wine, dessert, sweet	2 fl. oz	9.0	18.8
Wine, table, all types	3.5 fl. oz	9.6	11.5

Beverage Group	Serving Size (fl. oz)	Alcohol (Ethanol)	
		Weight (g)[a]	Volume (%)
Wine, table, red	3.5 fl. oz	9.6	11.5
Wine, table rose	3.5 fl. oz	9.6	11.5
Wine, table, white	3.5 fl. oz	9.6	11.5

[a] For each gram of alcohol, the caloric contribution of the alcohol alone is 7.0 kcal/g.

Source: Selected values from Pennington, J.A.T., *Bowes & Church's Food Values of Commonly Used Portions,* 15th ed., Harper & Row, New York, 1989, p. 258. With permission.

Purine-Yielding Foods

The drug, allipurinol (Lopurin®), largely prevents the formation of uric acid from purines and greatly reduces the need for low purine diets in those with a tendency to form uric acid stones. An occasional patient may be unwittingly consuming high amounts of purines and, thereby, reducing the benefits of the drug and requiring higher doses. Such a patient may benefit from counseling on avoiding high purine foods and from reinforcing of the need to maintain a high fluid intake sufficient to produce over 2 L of urine/d.

Very High In Purines: (1.50–8.25 mg/g)	High in Purines (0.5–1.5 mg/g)
Avoid even 1/2 cup or 100 g serving	**Limit to 1/2 cup or 100 g serving/d**
Anchovies	Fish, fresh or frozen
Canned fish, e.g.	Legumes, e.g.
Herring	Beans
Mackerel	Lentils
Sardines	Peas
Game meats, e.g.,	Meat, e.g.,
Deer or venison	Beef, veal
Gravies, especially *au jus*	Lamb
Meat extracts, e.g.	Pork
Bouillon	Shellfish, e.g.
Broth	Crab
Consommé	Lobster
Organ meats, e.g.	Oyster
Brains	Vegetables, e.g.
Kidneys	Asparagus
Liver	Cauliflower
Sweetbreads	Green Peas
Wheat germ and bran	Mushrooms
	Spinach
Very Low in Purines: (0-0.5 mg/g)	
Coffee and tea	

Very Low in Purines: (0-0.5 mg/g)
Breads and cereals without wheat germ or bran
Dairy products, e.g., butter, cheese, and milk
Eggs
Fruits and fruit juices
Margarines and salad dressings
Nuts
Candies, sugars, and soft drinks
Vegetables except as listed above
Soups made with vegetables and cream base.

Source: Adapted from Garrow, J.S. and James, W.P.T., Eds., *Human Nutrition and Dietetics*, 9th ed., Churchill Livingstone, Edinburgh, 1993, p. 617, and Pennington, J.A., *Bowes & Church's Food Values of Portions Commonly Used,* 17th ed., Lippincott, Philadelphia, 1998, p 391.

Nutrition Monitoring Screen

Mechanism of Deficiency	History	Check for Deficiency
Inadequate intake	Alcoholism	Kilocalories, protein, thiamin, niacin, folate, pyridoxine, riboflavin, magnesium
	Avoidance of fruit, vegetables, grains	Vitamin C, thiamin, niacin, folate
	Avoidance of meat, dairy products, eggs	Protein, vitamin B_{12}, Iron
	Constipation, hemorrhoids, diverticulosis	Dietary fiber
	Isolation, poverty, dental disease, food idiosyncrasies	Kilocalories, protein, B vitamins
	Weight loss	Kilocalories, B vitamins,
Inadequate absorption	Drugs (especially antacids, anticonvulsants, cholestyramine, laxatives, neomycin, alcohol)	See Chapter 6
	Malabsorption (diarrhea, weight loss, steatorrhea)	Vitamins A, D, K, kilocalories, protein, calcium, magnesium, zinc, folate
	Parasites	Iron, vitamin B_{12} (fish tapeworm)
	Pernicious anemia	Vitamin B_{12}
	Surgery	
	Gastrectomy	Vitamin B_{12}, iron, folate
	Intestinal resection	Vitamin B_{12} (if distal ileum), iron, others as in malabsorption
Decreased utilization	Drugs (especially anticonvulsants, antimetabolites, oral contraceptives, isoniazid, alcohol)	See Chapter 6
Increased losses	Alcohol abuse	Magnesium, zinc, thiamin
	Blood loss	Iron, folate

Mechanism of Deficiency	History	Check for Deficiency
Increased losses (*continued*)	Centesis (ascitic, pleural taps)	Protein
	Diabetes, uncontrolled	Kilocalories
	Diarrhea	Protein, zinc, electrolytes
	Draining abscesses, wounds	Protein, zinc
	Nephrotic syndrome	Protein, zinc
	Peritoneal dialysis or hemodialysis	Protein, water-soluble vitamins, Zinc
Increased requirements	Fever	Kilocalories
	Hyperthyroidism	Kilocalories
	Physiologic demands (infancy, adolescence, pregnancy, lactation)	See Dietary Reference Intakes
	Surgery, trauma, burns, infection	Kilocalories, protein, vitamin C, zinc, folate
	Tissue hypoxia	Kilocalories (inefficient utilization)
	Cigarette smoking	Vitamin C, folate

Source: Adapted from Weinsier R.L. and Morgan S.L., *Fundamentals of Clinical Nutrition,* Mosby-Yearbook, St. Louis, 1993, pp. 134–135. With permission.

Critical Points in Physical Assessment for Nutrition Status

A. Hair

Lackluster — Dull, dry, brittle, and wireless. Compare to local normal standards. Consider environmental and chemical causes.

Thinness, sparseness — Fine, silky, and sparse with wider gaps between hairs.

Straightness — Straight in cultural groups with normally curly hair. Other changes usually present.

Easy pluckability — Small clump can be pulled out with moderate force and no pain, especially on side of head. Generally occurs with other hair changes. Inspect comb or brush for excess shedding.

B. Face

Diffuse depigmentation — General lightening of skin color. In protein-calorie malnutrition this is most obvious centrally on the face.

Nasolabial seborrhea — Scaling with dry, greasy, gray, or yellowish threadlike material around the nostrils. Also on bridge of nose, eyebrows, and back of ears. Sebaceous gland ducts become plugged.

C. Eyes

Pale conjunctiva — Eyelid lining and whites of eyes are pale as are buccal mucosa (inner surface of cheeks). Mainly a symptom of anemia. Associated with iron, folate, or B12 deficiency.

Conjunctival xerosis — Inner lids and whites of eyes appear dull, dry, roughened, and pigmented. Hold lid open and rotate eyes to better identify. May look wrinkled with increased vascularity. Associated with vitamin A deficiency.

Corneal xerosis — Cornea (colored part of eye) becomes dull, milky, hazy, or opaque, especially the lower, central area. Associated with vitamin A deficiency.

Keratomalacia	Softening of part or all of cornea, usually bilaterally. Eyes become white or yellow gelatinous mass. No pain or discharge. Associated with riboflavin and niacin deficiency.
Angular palpebritis (blepharitis)	Corners of eyes become cracked and red. Often associated with angular stomatitis (see next). Eyelids are inflamed.

D. Lips

Angular stomatitis	Cracks, redness, and flaking at corners of the mouth. Important only if bilateral. Also results from poor dentures, herpes, and syphilis. Associated with riboflavin, niacin, iron, and pyridoxine deficiency.
Angular scars	White or pink scars at corners of the mouth from healed stomatitis (see preceding).
Cheilosis	Vertical cracks of lips, usually the center of the lower lip. Lips are red, swollen and inner mucosa appears to extend out onto the lip. May be ulcerated. Associated with riboflavin and niacin deficiency.

E. Tongue

Edema	Tooth pressure makes indentions along the edges of tongue.
Magenta tongue	Purplish red. Other changes may coexist.
Atrophic filiform papillae	Taste buds are atrophied. Tongue appears smooth pale and slick (even when slightly scraped). Associated with folate, niacin, riboflavin, iron, or B_{12} deficiency.
Glossitis	Tongue is beefy red, painful, and taste buds are atrophied. Usually hypersensitivity, burning, and even taste changes, especially when eating. Oral mucosa may also be red and swollen. Associated with niacin, folate, riboflavin, iron, B12, pyridoxine, and tryptophan deficiency.

F. Teeth

Mottled enamel	White or brownish patches in tooth enamel. May also be pitting of enamel. Most obvious in upper front teeth. If mild, paper-white spots are seen on tips and edges of teeth with gradual fading into normal coloration. If severe, there will be pitting or brown staining. Associated with fluorine excess.

G. Gums

Spongy, bleeding	Purplish or red, spongy and swollen. Usually bleed easily with slight pressure. Teeth must be present to occur.

H. Glands

Thyroid enlarged	May be visible or felt. More visible with head tipped back. Associated with iodine deficiency.
Parotid enlarged	Glands just below earlobes visible. Chronic, non-tender enlargement. Significant only if bilateral. Associated with protein deficiency.

I. Skin

Xerosis	General dryness with fine lines and shedding of branlike scales. Associated with vitamin A or essential fatty acid deficiency.

Follicular hyperkeratosis	Type 1: Spine-like plaques around mouths of hair follicles, especially on buttocks, thighs, elbow, and knees. Skin feels like sandpaper and looks like "gooseflesh." Doesn't disappear with rubbing. Associated with vitamin A or essential fatty acid deficiency. Type 2: (perifolliculosis) Similar except that mouths of hair follicles contain blood or pigment. Usually in adults on abdomen and thighs. Associated with vitamin C deficiency.
Petechiae, ecchymoses	Small red, purple, black, or blue hemorrhagic spots on skin and mucous membranes. Usually at pressure points. Associated with vitamin C and K deficiency.
Pellagrous dermatosis	Hyperpigmented areas bilaterally on body parts exposed to sunlight (cheeks, forearms, neck, etc.) Symmetrical with sharp edges. Acute: red, swollen with itching, cracking, burning, and exudate. Chronic: dry, rough, thickened, and scaly with brown pigmentation. Consider thermal, sun, or chemical burns and Addison's disease. Associated with niacin and tryptophan deficiency.
Flaky-paint dermatosis	Extensive hyperpigmented patches that peel off to leave hypopigmented skin or superficial ulcers. Especially on buttocks and back of thighs. Often bilateral.
Scrotal or vulval dermatosis	Often itchy, peeling lesions of skin of scrotum and vulva. May be secondary infection. Associated with riboflavin deficiency.

J. Nails

Koilonychia	Bilateral thin, concave spoon-shaped nails in older children and adults. Consider Plummer–Vinson syndrome (koilonychia, dysphagia, glossitis, and anemia), and clubbing from cardiopulmonary disease.

K. Subcutaneous Tissue

Edema	Bilateral swelling, usually of ankles and feet first. Press down on tissue for 3 seconds. Edematous tissue will pit. Occurs in conditions of sodium and water retention, pregnancy, protein-losing enteropathy, varicose veins, and stasis. Associated with thiamin and protein deficiency (serum albumin of less than 2.5 g/100 mL).
Subcutaneous fat	Measure with skinfold calipers. Decreased in protein-calorie malnutrition.

L. Muscular and Skeletal Systems

Muscle wasting	Evaluated with upper arm muscle measurements. Prominence of body skeleton. Excess folding of skin under buttocks. Decreased in protein-calorie malnutrition.
Craniotabes	Softening of the skull across the back and sides of head under one year of age. Associated with active vitamin D deficiency.
Frontal/parietal bossing	Round swelling or thickening of front and sides of head in infants. Head may be larger than normal. Generally bilateral. Associated with past vitamin deficiency.
Epiphyseal enlargement	Ends of long bones enlarge, especially at wrist, knees, and ankles. May be painless or tender. Consider trauma, congenital deformity, renal diesease, and malabsorption. Associated with active vitamin D deficiency if painless and vitamin C deficiency if painful.
Beading of ribs (rachitic rosary)	Small lumps on sides of chest wall on ribs. Consider renal rickets and malabsorption. Associated with active vitamin D and calcium deficiency.

Knocked-knees or bowed legs	Curve outward at knees. Legs are bowed outward. Consider congenital deformity. Associated with past vitamin D and calcium deficiency.
Diffuse or local skeletal deformities	Osteomalacia in adults. Bones may be tender.
Deformities of thorax	Pigeon chest and Harrison's sulcus (a horizontal depression along the lower border of the chest). Associated with past vitamin D deficiency.
Musculoskeletal hemorrhage	Bleeding into muscle. Can only be confirmed by special tests and clinical examination.

M. Internal Systems

Gastrointestinal:

| Hepatomegaly | Enlarged liver. Liver edge palpable more than 2 cm below costal margin. Feel abdomen with knees bent. Occurs with numerous medical conditions. Nonspecific but associated with protein deficiency and chronic malnutrition. |

Nervous:

Psychomotor change	Listless, apathetic. Associated with protein deficiency.
Mental confusion	Confusion and irritability. Associated with protein deficiency.
Sensory loss	Associated with thiamin deficiency; B6 toxicity.
Motor weakness	Inability to squat and then stand three to four times in a row. Associated with thiamin deficiency.
Loss of position sense	
Loss of vibratory sense	Tested with tuning fork. Significant only if bilateral. Consider peripheral neuropathy of other causes. Associated with thiamin and B12 deficiency.
Loss of ankle and knee jerks	Significant only if absolute and bilateral. Consider peripheral neuropathy of other causes. Associated with thiamin and B12 deficiency.
Calf tenderness	Squeeze calf muscle firmly between thumb and forefinger. Significant only if bilateral. Consider deep vein thrombosis and peripheral neuropathy of other causes. Associated with thiamin deficiency.

Cardiovascular:

| Cardiac enlargement | Enlarged heart. Generally not nutritional. May occur in anemia and beriberi (thiamin deficiency) |
| Tachycardia | Rapid heart rate (above 100). May occur in anemia or beriberi (thiamin deficiency) |

Source: Adapted from Grant, A., Nutritional Assessment Guidelines, Cutter Medical, Berkeley, CA, 1991. With permission.

Sample Questionnaire for Assessing Dietary Factors Affecting Potential for Biogenic Amines Interactions

Please check the frequency that best describes how often in a usual month that you eat or drink the following food items.

				0 = never 1 = once a month 4 = weekly 7 = daily
0	**1**	**4**	**7**	**Food Item Description**
__	__	__	__	1. Aged cheeses: cheddar, bleu, Roquefort, and dishes made from these.
__	__	__	__	2. Imported cheeses: Brie, Havarti, Cheshire, Stilton
__	__	__	__	3. Tap beer or Imported beer
__	__	__	__	4. Salami, summer sausage, dry sausages, mortadello, chorozio
__	__	__	__	5. Soy sauce and soy dishes (miso, bean paste, tofu)
__	__	__	__	6. Sauerkraut or other pickled vegetables
__	__	__	__	7. Yeast extract (e.g., Marmite®) or meat extract (e.g., Bovril®)
__	__	__	__	8. Wine: Circle all that apply: red, rose, white
__	__	__	__	9. Cottage or farmer's cheese
__	__	__	__	10. Yogurt or sour cream and dishes made with these
__	__	__	__	11. Pizza, lasagna, and other Italian dishes with cheese

Please circle how long between the time you purchase and freeze or prepare the following foods.

12.	Chicken or turkey	Same day	24 hours	48 hours	3–5 days	5–7 days
13.	Ground chicken or turkey	Same day	24 hours	48 hours	3–5 days	5–7 days
14.	Chicken livers	Same day	24 hours	48 hours	3–5 days	5–7 days
15.	Beef or pork liver	Same day	24 hours	48 hours	3–5 days	5–7 days
16.	Beef steak	Same day	24 hours	48 hours	3–5 days	5–7 days
17.	Pork or lamb chop/steak	Same day	24 hours	48 hours	3–5 days	5–7 days
18.	Roast beef or pork	Same day	24 hours	48 hours	3–5 days	5–7 days
19.	Ground beef or pork	Same day	24 hours	48 hours	3–5 days	5–7 days
20.	Leftover meat dishes	Same day	24 hours	48 hours	3–5 days	5–7 days
21.	Thawed chicken or turkey	Same day	24 hours	48 hours	3–5 days	5–7 days
22.	Leftover chicken or turkey	Same day	24 hours	48 hours	3–5 days	5–7 days
23.	Fish, fresh or thawed	Same day	24 hours	48 hours	3–5 days	5–7 days
24.	Seafood: shrimp or oyster	Same day	24 hours	48 hours	3–5 days	5–7 days

Do you read cartons for expiration date or sell by date for the following foods?

23.	Milk	Yes	No	Sometimes
24.	Cottage or farmer's cheese	Yes	No	Sometimes
25.	American or other processed cheese	Yes	No	Sometimes
26.	Yogurt or sour cream	Yes	No	Sometimes

Source: Adapted from Sweet, R.A. et al., *J. Clinical Psychiatry,* 56:196–201, 1995; Walker, S.E. et al., *J. Clinical Psychopharmacol.,* 16: 383–388, 1996. With permission.

General Dietary Screening for Food and Drug Reactions

Coumadin™ (warfarin): Please circle all the foods that you eat regularly or frequently.

Broccoli	Cabbage	Green leafy vegetables	Kale	Soybean oil
Brussel sprouts	Collard greens	Turnip greens	Spinach	

Diuretics: Lasix™ (furosemide), Bumex™ (bumetanide), HydroDiuril™ (hydrochlorothiazide). Please circle all the foods that you eat regularly or frequently.

Apricots	Broccoli	Dates	Mushrooms	Prunes	Sweet potatoes
Artichokes	Brussel sprouts	Dried beans	Nuts	Prune juice	Tomatoes
Asparagus	Cantaloupe	Figs	Oranges	Pumpkin	Tomato juice
Avocado	Carrots	Honeydew	Orange juice	Raisins	Winter squash
Banana	Chocolate	Milk	Potatoes	Spinach	Coffee

Guidelines for Estimating Energy Needs and Desirable Body Weight

DESIRABLE BODY WEIGHT DETERMINERS

Hamri Rule:

Females: 100 lbs + 5 lbs for each inch over 60 inches.
Males: 106 lbs + 6 lbs for each inch over 60 inches

Body Mass Index:

$$\text{Body Mass Index} = \frac{\text{Weight (Kg)}}{\text{Height}^2\ (M)}$$

BMI ≥ 25 indicates Obesity
BMI ≤ 16 indicates Severe Underweight

ENERGY NEEDS: ADULTS

General rule: 1 Kcal/kg/hour or 24 Kcal/kg/day

Harris–Benedict Equation Estimate of Resting Energy Requirements (REE)

For Female Patients:

$$REE = [655 + (9.6)(Wt/Kg) + (1.9)(Ht/cm) - (4.7)(Age/Yr)] \text{ Kcal}$$

For Male Patients:

$$REE = [66 + (13.8)(Wt/Kg) + (5)(Ht/cm) - (6.8)(Age/Yr)] \text{ Kcal}$$

ENERGY NEEDS: CHILDREN

General Guideline: 1000 kcal plus 100 Kcal for each year over one year.

WHO* Guidelines: Female 3–9 years $REE = [(22.5)(Wt/Kg) + 499] \text{ Kcal}$
10–17 years $REE = [(12.2)(Wt/Kg) + 746] \text{ Kcal}$
Male 3–9 years $REE = [(22.7)(Wt/Kg) + 495] \text{ Kcal}$
10–17 years $REE = [(17.5)(Wt/Kg) + 651] \text{ Kcal}$

* World Health Organization.

Competency Checklist for Nutrition Counselors

Needs Improvement	Not Tried Yet	Good	Performance Objective

Nutrition Information for Particular Patient

1. Counselor knows essential facts and rationale for prescribed diet

			1a. Knows all food categories of diet.
____	____	____	1a. Knows all food categories of diet.
____	____	____	1b. Comfortable with substitutions and rationale for food selection.
____	____	____	1c. Prepared to help patient adapt diet to his or her needs.

2. Counselor knows local eating pattern

____	____	____	2a. Grasp of regional customs and what foods are available.
____	____	____	2b. Familiar with restaurants and food/grocery chains.

3. At onset, assesses patient's knowledge of diet is adequate.

____	____	____	3a. Takes diet history/food frequency.
____	____	____	3b. Begins discussion of long-term goals. Explains diet and checks understanding
____	____	____	3c. Eliminates knowledge gaps of patient.
____	____	____	3d. Analyzes current eating behavior with patient.

Communication Skills

4. Sets appropriate tone through preparation, manner, and physical setting.

____	____	____	4a. Makes appointment for sufficient time and comfortable discussion.
____	____	____	4b. Arranges for private, quiet setting.
____	____	____	4c. Assesses patients literacy and language skills. Adapts if necessary.
____	____	____	4d. Shows interest in patient as individual.

Needs Improvement	Not Tried Yet	Good	Performance Objective
_____	_____	_____	4e. Makes patient feel at ease.
_____	_____	_____	4f. Indicates intentions to speak and to listen.

5. Prepares self and patient for continuing relationship over a specified period.

_____	_____	_____	5a. Initially explains the necessity of follow-up over time.
_____	_____	_____	5b. Outlines plans for working with patient: number of sessions, time, and method.

6. Uses principles of good communication.

_____	_____	_____	6a. Primarily uses open-ended questions.
_____	_____	_____	6b. Doesn't do too much of the talking.
_____	_____	_____	6c. Tolerates periods of silence.
_____	_____	_____	6d. Maintains a nonjudgmental, noncritical attitude toward patient's eating pattern/lifestyle.
_____	_____	_____	6e. Uses words patient understands.

7. Communicates interest and confidence nonverbally and verbally.

_____	_____	_____	7a. Shows poise and interest through posture and "body language."
_____	_____	_____	7b. Uses gestures and words to encourage to communicate freely, without putting words into patient's mouth.

Counseling Approaches

8. Aware that the change process is patient's responsibility.

_____	_____	_____	8a. Does not assume responsibility for changes or consequences.
_____	_____	_____	8b. Does not become too ego-involved in patient's eventual success or failure.

9. Aware of need for patient to recognize manageable goals.

_____	_____	_____	9a. Helps patient choose initial goal that is easily achieved.
_____	_____	_____	9b. Helps patient set specific short-term goals that are progressively more challenging.
_____	_____	_____	9c. Is able to help patient evaluate goals.
_____	_____	_____	9d. Helps patient avoid failure through too large or too many goals.

10. Aware of need to examine and anticipate obstacles that will interfere with progress.

_____	_____	_____	10a. Reviews with patient potential obstacles in social, personal, and physical environment.
_____	_____	_____	10b. Helps patient recognize potential or actual problems and encourages him to change environment.
_____	_____	_____	10c. Discusses how to deal with potential failure.

11. Defines own role of providing support and feedback.

_____	_____	_____	11a. Avoids taking the major responsibility.
_____	_____	_____	11b. Places responsibility for change on the patient.

Needs Improvement	Not Tried Yet	Good	Performance Objective
_____	_____	_____	11c. Is aware of own biases and belief systems, and is able to ignore them.

12. Able to evaluate progress toward stated goal.

Needs Improvement	Not Tried Yet	Good	Performance Objective
_____	_____	_____	12a. Is able to give patient feedback about progress.
_____	_____	_____	12b. Keeps notes in sufficient detail to depict patient's responsibilities and progress.
_____	_____	_____	12c. Measures progress by a combination of methods: food intake evaluation, biological measures, and subjective judgment with emphasis on changing behavior.

13. Encourages patient to get family and friends involved.

Needs Improvement	Not Tried Yet	Good	Performance Objective
_____	_____	_____	13a. Helps patient recognize influences; suggests he or she openly asks them for their support.
_____	_____	_____	13b. Suggests he or she ask them to participate in some way, sharing new tastes and habits, helping with food selection, and limiting inappropriate foods.
_____	_____	_____	13c. Helps patient cope with negative feedback through anticipating and rehearsing problem situations.
_____	_____	_____	13d. Helps patient evaluate which individuals are potentially supportive or negative.
_____	_____	_____	13e. Uses family and friends, but primary responsibility is patient's.

14. Understands that counselor's role is more than information giver or instructor.

Needs Improvement	Not Tried Yet	Good	Performance Objective
_____	_____	_____	14a. Acts as facilitator for patient.
_____	_____	_____	14b. Is appropriately assertive.
_____	_____	_____	14c. Resists "lecturing."

15. Aware of the need to keep the patient task-oriented.

Needs Improvement	Not Tried Yet	Good	Performance Objective
_____	_____	_____	15a. Recognizes delaying tactics and distractions.
_____	_____	_____	15b. Is able to redirect session toward specifics.

Index

T